Surgery of Conotruncal Anomalies

Francois Lacour-Gayet • Edward L. Bove
Viktor Hraška • Victor O. Morell
Thomas L. Spray
Editors

Surgery of Conotruncal Anomalies

Springer

Editors
Francois Lacour-Gayet
National Heart and Lung Institute
Imperial College
London
UK

Edward L. Bove
C.S. Mott Children's Hospital
University of Michigan
Ann Arbor, MI
USA

Viktor Hraška
German Pediatric Heart Center
Asklepios Klinik Sankt Augustin Gmb
Sankt Augustin
Germany

Victor O. Morell
University of Pittsburgh Medical School
Pittsburgh, PA
USA

Thomas L. Spray
Department of Cardiothoracic Surgery
Children's Hospital of Philadelphia
Philadelphia, PA
USA

ISBN 978-3-319-23056-6 ISBN 978-3-319-23057-3 (eBook)
DOI 10.1007/978-3-319-23057-3

Library of Congress Control Number: 2016931403

Springer Cham Heidelberg New York Dordrecht London

Printed on acid-free paper

Springer International Publishing AG Switzerland is part of Springer Science+Business Media (www.springer.com)

Foreword I

Welcome to one of the most fascinating challenges in all of clinical medicine—the conotruncal malformations—and their up-to-date management as described by many of the world's best congenital heart surgeons. The current surgical management of tetralogy of Fallot, truncus arteriosus, interrupted aortic arch, transposition of the great arteries, corrected transposition of the great arteries, double-outlet right ventricle, and double-outlet left ventricle are all presented.

Also included are brief presentations concerning the definition, genetics, embryology, pathology, classification, and echocardiographic diagnosis of these infundibulo-arterial malformations.

Boston, MA, USA | Richard Van Praagh

Foreword II

The index of this book reads as a "who's who" in congenital cardiac surgery. Before embarking on the surgical niceties of the conotruncal malformations, the first three chapters are dedicated to the definition, the embryology and the description of these anomalies. It is pleasing to be met at the entrance of this book by two scholars who devoted most of the past 50 years to the analysis and the teaching of malformed hearts to cardiologists and cardiac surgeons alike with a relentless enthusiasm, which transpires through their respective chapters. As expected from most academic endeavours, details of linguistics and terminology give rise to subtle disagreements that are actually rather pleasing for the reader. The third chapter is a well-written Cartesian tutorial of descriptive anatomy. The bulk of this textbook is a succession of chapters, each describing the surgical management of all varieties of conotruncal anomalies. The text is richly illustrated and this facilitates the understanding of the most complex surgical procedures. The challenges of risk-adjusted outcome analyses for rare lesions on a global scale are rightly discussed in one of the introductory chapters. The last chapter on genetics is an echo of the second chapter on embryology. They both highlight the direction of future research, which should aim at the prevention and the prenatal treatment of those congenital anomalies.

This book is a refreshing and up-to-date addition to the literature on the surgical management of congenital cardiac malformations, which will be welcomed by trainees and established heart surgeons as well as cardiologists interested in the field.

London, UK Marc de Leval

Contents

Contributors

Robert H. Anderson, BSc, MD, FRCPath Institute of Genetic Medicine, Newcastle University, Newcastle upon Tyne, UK

Emile Bacha, MD, FACS Division of Cardiac, Thoracic, and Vascular Surgery/ Pediatric and Congenital Cardiac Surgery, Cardiothoracic Department, New York Presbyterian-Columbia University Medical Center/Combined Morgan Stanley Children's Hospital of New York (CHONY) – Komansky Weill-Cornell Program, New York, NY, USA

Simon D. Bamforth, BSc (Hons), PhD Institute of Genetic Medicine, Newcastle University, Newcastle upon Tyne, UK

David J. Barron, MD, FRCP, FRCS(CT) Department of Paediatric Cardiac Surgery, Birmingham Children's Hospital, Birmingham, West Midlands, UK

Emre Belli, MD Department of Pediatric Cardiac Surgery, Hôpital Jacques Cartier, Massy, France

Edward L. Bove, MD Section of Pediatric Cardiovascular Surgery, Department of Cardiac Surgery, C. S. Mott Children's Hospital and Michigan Congenital Heart Center, University of Michigan, Ann Arbor, MI, USA

Nigel Andrew Brown, BSc, PhD Division of Biomedical Sciences, St George's Hospital Medical School, Institute of Medical and Biomedical Education, St George's University of London, London, UK

David Neil Campbell, MD Department of Pediatric Cardiovascular Surgery, The Children's Hospital Colorado Heart Institute, University of Colorado Denver Health Sciences Center, Aurora, CO, USA

Paul J. Chai, MD Department of Surgery, Morgan Stanley Children's Hospital of NY – Columbia University Medical Center, New York, NY, USA

Bill Chaudhry, MBBS, MRCP, PhD Institute of Genetic Medicine, Newcastle University, Newcastle upon Tyne, UK

Jose Pedro da Silva, MD Heart Surgery Service, Department of Cardiovascular Surgery, Hospital Beneficencia Portuguesa of São Paulo, Sao Paulo, Brazil

Joseph A. Dearani, MD Division of Cardiovascular Surgery, Department of Cardiovascular Surgery, Mayo Clinic, Rochester, MN, USA

Roberto M. Di Donato, MD Pediatric Cardiac Surgery, Prince Sultan Cardiac Center, Riyadh, Saudi Arabia

Yves d'Udekem, MD, PhD, FRACS Department of Cardiac Surgery, Royal Children's Hospital, Melbourne, VIC, Australia

Lucas Jon Eastaugh, MBBS, FRACP, FCSANZ Department of Cardiology, Royal Children's Hospital, Melbourne, VIC, Australia

Pirooz Eghtesady, MD, PhD Section of Pediatric Cardiothoracic Surgery, Department of Cardiothoracic Surgery, St. Louis Children's Hospital, St. Louis, MO, USA

Alain Fraisse, MD, Phd Pediatric Cardiology Department, Royal Brompton Hospital, London, UK

Michael A. Gatzoulis, MD Department of Cardiology, Royal Brompton Hospital, London, UK

The National Heart & Lung Institute, Imperial College, Adult Congenital Heart Centre and Centre for Pulmonary Hypertension, London, UK

Mohammed Said Ghanamah, MD Department of Cardiothoracic Surgery, St. Louis Children's Hospital, St. Louis, MO, USA

Olivier Ghez, MD Department of Pediatric Cardiac Surgery, Royal Brompton Hospital, London, UK

Robert A. Hanfland, MD Department of Pediatric Cardiothoracic Surgery, Children's Hospital of Colorado, Aurora, CO, USA

Deborah J. Henderson Institute of Genetic Medicine, Newcastle University, Newcastle upon Tyne, UK

Jennifer C. Hirsch-Romano, MD, MS Section of Pediatric Cardiovascular Surgery, Department of Cardiac Surgery, C. S. Mott Children's Hospital and Michigan Congenital Heart Center, University of Michigan, Ann Arbor, MI, USA

Takaya Hoashi, MD, PhD Department of Pediatric Cardiovascular Surgery, National Cerebral and Cardiovascular Center, Suita, Osaka, Japan

Lucile Houyel, MD Department of Congenital Cardiac Surgery, Centre Chirurgical Marie-Lannelongue, Marie-Lannelongue Hospital, Université Paris-Sud, Le Plessis-Robinson, France

Viktor Hraška, MD, PhD Department of Pediatric Cardiac Surgery, German Pediatric Heart Center, Asklepios Clinic Sankt Agustin, Sankt Augustin, Germany

Shengshou Hu, MD Department of Cardiovascular Surgery, National Heart Center and FuWai Cardiovascular Hospital, Beijing, PR China

Hajime Ichikawa, MD, PhD Department of Pediatric Cardiovascular Surgery, National Cerebral and Vascular Center, Suita, Osaka, Japan

Jeffrey P. Jacobs, MD Division of Cardiovascular Surgery, Department of Surgery, Johns Hopkins All Children's Heart Institute, Saint Petersburg, FL, USA

Koji Kagisaki, MD Department of Pediatric Cardiovascular Surgery, National Cerebral and Cardiovascular Center, Suita, Osaka, Japan

David Kalfa, MD, PhD Department of Pediatric Cardiac Surgery, Morgan Stanley Children's Hospital – New-York Presbyterian, Columbia University Medical Center, New York, NY, USA

Meriem Mostefa Kara, MD Department of Pediatric Cardiology, Centre de Référence Malformations Cardiaques Congénitales Complexes – M3C, Necker Hospital for Sick Children, Assistance Publique des Hopitaux de Paris, Paris, France

Université Paris Descartes, Sorbonne Paris Cité, Paris, France

Christian Kreutzer, MD Department of Pediatric Cardiac Surgery, Hospital Universitario Austral, Pilar, Province of Buenos Aires, Argentina

Hiromi Kurosawa, MD Cardiovascular Surgery, Tokyo Women's Medical University, Tokyo, Japan

Sakakibara Sapia Tower Clinic, Tokyo, Japan

Jikei University, Tokyo, Japan

Francois Lacour-Gayet, MD Department of Pediatric Cardiac Surgery, National Heart and Lung Institute, Royal Brompton Hospital, Imperial College University, London, UK

Brigitte Laforest, PhD Génétique Médicale & Génomique Fonctionnelle (GMGF), UMR_S910, Aix Marseille Université, Faculté de Médecine de la Timone, Marseille, France

Inserm, U910, Marseille, France

Shoujun Li, MD Pediatric Cardiac Surgery Center, National Center for Cardiovascular Disease and Fuwai Hospital, Chinese Academy of Medical Sciences, Peking Union Medical College, Beijing, PR China

Kai Ma, MD, PhD Pediatric Cardiac Surgery Center, National Center for Cardiovascular Disease and Fuwai Hospital, Chinese Academy of Medical Sciences, Peking Union Medical College, Beijing, PR China

Bohdan Maruszewski, MD Cardiothoracic Surgery, Children's Memorial Health Institute, Warsaw, Poland

Constantine Mavroudis, MD Johns Hopkins University School of Medicine, Johns Hopkins Children's Heart Surgery, Florida Hospital for Children, Orlando, FL, USA

Dominique Metras, MD Department of Cardio-Thoracic Surgery, Children's Hospital La Timone, University Marseille-Aix, Marseille, France

Timothy J. Mohun, PhD Division of Developmental Biology, MRC National Institute for Medical Research, London, UK

Claudia Montanaro, MD Department of Cardiology, Royal Brompton Hospital, London, UK

Victor O. Morell, MD Department of Cardiothoracic Surgery, University of Pittsburgh Medical School, Children's Hospital of Pittsburgh of UPMC, Pittsburgh, PA, USA

Peter Murín, MD Asklepios Clinic Sankt Augustin, German Pediatric Heart Center, Sankt Augustin, Germany

Michael O. Murphy, MA, MD, MRCP, FRCS Department of Congenital Cardiac Surgery, Guy's and St. Thomas' Hospital, London, UK

Richard G. Ohye, MD Section of Pediatric Cardiovascular Surgery, Department of Cardiac Surgery, C. S. Mott Children's Hospital and Michigan Congenital Heart Center, University of Michigan, Ann Arbor, MI, USA

Nilesh Oswal, MD Paediatric Cardiology Services, Royal Brompton and Harefield Hospitals Trust, London, UK

Ed Peng, FRCS(CTh)(UK) Department of Pediatric Cardiac Surgery, Children's Hospital of Colorado, Aurora, CO, USA

James A. Quintessenza, MD Division of Cardiac Surgery, Department of Cardiovascular Surgery, Johns Hopkins All Children's Heat Institute, All Children's Hospital, St. Petersburg, FL, USA

Olivier Raisky, MD, PhD Necker Hospital, Paris, France

Department of Pediatric Cardiac Surgery, APHP – Hôpital Universitaire Necker – Enfants Malades, University Paris Descartes, Sorbonne Paris Cité, Paris, France

Sameh M. Said, MD Department of Cardiovascular Surgery, Mayo Clinic, Rochester, MN, USA

Darryl Shore, MD Heart Division, Royal Brompton Hospital, London, UK

Department of Cardiac Surgery The National Heart & Lung Institute, London, UK

Ming-Sing Si, MD Department of Cardiac Surgery, Section of Pediatric Cardiovascular Surgery, C. S. Mott Children's Hospital and Michigan Congenital Heart Center, University of Michigan, Ann Arbor, MI, USA

Diane E. Spicer, BS Department of Pediatric Cardiology, University of Florida, Gainesville, FL, USA

Department of Pathology, Johns Hopkins All Children's Heart Institute, St. Petersburg, FL, USA

Thomas L. Spray, MD Division of Cardiothoracic Surgery, Department of Cardiothoracic Surgery, The Children's Hospital of Philadelphia, Philadelphia, PA, USA

Kalyani R. Trivedi, MD, FSCAI Pediatric Interventional Cardiology, University of Chicago Medical Center, Comer Children's Hospital, Chicago, IL, USA

Biological Sciences Division, Department of Pediatrics, The University of Chicago, Chicago, IL, USA

Andrew D.G. Van Praagh, PhD Preclinical Imaging Department of Bruker, Biospin Corporation, Billerica, MA, USA

Richard Van Praagh, MD, FACC, FAHA, AM(Hon), DrMedHC Professor of Pathology Emeritus, Harvard Medical School, Boston, MA, USA

Departments of Pathology, Cardiology, and Cardiac Surgery, Boston Children's Hospital, Boston, MA, USA

Pascal R. Vouhé, MD, PhD Necker Hospital, Paris, France

Department of Pediatric Cardiac Surgery, APHP – Hôpital Universitaire Necker – Enfants Malades, University Paris Descartes, Sorbonne Paris Cité, Paris, France

Neil Wilson Department of Pediatric Cardiology, Children's Hospital Colorado, Denver, CO, USA

Toshikatsu Yagihara, MD, PhD Department of Pediatric Cardiovascular Surgery, National Cerebral and Cardiovascular Center, Suita, Osaka, Japan

Stéphane Zaffran, PhD Medical Genetics & Functional Genomics, UMR_S910, Aix Marseille Université, Medical School of Marseille, Marseille, France

Laboratoire de Génétique Médicale et Génomique Fonctionnelle, Faculté de Médecin, Marseille, France

Génétique Médicale & Génomique Fonctionnelle (GMGF), UMR_S910, Aix Marseille Université, Faculté de Médecine de la Timone, Marseille, France

Inserm, U910, Marseille, France

Chapter 1
Definition of Conotruncal Anomalies

Richard Van Praagh

Abstract Conotruncal anomalies are malformations of the infundibulum (conus arteriosus) and great arteries (truncus arteriosus) that have abnormal ventriculo-arterial alignments and connections: tetralogy of Fallot, truncus arteriosus, interrupted aortic arch type B, transposition of the great arteries, double-outlet right ventricle, double-outlet left ventricle, anatomically corrected malposition of the great arteries. Normally related great arteries have complete right-left (R-L) asymmetry in the development and anatomy of the subarterial conal free walls, with involution of the subaortic conal free wall musculature and good growth and expansion of the subpulmonary conal free wall musculature.

All conotruncal anomalies lack this type of complete R-L conal free wall asymmetry. Solitus normally related great arteries (SNRGA) result from involution of the right-sided subaortic conal free wall and from simultaneous good growth and expansion of the left-sided subpulmonary conal free wall. Briefly, $SNRGA = OR + 4L$. The right-sided subaortic conal free wall muscular development is grade 0 (absent) and the left-sided subpulmonary conal free wall muscular development is grade 4 (normal). This is how the embryonic aortic switch is normally performed. The left-sided PA is carried superiorly, anteriorly, and rightward above the RV, away from the interventricular foramen, atop the developing subpulmonary conal free wall. Simultaneously, the right-sided Ao moves inferiorly, posteriorly, and leftward because the subaortic conal free wall is undergoing involution, thought to be due to apoptosis. Consequently, the aorta passes mostly through the interventricular foramen and normally comes into direct fibrous continuity with the developing mitral valve (MV), above the morphologically left ventricle (LV), thereby accomplishing the normal embryonic aortic switch. Eleven normal and abnormal developmental and anatomic conotruncal equations are presented in this chapter. From an evolutionary perspective, the conotruncal anomalies appear to represent physiologically unsuccessful attempts to perform the embryonic aortic switch. Conotruncal anomalies are infundibular malformations, causing the great arteries to be abnormally connected, abnormally aligned, and abnormally related in space.

R. Van Praagh, MD, FACC, FAHA, AM(Hon), DrMedHC
Professor of Pathology Emeritus, Harvard Medical School,
Boston, MA 02115, USA

Departments of Pathology, Cardiology, and Cardiac Surgery, Boston Children's Hospital,
300 Longwood Avenue, Boston, MA 02115, USA
e-mail: susan.boissonneault@cardio.chboston.org

F. Lacour-Gayet et al. (eds.), *Surgery of Conotruncal Anomalies*,
DOI 10.1007/978-3-319-23057-3_1

To summarize, the evolution of complete R-L asymmetry in the development of the subarterial conal free walls made possible the embryonic aortic switch. This in turn led to the development of solitus normally related great arteries: $SNRGA = 0R + 4L$. Its mirror-image isomer is: $INRGA = 4R + 0L$. Any other pattern of conal development results in a conotruncal malformation.

Keywords Conotruncal anomalies, infundibulo-arterial malformations • Abnormal ventriculo-arterial alignments • Abnormal ventriculo-arterial connections • Tetralogy of Fallot • Truncus arteriosus • Interrupted aortic arch • Transposition of the great arteries • Double-outlet right ventricle • Double-outlet left ventricle • Anatomically corrected malposition of the great arteries • Great arterial equations • Infundibuloarterial situs concordance and discordance

What Really Are The Conotruncal Malformations?

To be a conotruncal malformation, there must be anatomic anomalies of both the infundibulum (conus arteriosus) and the great arteries (truncus arteriosus) compared with the normal human heart. *Infundibulum* means funnel (Latin), and *conus arteriosus* means arterial cone (Latin). Infundibulum describes the inside anatomic appearance of this structure as it leads from the right ventricle (RV) into the main pulmonary artery (MPA). This structure really does look like a funnel leading from the RV into the MPA. Looking at an embryonic reconstruction from the outside, this same structure looks like a hollow cone between the RV below and the MPA above. So, *infundibulum* (funnel) describes the inside anatomic appearance, while *conus* (cone) describes the outside embryonic appearance of the same structure. Hence these terms are used interchangeably.

What Are Normally Related Great Arteries and How Did they Get That Way?

Following looping of the straight heart tube to the right forming a dextral or D-loop, the developing great arteries are both above the developing RV (Fig. 1.1) [2]. The developing semilunar valves are approximately side-by-side, with **the aortic valve to the right** and **the pulmonary valve to the left** (Fig. 1.1), reminiscent of the Taussig-Bing malformation.

Then normally, the right-sided subaortic infundibular free wall undergoes involution, due to apoptosis (programmed cell death) and migration of cells out of this area. Simultaneously, the left-sided subpulmonary infundibular free wall undergoes strong growth and expansion, elevating the pulmonary valve superiorly above the RV, and getting the developing pulmonary valve out of the way, well above the interventricular foramen (the normal embryonic ventricular septal defect). Elevating

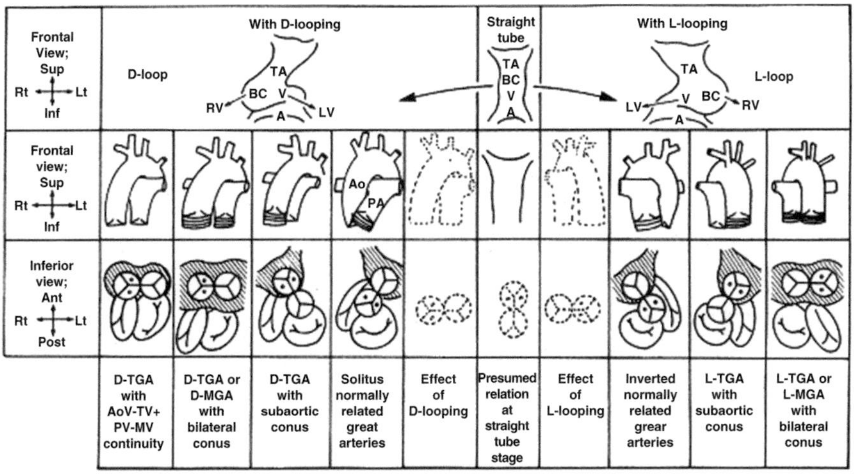

Fig. 1.1 Morphogenesis of normally and abnormally related great arteries, with ventricular D-loops and L-loops. Great arteries and infundibulum or conus arteriosus are shown from the front and from below. Subsemilunar conal musculature is indicated by cross hatching. Aortic valves are indicated by two coronary ostia, pulmonary valves by no coronary ostia. Mitral valves are bicuspid. Tricuspid valves have three leaflets. When great arteries and semilunar valves are depicted with broken lines, this means that these structures have not yet separated at straight tube or early D-loop or L-loop stages; they are so depicted for clarity of comprehension. For discussion, please see text. All of the diagrams in *row 3* showing the relationships between the semilunar and the atrioventricular valves are based on geometrically measured heart specimens; i.e., they are data-based, not hypothetical. **Abbreviations**: *A and Ant* anterior, *Ao* aorta, *AoV* aortic valve, *BC* bulbus cordis, *D-MGA* dextro-malposition of the great arteries, *D-TGA* dextro-transposition of the great arteries, *Inf* inferior, *Lt* left, *L-MGA* levo-malposition of the great arteries, *L-TGA* levo-transposition of the great arteries, *LV* morphologically left ventricle, *MV* mitral valve, *Post* posterior, *PA* main pulmonary artery, *PV* pulmonary valve, *Rt* right, *RV* morphologically right ventricle, *Sup* superior, *TA* truncus arteriosus, *TV* tricuspid valve, *V* ventricle (of the bulboventricular loop) (Reproduced from Van Praagh and Van Praagh [1] with permission of Elsevier)

the pulmonary valve and artery superiorly — above the interventricular foramen — facilitates the leftward movement of the aortic valve from above the RV to above the left ventricle (LV).

Strong growth of the left-sided subpulmonary conal free wall and involution of the right-sided subaortic conal free wall result in further dextral rotation of the developing great arteries. The aortic valve moves inferiorly, posteriorly and somewhat leftward, passing mostly through the interventricular foramen and coming into direct fibrous continuity with the developing mitral valve above the LV (Figs. 1.1 and 1.2) [2]. Simultaneously, the pulmonary valve moves reciprocally superiorly, anteriorly, and somewhat rightward above the RV (Figs. 1.1 and 1.2). This continuing dextral rotation goes from a side-by-side semilunar relationship, i.e., 90° rotation to the right relative to the sagittal plane, to the solitus normal semilunar interrelationship of approximately 150° dextrorotation relative to the sagittal plane (Figs. 1.1 and 1.2). The first 90° of dextrorotation of the developing semilunar valves appears to be due to D-loop formation of the heart tube.

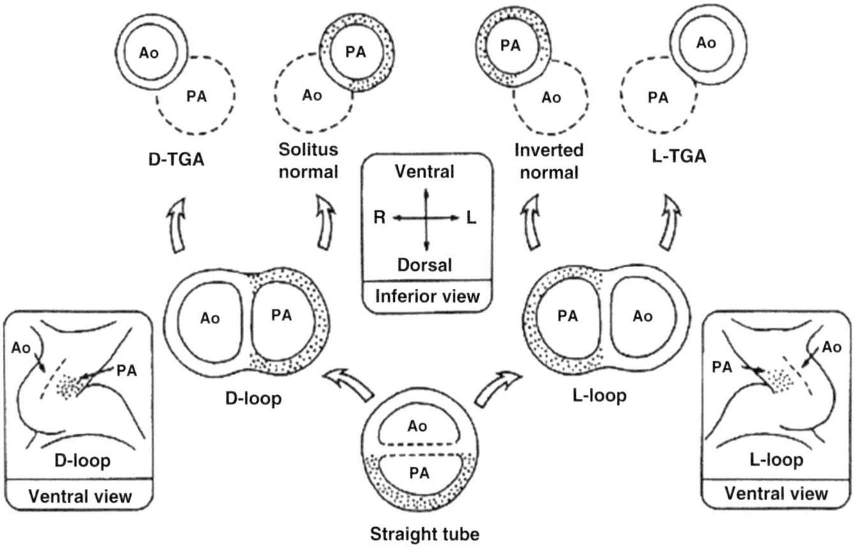

Fig. 1.2 Morphogenesis of normally related great arteries (solitus and inversus) is contrasted with that of transposition of the great arteries, D- and L-. Subpulmonary conal free wall is stippled. Subaortic conal free wall and conal septum are shown as clear (not stippled). Dashed circles indicate involution of subsemilunar conal free wall musculature. Arrows indicate progression of morphogenetic stages. Straight tube leading to D-loop ventricles and straight tube leading to L-loop ventricles are thought to be *different*, even though they are morphologically indistinguishable at this early stage. D-loop ventricles (solitus ventricles) and L-loop ventricles (inverted ventricles) do not arise from the same straight heart tube. Embryonic situs (solitus or inversus) is determined at, or shortly after fertilization. For discussion, please see text. *Abbreviations*: *Ao* aorta, *PA* main pulmonary artery, *D-TGA* dextro-transposition of the great arteries, *L-TGA* levo-transposition of the great arteries (Reproduced from Van Praagh [3] with permission of Elsevier)

The remaining 60° of normal dextrorotation of the semilunar valves appears to be due to complete right-left (R-L) asymmetry in the development of the subsemilunar conal free walls, which may be symbolized as follows: subaortic = grade 0 (0), and subpulmonary = grade 4 (4) (Figs. 1.1 and 1.2). The morphogenesis of solitus normally related great arteries (SNRGA) may be represented by the following equation: **SNRGA = 0R + 4L . In words, solitus normally related great arteries have complete R-L asymmetry in the development of the subarterial conal free walls. Normally, there is no right-sided subaortic conal free wall (0R) and (+) a well developed left-sided subpulmonary conal free wall (4L).**

This is the developmental and anatomic equation, or formula, or definition of solitus normally related great arteries. This is the *normal* conotruncal developmental and anatomic formula. This is the equation or formula of "Mother Nature's" normal aortic switch procedure. There is only one way to do it right (correctly), as above. There are many ways of doing it wrong (incorrectly), and they always result in a conotruncal malformation. A few examples follow.

In D-transposition of the great arteries (D-TGA), the development of the conal connector is the opposite of normal (Figs. 1.1 and 1.2): **the right-sided subaortic conal free wall develops well**, which may be symbolized as grade 4 (4), and **the left-sided subpulmonary infundibular free wall** typically undergoes complete involution, which may be symbolized as grade 0 (0).

So the conotruncal developmental and anatomic equation for typical **D-TGA is**:

$$\mathbf{D\text{-}TGA = 4R + 0L}$$

This equation has complete R-L asymmetry, but it is the opposite of the normal type of complete R-L asymmetry. So the wrong great artery gets switched. The right-sided aorta is elevated high above the RV, atop the developing subaortic conus; and the left-sided pulmonary artery is switched through the interventricular foramen and comes into direct fibrous continuity with the mitral valve above the left ventricle (LV), which is made possible by the involution (disappearance) of the left-sided subpulmonary infundibular free wall (Figs. 1.1 and 1.2).

Briefly, typical D-TGA has complete R-L conal free wall asymmetry that is the opposite of normal, so the wrong great artery, i.e., the pulmonary artery, gets switched embryologically. In other words, **D-TGA has subarterial conal free wall inversion (right-left reversal)** relative to what is normal in visceroatrial situs solitus.

The Taussig-Bing type of double-outlet right ventricle [4, 5] has a bilateral conus. Both the right-sided subaortic conal free wall and the left-sided subpulmonary conal free wall are well developed; neither has undergone involution (Fig. 1.1) [5]. Consequently both great arteries remain high above the RV, with no semilunar-atrioventricular valvar fibrous continuity, and with a subpulmonary ventricular septal defect (VSD) [4, 5].

The developmental and anatomic conotruncal equation for the Taussig-Bing malformation is:

$$\mathbf{Taussig\text{-}Bing\ DORV = 4R + 4L}$$

The Paul type of double-outlet left ventricle (DOLV) [6] has **no right-sided subaortic conal free wall** or septal musculature and **no left-sided subpulmonary conal free wall** or septal musculature, facilitating aortic-mitral and pulmonary-mitral direct fibrous continuity. The ventricular septum was intact [6]. The developmental and anatomic conotruncal equation for the Paul type of DOLV [6] is:

$$\mathbf{Paul\ type\ of\ DOLV = 0R + 0L}$$

Typical tetralogy of Fallot (TOF) is:

$$\begin{aligned}\mathbf{TOF} &\mathbf{= 0R + 1L, or}\\ &\mathbf{= 0R + 2L, or}\\ &\mathbf{= 0R + 3L.}\end{aligned}$$

In TOF, the left-sided subpulmonary conus is underdeveloped in 3 dimensions and hence is obstructive. TOF is a subnormality. In TOF, the conal septum may be normal, underdeveloped, or absent. **1L means that a small amount of subpulmonary conus is present, but unexpanded, and hence pulmonary outflow tract atresia is present. 2L means severe stenosis of the pulmonary outflow tract. 3L means mild to moderate stenosis of the pulmonary outflow tract. 4L means normal development with no stenosis of the pulmonary outflow tract**.

Truncus arteriosus type A1 [7] is a TOF with pulmonary infundibular and valvar atresia, plus an aortopulmonary septal defect or AP window (APW).

$$\textbf{Truncus arteriosus type A1} = \textbf{0R} + \textbf{1L} + \textbf{APW}$$

Type A means that a subtruncal ventricular septal defect (VSD) is present.

Truncus arteriosus type A2 [7, 8] is TOF with pulmonary infundibular and valvar atresia, with absence of the main pulmonary artery (MPA), and origin of the right pulmonary artery (RPA) and of the left pulmonary artery (LPA) from the ascending aorta (from the aortic sac) [8]. The equation for truncus arteriosus type A2 is:

$$\textbf{Truncus Arteriosus type A2} = \textbf{0R} + \textbf{1L} - \textbf{MPA}$$

Because the MPA is absent, the RPA and the LPA remain in their site of origin — arising from the aortic sac, because there is no main pulmonary artery on to which they would normally migrate. This is also why there is no remnant of the aortopulmonary septum.

We think that the conventional understanding of truncus arteriosus is wrong [7, 8], i.e., that truncus is caused by a failure of downgrowth of the trunco-conal septum. Instead, truncus appears to be closely related to TOF. Truncus arteriosus type A1 is a common aortopulmonary trunk (i.e., a truncus arteriosus communis). But truncus arteriosus type A2 is a solitary aortic trunk (i.e., a truncus aorticus solitarius). This is why we refer to **truncus arteriosus**, but not to truncus arteriosus *communis*, because type A2 is a *solitary aortic* trunk, not a *common arterial* trunk.

In hearts with a ventricular L-loop, the developmental and anatomic conotruncal equations or formulas are inverted, or right-left reversed (Figs. 1.1 and 1.2).

Anatomically corrected malposition of the great arteries (**ACM**) is a rare type of conotruncal anomaly in which there is a malposition of the great arteries, but in which the great arteries nonetheless arise above the morphologically appropriate ventricles, aorta above the LV and pulmonary artery above the RV. In this sense, the malposition of the great arteries is "anatomically corrected." This is possible because *the abnormal conotruncus and the ventricles twist in opposite directions* [9]. In patients with visceroatrial situs solitus, there are two anatomic types: *ACM* {*S,D,L*} and *ACM* {*S,L,D*}.

In ACM {**S,D,L**}, as the segmental anatomy indicates, there is visceroatrial situs solitus, concordant D-loop ventricles, and L-malposition of the great arteries. The malposed aorta is anterior and to the left above the LV, and the malposed pulmonary artery is posterior and to the right above the RV. So, ACM {S,D,L} is corrected both anatomically and physiologically. Surgically, ACM {S,D,L} may just require VSD closure.

In ACM {S,L,D}, as the segmental anatomy indicates, there are discordant L-loop ventricles associated with D-malposed great arteries. Although the great arteries are *anatomically* corrected, they are *physiologically* uncorrected. Surgically, ACM {S,L,D} may benefit from an atrial switch operation.

In ACM, there is ventriculoarterial concordance, but the great arteries are *not* normally related. In ACM, the conus is either bilateral (subaortic and subpulmonary), or subaortic only with pulmonary-atrioventricular valvar fibrous continuity [9]. Thus, **ventriculoarterial concordance** does not always mean normally related great arteries (solitus or inversus) because anatomically corrected malposition of the great arteries also has VA concordance. For more information on ACM, please see Chap. 33.

Interrupted aortic arch (IAA) may be regarded as "anti-tetralogy"—the opposite of tetralogy of Fallot [10]. In TOF, the conal septum is displaced anteriorly, superiorly, and leftward, with narrowing of the pulmonary outflow tract and typically with a large subaortic VSD. In IAA type B (distal to the left common carotid artery), the conal septum is displaced inferiorly and posteriorly, too close to the mitral valve, resulting in a narrowed subaortic outflow tract and a large subpulmonary VSD. IAA may have excessive dextral rotation at the semilunar valve level, accounting for the conal septal malalignment, whereas TOF has deficient dextral rotation at the semilunar valves, which also accounts for the conal septal malalignment in typical TOF.

The etiology of the conotruncal anomalies is now undergoing intensive investigation. Molecular genetic evidence suggests that malformations of right-left development may be caused by one or more mutations in the Nodal cascade [2], the anterior heart field [10], the neural crest cells [10], the Pax 3 gene [10], and Pit x2c [11]. Rapid dextral rotation at the conotruncal junction between Carnegie stages 15 and 19 has been observed in normal mice, but fails to occur in mouse models of DORV, truncus, and TGA [12].

The conotruncal equations or formulas are presented here in print for the first time. They help to provide a quantitative approach to the definition and understanding of the many different anatomic types of conotruncal malformation.

Spiral Versus Straight Great Arteries

In TGA, why are the great arteries straight, or parallel, or uncrossed, whereas with normally related great arteries, the great arteries are spiral, or twisted about each other? It used to be thought (Quain, 1844 [13]) that TGA results from straight downgrowth of the truncoconal septum that separates the great arteries and the ventricular outflow tracts; whereas with normally related great arteries, the truncoconal septum grows down from the aortic arch 4/6 junction in a spiral or twisted fashion.

We now think that it's a matter of simple developmental and anatomic geometry: i.e., the difference between the highly variable semilunar spatial relationship proximally, and the fixed aorticopulmonary relationship distally between the aortic arch and the pulmonary arterial bifurcation. As long as it is present (i.e., not absent), the aorta is always anterior (ventral) and superior (cephalad) relative to the pulmonary arterial bifurcation, because this is the fixed relationship between embryonic aortic arches 4 and pulmonary arterial arches 6. This is why the aorta always arches over the pulmonary artery bifurcation.

So, the aorto-pulmonary relationship distally is a *constant*: aorta anterior and superior, pulmonary artery posterior and inferior. But, the semilunar valvar interrelationship proximally is a *variable* (Fig. 1.1).

Looping of the heart tube to the right usually carries the developing aortic valve to the right of the developing pulmonary valve, in an approximately side-by-side relationship (Fig. 1.1). Then this side-by-side semilunar relationship may be modified in various ways by development (growth or involution) of the subsemilunar conal free walls. With solitus normally related great arteries, the right-sided subaortic conal free wall involutes (disappears), and consequently the aortic valve moves inferiorly, posteriorly and leftward (Fig. 1.1). The left-sided subpulmonary conal free wall grows well, and consequently the pulmonary valve is carried superiorly, anteriorly, and rightward (Fig. 1.1).

In D-TGA, the aortic valve moves superiorly and anteriorly, while the pulmonary valve moves inferiorly and posteriorly, because of reversed right-left development (inversion) of the subsemilunar conal free walls (Fig. 1.1). In this diagram (Fig. 1.1), the D-transposed aortic valve is only 30° to the right of the sagittal (antero-posterior) plane. In contrast, the normally related aortic valve is 150° to the right of the sagittal plane (Fig. 1.1).

Thus, normally related great arteries (Fig. 1.1) have much more untwisting to do than do transposed great arteries. In this case (Fig. 1.1): 150° − 30° = 120° difference. This is why normally related great arteries look as though they are twisting about each other; in fact, they are **untwisting** about each other. Normally related great arteries have approximately 150° of dextral rotation to undo. This is also why transposed great arteries look parallel, or straight, or uncrossed — because they have so little rightward twisting to undo between the semilunar valves below, and the aortic arch and pulmonary bifurcation above — compared with the untwisting done by normally related great arteries (Fig. 1.1): only 30° compared with 150°. Thus, in this heart specimen with D-TGA, the great arteries have only 20 % as much untwisting to do as do normally related great arteries (30°/150° × 100). 80 % of the untwisting has been abnormally accomplished by the R-L reversed (inverted) development of the subarterial conal free walls.

An equation for magnitude of the untwisting of the great arteries is as follows: **Untwisting of Ao and PA = $R_v - R_{Ao\,\&\,PA}$**[1]

[1] Ao, aorta; PA, main pulmonary artery; R_v, rotation of semilunar valves (V) relative to the antero-posterior (AP) plane; $R_{Ao\,\&\,PA}$ rotation of the aortic arch and pulmonary bifurcation relative to the AP plane; measurements in degrees (°).

The morphogenesis of normally related great arteries and transposition of the great arteries is contrasted in Fig. 1.2. The "engines" controlling semilunar morphogenesis are thought to be (Figs. 1.1 and 1.2): (1) ventricular loop formation (the first approximately 90° relative to the sagittal plane); and (2) subsemilunar conal free wall development (variations from a side-by-side relationship). When the subsemilunar conal free walls are equally developed bilaterally (equally well developed as in the Taussig-Bing malformation [4, 5], or equally deficient as in the Paul type of double-outlet left ventricle) [6], the semilunar relationship is approximately side-by-side, aortic valve to the right and pulmonary valve to the left, when D-loop ventricles are present.

In the so-called conotruncal malformations, the great arteries *per se* are almost always normally developed. The only exception is truncus arteriosus. The so-called conotruncal malformations, from a developmental viewpoint, are almost all infundibular or conal malformations only (Fig. 1.1 and 1.2). The anatomic anomalies of the great arteries are secondary to the primary developmental anomalies of the **conal connector**. This is why these normally formed great arteries are abnormally connected with the underlying ventricles and atrioventricular canal, resulting in abnormal ventriculo-arterial *alignments*. This is also why abnormally connected and therefore abnormally aligned great arteries are also abnormally related great arteries, i.e., abnormally related relative to external spatial coordinates (right-left, anterior-posterior, and superior-inferior). The designation *conotruncus* serves as a helpful reminder that the conus arteriosus belongs with the great arteries, i.e., that the conus is not an intrinsic part of either ventricle, or of both ventricles. The conus arteriosus is the great arteries' connecting segment. That is why abnormally, the subarterial conus can override the ventricular septum to any degree, from mostly or entirely above the RV, to mostly or entirely above the LV — because the conus is really an intrinsic part of neither ventricle.

The great arteries do not *connect* with the ventricles directly, tissue to tissue, because of the interposition of the conus. [Note the active voice of the verb *connect*.]

Instead, the great arteries *are connected* with the ventricles (ventricular sinuses or inflow tracts) in many different ways by the conal connector. [Note the passive voice of the verb *are connected*.] This distinction is made in the interests of anatomic accuracy.

Consequently, we talk and write about ventriculoarterial *alignments* (not ventriculoarterial *connections*) because, accurately speaking, the ventricles do not connect with the great arteries, because of the interposition of the conus. Only the VA alignments can be described as concordant, or discordant, or double-outlet, etc. The conal connections cannot be so described.

This anatomically based distinction between *alignments* and *connections* is not a semantic quibble. This distinction has nothing to do with verbal preferences. **An accurate understanding of the normal and abnormal anatomy of the conus arteriosus is the key to an accurate understanding of the conotruncal anomalies**. The conus is not "just part of the RV." The conus is much more interesting than that (Tables 1.1 and 1.2).

Table 1.1 Normally and abnormally related great arteries correlated with right-left conal free wall development: grades 0–4

Relation between great arteries	Right-sided conal free wall	Left-sided conal free wall
D-loop ventricles	*AoV right-sided*	*PV left-sided*
Normal	0	4
Tetralogy	0	1/2/3
Truncus	0	1
D-TGA	4	0
DORV	4	4
DOLV	0	0/1/2
L-loop ventricles	*PV right-sided*	*AoV left-sided*
Inverted normal	4	0
Inverted TOF	1/2/3	0
L-TGA	0	4
Inverted DORV	4	4

Abbreviations: *D-loop* heart tube that has folded or looped in a rightward or dextral direction, *DOLV* double-outlet left ventricle, *DORV* double-outlet right ventricle, *D-TGA* dextro-transposition of the great arteries, *L-TGA* levo-transposition of the great arteries, *L-loop* heart tube that has looped in a levo or leftward direction. Grades of subarterial conal free wall development: *0* absent, *1* present but atretic, *2* severe stenosis, *3* mild stenosis, *4* normally well developed & not stenotic, *TOF* tetralogy of Fallot; other abbreviations as previously

Table 1.1 correlates normally and abnormally related great arteries with right-left subarterial conal free wall development, with D-loop ventricles and with L-loop ventricles.

Table 1.2 presents 11 conotruncal or infundibuloarteiral equations, with ventricular D-loops and with ventricular L-loops. It should be understood that there are many more than 11 equations; these are just examples. The equation concerning an individual case should precisely reflect the subarterial conal free wall anatomy of that patient, and such anatomy is highly variable.

The anatomic and developmental equations presented in Table 1.2 may be used as **quantitative indices of the size of the subarterial conal free walls** as follows: A quantitative index of the size of the conal free wall = the distance between the semilunar valve (SLV) above and the atrioventricular valve (AVV) below (in mm or cm). These are measurements of the "height" of the conal musculature that separates (or does not separate) the semilunar valves above from the atrioventricular valves below.

Why is inverted truncus arteriosus not included in Table 1.2? Because we have never seen truncus arteriosus in situs inversus totalis. Table 1.2 is data-based (not "conceptual"). There are many more anatomic variations than are represented by these 11 equations (Table 1.2); these equations are examples of some of the more common anatomic data.

Anatomic types of human heart are presented diagrammatically in Fig. 1.3 **in terms of segmental sets, AV and VA alignments, and conal connections.**

Conotruncal (infundibuloarterial) malformations are shown in rows 5–8 inclusive (Fig. 1.3): TGA, row 5; ACM, i.e., anatomically corrected malposition of the great arteries, row 6; DORV, row 7; and DOLV, row 8.

Table 1.2 Normal and abnormal infundibuloarterial equations

With D-loop ventricles, Ao Rt & PA Lt
1. Solitus NRGA = 0R + 4L
2. TOF = 0R + 1L, or
= 0R + 2L, or
= 0R + 3L
3. Truncus Arteriosus
Type A1 = 0R + 1L + APW
Type A2 = 0R + 1L – MPA
4. D-TGA = 4R + 0L
5. TGA {S, D, L} = 2R + 4L[a]
6. DORV, Taussig-Bing type = 4R + 4L
7. DOLV, Paul type = 0R + 0L
With L-loop ventricles, PA Rt & Ao Lt
8. Inverted NRGA = 4R + 0L
9. Inverted TOF = 1R + 0L, or
= 2R + 0R, or
= 3R + 0L
10. L-TGA = 0R + 4L
11. Inverted DORV = 4R + 4L

Abbreviations: *Ao* aorta, *DOLV* double-outlet left ventricle, *DORV* double-outlet right ventricle, *APW* aortopulmonary window, *D-TGA* dextro-transposition of the great arteries, *Lt* left-sided, *L-TGA* levo-transposition of the great arteries, *MPA* main pulmonary artery, *NRGA* normally related great arteries, *PA* main pulmonary artery, *Rt* right-sided, *TOF* tetralogy of Fallot, +, and, –, without. TOF = 0R + *1L* means TOF with pulmonary outflow tract atresia. TOF = 0R + *2L* means TOF with severe pulmonary outflow tract stenosis. TOF = 0R + *3L* means TOF with mild to moderate pulmonary outflow tract stenosis

[a]In TGA {S, D, **L**}, as the segmental anatomic diagnosis indicates, the subaortic conal freewall is left-sided, and the subpulmonary conal free wall is right-sided

Figure 1.3 depicts some, but by no means all, of the anatomic types of human heart.

So, what really are conotruncal or infundibuloarterial malformations?

From the anatomic standpoint, as the name *conotruncal* or *infundibuloarterial* indicates, such malformations have anomalies both of the infundibulum (conus) and of the great arteries (truncus arteriosus) that may be expressed verbally, or diagrammatically (Figs. 1.1, 1.2 and 1.3), or symbolically with infundibuloarterial equations (Table 1.2).

Isolated semilunar valvar anomalies — such as congenital pulmonary stenosis or congenital aortic regurgitation — are *not* regarded as conotruncal anomalies because neither the conus, nor the truncus is malformed.

One may harbor some doubts regarding the accuracy of excluding isolated semilunar valvar anomalies because the aortic and the pulmonary valves are located right at the cono-truncal or infundibulo-arterial junction. Nonetheless, it is difficult to

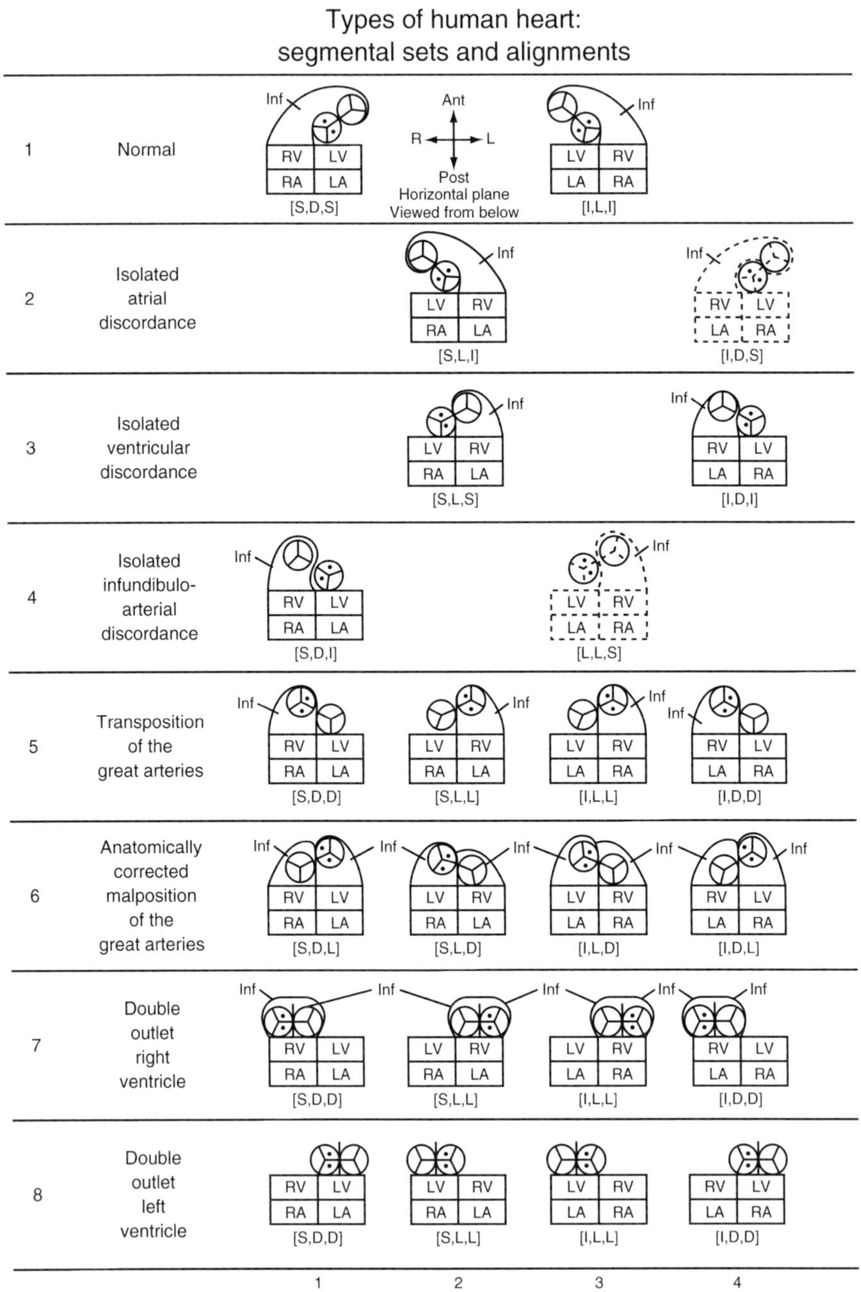
Types of human heart:
segmental sets and alignments
1 Normal
[S,D,S]
Ant
R
L
Post
Horizontal plane
Viewed from below
[I,L,I]
2 Isolated atrial discordance
[S,L,I]
[I,D,S]
3 Isolated ventricular discordance
[S,L,S]
[I,D,I]
4 Isolated infundibulo-arterial discordance
[S,D,I]
[L,L,S]
5 Transposition of the great arteries
[S,D,D]
[S,L,L]
[I,L,L]
[I,D,D]
6 Anatomically corrected malposition of the great arteries
[S,D,L]
[S,L,D]
[I,L,D]
[I,D,L]
7 Double outlet right ventricle
[S,D,D]
[S,L,L]
[I,L,L]
[I,D,D]
8 Double outlet left ventricle
[S,D,D]
[S,L,L]
[I,L,L]
[I,D,D]
Inf
RV
LV
RA
LA
1
2
3
4

Fig. 1.3 Types of human heart in terms of segmental sets (combinations), AV and VA segmental alignments (what opens into what), and subarterial conal connections or infundibulum (*Inf*). All of the heart diagrams are shown as viewed from below, similar to a subxiphoid 2 D echocardiogram. Cardiotypes shown in broken lines had not been documented when this diagram was made. The aortic valve is indicated by the coronary ostia. The pulmonary valve is indicated by the absence of coronary ostia. Braces { } mean "the set of". Columns 1–4 are arranged in terms of **atrioventricular (AV) concordance and discordance. All of the heart diagrams in column 1 have AV concordance**. The morphologically right atrium (RA) opens into the morphologically right ventricle (RV), and the morphologically left atrium (LA) opens into the morphologically left ventricle (LV) because the viscera and atria are in situs solitus, i.e., {S,-,-} and a ventricular D-loop is present, i.e., {S,D,-}. Also important is that all 4 cardiac chambers are well developed. If the RV sinus (inflow) is absent, for example, then both atria can open into the LV, resulting in double-inlet single LV with an infundibular outlet chamber. **All of the hearts diagrammed in column 2 have AV discordance**, right-sided RA opening into right-sided LV and left-sided LA opening into left-sided RV, because the viscera and atria are in situs solitus, but a ventricular L-loop is present, i.e., {S,L,-}. **All of the hearts in column 3 have AV concordance** because the viscera and atria are in situs inversus, i.e., {I,-.-} and a ventricular L-loop is present, i.e., {I,L,-}. The left-sided RA opens into the left-sided RV and the right-sided LA opens into the right-sided LV. **All the hearts in column 4 have AV discordance** because the viscera and atria are in situs inversus, i.e., {I,-,-}, but D-loop ventricles are present, i.e., {I,D,-}. **The 8 rows are organized in terms of the type of ventriculo-arterial (VA) alignment that is present. Row 1** shows the solitus normal heart, i.e., {S,D,S} and the inverted normal heart, i.e., {I,L,I}. Both have AV and VA concordance, and a well developed subpulmonary infundibulum (Inf) and no subaortic infundibular free wall—permitting aortic-mitral fibrous continuity. **Rows 2, 3, and 4** show solitus and inversus normally related great arteries with rare segmental sets: {S,L,I}, {S,L,S}, {I,D,I}, and {S,D,I}. **The conotruncal or infundibuloarterial anomalies are depicted in rows 5–8**. Some of the anatomic types of transposition of the great arteries are shown in *row 5*, anatomically corrected malposition of the great arteries in *row 6*, double-outlet right ventricle in *row 7*, and double-outlet left ventricle in *row 8*. **Visceroatrial situs ambiguus** with the heterotaxy syndromes of asplenia, polysplenia, and normally formed but right-sided spleen were intentionally omitted. Atrial situs ambiguus is not a third anatomic type of atrial situs; instead, atrial situs ambiguus, i.e., {A,-,-} means that the type of atrial situs is morphologically uncertain, or unknown. The atrioventricular valves are not depicted because they typically correspond to the ventricle of entry (not to the atrium of exit): tricuspid valve enters RV, and mitral valve enters LV. **The *segmental* method of diagnosis is *sequential***, i.e., it proceeds in a veno-arterial sequence, i.e., {atria, ventricles, great arteries}, as, for example, in TGA {S,D,D}. **VA concordance** does not always mean normally related great arteries. Anatomically corrected malposition of the great arteries (*row 6*) also has VA concordance. **Tetralogy of Fallot** has a subpulmonary conus, with absence of the subaortic conal free wall, like normally related great arteries {S,D,S} and {I,L,I} (*row 1*). However the subpulmonary conus is undeveloped, and hence is stenotic or atretic. **Truncus arteriosus** typically is tetralogy of Fallot with pulmonary outflow tract atresia, with additional malformations such as aortopulmonary septal defect (AP window) (type 1), or absence of the main pulmonary artery with origin of the right and left pulmonary artery branches from the ascending aorta (i.e., from the aortic sac) (type 2), or absence of a proximal portion of a pulmonary artery branch, with that lung being supplied by a ductus-like collateral artery (type 3), or interrupted aortic arch with a small ascending aortic component and a large main pulmonary artery component with a large patent ductus arteriosus supplying the descending thoracic aorta (type 4). Rarely, truncus arteriosus can arise above the RV, with a well developed subarterial conus arteriosus, preventing truncal-mitral or truncal-tricuspid fibrous continuity. It looks like a type 2 truncus with a subarterial muscular conus arteriosus arising above the RV. The general anatomic definition of truncus arteriosus is: one great artery arising from the base of the heart that gives rise to the coronary arteries (at least one), the pulmonary artery branches (at least one), and the brachiocephalic arteries. This definition permits the inclusion of multiple different anomalies. This is also true of most of the other conotruncal anomalies (rows 5–8, inclusive) (Reproduced from Foran et al. [14], with permission of Elsevier)

regard isolated aortic valvar and isolated pulmonary valvar anomalies as conotruncal or infundibuloarterial malformations when both the infundibulum (conus) and the great arteries (truncus) are normally formed anatomically.

Interrupted aortic arch (IAA) also merits explanation. **IAA type A** (the interruption being distal to the left subclavian artery) is *not* considered to be a conotruncal anomaly because the infundibulum typically is normally formed.

However, **IAA type B** is considered to be a conotruncal malformation because the infundibulum typically is malformed. The conal septum is malaligned postero-inferiorly — too close to the mitral valve — resulting in stenosis of the outflow tract from the LV to the ascending aorta, and also resulting in a large subpulmonary VSD. So IAA type A and IAA type B are very different malformations.

If this seems a little strange, it may be helpful to recall that cyanotic congenital heart disease has many different anatomic causes. IAA is a secondary malformation, not a primary one. In other words, IAA typically appears to be a secondary effect, not a primary cause. More specifically, IAA usually appears to be the result of reduced anterograde blood flow in the aortic arch. There are a variety of different anatomic malformations that can critically reduce anterograde aortic arch blood flow, predisposing to IAA, either type A or type B. IAA type C (distal to the right common carotid artery) is a rare form, that may have a different causation.

The so-called conotruncal or infundibuloarterial malformations are fascinating from a developmental (embryologic and genetic) viewpoint:

Almost all of the conotruncal malformations are conal or infundibular anomalies *only*. The great arteries (truncus arteriosus) are normally formed *per se*.

The only conotruncal anomaly in which the great arteries are abnormally formed is truncus arteriosus. In type 1, an aortopulmonary (AP) window is present [7]. In type 2, the main pulmonary artery appears to be absent.

Why then, do the great arteries look so abnormal anatomically, as for example, in TGA?

Because the conal connector is malformed. The subarterial infundibular free walls form the platforms on which the great arteries stand. If these subarterial platforms are malformed, then the great arteries are abnormally related (Figs. 1.1, 1.2 and 1.3), the ventriculo-arterial alignments are abnormal (Figs. 1.1 and 1.3), and the ventriculo-arterial connectors (the platforms) are abnormal (Fig. 1.2, Tables 1.1 and 1.2).

Abnormally related great arteries are abnormally connected great arteries.

The truncoconal malseptation hypothesis is wrong [13], i.e., spiral truncoconal septation results in normally related great arteries; whereas straight downgrowth of the truncoconal septum results in TGA, etc.

If ever you see an AP window in a conotruncal anomaly (apart from truncus), you should report it because AP windows are rare in non-truncus infundibulo-arterial anomalies. If conotruncal anomalies were caused by truncoconal malseptation, definite anatomic evidence of such malseptation (like an AP window) should be common. But in fact, such anatomic evidence is vanishingly rare.

At the present time, most cardiologists and cardiac surgeons understand that tetralogy of Fallot is basically an infundibular anomaly. But at the present time, most informed observers do not understand that the same is true of TGA, ACM, DORV, and DOLV, that the great arteries in all of these anomalies are normally formed *per se*, and that the malformation is at the infundibular or conal level. Since congenital heart disease is named, defined, and diagnosed *anatomically* (not physiologically, embryologically, or genetically), the term conotruncal anomalies is *anatomically* correct: the infundibulum is the site of the *primary* developmental and anatomic malformations, and the great arteries are the site of the *secondary* anatomic malformations.

Normal development of the infundibulum (conus arteriosus) is "Mother Nature's" way of performing the embryonic aortic switch procedure [2].

The infundibulum is basically a muscular structure, whereas the aortic and pulmonary valves are fibroelastic, similar to the great arteries. This may explain why it is possible for anomalies of the aortic and pulmonary valves to occur, without associated malformations either of the infundibulum or of the great arteries.

Infundibuloarterial or conotruncal equations, published here for the first time (Table 1.2), are a step in the direction of a more quantitative understanding of the development and the anatomy of normally and abnormally related great arteries.

Attention is focused on the subarterial infundibular *free walls* (rather than on truncoconal septation). It is important for current embryologic and genetic investigators to understand where the problem is located [12].

The infundibulum or conus arteriosus is an independent variable. The infundibulum can be located above either, or both ventricles, and the infundibulum can be beneath either, or both great arteries.

It is important to understand that the infundibulum is not "just part of the right ventricle." Instead, it is an independent connecting cardiac segment of the great arteries that is of major developmental and anatomic importance [2].

What About TGA {S,D,L}? [15]

In this form of TGA, as the segmental diagnsosis indicates, there is visceroatrial situs solitus, D-loop ventricles, and L-TGA, with AV concordance and VA discordance. The transposed aortic valve lies anteriorly and to the *left* relative to the transposed pulmonary valve that lies posteriorly and to the *right*. The right-sided RV ejected into the left-sided and anterior transposed Ao, and the left-sided LV ejected into the right-sided and posterior transposed PA.

Where Is the Subaortic Conal free Wall? And Where Is the Subpulmonary Conal Free Wall?

Ask the semilunar valves, because the subarterial conal free walls lie immediately beneath the semilunar valves. So, the subaortic conal free wall is anterior and to the left (beneath the aortic valve), and the subpulmonary conal free wall is posterior and to the right (beneath the pulmonary valve).

As the segmental anatomic diagnosis (TGA {S,D,L}) indicates, the ventricles looped to the right, but the conotruncus twisted to the left, like a backwards S (Ƨ). So, there is malrotation of the bulboventricular loop.

Usually, the bulboventricular loop is like the letter C: both the ventricles and the conotruncus twist in the same direction, to the right, as in TGA {S,**D**,**D**}.

Similarly, when the bulboventricular loop is inverted, as in TGA {S,**L**,**L**}, the ventricles and the conotruncus both twist in the same direction, to the left, like a backwards C (Ɔ).

But, TGA {S,**D**,**L**} is uncommon because the ventricles and the conotruncus have twisted in opposite directions — ventricles to the right, and infundibulum and great arteries to the left.

The segmental anatomic diagnosis indicates how this conotruncal equation should be written: $\text{TGA}\{\text{S, D, L}\} = 2\text{R} + 4\text{L}$ (Table 1.2, Eq. 8). The segmental anatomic diagnosis — TGA {S,D,**L**} indicates that the well developed subaortic conal free wall is left-sided, i.e., 4L. The subpulmonary conal free wall is right-sided and is often present, but underdeveloped and hence stenotic, i.e., 2R. Hence, the infundibuloarterial equation for TGA {S,D,L} often equals 2R+4L [15].

Great Arterial Switch Procedures

Normally, in "Mother Nature's" embryonic arterial switch procedure, only *one* great artery — the aorta — gets switched from the RV to the LV (Fig. 1.4). Even abnormally, as in TGA, only one great artery gets switched — the pulmonary artery.

Fig. 1.4 Dissected embryonic human hearts, great arteries removed above the semilunar valve level to expose the morphogenetic movements of the developing aortic valve (*AoV*) and pulmonary valve (*PV*). The atrial free walls have been removed to expose the division of the common atrioventricular valve (*CAVV*) into the mitral valve (*MV*) and the tricuspid valve (*TV*). View of the hearts from behind and above. The anterior (ventral) surface is towards the top of the page. The posterior (dorsal) surface is towards the bottom of the page. The right (*Rt*) surface is towards the viewer's right hand. The left (*Lt*) surface is towards the viewer's left hand. The Roman numerals indicate Streeter's horizons (stages). Horizon XV corresponds to an embryonic age (age since fertilization) of 30–32 days. Take Streeter's horizon (*XV*) and double it (30 days); that is when the horizon starts. Each horizon is 2 days long. Therefore, Streeter's horizon 15 corresponds to a stage that begins at 30 days of age and ends at the end of 32 days. Horizon XV1a indicates the first half of this horizon, i.e., day 32. Horizon XV1b means the last half of this horizon, i.e., day 33. (*ant.* anterior, *DORV* double-outlet right ventricle, *NRGA* normally related great arteries, *TOF* tetralogy of Fallot. NRGA undergo approximately 150° of dextrorotation relative to the sagittal plane at the semilunar valves. In contrast, abnormally connected great arteries with conotruncal malformations undergo much less dextrorotation at the level of the semilunar valves, i.e., much less than 150° dextrorotation. NRGA untwist through approximately 150° levorotation as they go from the semilunar valves below to the aortic arch and pulmonary arterial bifurcation above. Abnormally related great arteries have much less untwisting (i.e., levorotation) to do than do normally related great arteries — because abnormally related great arteries have undergone far less dextrorotation at the semilunar valve level and consequently have far less untwisting to do than do normally related great arteries. This is why the great arteries in TGA appear parallel, or straight, or uncrossed when compared with normally related great arteries, because normally related great arteries have much more leftward untwisting to do. Note also that the common AV valve normally starts to undergo septation into the mitral and tricuspid valves when the human embryo is 34–36 days of age (Modified from Asami [16], with permission of Wiley)

Only human cardiac surgeons routinely switch *both* great arteries for patients with TGA. Rarely, Mother Nature does do an embryonic double great arterial switch, as in DOLV (Table 1.2).

Morphogenetic Movement of the Great Arteries

Thus far, I have emphasized the importance of the pathologic anatomy and the pathologic development of the subarterial conal free walls (Tables 1.1 and 1.2), because this is what appears to cause abnormally related great arteries (Figs. 1.1, 1.2 and 1.3).

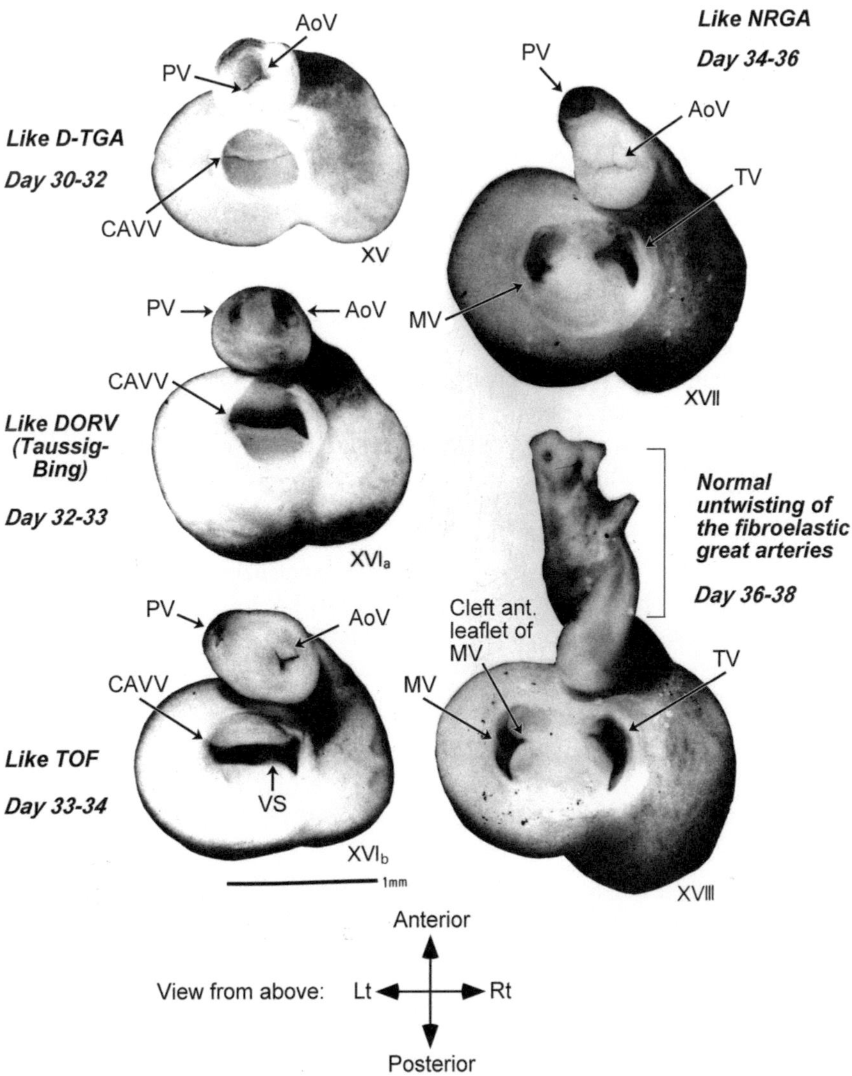

Let us look at these normal and abnormal relationships between the great arteries in greater detail. **During normal development, the morphogenetic movements of the developing semilunar valves and great arteries are very real and very important** (**Fig**. 1.4) [16].

By 30–32 days of age in utero, the semilunar interrelationship of the human embryo looks like D-TGA The developing aortic valve (AoV) is anterior and to the right relative to the developing pulmonary valve (PV) which is posterior and to the left (Fig. 1.4, top, left). The rotation of the semilunar valves relative to the sagittal plane is 50° to the right (50° dextrorotation).

By 32–33 days of age in utero, the semilunar valves are side-by-side, AoV to the right and PV to the left – reminiscent of the Taussig-Bing malformation (Fig. 1.4, left, middle). The aortic and pulmonary valves now display 90° dextrorotation relative to the sagittal plane.

By 33–34 days of age, the semilunar valves of the human embryo resemble that of tetralogy of Fallot (Fig. 1.4, left, bottom). The AoV is mildly posterior and right-sided, whereas the PV is mildly anterior and left-sided. The semilunar valves have now rotated 110° to the right relative to the sagittal plane (110° dextrorotation). The AoV is beginning to be switched into the LV.

By 34–36 days of age (Fig. 1.4, top, right), normally related great arteries appear to have been achieved. The AoV is posterior on the right and the PV is anterior on the left. The semilunar valves have undergone 155° rotation to the right relative to the sagittal plane (155° dextrorotation).

By 36–38 days of age in utero (Fig. 1.4, right, bottom), the normal human great arteries are seen to be untwisting, to undo the approximately 150° of dextrorotation that makes possible to normal human aortic switch from above the RV to above the LV.

This elegant study by Asami [16] also shows the normal fusion of the superior and inferior endocardial cushions of the common atrioventricular valve (CAVV) above the ventricular septum (VS) to form the mitral valve (MV) and the tricuspid valve (TV). The cleft in the anterior leaflet of the MV is still incompletely fused.

The Roman numerals indicate Streeter's horizons: XV, XV1a, XV1b, XV11, and XV111 (Fig. 1.4).

The fifth week of gestation, when the mother is just realizing that she is pregnant, is when the embryonic human aortic switch normally occurs (Fig. 1.4).

What is responsible for these morphogenetic movements of the Ao and the PA?

The development of the subarterial conal free walls (Figs. 1.1, 1.2 and 1.3). "Development" includes growth and expansion, as well as involution and disappearance.

Cardiovascular Evolution

When did life come ashore and what made it possible? [2, 11]. Our phylum Chordata goes back to ancient fish of the Ordovician and upper Devonian periods, 500 million to 345 million years ago. These fish had a single ventricle, from which our left ventricle (LV) is derived.

Amphibia evolved 345–325 million years ago during the Carboniferous period. They had lungs and so could breathe air, but they had no right ventricle.

Some amphibia evolved into fully terrestrial animals, the Amniota — animals with an amniotic sac in which the embryo and fetus could float and "swim", like our piscine ancestors. Amphibia have to return to the water to breed, but the amniotes were fully terrestrial.

Some amniotes evolved into reptiles. Others evolved into birds — feathered reptiles — like *archeopterix*. Still other reptiles evolved into mammals — furry or hairy reptiles. Mammals evolved during the Jurassic period, about 180 million years ago.

Although fish and amphibia do not have a right ventricle (RV), the higher reptiles (crocodiles and alligators), birds, and mammals normally all do. The comparatively recently evolved RV is only about 36 % as old as the LV: 180 million vs at least 500 million years old, respectively. The RV is the lung pump. Most permanent air-breathers have an RV.

The development of the RV sinus (body, or inflow tract) was the second, key, cardiovascular evolutionary adaptation that helped to make it possible for us to become permanent land-living and air breathing vertebrates.

The embryonic aortic switch was achieved by complete right-left asymmetry in the development of the subarterial conal free walls, with involution of the right-sided subaortic conal free wall, and good development of the left-sided subpulmonary conal free wall [2]. Following normal D-loop formation: $\text{NRGA} = 0\text{R} + 4\text{L}$.

Any other development of the conal connector results in a conotruncal malformation [2].

The third evolutionary cardiovascular adaptation that facilitated permanent land-living and air-breathing was cardiovascular septation that separated the unoxygenated and the oxygenated blood streams.

To summarize, the evolution of complete R-L asymmetry in the development of the subarterial conal free walls made possible the embryonic aortic switch. This in turn led to the development of solitus normally related great arteries — one of the most important evolutionary cardiovascular adaptations that helped to make possible permanent land-living and air-breathing:

$$\text{SNRGA} = \text{OR} + 4\text{L}.$$

It's mirror-image isomer is:

$$\text{INRGA} = 4\text{R} + 0\text{L}.$$

Any other pattern of conal development results in a conotruncal malformation (Table 1.2).

Infundibulo-Arterial (IA) Situs Concordance and Discordance

The following are newly understood basic principles:

1. When the pattern of anatomic organization, or situs, of the subarterial infundibulum and of the great arteries are concordant (the same), the great arteries are normally related.
2. When the pattern of anatomic organization, or situs, of the subarterial infundibulum and of the great arteries are discordant (different), the great arteries are abnormally related.

Examples of these basic principles follow (Fig. 1.1 and Table 1.1):

$$\mathbf{SNRGA = 0R + 4L.} \tag{1.1}$$

In solitus normally related great arteries, the subarterial infundibular situs formula is 0R+4L, as in the above equation. This is the normal solitus infundibular formula or "recipe". The great arteries also are in situs solitus. The aortic valve is to the right of the pulmonary valve. Hence, in SNRGA, **IA situs analysis is solitus-solitus**; i.e., IA situs concordance is present.

$$\mathbf{INRGA = 4R + 0L} \tag{1.2}$$

In inverted normally related great arteries (INRGA), the subarterial infundibular formula is 4R+0L. This is the normal inverted infundibular formula. The great arteries also are in situs inversus; the aortic valve is to the left of the pulmonary valve. Thus, **IA situs analysis is inversus-inversus.** Hence, in INRGA, there is IA situs concordance, both inverted.

$$\mathbf{TGA\{S, D, D\} = 4R + 0L} \tag{1.3}$$

In typical transposition of the great arteries with solitus viscera and atria, D-loop (solitus) ventricles, and D-TGA, with atrioventricular (AV) alignment concordance and ventriculoarterial (VA) alignment discordance, the subarterial situs formula is 4R+0L. This is the same formula as in INRGA; please compare with Eq. (1.2) above. But the D-transposed great arteries are in situs solitus; the aortic valve is to the right of the pulmonary valve.

So, **in typical D-TGA, IA situs analysis is inversus-solitus.** Hence, in typical D-TGA, there is IA situs discordance.

Note: There is an important difference between *situs* concordance or discordance, and *alignment* concordance or discordance – that some of our colleagues call *connection* concordance or discordance.

Situs concordance or discordance refers to the pattern of anatomic organization of adjacent cardiac segments, which may be *solitus* (normal), or *inversus* (a mirror-image of solitus). *Situs ambiguus* (uncertain or unknown pattern of anatomic organization) is not a specific type of situs; it means situs not diagnosed.

Alignment concordance or discordance indicates what opens into what, and whether it is anatomically normal or not. The morphologically right atrium (RA) opening into the morphologically right ventricle (RV) is a concordant (or appropriate) atrioventricular (AV) alignment; whereas RA opening into the morphologically left ventricle (LV) is a discordant (inappropriate, anatomically abnormal) AV alignment.

Thus, *situs* concordance/discordance and *alignment* concordance/discordance are different concepts.

$$\mathbf{TGA\{S,L,L\} = 0R + 4L} \tag{1.4}$$

The classical form of congenital physiologically corrected transposition of the great arteries with solitus viscera and atria, L-loop (inverted) ventricles, and L-TGA, with AV alignment discordance and VA alignment discordance has an infundibular situs formula of the solitus normal type (compare with Eq. 1.1 above). But the great arteries in L-TGA are inverted; the aortic valve is to the left of the pulmonary valve. **In typical L-TGA, IA situs analysis is solitus-inversus, hence discordant.**

$$\mathbf{Taussig\text{-}Bing\ DORV\{S,D,D\} = 4R + 4L} \tag{1.5}$$

In the Taussig-Bing type of double-outlet right ventricle [4, 5] with solitus viscera and atria, D-loop (solitus) ventricles, and D-malposition of the great arteries, the subarterialinfundibular situs formula is 4R+4L, which is neither that of infundibular situs solitus, Eq. (1.1) above, nor that of infundibular situs inversus, Eq. (1.2) above. This infundibular situs formula (4R+4L) is one type of infundibular situs ambiguus. The aortic valve is to the right of the pulmonary valve; hence the great arteries are in situs solitus. Hence, the **IA situs analysis is ambiguus – solitus, which is nonconcordant.**

$$\mathbf{Paul\ DOLV\{S,D,D\} = 0R + 0L} \tag{1.6}$$

In the Paul type of DOLV [6], the infundibular situs formula (0R+0L) is different from both the normal solitus infundibular formula (0R+4L) of Eq. (1.1) above, and from the normal inverted infundibular formula (4R+0L) of Eq. (1.2) above. Consequently, the infundibular situs formula of the Paul type of DOLV (0R+0L) is a second anatomic type of infundibular situs ambiguus.

In the Paul type of DOLV, the great arteries are in situs solitus, with the aortic valve to the right of the pulmonary valve, as is indicated by the third element of the segmental situs anatomy: {S,D,**D**}.

In the Paul type of DOLV, IA analysis is ambiguus – solitus, which is nonconcordant.

In anatomically corrected malposition of the great arteries (ACM) (Fig. 1.3), the subarterial infundibulum can be subaortic only, or bilateral (subaortic and subpulmonary) [9].

$$\mathbf{ACM\{S,D,L\} = 0R + 4L} \tag{1.7}$$

In this anatomic type of ACM, the infundibular situs formula is of the solitus normal type (0R+4L), similar to Eq. (1.1). But the great arteries are inverted, with the aortic valve to the left of the pulmonary valve: {S,D,**L**}. Consequently, **IA analysis is solitus-inversus, i.e., discordant.**

If a bilateral conus (subaortic and subpulmonary) were present, IA analysis would be ambiguus–inversus, i.e., abnormal – even though in ACM, there is ventriculoarterial (VA) *alignment* concordance, by definition (Fig. 1.3). Thus, IA *situs* analysis indicates that an infundibuloarterial (or conotruncal) anomaly is present, whereas VA *alignment* analysis is concordant ("normal"). In ACM, the ventricles loop in one direction (say to the right) and the infundibular and the arterial segments (the conotruncus) twist in the opposite direction (say to the left), as in ACM {S,**D**,**L**}.

Both IA situs analysis and VA alignment analysis are accurate, but different.

In Eqs. (1.1) and (1.2) (Table 1.2), the subarterial infundibular situs and the great arterial situs are the same, typically resulting in normally related great arteries (solitus and inversus).

In Eqs. (1.3), (1.4), (1.5), (1.6), and (1.7) inclusive (Table 1.2), the infundibular situs and the great arterial situs are different, predictably resulting in abnormally related great arteries (D-TGA, L-TGA, DORV, DOLV, and ACM).

Is it possible to have infundibuloarterial (conotruncal) anomalies when the situs of the subarterial infundibulum and of the great arteries are the same?

Yes. Tetralogy of Fallot (TOF) and truncus arteriosus (TA) are familiar examples (Table 1.2)**.**

TOF {S,D,S} is characterized by variable underdevelopment of the normal or solitus type of subpulmonary infundibulum:

$$\mathbf{TOF\{S,D,S\} = 0R + 1L} \tag{1.8}$$

Grade 1 development of the left-sided subpulmonary infundibulum (0R+**1L**) indicates extreme underdevelopment and *atresia* of the left-sided subpulmonary infundibulum.

$$\mathbf{TOF\{S,D,S\} = 0R + 2L} \tag{1.9}$$

Grade 2 development of the left-sided subpulmonary infundibulum (0R+**2L**) indicates severe underdevelopment of the left-sided subpulmonary infundibulum with severe pulmonary outflow tract stenosis.

$$\mathbf{TOF\{S,D,S\} = 0R + 3L} \tag{1.10}$$

Grade 3 development of the left-sided subpulmonary infundibulum (0R+**3L**) indicates mild to moderate underdevelopment of the left-sided subpulmonary infundibulum, with mild to moderate pulmonary outflow tract stenosis.

In all three equations (1.8, 1.9, and 1.10, inclusive), the infundibular situs formulas are of the normal solitus type (0R + 4L), but with underdevelopment of the left-sided subpulmonary conus (infundibulum). The great arteries are of the solitus (normal) type, as the segmental anatomy indicates: TOF {S,D,**S**}.

Hence, in TOF, IA situs analysis is solitus-solitus, i.e., concordant.

Truncus arteriosus (TA) we think is TOF with pulmonary outflow tract atresia, with additional anomalies of the great arteries (Table 1.2) [7, 8].

$$\mathbf{TA\{S,D,S\} = 0R + 1L + APW} \tag{1.11}$$

This is what we call **TA type A1**. Type A indicates that a subtruncal ventricular septal defect (VSD) is present. Type 1 means that an aortopulmonary septal remnant is present, with an aortopulmonary septal defect or aortopulmonary window (APW).

$$\mathbf{TA\{S,D,S\} = 0R + 1L - MPA} \tag{1.12}$$

This is what we call truncus arteriosus type A2. Type A indicates that a subtruncal VSD is present. Type 2 means that there is no aortopulmonary (AP) septal remnant. We think that in TA type A2, the main pulmonary artery (MPA) is absent. This may explain why there is no AP septal remnant. The right pulmonary artery (RPA) and the left pulmonary artery (LPA) normally arise from the aortic sac on the dorsal aspect of the ascending aorta. Then, the LPA and the RPA normally migrate leftward on to the MPA. But in TA type A2, if the MPA is absent, the RPA and the LPA must remain in the aortic sac on the dorsal aspect of the ascending aorta. The RPA and the LPA have nowhere to migrate to.

This appearance in TA type A2 usually has been interpreted as a failure of the AP septum to develop.

However, it is helpful to remember that in TOF with pulmonary outflow tract atresia ("tet-atresia"), absence of the MPA does occur. And that the starting position of the RPA and the LPA is the aortic sac, on the dorsal aspect of the aorta. If the MPA is absent, the RPA and LPA have nowhere to migrate to.

We found that we could not tell "tet-atresia" from TA by examining the RV outflow tract. Both are very similar. Only when we allowed ourselves to look at the great arteries could we tell "tet atresia" (TOF) from TA. Consequently, we think that TOF and TA are very closely related, and that the classical concept of TA (absence of the AP and infundibular septa) is wrong. Also, we have never seen the classical four-leaflet truncal valve predicted by the classical hypothesis. Instead, the truncal valve looks like, and measures like, the aortic valve [7, 8].

In TA, IA situs analysis is solitus-solitus, i.e., concordant, like TOF.

Conclusions

The conotruncus or infundibuloarterial cardiovascular segment is a two-part system. The infundibulum (or conus arteriosus) and the great arteries (truncus arteriosus) are both critically important in determining the anatomic diagnosis. The development of normal and abnormal infundibuloarterial equations (Table 1.2) and infundibuloarterial (IA) situs analysis have been particularly helpful.

Understanding the anatomic type of conotruncus is a *systems* or *relationship* diagnosis between the conus (infundibulum) and the truncus (great arteries). It's not just one thing. Instead, it's the relationship between two different things. That's why the situs of the infundibulum and the situs of the great arteries are so important, as revealed by infundibulo-arterial (IA) situs analysis.

Do the infundibulum and the great arteries fit together normally?

Yes, if both have the same pattern of anatomic organization, the same situs, i.e., yes, if situs concordance is present.

No, if the patterns of anatomic organization, the situs[2] of the infundibulum and of the great arteries are different, i.e., no, if situs discordance, or nonconcordance is present.

Can an embryonic arterial switch procedure be performed from above the right ventricle to above the left ventricle, and if so, how?

When the usual ventricular D-loop is present, the following can occur (Figs. 1.1 and 1.2):

1. If the right-sided subaortic conal free wall involutes, the aorta is switched into the left ventricle and normally related great arteries result.
2. If the left-sided subpulmonary conal free wall involutes, the pulmonary artery is switched into the left ventricle, resulting in typical D-transposition of the great arteries.
3. If neither the right-sided subaortic conal free wall nor the left-sided subpulmonary conal free wall involutes, then neither the aorta nor the pulmonary artery is switched into left ventricle, resulting in double-outlet right ventricle.
4. If both the right-sided subaortic conal free wall and the left-sided subpulmonary conal free wall involute or fail to develop, then both the aorta and the pulmonary artery can be switched into the left ventricle, resulting in double-outlet left ventricle.

Acknowledgement I would like to thank Paul M. Weinberg, M.D. for his help in simplifying the notation of the infundibularterial equations.

---

[2] *Situs* is both singular and plural. *Situs, sitūs* is a fourth declension Latin masculine noun.

References

1. Van Praagh R, Van Praagh S. Isolated ventricular inversion. A consideration of the morphogenesis, definition, and diagnosis of nontransposed and transposed great arteries. Am J Cardiol. 1966;17:395–406.
2. Van Praagh R. The cardiovascular keys to air-breathing and permanent land-living in vertebrates: the normal human embryonic aortic switch procedure produced by complete right-left asymmetry in the development of the subarterial conal free walls, and the evolution of the right ventricular sinus. Kardiochirurgia i Torakochirurgia Polska. 2011;8:1–22.
3. Van Praagh R. The importance of segmental situs in the diagnosis of congenital heart disease. Semin Roentgenol. 1985;20:254–71.
4. Taussig HB, Bing RJ. Complete transposition of the aorta and a levoposition of the pulmonary artery: clinical, physiological, and pathological findings. Am Heart J. 1949;37:551–9.
5. Van Praagh R. What is the Taussig-Bing malformation? Circulation. 1968;38:445–9.
6. Paul MH, Muster AJ, Sinha SN, Cole RB, Van Praagh R. Double-outlet left ventricle with an intact ventricular septum. Clinical and autopsy diagnosis and developmental implications. Circulation. 1970;41:129–39.
7. Van Praagh R, Van Praagh S. The anatomy of common aorticopulmonary trunk (truncus arteriosus communis) and its embryologic implications. A study of 57 necropsy cases. Am J Cardiol. 1965;16:406–25.
8. Vizcaino A, Campbell J, Litovsky S, Van Praagh R. Single origin of right and left pulmonary artery branches from ascending aorta with nonbranching main pulmonary artery: relevance to a new understanding of truncus interiosus. Pediatr Cardiol. 2002;23:230–4.
9. Van Praagh R, Durnin RE, Jockin H, Wagner HR, Korns M, Garbedian H, Ando M, Calder AL. Anatomically corrected malposition of the great arteries {S,D,L}. Circulation. 1975;51:20–31.
10. Kreutzer J, Van Praagh R. Comparison of left ventricular outflow tract obstruction in interruption of the aortic arch and in the coarctation of the aorta, with diagnostic, developmental, and surgical implications. Am J Cardiol. 2000;86:856–62.
11. Van Praagh R. The evolution of the human heart and its relevance to congenital heart disease. Kardiochirurgia i Torakochirurgia Polska. 2011;8(4):427–31.
12. Bajolle F, Zaffran S, Kelly RG, Hadchouel J, Bonnet D, Brown NA, Buckingham ME. Rotation of the myocardial wall of the outflow tract is implicated in the normal positioning of the great arteries. Circ Res. 2006;98:421–8.
13. Quain R: Cited by Peacock TB: On malformations, etc. of the human heart, with original cases. London: Churchill; 1858. p. 116. Birmingham, Alabama, The Classics of Medicine Library, 1981, Gryphon Editions Limited.
14. Foran RB, Belcourt C, Nanton MA, Murphy DA, Weinberg AG, Liebman J, Castañeda AR, Van Praagh R. Isolated infundibuloarterial inversion {S, D, I}: a newly recognized form of congenital heart disease. Am Heart J. 1988;116:1337–50.
15. Houyel L, Van Praagh R, Lacour-Gayet F, Serraf A, Petit J, Bruniaux J, Planché C. Transposition of the great arteries {S, D, L}: pathologic anatomy, diagnosis, and surgical management of a newly recognized complex. J Thorac Cardiovasc Surg. 1995;110:613–24.
16. Asami I. Partitioning of the arterial end of the human heart. In: Van Praagh R, Takao A, editors. Etiology and Morphogenesis of Congenital Heart Disease. Mt. Kisco/New York: Futura Publishing Co; 1980. p. 51–61.

Chapter 2
Development and Maldevelopment of the Ventricular Outflow Tracts

Robert H. Anderson, Simon D. Bamforth, Diane E. Spicer, Deborah J. Henderson, Bill Chaudhry, Nigel Andrew Brown, and Timothy J. Mohun

Abstract In this chapter, we provide an account of cardiac development that, hopefully, will underscore the understanding of the surgical anatomy of the lesions to be contained within the overall book. The book alleges coverage of the surgical treatment of "conotruncal anomalies". It is our belief that one of the lesions to be considered, namely congenitally correct transposition, requires abnormal looping of the developing heart tube as the primary abnormal developmental event. To put this lesion into context, therefore, we begin our account with a brief review of formation and looping of the heart tube. We then concentrate on the normal and abnormal development of the ventricular outflow tracts, although we question whether development is best considered in terms of the "conus" as opposed to the "truncus". It is anatomically more accurate to address development of the outflow tract in terms of its proximal, intermediate, and distal components, and to consider these intrapericardial parts separately from the extrapericardial arterial pathways, which develop within the pharyngeal mesenchyme. The tripartite approach to development then permits rational explanations to be provided for formation of the ventricular outflow tract, the arterial valves and their supporting sinuses, and the intrapericardial arterial trunks. This approach to normal development permits analyses to be made of the

R.H. Anderson, BSc, MD, FRCPath (✉) • S.D. Bamforth, BSc (Hons), PhD
D.J. Henderson, BSc, PhD • B. Chaudhry, MBBS, MRCP, PhD
Institute of Genetic Medicine, Newcastle University, Newcastle upon Tyne, UK
e-mail: sejjran@ucl.ac.uk

D.E. Spicer, BS
Department of Pediatric Cardiology, University of Florida, Gainesville, FL, USA

Department of Pathology, Johns Hopkins All Children's Heart Institute, St. Petersburg, FL, USA

N.A. Brown, BSc, PhD
Division of Biomedical Sciences, St George's Hospital Medical School, Institute of Medical and Biomedical Education, St George's University of London, London, UK

T.J. Mohun, PhD
Division of Developmental Biology, MRC National Institute for Medical Research, London, UK

F. Lacour-Gayet et al. (eds.), *Surgery of Conotruncal Anomalies*,
DOI 10.1007/978-3-319-23057-3_2

lesions afflicting the different components, such as aortopulmonary windows, common arterial trunk, arterial valvar malformations, tetralogy of Fallot, double outlet right ventricle, and discordant ventriculo-arterial connections.

Keywords Conotruncal anomalies • Embryology • Intrapericardial arterial trunks • Arterial roots • Ventricular outflow tracts • Tetralogy of Fallot • Common arterial trunk • Double outlet right ventricle • Interrupted aortic arch

Introduction

The book in which this review will appear is entitled "Surgery for conotruncal anomalies". We have difficulties, however, when we are asked to address the development of these various lesions. In the first place, in our opinion, the major developmental problem in one of the entities to be discussed, specifically congenitally corrected transposition, reflects abnormal formation of the ventricular loop, as opposed to an initial problem involving the outflow tract. In the second place, to the best of our knowledge, there is, as yet, no consensus as to which lesions should, or should not, be grouped under the banner of the "conotruncal" malformations. There is also, currently, a lack of agreement amongst those who investigate the developing heart as to the precise definition of the "conus", as opposed to the "truncus". When used to describe postnatal hearts, the "conus" is usually considered to represent the infundibular musculature which supports the leaflets of the arterial valves. "Truncus" is less frequently used to describe components of the postnatal heart, but we presume it should be considered synonymous with the intrapericardial arterial trunks. If this is the case, we are left with another problem. In which of these components are we to include the arterial valves, and their supporting valvar sinuses? And from which developmental component are they presumed to have developed? Since the arterial roots develop within the central part of the embryonic ventricular outflow tract, should not they, when malformed, be included in groupings of conotruncal anomalies?

Faced with all these uncertainties, rather than discussing the development of "conotruncal anomalies", we will use this chapter to provide a review of our current understanding of the development, and maldevelopment, of the outflow tract of the heart. We will show how its initially common lumen is septated into aortic and pulmonary channels. With ongoing development, however, the septated structure becomes separated into discrete systemic and pulmonary pathways, each with its own walls [1, 2]. The essence of the normal postnatal heart, therefore, is that there is very little separating the outflow tracts that is septal [3]. With regard to the initially common outflow tract, we will describe the development of its proximal, intermediate, and distal components, showing how analysis in such tripartite fashion then facilitates the understanding of abnormal development. We begin our account, however, with a short review of the morphological changes that occur during formation of the heart tube. It is an appreciation of these early changes that permits understanding of the morphogenesis of lesions such as congenitally corrected transposition.

Early Development of the Heart Tube

Most embryologic textbooks continue to explain cardiac development on the basis of twisting and septation of an initial linear heart tube. This concept was based on the presumption that all parts of the definitive heart were represented within the initial tube. It had long been suggested, however, that cells derived from the splanchnic mesoderm within the embryonic disc were added continuously at both its venous and arterial poles [4–6]. These concepts have now been validated by rigorous molecular studies [7–9]. The source of the new material has been called the second heart field, with the first heart field presumed to produce the initial linear tube. The morphological differences between this purported second field, the presumptive primary field, and potentially still more "fields", have yet adequately to be defined [10]. It is the confirmation that cells are added continuously to the heart tube during its development that has revolutionised our understanding of the formation of the postnatal heart.

The heart-forming cells are part of the mesodermal layer of the embryonic disc, this layer being formed by migration through the primitive streak during the process of gastrulation. The migrating cells initially give rise to two heart-forming regions, the cardiac mesoderm, positioned on either side of the midline. As development proceeds, they join across the midline to form a crescent-shaped area, part of which then becomes a tube. This transformation is a complex procedure. Concomitant with infolding of the gut, and folding of the body walls, the parts of the crescent initially positioned peripherally become the ventral part of the definitive heart tube. The remainder of the cardiac mesoderm, which has not formed the initial tube, represents the so-called secondary heart field [7–9]. It is the addition of these cells to the cranial pole of the initial heart tube that provides the material for formation of the right ventricle and outflow tract. Proper development and migration of this component of the initial cardiac crescent, therefore, is fundamental for normal formation of the ventricular outflow tracts. The tissues entering, and then reinforcing, the arterial pole are directly adjacent to the pharyngeal mesoderm, in which are formed the pharyngeal arches. The second heart field is responsible for providing not only the myocardial components of the right ventricle and outflow tract, but also the non-myocardial intra-pericardial arterial trunks, along with their valves and sinuses. As we will describe, an important aspect of development is the regression of the border between the myocardial and non-myocardial components when judged relative to the margins of the pericardial cavity.

When first seen, the initial heart tube is straight (Fig. 2.1a). It is with the addition of the material from the heart-forming areas, which enter at the venous as well as

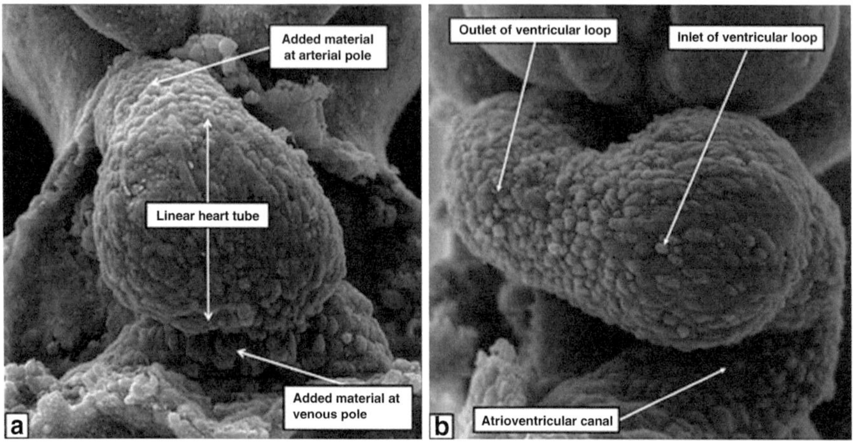

Fig. 2.1 The scanning electron microscopic images show how, with addition of new material from the heart-forming areas, the initial linear heart tube (**a**) lengthens and forms its ventricular loop (**b**). The images are from embryonic mouse hearts early and late during the 8th day of development, equivalent to about 5 weeks of development in man

the arterial pole, that it quickly becomes S-shaped. The process of elongation is known as looping (Fig. 2.1b). The initial component of the linear tube eventually forms little more than the body and septum of the definitive left ventricle [11]. During looping, the lumen of the tube, throughout its length, is lined with cardiac jelly. Its walls are made up of so-called primary myocardium. Subsequent to looping, there is expansion of the lumen in what can now be recognised as its atrial and ventricular components. The atrial expansions are bilateral, and form the primordiums of the right and left atrial appendages (Fig. 2.2a). The expansions in the ventricular loop, in contrast, occur in series, with the pouch developing from the inlet of the loop eventually becoming the apical component of the left ventricle, and that growing from the outlet becoming the apical part of the right ventricle (Fig. 2.2b). The processes that produce the expansions of the cavities of the atrial component, and of the inlet and outlet parts of the ventricular loop, are known as ballooning [12]. The walls of these expanded components have different molecular phenotypes when compared to those of the initial heart tube. They can be described as being made of chamber, or secondary, myocardium. It is the appendages, and the apical components, derived from this chamber myocardium, which give the atrial and ventricular chambers their morphological specificity in the postnatal heart. As these parts expand from the original solitary lumen of the linear tube, so the cardiac jelly becomes confined to the atrioventricular canal and the developing outflow tract. In these regions, by the process known as endothelial-to-mesenchymal transformation [13], the jelly becomes converted into endocardial cushions, with cells derived from the neural crest migrating into the cushions formed within the outflow tract. The atrioventricular cushions face each other in superior and inferior fashion within the atrioventricular canal (Fig. 2.3a). The outflow cushions, in contrast, extend through the larger part of the outflow tract, spiralling as they are traced towards the pericar-

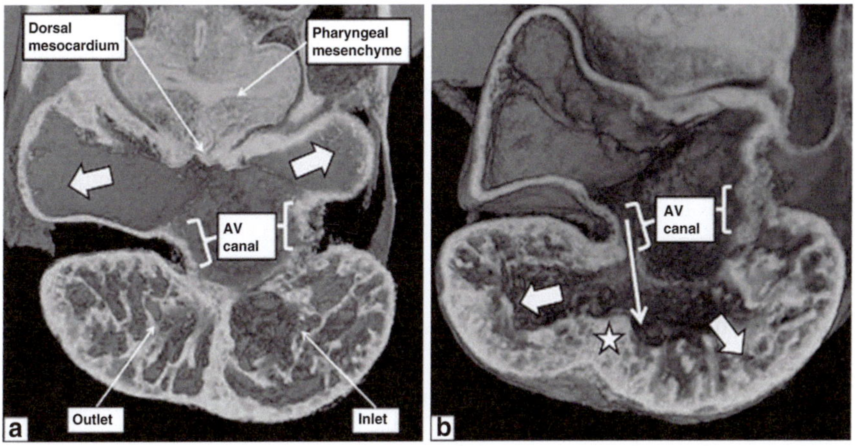

Fig. 2.2 The images are taken from an episcopic dataset prepared from a developing mouse sacrificed during the 10th day of embryonic development. The *left hand panel* (**a**) shows how the cavity of the atrial component is ballooning bilaterally to form the primordiums of the atrial appendages (*large white arrows*). The *right hand panel*, from the same dataset, shows how the apical components of the inlet and outlet components of the ventricular loop are ballooning (*large white arrows* in **b**) to form the apical components of what will become the left and right ventricles, respectively. Note that the process of ballooning produces the primordium of the apical muscular septum (*star* in **b**). Note also that the atrioventricular (AV) canal initially is supported exclusively by the inlet component of the ventricular loop (*long white arrow*)

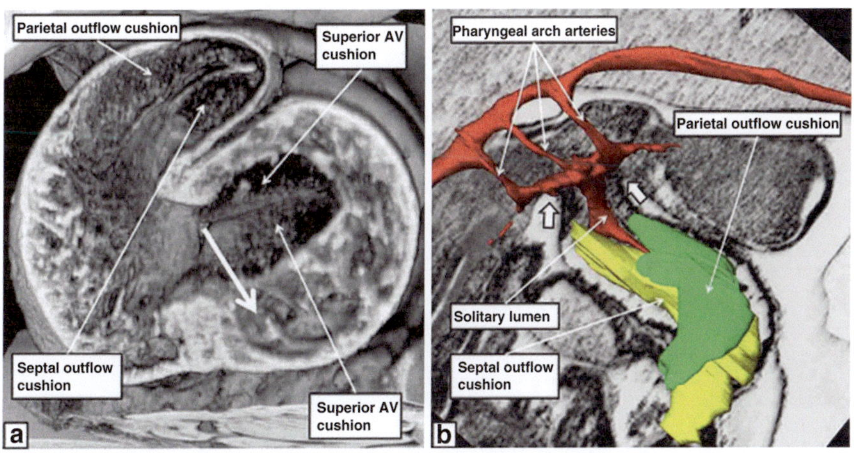

Fig. 2.3 The images are from episcopic datasets from embryonic mice at day 10.5 (**a**) and early on 11.5 (**b**). They show how the cardiac jelly, which initially lined the entirety of the solitary lumen of the heart tube, has become changed by the process of endothelial-to-mesenchymal transformation to form cushions in the atrioventricular canal and outflow tract. Panel (**a**) shows how the cavity of the atrioventricular canal initially opens exclusively to the developing left ventricle (*white arrow*), with the newly formed cushions facing each other in supero-inferior locations. Panel (**b**) shows the spiralling outflow cushions, which stop short of the margins of the pericardial cavity (*large white arrows*). At the margins of the pericardial cavity, the solitary lumen of the distal outflow tract becomes continuous with the pharyngeal arch arteries, which extend bilaterally through the third, fourth, and sixth arches to join the descending aorta. The ventral manifold that supplies the arch arteries is known as the aortic sac

dial margins. When the outflow tract is first formed, the cardiac jelly lining the lumen extends to the margins of the pericardial cavity. Subsequent to formation of the outflow cushions, their distal tips stop short of the pericardial margins (Fig. 2.3b). This change reflects the ongoing migration of new tissues into the heart from the heart-forming areas. The newly added material is non-myocardial. As we will describe, it forms the walls of the intrapericardial arterial trunks [1, 2], and eventually also forms the arterial valvar sinuses.

Expansion of the Atrioventricular Canal

Subsequent to looping, and ballooning of the chamber myocardium, the atrioventricular canal is supported exclusively by the inlet component of the ventricular loop, while the outflow tract arises exclusively from the outlet component (Fig. 2.3a). The default option for the developing heart, therefore, is double inlet left ventricle, and double outlet right ventricle. This arrangement is rarely seen in clinical practise, but was recently produced by Scambler and his colleagues, working in the Institute of Child Health in London, in a mouse they modified by perturbing the chd7 gene (Fig. 2.4). Formation of the four-chambered heart, with proper septation of its components, requires appreciable remoulding of the lumen of the heart directly related to the inner heart curvature, the walls of this part still being formed of primary myocardium. This, in turn, produces marked remodelling of the embryonic interventricular foramen. In the stage shown in Fig. 2.3a, and in the abnormal heart

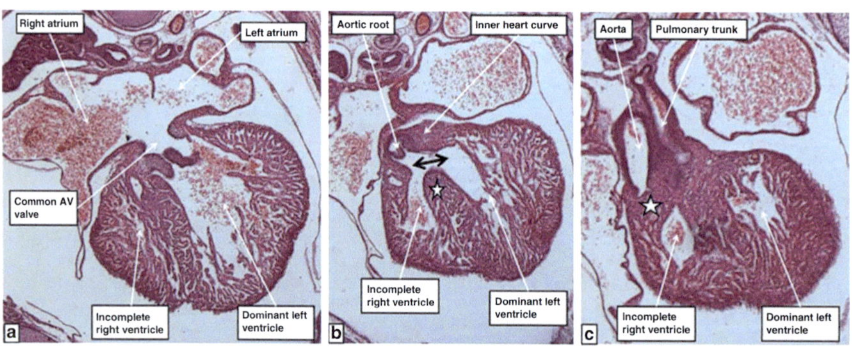

Fig. 2.4 The images show histological sections, stained using haematoxylin and eosin, and cut in the four-chamber plane, of a mouse with perturbation of the chd7 gene prepared by Professor Peter Scambler, from the Institute of Child Health, University College, London. Panel (**a**) shows double inlet through a common atrioventricular (AV) valve to the dominant left ventricle. Panel (**b**) shows the interventricular communication (*double headed arrow*), which is roofed by the musculature of the inner heart curvature, and floored by the crest of the apical muscular septum (*star*). Panel (**c**) shows double outlet from the incomplete right ventricle, with spiralling arterial trunks. The arterial roots are separated by the muscular outlet septum (*star*), which because of the double outlet is an exclusively right ventricular structure. The abnormal heart is directly comparable with situation during development of the normal heart as shown in Fig. 2.3a

shown in Fig. 2.4b, the foramen is floored by the developing apical ventricular septum, but roofed by the inner heart curvature. At these stages, the atrioventricular canal, now separated into right and left halves by formation of the cushions, opens to the left of the muscular ventricular septum (Fig. 2.3a). The roof of the developing right ventricle, however, is already in continuity with the floor of the right atrium at the right margin of the canal, even though its rightward orifice carries the atrial blood into the left ventricle (Fig. 2.5a). The key step in connecting the right atrium directly to the right ventricle, therefore, is rightward expansion of the atrioventricular canal. This occurs, in the mouse, during the eleventh embryonic day (Fig. 2.5b), which is equivalent, in humans, to around 6 weeks of development subsequent to the last menstrual period. Subsequent to the expansion of the canal, the right atrioventricular orifice provides a direct connection between the cavities of the right atrium and the developing right ventricle.

As already emphasised, the expansion also remodels the margins of the initial interventricular communication. Prior to any expansion, all the atrial blood had to pass through the interventricular communication so as to reach the outflow tract (Fig. 2.6a). Subsequent to expansion, part of the initial boundary of the communication surrounds the newly-formed right atrioventricular junction (Fig. 2.6b). The outflow tract, however, remains supported exclusively by the right ventricle at this stage. The stream of blood flowing from the developing left ventricle, therefore, must still traverse the remaining interventricular part of the communication so as to

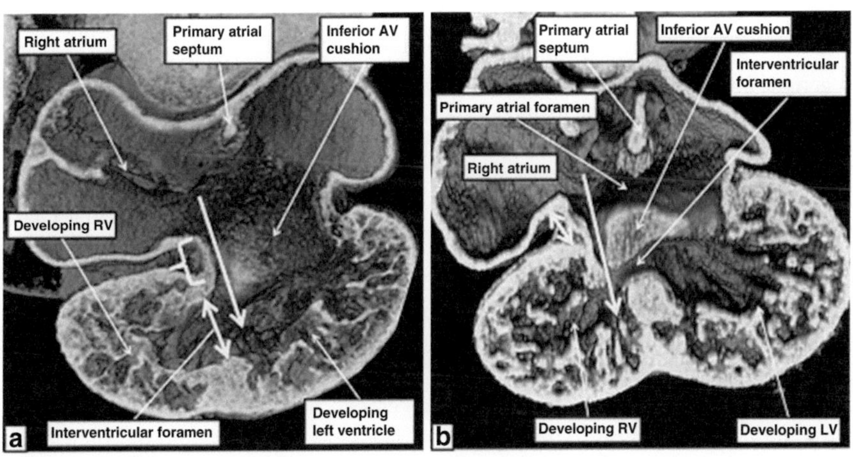

Fig. 2.5 The images show the expansion of the atrioventricular canal that takes place during the 11th day of development in the mouse. Panel (**a**) shows the situation at embryonic day 10.5. Although the cavity of the right atrium is draining to the developing left ventricle (*long white arrow*), the floor of the right atrium is already continuous with the roof of the right ventricle through the right margin of the atrioventricular canal (*white bracket*). Panel (**b**) shows that, by the middle of the 11th day of development, the canal has expanded such that the right atrium now connects directly with the right ventricle. The interventricular foramen now carries left ventricular blood to the outflow tract, which remains supported above the developing right ventricle (See Fig. 2.6)

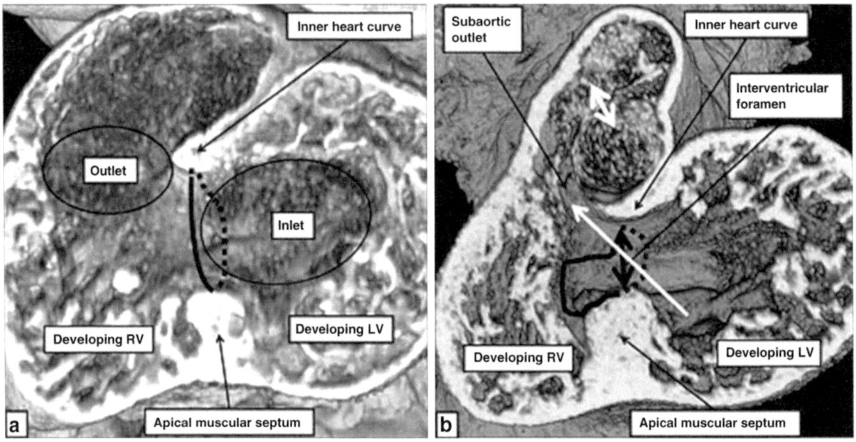

Fig. 2.6 The images show how expansion of the atrioventricular canal is also responsible for remoulding of the embryonic interventricular communication. At embryonic day 10.5 (panel **a**), all the blood entering through the inlet has to traverse the interventricular foramen so as to reach the outlet. After expansion of the canal during the eleventh embryonic day (Panel **b**), it is only the left ventricular blood that must traverse the foramen so as to reach the developing subaortic outlet (*long white arrow*). Note how the outflow cushions are lying edge to edge, (*double headed white arrow*), potentially separating the subaortic and subpulmonary outlets. Part of the initial interventricular foramen now surrounds the right atrioventricular junction (*solid black border* in Panel **b**). The dotted black lines in both panels mark the ventral extent of the embryonic interventricular communication

reach the aortic outflow tract, which is now formed within the outflow tract by apposition of the proximal ends of the spiralling outflow cushions. This arrangement in the developing heart is analogous to double outlet right ventricle in the congenitally malformed heart.

An understanding of the consequence of expansion of the atrioventricular canal also provides the explanation for the formation of discordant, as opposed to concordant atrioventricular connections. As can be seen from Figs. 2.4 and 2.5, rightward expansion of the atrioventricular canal brings the cavity of the right atrium into direct continuity with that of the developing right ventricle. After the completion of septation, therefore, the atrial chambers will be connected in concordant fashion with their respective ventricles. This arrangement, however, can only occur when the ventricular loop turns to the right, as shown in Fig. 2.1b. Should the ventricular loop turn to the left, rather than the right, then the outflow tract will also be positioned leftward relative to the atrioventricular canal (Fig. 2.7). In this setting, presuming the presence of usual atrial arrangement, the embryonic interventricular communication will be related to the leftward margin of the canal, which can only expand in leftward direction. And, subsequent to such leftward expansion, it is the cavity of the left atrium which is brought into connection with that of the developing right ventricle, leaving the cavity of the right atrium in communication with the developing left ventricle. It is leftward looping of the developing heart tube,

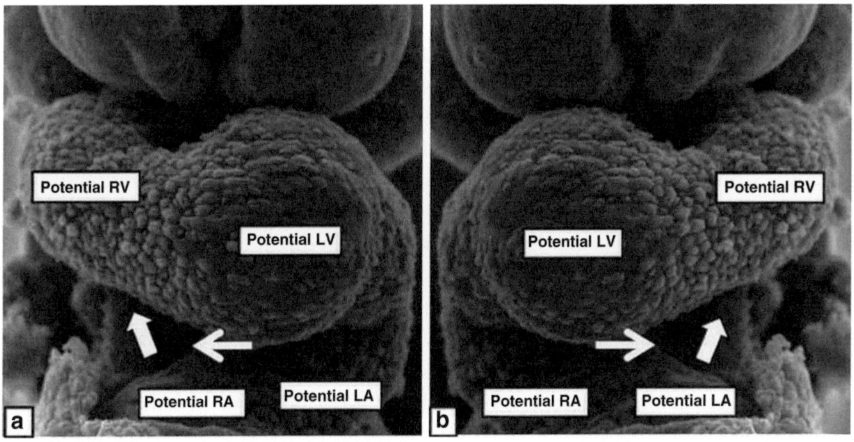

Fig. 2.7 The images show the consequence of leftward looping of the ventricular component of the heart tube subsequent to expansion of the atrioventricular canal. Panel (**a**) shows the usual situation, in which rightward expansion, shown by the *thinner white arrow*, permits the cavity of the developing right atrium (*solid white arrow*) to make contact with the cavity of the developing right ventricle, thus producing concordant atrioventricular connections. Panel (**b**) shows that, after leftward looping of the tube, produced artifactually in this figure by mirror-imaging the normal situation, it is the cavity of the developing left atrium that will be brought into communication with the cavity of the right ventricle, leaving the right atrium in communication with the left ventricle, and hence producing discordant atrioventricular connections

therefore, which sets the scene for the formation of discordant atrioventricular connections. Such discordant atrioventricular connections are usually associated with discordant ventriculo-arterial connections, producing the combination known as congenitally corrected transposition. Discordant atrioventricular connections, nonetheless, can also be found with double outlet right ventricle, or rarely with concordant ventriculo-arterial connections [14]. Hence, all of the changes that produce malformations of the outflow tracts, which we will describe below, can be found in association with leftward, rather than rightward, ventricular looping. It is the abnormal leftward looping of the ventricular component of the heart tube, nonetheless, that is the key feature in the morphogenesis of congenitally corrected transposition (Fig. 2.7).

Normal Development of the Outflow Tract

Subsequent to expansion of the atrioventricular canal, the outflow tract remains supported exclusively by the developing right ventricle (Fig. 2.6b). Although the outflow cushions have now formed throughout its length in spiralling fashion (Fig. 2.3b), as yet they have not fused together. The outflow tract, therefore, retains a potentially common lumen, although apposition of the unfused cushions will already have potentially separated the putative aortic and pulmonary channels. Ongoing normal development results in initial septation of the lumen by fusion of the cushions. Normal development, however, also requires that, distally, the newly septated pulmonary channel feeds the pulmonary arteries, which are canalising in the pharyngeal mesenchyme, and arise from the floor of the aortic sac. The aortic channel will be placed in communication with the systemic components of the pharyngeal arch arteries, which arise from the cranial component of the sac. The completion of normal development also requires expansion proximally of the base of the outflow tract. This is needed to bring the aortic channel into direct communication with the left, rather than the right, ventricle.

To understand all these processes, it is necessary to consider the changes that occur from the stage at which the outflow tract, with its lining of endocardial jelly, initially has exclusively muscular walls. This situation is found subsequent to looping of the ventricular component of the heart tube, but prior to ballooning of the apical ventricular components. At this early stage, which is found at the beginning of the tenth embryonic day of development in the mouse, equivalent to about 5 weeks of development in man, the outflow tract is supported exclusively by the outlet component of the ventricular loop. It extends in serpentine fashion towards the pharyngeal mesenchyme, with its lumen becoming continuous with the origins of the pharyngeal arch arteries at the margins of the pericardial cavity. The arrangement is comparable in man and mouse (Fig. 2.8) [1, 2].

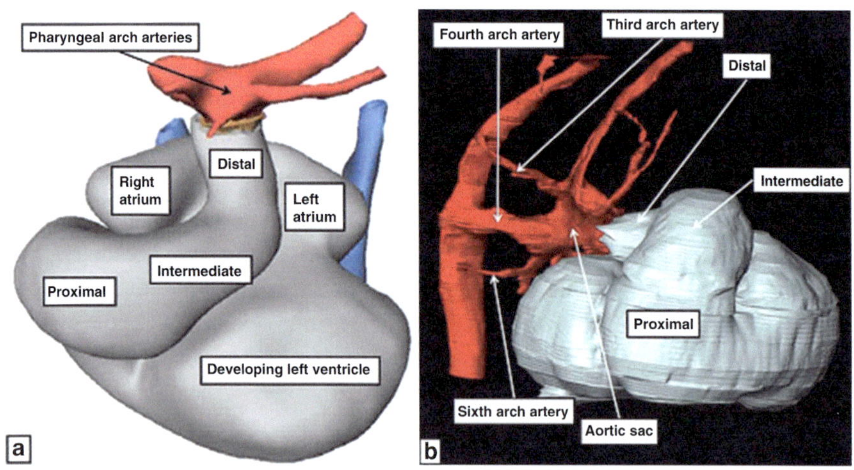

Fig. 2.8 The images show reconstruction of the developing heart at Carnegie stage 13 in the human (Panel **a**), and on the 11th day of development in the mouse (Panel **b**). The human specimen, modified from the study of Sizarov and colleagues [2], is shown from the front, while the mouse heart is shown from the right side. The sections from which the images were reconstructed in the human heart had been stained to visualise myocardium, which is shown in silver. The sections from the murine heart were coloured to match the human arrangement. The entirety of the outflow tract at these stages has myocardial walls, which extend to the margins of the pericardial cavity. The tract itself runs a serpentine course, with obvious proximal, intermediate, and distal components. Note the sets of arteries, shown in red, running through the pharyngeal mesenchyme. They take origin from the aortic sac

The arteries running through the pharyngeal mesenchyme are often illustrated as arising in five symmetrical pairs, taking origin from a ventral aortic sac. By the beginning of the 11th day of development in the mouse, the aortic sac is better considered as having bilateral cranial and caudal components. The cranial component is the systemic part, branching on each side to form the third and fourth pairs of arch arteries (Fig. 2.9a). The caudal part of the sac gives rise to the sixth arch arteries (Fig. 2.9b), with the right and left pulmonary arteries arising from these arteries shortly after they have emerged from the floor of the sac, the pulmonary arteries themselves canalising within the pharyngeal mesenchyme. At this stage, therefore, it is the dorsal wall of the pharyngeal mesenchyme that represents the future aortopulmonary septum, separating the cranial systemic and caudal pulmonary components of the sac (Fig. 2.9b).

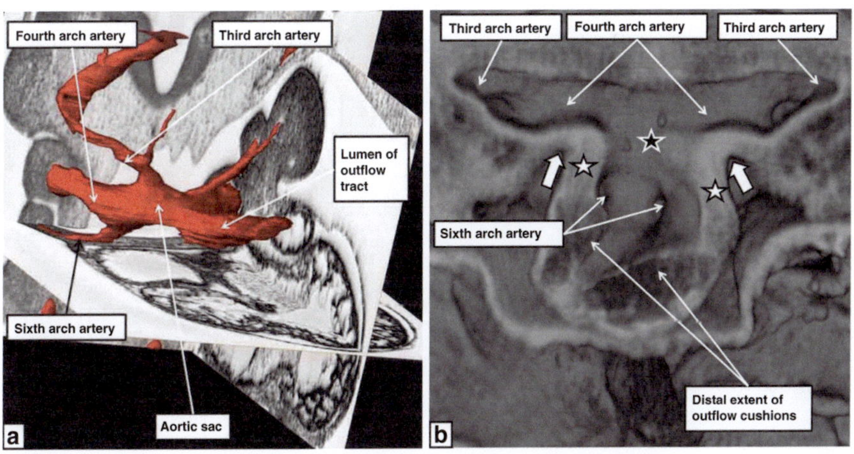

Fig. 2.9 The images show the origin of the pharyngeal arch arteries from the aortic sac. As is shown in Panel (**a**), the same heart as in Fig. 2.8b, the solitary lumen of the outflow tract becomes continuous with the aortic sac at the margins of the pericardial cavity. The junctions between the outflow tract and the aortic sac are shown by the *large white arrows* in Fig. 2.9b, which is a frontal section from an episcopic dataset from a mouse heart early on the 11th day of development. By now, non-myocardial tissue has begun to enter the distal margins of the outflow tract (*white stars with black borders*). The ends of the outflow cushions have regressed from the pericardial margins, as shown in Fig. 2.3B, and are confluent with the distal myocardial border. The arteries of the third and fourth aortic arches arise from the cranial part of the sac, while the arteries of the sixth arches take origin from the caudal part, as shown in Fig. 2.9b. The dorsal wall of the sac (*black star with white borders*) is the effective aortopulmonary septum

Remodelling of the Distal Outflow Tract

As we have emphasised, when first formed the outflow tract has exclusively myocardial walls. It is the addition of the new non-myocardial tissue to the walls of the outflow tract by ongoing migration from the cardiac mesoderm in the pharyngeal mesenchyme that is associated with regression of the distal extent of the myocardium relative to the margins of the pericardial cavity. When first seen within the pericardial cavity, the non-myocardial tissue forms spurs located cranially and caudally. These areas then rotate to become the right-sided and left-sided parietal walls of the intrapericardial arterial trunks. The right-sided wall, destined to become the parietal wall of the intrapericardial aorta, extends lengthwise in cranial-to-caudal fashion. The left-sided wall, destined to be part of the pulmonary trunk, has greater length in ventro-caudal direction. As the non-myocardial tissues enter the pericardial cavity to form the parietal walls of the intrapericardial arterial trunks, so the dorsal wall of the aortic sac protrudes ventrally, dividing the lumen of the distal outflow tract. This protrusion is the first proper aortopulmonary septum (Fig. 2.10).

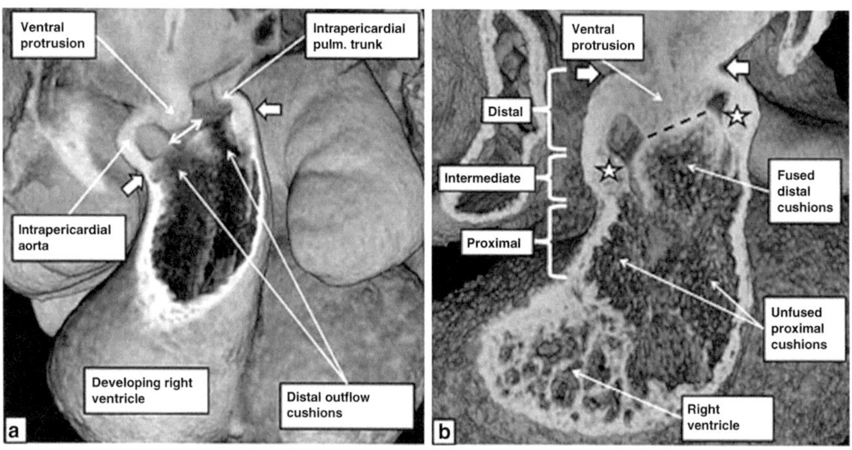

Fig. 2.10 The images, in comparable short axis planes, are from datasets prepared from mice during the 11th (Panel **a**) and 12th (Panel **b**) days of embryonic development. In Panel (**a**), the *arrows* mark the regressing level of the myocardial boundary relative to the margins of the pericardial cavity. The ongoing addition of new material from the heart-forming areas has produced the parietal walls of the intrapericardial arterial trunks. As shown in Panel (**b**), these walls now occupy the distal component of the outflow tract. The intrapericardial aortic and pulmonary channels are separated centrally by further ingrowth ventrally of the dorsal wall of the aortic sac. This ventral protrusion is the first indication of aortopulmonary septation, with the space between it and the distal margins of the outflow cushions functioning as an aortopulmonary foramen (*double headed white arrow* in Panel **a**). By the 12th day of development (Panel **b**), the protrusion has fused with the distal end of the outflow cushions (*black dashed line*), the cushions themselves also having fused edge-to-edge at this stage. The proximal cushions, however, remain unfused. By this stage, it is now possible to recognise the intermediate part of the outflow tract due to the formation at its parietal margins of intercalated cushions (*stars*). The *large white arrows* in Panel (**b**) show the margins of the pericardial cavity

It obtrudes into the pericardial cavity in oblique fashion, placing the cranial origins of the fourth arch arteries in rightward and superior position relative to the caudal and leftward openings of the sixth arch arteries.

There is concomitant remodelling of the pharyngeal arch arteries, producing regression of the rightward and dorsal components of the initially bilateral channels. This means that, for the sixth arch arteries, the left-sided channel becomes the arterial duct. The right-sided sixth arch artery disappears, meaning that the developing left-sided intrapericardial pulmonary channel feeds both extrapericardial pulmonary arteries. Similar changes to the third and fourth arch arteries, with regression of the right-sided dorsal aorta, leave the left fourth arch artery as the extrapericardial arch of the aorta. Within the distal outflow tract, the ventral growth of the protrusion, which separates extrapericardially the aortic and pulmonary components of the aortic sac, had brought its leading edge towards the distal ends of the outflow cushions. The cushions themselves have moved proximally relative to the margins of the pericardial cavity concomitant with the regression of the distal myocardial boundary. Their distal parts have now also fused, dividing the intermediate component of the outflow tract into separate aortic and pulmonary channels. The space between the leading edge of the protrusion, and the distal end of the fused cushions, therefore, is an embryonic aortopulmonary foramen. It is failure to close this foramen that will result in persistence postnatally of an aortopulmonary window (Fig. 2.11).

We know from molecular analysis of developing human [2] and mouse [1] hearts that the non-myocardial tissues replacing the myocardial walls of the distal outflow tract are derived from the cardiac mesoderm. The core of the ventral protrusion is also derived from the second heart field. The protrusion, however, is capped by a layer of cells that have migrated into the pericardial cavity from the neural crest

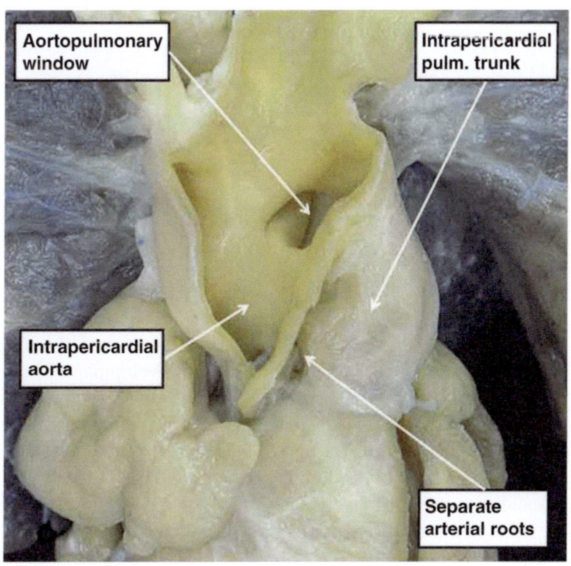

Fig. 2.11 The image shows an aortopulmonary window, well explained on the basis of failure of closure of the embryonic aortopulmonary foramen. Note that the arterial roots are separated, as are the ventricular outflow tracts, confirming that septation of the intermediate and proximal components of the outflow tract has proceeded in normal fashion

[15]. The outflow cushions, which spiral throughout the full extent of the outflow tract, are also populated by large numbers of cells derived from the neural crest. Separation of the cavities of the intrapericardial aorta and the pulmonary trunk, therefore, is dependent on the fusion of tissues derived from the neural crest. But, having served to fuse together the protrusion and the distal extent of the outflow cushions, the cells from the neural crest become increasingly insignificant. Their line of fusion is eventually seen as a longitudinal seam between the walls of the intrapericardial arterial trunks (Fig. 2.12a). By the 12th day of development in the mouse, the trunks themselves have acquired their own discrete walls, with no septal structures then interposing between them (Fig. 2.12b).

By the time the ventral protrusion of the dorsal wall of the aortic sac has fused with the distal end of the outflow cushions, thus separating the intrapericardial arterial trunks, the right-sided components of the pharyngeal arch arteries have largely regressed. As already described, these right-sided structures initially, together with their left-sided counterparts, encircled the developing tracheo-esophageal pedicle (Fig. 2.13a). By the 12th day of development, therefore, the left-sided artery of the fourth arch is recognisable as the extrapericardial aortic arch, with the ventral third and fourth arch arteries contributing to the brachiocephalic and left common carotid arteries (Fig. 2.13b). It is fusion of the ventral protrusion from the dorsal wall of the aortic sac with the distal ends of the cushions that has placed the aortic arch into continuity with the intrapericardial aorta. The same process places the left-sided

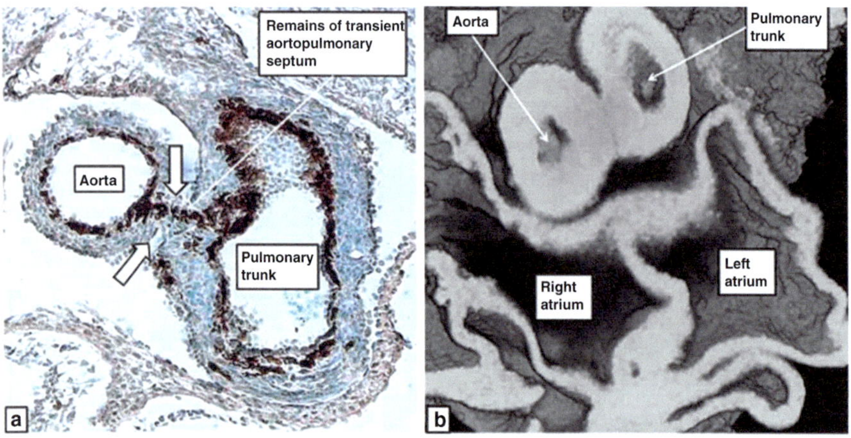

Fig. 2.12 The images show short axis sections across the intrapericardial arterial trunks from mouse hearts at the 12th day of embryonic development. The image in panel (**a**) comes from a mouse genetically modified so as to show, in brown, all the cells derived from the neural crest. The neural crest cells, at this stage, form the endothelial linings of both intrapericardial trunks, but also produce a seam marking the site of the ventral protrusion (*white arrows* in panel **a**), which fused with the distal ends of the outflow cushions to close the embryonic aortopulmonary foramen. This tissue disappears completely during the 12th day of development, so that, as shown in Panel (**b**), the aorta and pulmonary trunk each have their discrete walls, with no septal structures between them

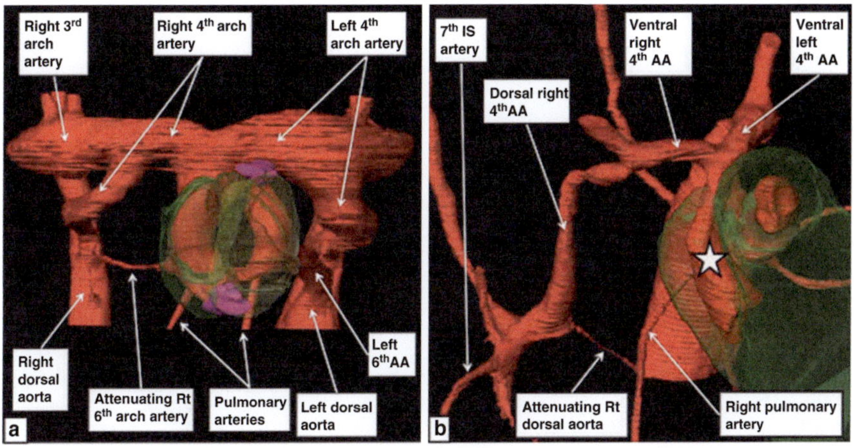

Fig. 2.13 The images are prepared by reconstructing the pharyngeal arteries from episcopic datasets prepared from embryonic mice sacrificed during the 11th (panel **a**) and 12th (panel **b**) days of intrauterine development. Panel (**a**) shows a frontal view, whereas panel (**b**) is shown as seen obliquely from the right. Panel (**a**) shows the beginning of regression of the right (Rt) sixth arch artery, leaving the pulmonary arteries fed from the pulmonary trunk. Panel (**b**) shows how, subsequent to regression of the caudal part of the descending aorta, the right seventh intersegmental (IS) artery becomes the subclavian artery, fed by the ventral right fourth arch artery (AA), which becomes the brachiocephalic artery. The *green* transparent shadings show the extent of the pericardial cavity, with the *star* in panel (**b**) showing the intrapericardial aorta. The pink structures on panel (**a**) are the intercalated cushions

sixth arch artery, now recognisable as the arterial duct, into continuity with the intrapericardial pulmonary trunk. As explained above, the regression of the right-sided sixth arch artery, leaves the pulmonary trunk feeding the right and left pulmonary arteries, which can now be seen arising from the base of the extrapericardial aortic sac (Fig. 2.13a). During these processes, the seventh cervical intersegmental arteries have migrated cranially to form the subclavian arteries. As part of the remoulding, the right subclavian artery incorporates the dorsal part of the right fourth arch artery as it takes origin from the brachiocephalic artery (Fig. 2.13b). Abnormal attenuation or disappearance of the different parts of this initially bilateral system of arteries explains all the various forms of arch interruption and vascular rings.

Remodelling of the Intermediate Component of the Outflow Tract

It is the appearance of additional cushions, known as the intercalated cushions [16], that makes it possible, as shown in Fig. 2.10b, to identify directly the distal, intermediate, and proximal parts of the developing outflow tract. Within the intermediate

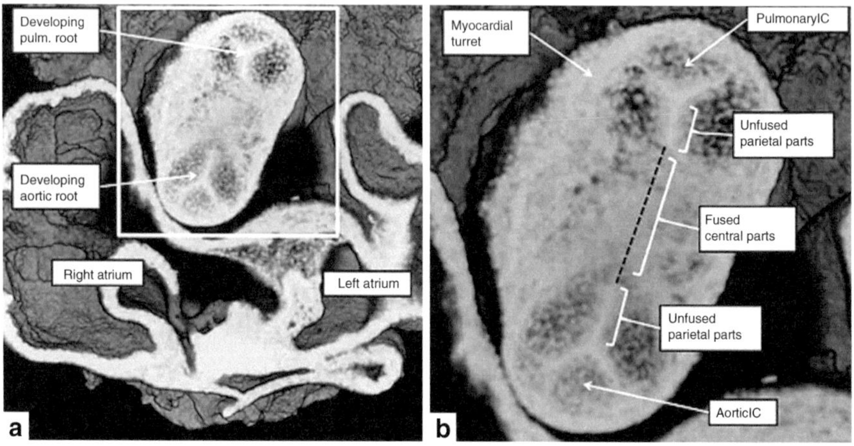

Fig. 2.14 (**a**) Is a cut in short axis through a dataset from an embryonic mouse heart at embryonic day 12.5. It has sectioned through the intermediate part of the outflow tract, along with the atrial chambers. The enlargement of the boxed area of (**a**), as shown in (**b**), reveals how the interdigitation of the newly formed intercalated cushions (*IC*) with the unfused parietal ends of the central cushions provides the basis for formation of the aortic and pulmonary roots

part, the central components of the major outflow cushions have fused together. The parietal ends of the cushions remain unfused. It is this parietal lack of fusion, together with the formation of the intercalated cushions, which produces the primordiums of the developing arterial roots (Fig. 2.14). As the central parts of the cushions fuse to divide the intermediate part of the outflow tract into the aortic and pulmonary roots, the intermediate part itself is still encased within a turret of myocardium. The process of fusion is dependent on the presence of cells derived from the neural crest (Fig. 2.15a) [15]. As was the case with the distal outflow tract, once fusion has taken place, the area occupied by the material derived from the neural crest becomes increasingly insignificant. The material initially responsible for septation disappears as the aortic and pulmonary roots separate one from the other. The process of separation is in a plane at right angles to the line of fusion between the central cushions. Prior to the completion of separation of the roots, however, excavation of the distal ends of the cushions produced the valvar leaflets and their hinges (Fig. 2.15b). This excavation is within the surrounding turret of myocardium, so that the leaflet hinges are supported by the outflow tract musculature (Fig. 2.15c).

With continuing development through the fourteenth and fifteenth embryonic days in the mouse, there is continuing growth proximally of non-myocardial tissues derived from the second heart field (Fig. 2.16b). These new walls produce the valvar sinuses, which support in semilunar fashion the valvar leaflets derived by excavation of the outflow cushions. Because of the presence of the myocardial turret, the leaflets are initially hinged exclusively from myocardium in both the aortic and pulmonary roots (Fig. 2.16a), the support for the adjacent leaflets provided by the newly formed muscularised infundibulum (Fig. 2.15c). By the stage of the comple-

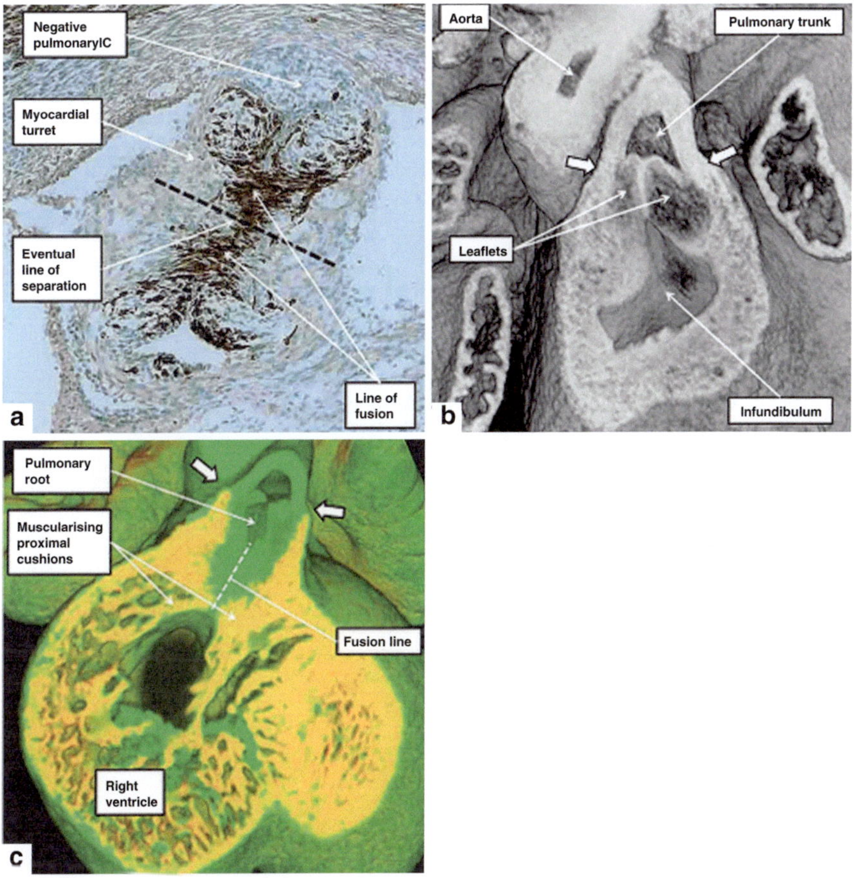

Fig. 2.15 The images show the initial steps in formation of the arterial roots. (**a**) Is a section from a developing mouse heart at embryonic day 12.5 genetically modified to show the presence of cells derived from the neural crest, which are stained brown. The neural crest cells mark the line of fusion between the major outflow cushions. Note that the cells derived from the neural crest also populate the distal ends of both major cushions, and the aortic intercalated cushion, but not the pulmonary intercalated cushion. The roots will eventually separate at right angles to the plane of fusion of the major cushion, as shown by the black dashed line. Panel (**b**) shows a frontal section through the developing pulmonary root at embryonic day 13.5. The ends of the cushions are beginning to excavate so as to form the valvar leaflets and their hinges. Panel (**c**) is from another heart, in which myocardium has been marked, and is coloured in dense yellow. It shows how, as cushions excavate to form the valvar leaflets, they remain encased in the turret of myocardium. Note, however, that the myocardial cells are beginning to populate the proximal cushions to form the subpulmonary infundibulum. The *large white arrows* in panels (**b**, **c**) mark the distal extent of the myocardial walls of the outflow tract

tion of excavation of the leaflets, the aortic root has been transferred to the left ventricle. The persisting component of the embryonic interventricular foramen is closed by formation of the membranous septum, which is derived from the rightward tubercles of the atrioventricular cushions. The proximal parts of the outflow

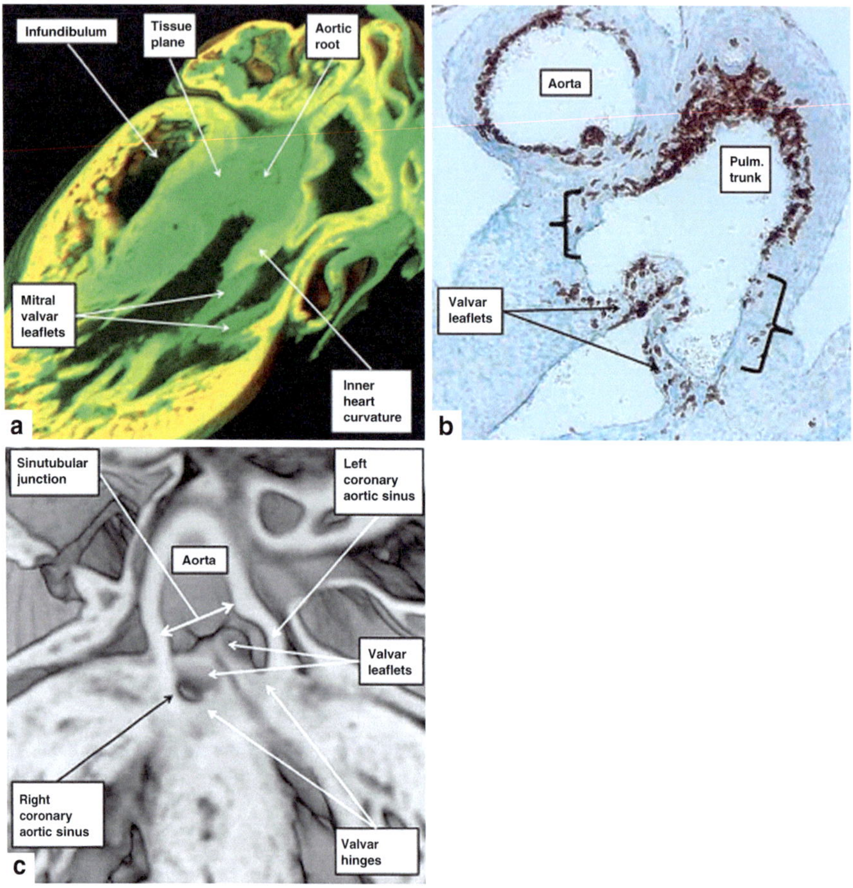

Fig. 2.16 The images show the continuing stages in formation of the arterial valves. Panel (**a**) is from a mouse heart at embryonic day 15.5 in which myocardium has been marked by deep *yellow colour*, although penetration of the colouring agent has not been complete. It shows, nonetheless, that the aortic root remains at this stage enclosed within a myocardial turret. Note, however, that a tissue plane has now developed centrally between the aortic root and the infundibulum. Panel (**b**), which shows the pulmonary valve from a mouse at embryonic day 15.5 genetically modified to show neural crest cells in brown, reveals how the leaflets, marked in brown, are supported by the developing sinuses (*brackets*). The sinuses, however, are not derived from the neural crest, but instead have continued to grow from the second heart field. Panel (**c**), which is a frontal section through the aortic root at embryonic day 16.5, shows that the simple excavation of the cushions has produced the semilunar leaflets of the aortic valve, which remain at this stage exclusively hinged from the myocardial walls. Only later will the myocardial inner heart curve be converted to the fibrous region of continuity between the leaflets of the aortic and mitral valves

cushions, muscularising to form the right ventricular infundibulum, have also been brought into line with the apical part of the muscular septum as the aortic root is transferred to the left ventricle. Conventional wisdom suggests that a discrete anatomic annulus is formed to support the leaflets of the arterial valves [17]. In reality, the leaflets adopt a semilunar shape as they are excavated from the distal tips of the outflow cushions, with the new tissue from the second heart field growing in between the excavating margins to form the valvar sinusal walls. There is no ring-like "annulus" as such formed to support the valvar leaflets. Instead, they are simply hinged from the arterial roots in semilunar fashion (Fig. 2.16c).

Development of the Proximal Outflow Tract

The transfer of the aorta to the left ventricle involves alignment of the muscularising proximal outflow cushions with the apical muscular ventricular septum. When the distal parts of the outflow cushions initially fused to separate the developing arterial roots, the proximal cushions were unfused (Fig. 2.9b). It is with continuing development that the proximal ends of the cushions fuse, thus forming an arch across the cavity of the outflow of the right ventricle, with the cushions themselves attached septally and parietally (Fig. 2.17a). At the stage when the ventral protrusion has fused with the distal cushions so as to separate the intrapericardial arterial trunks, and the distal cushions have themselves fused to separate the developing arterial roots, it becomes possible to recognise a distinct whorl of condensed mesenchyme

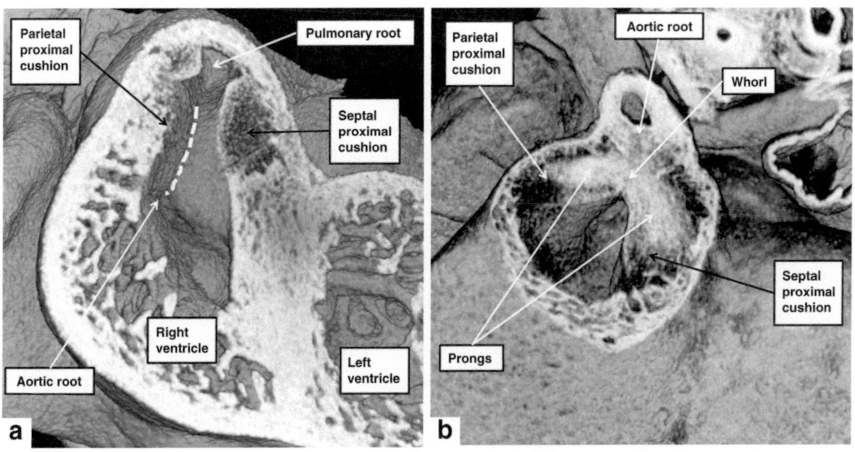

Fig. 2.17 The images are from an episcopic dataset from a fetal mouse in the 12th day of development. Panel (**a**) shows the developing right ventricle viewed from the front having removed the Parietal wall. Both the aortic and pulmonary outflow tracts, at this stage, are supported by the developing right ventricle. They are separated by the fusing proximal parts of the outflow cushions, with the white dashed line showing the zone of fusion. Panel (**b**) is a section taken through the fused central parts of the cushions. It shows the columns of condensed mesenchyme within the cushions that form the so-called "prongs" of the alleged aortopulmonary septal complex. As can be seen, the cushions, along with the contained prongs, will separate the developing ventricular outflow tracts. The intrapericardial aorta and pulmonary trunk are already separated at this stage of development

at the site of fusion between the protrusion and the distal ends of the outflow cushions. This condensed mesenchyme corresponds with the location of the cells derived from the neural crest cells, which are necessary to produce the process of fusion [15]. The areas of condensed mesenchyme can then be traced as prongs into the fusing proximal cushions (Fig. 2.17b). Previous observers have correlated these structures with a so-called aortopulmonary septal complex [18]. The columns, however, are never interposed between the walls of the intrapericardial aorta and pulmonary trunk. The changes affecting the proximal cushions involve the migration of cardiomyocytes from the parietal walls into the parts which contain the prongs [19], this process producing the subpulmonary infundibular myocardial sleeve (Fig. 2.15c). Having muscularised, the developing infundibulum then separates itself from the aortic root to form a free-standing muscular sleeve. It is the ventral protrusion from the dorsal wall of the aortic sac, therefore, that is the embryonic aortopulmonary septum [20].

The key feature in the completion of normal ventricular septation, and the final process in remodelling of the outflow tract, is the transfer of the aortic root to the left ventricle. This takes place, in the mouse, during the thirteenth embryonic day. As the aorta moves to achieve its definitive position above the left ventricle, so there is further reorientation of the initial embryonic interventricular communication. We have already described how the dorsal part of the communication comes to surround the right atrioventricular orifice during expansion of the atrioventricular canal (Fig. 2.6b). Transfer of the aortic root to the left ventricle then means that the ventral part of the initial communication becomes reorientated so as to form the left ventricular outlet (Fig. 2.18a).

Transfer of the root to the left ventricle brings the leading edge of the arch formed by the proximal outflow cushions into better alignment with the crest of the muscular septum. This process also brings the rightward components of the fused atrioventricular cushions into apposition with the septal attachment of the fused proximal outflow cushions (Fig. 2.18b). As these endocardial structures come together to close the embryonic interventricular communication, thus walling the aortic root into the left ventricle, so has the surface of the proximal outflow cushions become muscularised [19] to form the free-standing subpulmonary infundibulum (Figs. 2.15c and 2.18c). Subsequent to commitment of the aortic root to the left ventricle by formation of the membranous part of the septum (Fig. 2.19a), the central part of the fused proximal cushion is transformed into the tissue plane that separates the free-standing infundibulum from the aortic root (Fig. 2.19b).

Maldevelopment of the Outflow Tract

As we have explained throughout our review, we find it less than optimal to seek to explain normal development in terms of the "conus" and the "truncus". When Kramer introduced these terms [16], his intentions were to improve communication. This has not proved to be the case. As we will show, far better correlations between

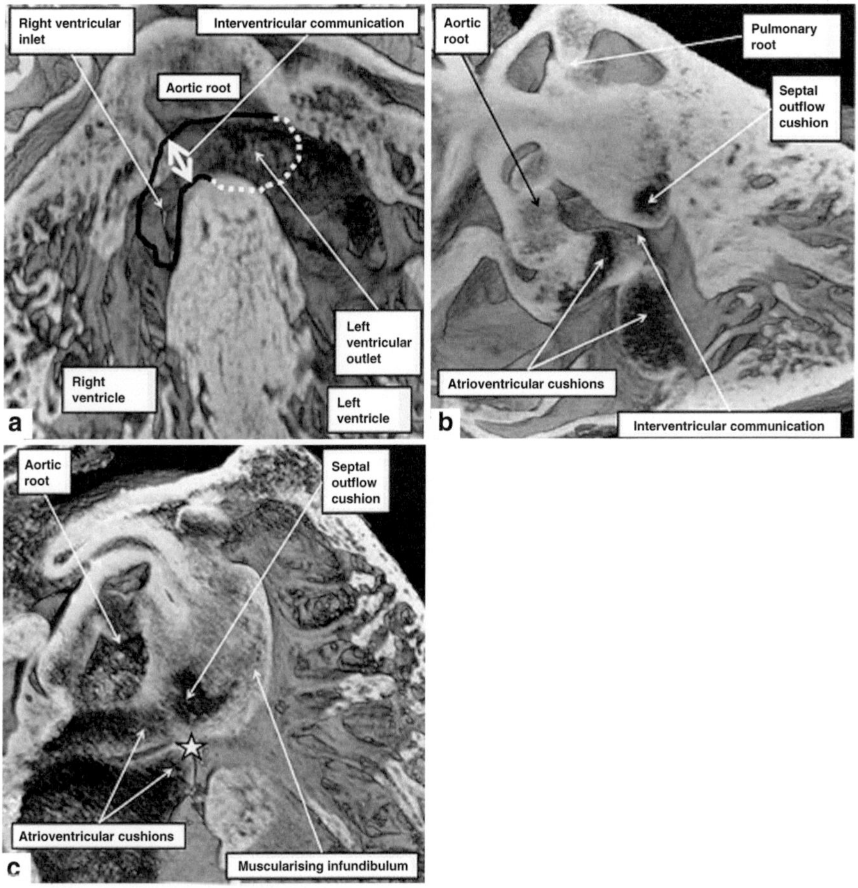

Fig. 2.18 Panel (**a**) shows a frontal section through the aortic root in a mouse at the beginning of the thirteenth embryonic day of development. The root is being transferred to the left ventricle, but at this stage is overriding the crest of the muscular ventricular septum. The *black line* shows how part of the initial interventricular communication came to surround the right atrioventricular orifice subsequent to expansion of the atrioventricular canal. The *white dotted line* shows how the ventral part of the original communication is now becoming the outlet for the left ventricle. The *double headed white arrow* shows the persisting communication, which can now be closed. As is shown in panel (**b**), closure is achieved by the rightward tubercles of the atrioventricular cushions coming into apposition with the proximal septal outflow cushion as the root moves into the left ventricle. Panel (**c**) then shows that, as the interventricular communication (*star*) is closed, so the surface of the fused proximal cushions muscularises to become the free-standing subpulmonary infundibulum

developmental changes and morphological findings can be provided when congenital cardiac malformations are assessed on the basis of abnormal development of the extrapericardial systemic and pulmonary channels, and then in terms of maldevelopment of the distal, intermediate, and proximal components of the outflow tract. It is an understanding of the remoulding of the extrapericardial pharyngeal arch

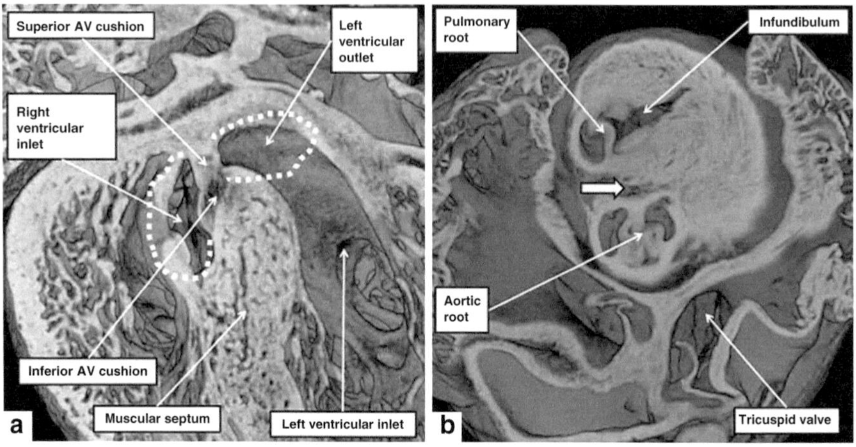

Fig. 2.19 Panel (**a**) shows how, by the end of the 13th day of development in the mouse, the rightward tubercles of the atrioventricular endocardial cushions have fused to close the remaining embryonic interventricular communication, thus forming the membranous part of the septum. The *white dotted lines* show how the boundaries of the initial communication now surround the inlet of the right, and the outlet of the left ventricle. Panel (**b**) shows how, by the time of birth in the mouse, a plane of separation has developed between the pulmonary infundibulum and the aortic root. This means that, in the postnatal heart, there is hardly any recognisable outlet septum

arteries that provides rational explanations for the abnormal patterns of branching that accompany so many of the intrapericardial lesions. Edwards [21] showed how all of these lesions could adequately be explained on the basis of the initial symmetry of the arteries running throught the pharyngeal arches. His concept still retains its validity. Interruption or persistence between the various segments of the double arch, coupled with the disappearance or persistence of unilateral or bilateral arterial ducts, explains the multiple variations producing vascular rings, and also account for isolation of the brachiocephalic arteries [22]. Space does not permit discussion of all these variants, but abnormal patterns of branching of the extrapericardial arteries are frequently found in association with the malformations on which we will now concentrate.

Malformations of the Distal Outflow Tract

We have already discussed the most obvious lesion resulting from maldevelopment of the distal outflow tract, namely the aortopulmonary window (Fig. 2.11). The location of this lesion exemplifies the advantages of approaching development, and initial septation, in terms of the three components of the outflow tract. The lesion represents failure of fusion of the spur that protrudes ventrally from the pharyngeal mesenchyme with the distal ends of the outflow cushions. The presence of separate arterial roots, however, along with the normal septation of the ventricles, indicates that division of the intermediate and proximal parts of the outflow tract has proceeded in normal fashion. It is also easy to provide an explanation for the frequent finding of anomalous origin of the right pulmonary artery from the aorta in the setting of aortopulmonary window [23]. An abnormal orientation of the ventral protrusion can leave the right pulmonary artery, which takes its origin from the base of the aortic sac, in communication with the aortic component of the distal outflow tract. Such abnormal protrusion of the dorsal wall of the aortic sac, but in the setting of subsequent appropriate fusion with the distal cushions, then provides a rational explanation of anomalous origin of the right pulmonary artery from the ascending aorta [24], another lesion which is difficult to explain using conventional approaches to development of the outflow tract. When assessing the latter lesion, the presence of a normal right ventricular infundibulum, supporting the pulmonary trunk means that such anomalous origin of the right pulmonary artery should not be described in terms of "hemitruncus".

Anomalous Development of the Intermediate Part of the Outflow Tract

It is the arterial roots that are derived from the intermediate part of the outflow tract, with normal fusion of the major outflow cushions required to separate the aortic from the pulmonary root. Failure of fusion of the major outflow cushions results in persistence of a common ventriculo-arterial junction. This is the phenotypic feature of common arterial trunk, a lesion often described in terms of "persistent truncus arteriosus". This usage in itself points to further problems in the use of "truncus" as opposed to "conus", since unless it is presumed that the arterial roots are derived from the embryonic "truncus", the lesion would need to be described as "persistent conus arteriosus". Since the common ventriculo-arterial junction is the defining feature of the lesion, persistent conus arteriosus would, perhaps, be a more appropriate "traditional term". Describing the lesion in terms of common arterial trunk, however, removes the need for such debates. The morphogenesis of the entity has also generated controversy. Van Praagh and Van Praagh [25] suggested, on the basis of analysis of autopsied examples of the lesion, that the entity reflected failure of growth, during development, of the subpulmonary conus. They suggested that, in essence, the truncal root was no more than the persisting aortic root. Van Mierop and his colleagues [26], in contrast, produced embryological evidence, having studied the development of the outflow tract in Keeshond dogs, that the malformation reflected failure of fusion of the major outflow cushions. Our own observations endorse the concept of failure of fusion of the outflow cushions. We have been able to examine mice genetically modified by knocking out the Tbx1 gene. All of these mice have common arterial trunks, defined on the basis of a solitary arterial trunk that exits from the base of the heart through a common ventriculo-arterial junction, which supply directly the systemic, pulmonary, and coronary arteries (Fig. 2.20a).

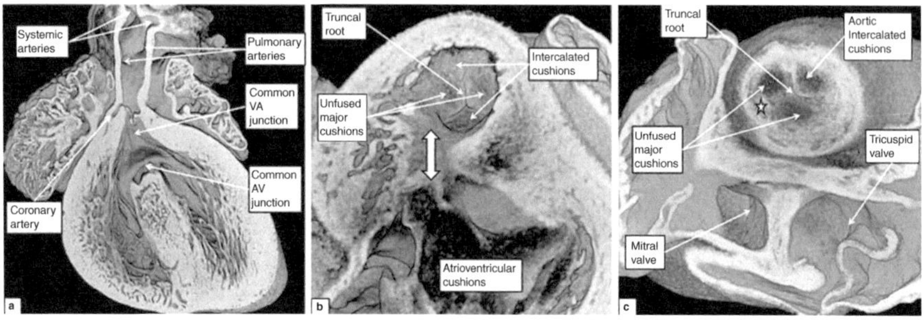

Fig. 2.20 The images show common arterial trunks in mice genetically modified by knocking out the Tbx1 gene. Panel (**a**) shows an embryonic mouse in the 17th day of development, in which the arterial trunk, exiting through and common ventriculo-arterial (*VA*) junction, divides to supply coronary, systemic, and pulmonary arteries. This mouse also has a common atrioventricular (*AV*) junction. Panels (**b**, **c**) are from mice at the 13th day of embryonic development. Panel (**b**), a short axis cut viewed from the ventricular apexes, shows undivided major cushions and two intercalated cushions, giving the template for formation of a quadrifoliate truncal valve. The *double headed white arrow* shows the interventricular communication. In Panel (**c**), viewed from above, the pulmonary intercalated cushion (*star*) is grossly hypoplastic, setting the scene for formation of a truncal root with three sinuses and leaflets (Mice kindly provided by Dr Robert Kelly, University of Marseilles, France)

Examination of knock-out embryos obtained during the 13th day of embryonic development, when as we have seen the arterial roots have normally separated one from the other, reveals failure of fusion of the major outflow cushions. In many instances, we are also able to identify the presence of both intercalated cushions, this arrangement providing the template for formation of common arterial trunk with quadrifoliate truncal valves and sinuses (Fig. 2.20a). In other embryos, however, the pulmonary intercalated cushion is markedly hypoplastic, producing the situation in which the valve will eventually develop with three rather than four sinuses and leaflets (Fig. 2.20b). In none of the Tbx1 null mice has there been any formation of the ventral protrusion from the dorsal wall of the aortic sac, so that the common trunk shows no division of the intrapericardial aortic and pulmonary pathways (Fig. 2.20a). We have now also identified common arterial trunks in mice genetically modified by perturbing the furin enzyme. In these mice, there is extensive separation of the intrapericardial pathways, with good formation of the ventral protrusion. Some of these mice have well separated intrapericardial arterial pathways, but with dominance of the aortic component (Fig. 2.21a). Others have hypoplasia of the aortic component, interruption of the extrapericardial aortic pathways, and persistence of the arterial duct, which supplies the descending aorta through a dominant pulmonary component of the trunk (Fig. 2.21b). These findings correlate well with the suggestions that, rather than analysing clinical examples of common trunk as suggested by Collett and Edwards [27], it is better simply to consider the lesion in terms of aortic as opposed to pulmonary domi-

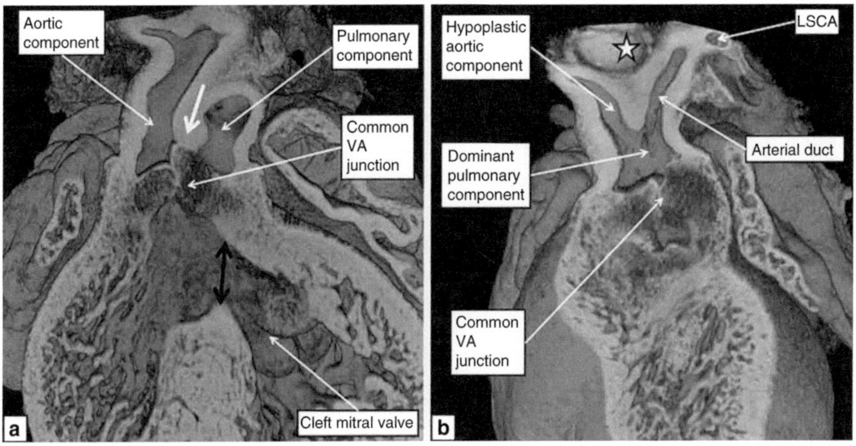

Fig. 2.21 The images show common arterial trunks, defined on the basis of the common ventriculo-arterial (VA) junction in two mice genetically modified by perturbing the furin enzyme. In the heart shown in Panel (**a**), the aortic component of the common trunk is dominant, with extensive separation of the intrapericardial pathways produced by formation of the ventral protrusion from the dorsal wall of the aortic sac (*white single headed arrow*). The trunk arises predominantly from the right ventricle, so the left ventricular outlet is the embryonic interventricular communication (*double headed black arrow*). Note the cleft mitral valve. Panel (**b**) shows another heart with separation of the arterial intrapericardial pathways, but with dominance of the pulmonary component of the trunk, which continues through the patent arterial duct to supply the descending aorta and the left subclavian artery (LSCA). The aortic arch is interrupted (*star*), and the ascending aortic component of the trunk is hypoplastic

nance [25], but then to describe precisely the pattern of the aortic and pulmonary branches [28].

Once we appreciate that the arterial roots are also developed from the intermediate component of the outflow tract, we can justifiably include lesions of the arterial valves as outflow tract malformations. It remains a mystery why these lesions should not be considered "conotruncal" malformations. If we look again at Fig. 2.14b, we can then provide a logical explanation for arterial valves with two, as opposed to three, leaflets. Bicuspid aortic valve, along with prolapse of the mitral valve, is the commonest congenital cardiac malformation. As shown in Fig. 2.14b, the distal parts of the major outflow cushions, during normal development, do not fuse throughout the area of the apposition of their edges. Sans-Coma and his colleagues, who studied a colony of Syrian hamsters with naturally occurring bicuspid aortic valves, revealed in elegant fashion the reason for the bicuspidity [29]. They found exuberant fusion of the major outflow cushions on the aortic side of the separating arterial roots. In the presence of such complete fusion of the major cushions, subsequent excavation resulted in an aortic root with two sinuses and two leaflets. The larger leaflet then represented conjunction of the leaflets that, normally, would have guarded the aortic valvar sinuses giving rise to the coronary arteries. As the group from Malaga then showed subsequently [30], fusion during development between the parietal major outflow cushion and the aortic intercalated cushion provides an equally convincing explanation for the variant of bicuspid aortic valve in which the conjoined leaflet is formed by the right coronary and non-coronary aortic leaflets. As Phillips and colleagues have subsequently shown [31], the degree of population of the developing cushions by cells derived from the neural crest can also be significant in producing animals with bicuspid arterial valves, with the bicuspidity reflecting hypoplasia of one of the cushions, rather than exuberant fusion.

Abnormal Development of the Proximal Outflow Tract

As we have shown, it is the proximal outflow tract, if development proceeds normally, that is separated to provide the ventricular outlets. This requires the migration of cardiomyocytes into the proximal outflow cushions so as to produce the free-standing right ventricular infundibulum [19]. Normal development, however, also requires the removal of myocardium from the left ventricular outlet subsequent to closure of the embryonic interventricular communication. This is because, as shown in Fig. 2.16a, the aortic valvar leaflets continue to be supported by a muscular infundibulum, or "conus", at the time of the completion of ventricular septation. Both of these features are significant as we seek clues to the maldevelopment of the proximal outflow tract.

Subsequent to ventricular looping, the default option for the developing heart is double outlet from the right ventricle. At the time of fusion of the proximal outflow cushions, this process producing the arch above the cavity of the right ventricle, and which occurs in the mouse heart during the 12th day of embryonic development, equivalent to about 6 weeks of development in humans, the proximal outflow cushions are mesenchymal structures packed with cells derived from the neural crest. Should there be failure to convert the cushions into the muscular subpulmonary infundibulum during ongoing development, and the ventricular septum itself fail to close, then a channel will persist between the ventricles which is roofed by the remnants of the mesenchymal outflow cushions. We have now encountered precisely this lesion in our mouse embryos in which we perturbed the furin enzyme. The result is a doubly committed interventricular communication, roofed by continuity between the remnants of the proximal cushions. These structures support cranially the intermediate cushions, which have fused in appropriate fashion to produce normally formed and separated arterial roots. The structure that is missing is the muscularised subpulmonary infundibulum (Fig. 2.22).

In the lesion illustrated in Fig. 2.22, the ventriculo-arterial connection is one of double outlet from the right ventricle. The interventricular communication is directly beneath both arterial roots, and hence is doubly committed. Had the aortic root been transferred to the left ventricle, however, the heart would have shown a

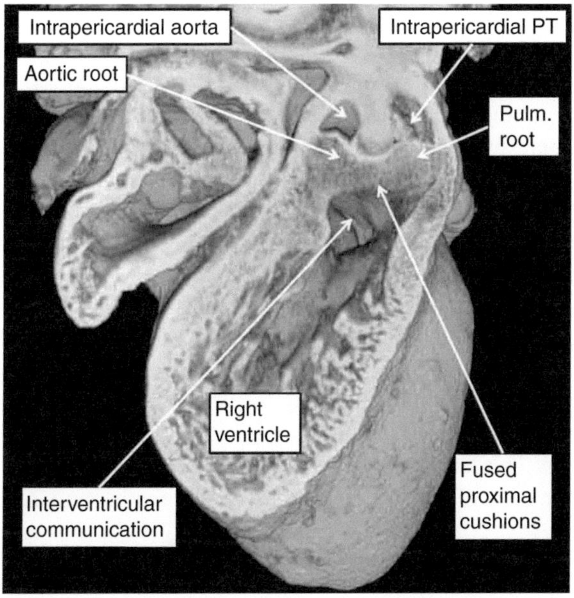

Fig. 2.22 The image is from another mouse in which the furin enzyme has been genetically modified. As shown by the separate nature of the intrapericardial arterial trunks, and the separate arterial roots, septation and separation of the distal and intermediate parts of the outflow tract has proceeded in normal fashion. The proximal outflow cushions have fused, but then failed to muscularise. Thus, the embryonic interventricular communication is roofed by the fused cushions. The arterial roots remain above the right ventricle, so the ventriculo-arterial connection is one of double outlet

doubly committed and juxta-arterial ventricular septal defect with concordant ventriculo-arterial connections. Such defects, with the phenotypic feature of a common ventriculo-arterial junction divided into aortic and pulmonary valvar orifices, have more in common with common arterial trunk than with the other phenotypic variants of ventricular septal defect. And, had transfer to the left ventricle been exuberant, the end result would have been double outlet from the left ventricle. This spectrum, in the setting of failure of muscularisation of the subpulmonary infundibulum, was described by Brandt and colleagues [32] as "double outlet both ventricles". It is similar spectrums existing in the setting of spiralling as opposed to parallel arterial trunks that provide the basis for understanding the different hearts that can exist with the ventriculo-arterial connection of double outlet right ventricle [33].

This is because double outlet right ventricle does not represent a specific phenotype, but rather is made up of a group of hearts exhibiting the same ventriculo-arterial connection. It became customary in the past to demand bilateral "conuses" so as to permit the diagnosis of double outlet right ventricle. Such an approach, however, is a direct abrogation of the most important principle established to clarify the analysis of congenitally malformed hearts, namely the morphological method.

Propounded by Van Praagh and colleagues [34], this principle stated that one variable feature in the heart should not be determined on the basis of another feature that is itself variable. Thus, in the setting of double outlet ventriculo-arterial connection, infundibular morphology is itself variable, and should therefore be disqualified as a criterion for diagnosis. As we have shown, there is no justification for considering the persistence of infundibulums bilaterally as being a feature of the right ventricle, since the normally developing heart still possesses bilateral infundibulums, or conuses, when the aorta is walled into the left ventricle at the time of closure of the embryonic interventricular communication (Fig. 2.16a).

We have also emphasised, nonetheless, that double outlet is the default option for the developing heart. While both arterial trunks remain supported by the developing right ventricle, the interventricular communication represents the outlet for the developing left ventricle. As is revealed in Fig. 2.23, the interventricular communication is in a different plane from that representing the locus for subsequent ventricular septation. This latter plane extends between the base of the proximal outflow cushions and the crest of the apical muscular ventricular septum. As the aortic root

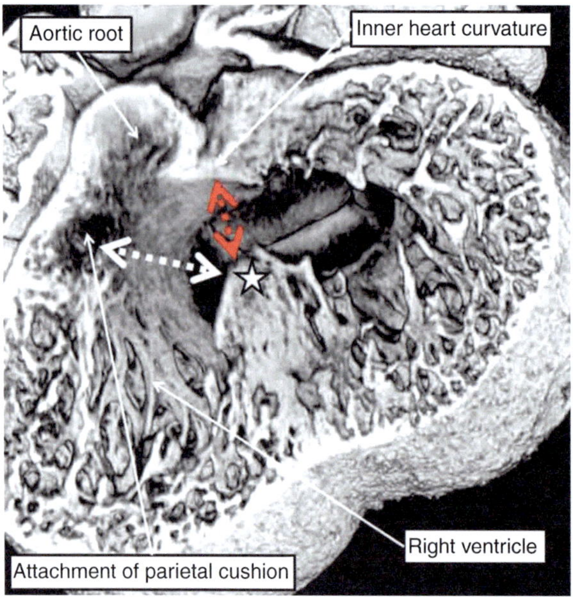

Fig. 2.23 The image shows a tilted ventral four-chamber cut through a dataset obtained from a mouse early during the 12th day of embryonic development. The aortic root remains supported in its entirety by the developing right ventricle. The inner heart curvature separates the arterial roots from the atrioventricular canal, equivalent to bilateral conuses in the postnatal heart. The image shows that the interventricular communication (*double headed red arrow*) provides the outlet for the developing left ventricle. It is bounded by the crest of the apical muscular ventricular septum (*star*) and the inner curve. It is not, however, a ventricular septal defect, since the plane of putative ventricular septation is shown by the *double headed white arrow*. By analogy, it is this plane that would be closed by a surgeon working in a postnatal heart so as to tunnel the aortic root into the left ventricle

is transferred to the left ventricle during normal development, so this plane is brought into alignment with the apical septum, and is finally closed by formation of the membranous part of the septum (Fig. 2.19a).

It is incorrect, therefore, to describe the channel between the ventricles in the setting of double outlet right ventricle as a “ventricular septal defect”. The space can never be closed, since it is an obligate part of the systemic circulation. Distinction between the plane of putative ventricular septation, and the plane of the geometric interventricular communication, also provides a pragmatic means of distinguishing between double outlet right ventricle as opposed to concordant or discordant ventriculo-arterial connections. If the surgeon, in the operating room, considers that he or she has closed the “defect”, then the patient must have had concordant or discordant ventriculo-arterial connections. If the patient had double outlet right ventricle, then the surgeon will have needed to tunnel the “defect” to one or other ventricular outflow tract.

The different phenotypes that can be found within the group of hearts having double outlet ventriculo-arterial connection, therefore, depend on the specific intracardiac anatomy. If the outflow cushions develop so as to produce spiralling of the arterial trunks, which is usually the case, then double outlet connection from the right ventricle can exist in the spectrums of either tetralogy of Fallot or the Eisenmenger defect. The difference between these entities depends on whether or not there is muscular sub-pulmonary obstruction. In both phenotypes, the septal outflow cushion will be inserted cephalad relative to the interventricular communication. So as to produce tetralogy, there will also need to be an abnormal relationship between the malaligned septal outflow cushion and the septo-parietal trabeculations, with the latter derived by compaction of the trabecular layer of the right ventricular wall. Such an abnormal relationship between the malaligned outflow cushions and the septoparietal trabeculations will also be the substrate for development of tetralogy of Fallot in the setting of concordant ventriculo-arterial connections, but in this instance with greater commitment of the overriding aortic root to the left ventricle. The more frequent variant of tetralogy, therefore, that with effectively concordant ventriculo-arterial connections, is no more than the end of the spectrum of transfer of the aorta into the left ventricle, but with malalignment of the outflow cushions, and abnormal formation of the septoparietal trabeculations. We have already discussed, and illustrated, the phenotype of double outlet produced by failure of formation of the subpulmonary muscular infundibulum (Fig. 2.22). This variant typically co-exists with spiralling arterial trunks, but can also be found with parallel arterial trunks.

It is the formation of the intrapericardial arterial trunks in parallel rather than spiral fashion that underscores the third variant of double outlet right ventricle. The developmental process resulting in this variant will also be responsible for producing transposition, better described as discordant ventriculo-arterial connections. Quite some time ago, Van Mierop and colleagues [20] showed how the outflow cushions, if fusing in straight rather than spiral fashion, would produce discordant ventriculo-arterial connections. We have now confirmed that the cushions fuse in such parallel fashion in mice in which the gene for Pitx2 has been knocked out.

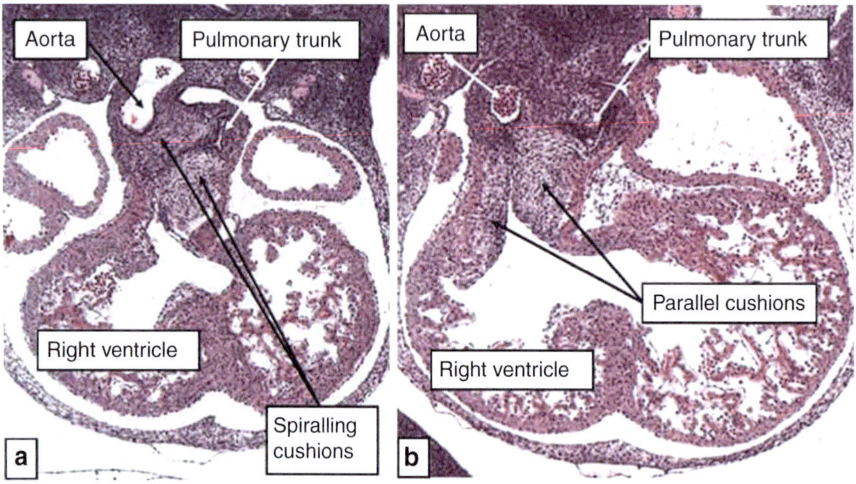

Fig. 2.24 The images compare the orientation of the developing arterial trunks in wild-type mice (Panel **a**) and mice in which the Pitx2 gene has been knocked out (Panel **b**). As can be seen, the wild-type mice show the typical spiralling pattern of the outflow cushions, while the knock-out animals have parallel cushions. The knock-out mice all develop hearts showing the Taussig-Bing malformation

These mice show the spectrum of double outlet that extends from discordant ventriculo-arterial connections to double outlet right ventricle with subpulmonary interventricular connection, the spectrum also being well described as the Taussig-Bing malformation [35]. The key consequence of parallel development of the arterial trunks is that, subsequent to fusion of the ventral protrusion with the distal ends of the cushions, the rightward outflow tract arising from the right ventricle is connected with the cranial component of the aortic sac, which feeds the systemic channels. The leftward and posterior part of the proximal outflow tract is then connected to the pulmonary component of the aortic sac. This part is closest to the embryonic interventricular communication. Thus, when the proximal outflow tract is transferred to the left ventricle, the end result will be to produce discordant ventriculo-arterial connections (Fig. 2.24). This arrangement will co-exist with an intact ventricular septum should the atrioventricular cushions subsequently close the embryonic interventricular communication.

It is potentially possible for the orientation of the ventral protrusion from the dorsal wall of the aortic sac to produce still further variations in the panoply of abnormal ventriculo-arterial connections. In the normal situation, the protrusion grows so as to join the systemic component of the aortic sac with the rightward channel in the distal outflow tract. If, however, the protrusion grows with reciprocal angulation, then it is feasible for the systemic component of the sac to be joined to the leftward distal channel. This would then place the pulmonary component of the sac in communication with the rightward channel of the distal outflow tract. These alternative processes are able to provide an explanation for the rare situations in which hearts are formed with concordant ventriculo-arterial connections, but with parallel arterial trunks, so-called "anatomically corrected malposition". Variations in the formation of the infundibular components can then explain all the different forms of this lesion [36].

Conclusions

Almost a century has now passed since Maude Abbott, the first pathologist to provide a comprehensive analysis of congenitally malformed hearts, argued that understanding of ontogenesis could aid in the appreciation of the abnormal anatomy [37]. At the time of her writing, the evidence available regarding cardiac development was insufficiently robust to substantiate her opinion. All has changed over the past two decades. The advent of episcopic microscopy [38] now makes it possible to analyse the changes occurring in the developing heart with just as much accuracy as the clinician using computed tomography or magnetic resonance imaging. As we have shown, this technique, combined with the advances made in genetic manipulation of mice, permits us to make direct correlations between the developing heart and congenitally malformed hearts with abnormalities of their outflow tracts. In our opinion, the evidence now shows that the time has come to move away from analysis of so-called "conotruncal anomalies". The normal outflow tract can better be analysed in terms of the changes occurring in its proximal, intermediate, and distal components, along with the extrapericardial arterial trunks. Congenital cardiac malformations can then be analysed and compared in similar tripartite fashion. The knowledge accruing from these studies shows that congenitally corrected transposition depends on abnormal ventricular looping, although this is then combined with abnormal development of the outflow tracts. Abnormal development of the outflow tracts themselves now permits realistic concepts to be advanced to explain the morphogenesis of aortopulmonary window, common arterial trunk, tetralogy of Fallot, transposition, and the various forms of double outlet right ventricle. The findings regarding development, however, also show that lesions afflicting the arterial roots should now be included within the group of outflow tract malformations, since these components occupy a crucial location in the middle of the developing outflow tract.

Acknowledgements We are indebted to Professor Pete Scambler from the Institute of Child Health, University College, London, who has permitted us to use images obtained from mice engineered in his department. We also thank Dr Robert Kelly, University of Marseilles, for ongoing discussion regarding the Tbx1 knock-out mice.

References

1. Anderson RH, Chaudhry B, Mohun TJ, Bamforth SD, Hoyland D, Phillips HM, Webb S, Moorman AF, Brown NA, Henderson DJ. Normal and abnormal development of the intrapericardial arterial trunks in humans and mice. Cardiovasc Res. 2012;95:108–15.
2. Sizarov A, Lamers WH, Mohun TJ, Brown NA, Anderson RH, Moorman AF. Three-dimensional and molecular analysis of the arterial pole of the developing human heart. J Anat. 2012;220:336–49.
3. Webb S, Qayyum SR, Anderson RH, Lamers WH, Richardson MK. Septation and separation within the outflow tract of the developing heart. J Anat. 2003;202:327–42.
4. Patten BM, Kramer TC. The initiation of contractions in the embryonic chicken heart. Am J Anat. 1933;53:349–75.
5. Viragh SZ, Challice CE. Origin and differentiation of cardiac muscle cells in the mouse. J Ultrastruct Res. 1973;42:1–24.
6. Arguello C, De la Cruz MV, Gomez CS. Experimental study of the formation of the heart tube in the chick embryo. J Embryol Exp Morphol. 1975;33:1–11.
7. Kelly RG, Brown NA, Buckingham ME. The arterial pole of the mouse heart forms from Fgf10-expressing cells in pharyngeal mesoderm. Dev Cell. 2001;1:435–40.
8. Mjaatvedt CH, Nakaoka T, Moreno-Rodriguez R, Norris RA, Kern MJ, Eisenberg CA, Turner D, Markwald RR. The outflow tract of the heart is recruited from a novel heart-forming field. Dev Biol. 2001;238:97–109.
9. Waldo KL, Kumiski DH, Wallis KT, Stadt HA, Hutson MR, Platt DH, Kirby ML. Conotruncal myocardium arises from a secondary heart field. Development. 2001;128:3179–88.
10. Moorman AFM, Christoffels VM, Anderson RH, van den Hoff MJB. The heart-forming fields – one or multiple? Phil Trans R Soc B. 2007;362:1257–65.
11. Aanhaanen WT, Brons JF, Dominguez JN, et al. The Tbx2+ primary myocardium of the atrioventricular canal forms the atrioventricular node and the base of the left ventricle. Circ Res. 2009;104:1267–74.
12. Moorman AFM, Christoffels VM. Cardiac chamber formation: development, genes, and evolution. Physiol Rev. 2003;83:1223–67.
13. Eisenberg LM, Markwald RR. Molecular regulation of atrioventricular valvuloseptal morphogenesis. Circ Res. 1995;77:1–6.
14. Tenorio de Albuquerque A, Rigby ML, Anderson RH, Lincoln C, Shinebourne EA. The spectrum of atrioventricular discordance. A clinical study. Br Heart J. 1984;51:498–507.
15. Kirby ML, Gale TF, Stewart DE. Neural crest cells contribute to normal aorticopulmonary septation. Science. 1983;220:1059–61.
16. Kramer TC. The partitioning of the truncus and conus and the formation of the membranous portion of the interventricular septum in the human heart. Am J Anat. 1942;71:343–70.
17. Hinton Jr RB, Alfieri CM, Witt SA, Glascock BJ, Khoury PR, Benson DW, Yutzey KE. Mouse heart valve structure and function: echocardiographic and morphometric analyses from the fetus through the aged adult. Am J Phys Heart Circ. 2008;294:H2480–8.
18. Bartelings MM, Gittenberger-de Groot AC. The outflow tract of the heart – embryologic and morphologic correlations. Int J Cardiol. 1989;22:289–300.
19. van den Hoff MJB, Moorman AFM, Ruijter JM, et al. Myocardialization of the cardiac outflow tract. Dev Biol. 1999;212:477–90.
20. Van Mierop LHS, Alley RD, Kausel HW, Stranahan A. Pathogenesis of transposition complexes. 1. Embryology of the ventricles and great arteries. Am J Cardiol. 1963;12:216–25.
21. Edwards JE. Anomalies of the derivatives of the aortic arch system. Med Clin North Am. 1948;32:925–48.
22. Yoo SJ, Bradley TJ. Vascular rings, pulmonary arterial sling, & related conditions. In: Anderson RH, Baker EJ, Penny D, Redington AN, Rigby MJ, Wernovsky G, editors. Paediatric cardiology. 3rd ed. Philadelphia: Elsevier; 2010. p. 967–90.

23. Kiran VS, Singh MK, Shah S, John C, Maheshwari S. Lessons learned from a series of patients with missed aortopulmonary windows. Cardiol Young. 2008;18:480–4.
24. Fong LV, Anderson RH, Siewers RD, Trento A, Park SC. Anomalous origin of one pulmonary artery from the ascending aorta: a review of echocardiographic, catheter, and morphological features. Br Heart J. 1989;62:389–94.
25. Van Praagh R, Van Praagh S. The anatomy of common aorticopulmonary trunk (truncus arteriosus communis) and its embryologic implications. A study of 57 necropsy cases. Am J Cardiol. 1965;16:406–25.
26. Van Mierop LHS, Patterson DF, Schnarr WR. Pathogenesis of persistent truncus arteriosus in light of observations made in a dog embryo with the anomaly. Am J Cardiol. 1978;41:755–62.
27. Collett RW, Edwards JE. Persistent truncus arteriosus; a classification according to anatomic types. Surg Clin North Am. 1949;29:1245–69.
28. Russell HM, Jacobs ML, Anderson RH, Mavroudis C, Spicer D, Corcrain E, et al. A simplified categorization for common arterial trunk. J Thorac Cardiovasc Surg. 2011;141:645–53.
29. Sans-Coma V, Fernandez B, Duran AC, et al. Fusion of valve cushions as a key factor in the formation of congenital bicuspid aortic valves in Syrian hamsters. Anat Rec. 1996;244:490–8.
30. Fernandez B, Duran AC, Fernandez-Gallego T, et al. Bicuspid aortic valves with different spatial orientation of the leaflets are distinct etiological entities. J Am Coll Cardiol. 2009;54:2312–8.
31. Phillips HM, Mahendran P, Singh E, Anderson RH, Chaudhry B, Henderson DJ. Neural crest cells are required for correct positioning of the developing outflow cushions and pattern the arterial valve leaflets. Cardiovasc Res. 2013;99:452–60.
32. Brandt PWT, Calder AL, Barratt-Boyes BG, Neutze JM. Double outlet left ventricle, morphology, cineangiocardiographic diagnosis and surgical treatment. Am J Cardiol. 1976;38:897–909.
33. Capuani A, Uemura H, Ho SY, Anderson RH. Anatomic spectrum of abnormal ventriculoarterial connections – surgical implications. Ann Thorac Surg. 1995;59:352–60.
34. Van Praagh R, David I, Wright GB, Van Praagh S. Large RV plus small LV is not single RV. Circulation. 1980;61:1057–8.
35. Stellin G, Zuberbuhler JR, Anderson RH, Siewers RD. The surgical anatomy of the Taussig Bing malformation. J Thorac Cardiovasc Surg. 1987;93:560–9.
36. Cavalle-Garrido T, Bernasconi A, Perrin D, Anderson RH. Hearts with concordant ventriculoarterial connections but parallel arterial trunks. Heart. 2007;93:100–6.
37. Abbott ME. Atlas of congenital cardiac disease. New York: American Heart Association; 1936. p. 2.
38. Mohun TJ, Weninger WJ. Imaging heart development using high-resolution episcopic microscopy. Curr Opin Genet Dev. 2011;21:573–8.

Chapter 3
Anatomy of Conotruncal Anomalies

Lucile Houyel and Meriem Mostefa Kara

Abstract In this chapter, we provide an extensive description of the anatomic features of the various anomalies affecting the outflow tract of the heart (conotruncal defects or outflow tract defects) including tetralogy of Fallot (TOF) and its variants, common arterial trunk (CAT), interrupted aortic arch (IAA), various anatomic forms of double-outlet right ventricle (DORV), transposition of the great arteries (TGA) and congenitally corrected transposition of the great arteries (cc-TGA). These anomalies can be divided in two groups according to their embryologic origin, those due primarily to a lack of migration of the cardiac neural crest cells, and those due primarily to a perturbation of the laterality genes. The embryologic basis of this grouping is comforted by the anatomic differences between the two groups regarding the ventricular septal defect (VSD) and the coronary arteries pattern, as well as the course of the proximal great vessels.

The VSD is always present and always of the outlet type in neural crest defects, although there are differences regarding its postero-inferior and superior rims. These differences suggest an anatomic continuum from TOF to IAA type B rather than distinct physiological phenotypes, related to various degrees of abnormal rotation of the outflow tract during heart development, incomplete in TOF, TOF with pulmonary atresia and DORV, absent in CAT, excessive in IAA type B. On the other hand, TGA is not always associated with a VSD, and when present, this VSD can be of any type (outlet, inlet, muscular, central membranous). The position of the coronary orifices on the aortic or truncal circumference depends on the rotation of the aorta, but also on the spatial relationship between the two great vessels, which accounts for the high frequency of coronary abnormalities in conotruncal defects.

L. Houyel, MD (✉)
Department of Congenital Cardiac Surgery, Centre Chirurgical Marie-Lannelongue, Marie-Lannelongue Hospital, Université Paris-Sud,
133 avenue de la Resistance, Le Plessis-Robinson 92350, France
e-mail: l.houyel@ccml.fr

M. Mostefa Kara, MD
Department of Pediatric Cardiology, Centre de Référence Malformations Cardiaques Congénitales Complexes – M3C, Necker Hospital for Sick Children, Assistance Publique des Hopitaux de Paris, Paris, France

Université Paris Descartes, Sorbonne Paris Cité, Paris, France

F. Lacour-Gayet et al. (eds.), *Surgery of Conotruncal Anomalies*,
DOI 10.1007/978-3-319-23057-3_3

The great vessels emerge from the heart in a spiraling fashion in cardiac neural crest defects, but are parallel in TGA and cc-TGA.

Congenitally corrected transposition of the great arteries includes as part of its phenotype a malformation of the outflow tract (ventriculo-arterial discordance). However, the major determinant of this laterality defect is the atrioventricular discordance, which puts it in a class of its own. In this complex malformation, the VSD is not constant and usually opens both in the outlet and in the inlet of the left ventricle, which, among other characteristics such as the abnormal location of the conduction tissue and the frequency of right ventricle and tricuspid valve anomalies, underlines its differences with the conotruncal defects mentioned above.

Keywords Conotruncal anomalies • Anatomy • Outflow tract • Tetralogy of Fallot • Pulmonary atresia • Common arterial trunk • Double outlet right ventricle • Interrupted aortic arch • Transposition of the great arteries • Congenitally corrected transposition of the great arteries

Introduction

The term "conotruncal defects" encompasses very different morphologic entities, having in common an abnormal development of the outflow tract of the heart. Within this large group of defects, two classes can be distinguished [1]: those with "normally related great arteries", and transposition of the great arteries (TGA). Congenitally corrected transposition of the great arteries (ccTGA) is usually not included in the group of conotruncal defects [1] and has been considered by various authors either an anatomic form of TGA, or a situs or looping abnormality [2, 3]. We chose to divide the conotruncal, or outflow tract, defects in two groups according to their currently presumed developmental origin.

The first group is due to a lack of migration of cardiac neural crest cells, leading to a lack of addition of cardiomyocytes by the anterior part of the second heart field to the developing outflow tract [4]. These "cardiac neural crest defects" include tetralogy of Fallot (TOF) and its anatomic variants (including TOF with pulmonary atresia and with absent pulmonary valve), common arterial trunk (CAT), certain anatomic forms of interrupted aortic arch (IAA), and certain anatomic forms of double-outlet right ventricle (DORV). These defects might be due to a disturbance of the "alignment" aspect of wedging [1]. The majority of these defects are strongly associated with Di George syndrome and 22q11 microdeletion.

The second group, although involving the same region of the heart, is now considered to be primarily due to disorders of the laterality genes: transposition of the great arteries (TGA) and congenitally corrected TGA. There is now increasing evidence, based on epidemiologic, experimental and genetic data, that TGA, ccTGA and heterotaxy could share as a common genetic origin, a perturbation of the laterality genes such as ZIC3, CFC1, NODAL [5–7]. These defects might be due to a disturbance of the "rotational" aspect of wedging [1].

Cardiac Neural Crest Defects

Tetralogy of Fallot

Anatomic Features of Tetralogy of Fallot

The first description of the anomaly now known as tetralogy of Fallot (TOF) was provided by Niels Stensen in 1671, in a fetus with ectopia cordis [8]. But it was Etienne-Louis- Arthur Fallot in 1888 who accurately detailed this malformation that he called the "maladie bleue" or blue disease [9]. The term "tetralogy of Fallot" was coined by Maude Abbott in 1924 [10].

The tetralogy of Fallot is classically described as the association of four anatomic features:

- pulmonary outflow tract obstruction
- ventricular septal defect (VSD)
- aortic overriding
- right ventricular hypertrophy

However, the mechanism of this tetrad is unequivocal: hypoplasia and failure of normal growth of the subpulmonary infundibulum or conus [8] due to "anterocephalad malalignment and deviation of the insertion of the muscular outlet septum relative to the limbs of the septomarginal trabeculation (septal band), coupled with an abnormal arrangement of the septoparietal trabeculations" [11]. Figure 3.1 compares the anatomy of the right ventricular outflow tract in a normal heart (Fig. 3.1a) and in a heart specimen with tetralogy of Fallot (Fig. 3.1b).

The Pulmonary Outflow Tract Obstruction

The obstruction is produced by the squeeze between the malaligned outlet (conal, infundibular) septum and the hypertrophied septoparietal trabeculations [11]. The infundibulum is narrow and hypoplastic in its three dimensions [8, 11] but the length of the outlet septum is highly variable, often normal but sometimes superior or inferior to normal [8, 11].

Because of the malalignment between the outlet septum and the ventricular septum, the conal septum is no more an interventricular structure but is an entirely right ventricular structure [11]. This anatomic characteristic is constant in all cardiac neural crest defects except for IAA.

The diminished amount of blood flow through the pulmonary outflow tract due to the subpulmonary obstruction often leads to a certain degree of valvar annulus hypoplasia (with often a bicuspid pulmonary valve) and of hypoplasia of pulmonary trunk and branches.

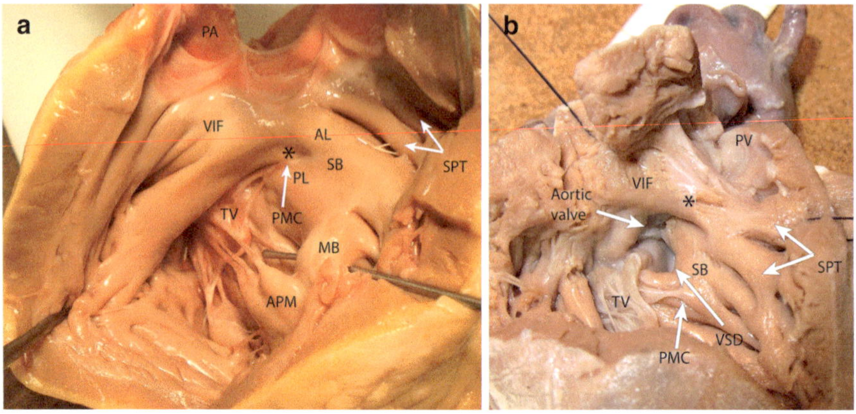

Fig. 3.1 Anatomy of the right ventricular outflow tract in a normal heart (**a**) and in a heart with a tetralogy of Fallot (**b**). (**a**) The right ventricle in a normal heart. The ventriculo-infundibular fold (*VIF*, grouping together parietal band and subpulmonary conus) is a muscular band, which separates the anterior leaflet of the tricuspid valve (*TV*) from the leaflets of the pulmonary valve (*PA*) in the normal heart. The left extremity of the VIF represents the upper part of the ventricular septum: the outlet (or conal) septum (*asterisk*), which is fused with the upper extremity of the septal band (*SB*, or septomarginal trabeculation), between its two limbs, anterior (*AL*) and posterior (*PL*). The septoparietal trabeculations (*SPT*, *double arrow*) are anterior to the septal band. In the normal heart, the posterior limb of the septal band, which carries the papillary muscle of the conus (*PMC*, *arrow* or muscle of Lancisi) and its attachments, is not fused with the VIF, but is separated from it by the atrioventricular part of the membranous septum, connecting the anterior leaflet of the tricuspid valve with the leaflets of the aortic valve. The interventricular part of the membranous septum connects the septal leaflet of the tricuspid valve with the right coronary and the non-coronary leaflets of the aortic valve. The septal band continues with the moderator band (*MB*), then with the anterior papillary muscle of the tricuspid valve (*APM*). (**b**) The right ventricle in a specimen with tetralogy of Fallot. The outlet septum (*asterisk*) is not fused with the septal band, leaving the outlet ventricular septal defect (*VSD*) between the two limbs of the septal band (*SB*). In this specimen, the anterior leaflet of the tricuspid valve (*TV*) is in fibrous continuity with the leaflets of the aortic valve. The septoparietal trabeculations (*SPT*) are hypertrophied. *PMC* papillary muscle of the conus, *PV* pulmonary valve, *VIF* ventriculo-infundibular fold

The Ventricular Septal Defect

The ventricular septal defect is, like in all cardiac neural crest defects, an outlet malalignment defect (outlet VSD), located between the two limbs of the septal band [12]. This type of VSD is due to the failure of the outlet septum to fuse with the primitive ventricular septum during the last phase of cardiac looping. This fusion normally leads to the transfer of the aorta towards the left ventricle, and to the wedging of the aortic valve between the tricuspid and the mitral valve [13]. The inferior margin of the outlet VSD is thus formed by the upper extremity of the septal band, and its superior margin by the outlet septum on the left and the aortic valve on the right. Therefore, the plane of the deficient ventricular septation (between the malaligned outlet septum and the upper extremity of the ventricular septum) is not the same than the plane of the ventricular septum itself, which serves as an egress for the left ventricle. This leads some authors to describe this type of defect as an "interventricular communication" rather than a "ventricular septal defect" [14].

Although the constant characteristic of this type of VSD is its location between the two limbs of the septal band, some anatomic variants exist:

- Frequently the outlet VSD extends towards the membranous septum (outlet malalignment VSD with fibrous postero-inferior rim, Fig. 3.1b). The posterior limb of the septal band is hypoplastic, permitting fibrous continuity between the tricuspid valve and the leaflets of the aortic valve [8, 11]. In a series of 71 anatomic specimens with TOF, including eight with absent pulmonary valve, we found such a fibrous extension in 66 % of cases [12]. When present, this fibrous continuity always involves the anterior tricuspid leaflet, which distinguishes this outlet VSD from a central membranous VSD, in which this continuity involves the septal leaflet of the tricuspid valve [12].
- When the posterior limb of the septal band is fused with the ventriculo-infundibular fold or parietal band (outlet malalignment VSD with entirely muscular borders), the muscular postero-inferior rim prevents aortic-tricuspid continuity and protects the conduction tissue against surgical injury.
- The VSD can be doubly committed or juxta-arterial (Fig. 3.2a), the outlet septum being then extremely hypoplastic, reduced to a fibrous remnant between the aortic and the pulmonary valve [8].
- The VSD can also extend towards the inlet septum when TOF is associated with an atrioventricular septal defect.
- Multiple VSDs can be present, usually muscular VSDs.

The Overriding of the Aorta

Aortic overriding, or dextroposition of the aorta, is also a consequence of the anterior deviation of the outlet septum. The subpulmonary infundibulum hypoplasia leads to an abnormal location of both aortic and pulmonary valves: the aortic valve is abnormally right-sided, superior and anterior, the pulmonary valve is reciprocally left-sided, inferior and posterior [8]. In TOF, aortic-mitral fibrous continuity is preserved but, contrarily to the normal heart in which both left coronary and non coronary aortic valve leaflets are in fibrous continuity with the anterior leaflet of the mitral valve, only the left coronary leaflet retains this continuity. Dextroposition of the aorta can then be considered a failure to achieve a completely normal wedging of the aortic valve between the tricuspid and mitral valves.

The Right Ventricular Hypertrophy

Right ventricular hypertrophy is a hemodynamic consequence of the right outflow tract obstruction. It is a postnatally acquired lesion and is not really part of the congenital defect.

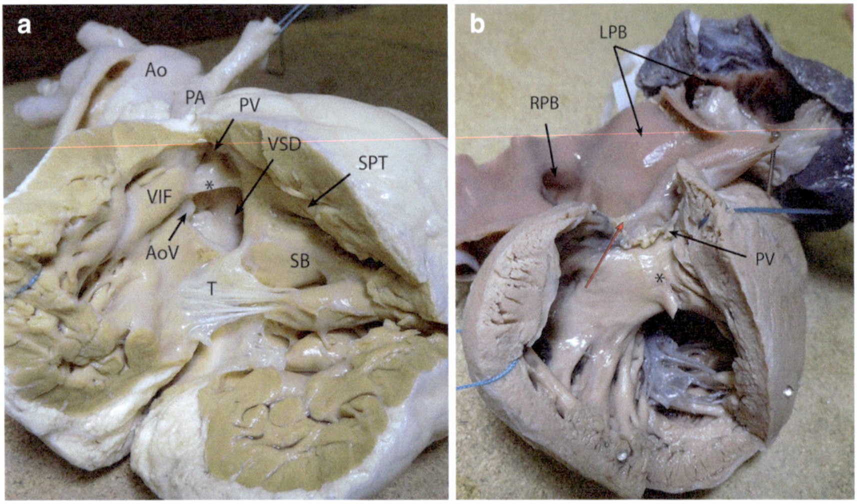

Fig. 3.2 Anatomy of the right ventricular outflow tract in two anatomic forms of tetralogy of Fallot: with doubly committed VSD (**a**) and with absent pulmonary valve (**b**). (**a**) The outlet septum (*asterisk*), reduced to a fibrous remnant, is deviated anteriorly, creating subpulmonary obstruction. The pulmonary valve (*PV*) annulus is small and the valve is bicuspid. The outlet ventricular septal defect (*VSD*) is cradled between the two limbs of the septal band (*SB*). The aortic valve (*AoV*), seen through the VSD, is overriding the ventricular septum. *Ao* aorta, *PA* pulmonary artery, *SPT* septoparietal trabeculations, *VIF* ventriculo-infundibular fold. (**b**) Tetralogy of Fallot with absent pulmonary valve: the pulmonary annulus is hypoplastic and lined with small, nodular, pulmonary valve (*PV*) remnants. In addition, there is a fibrous supravalvular stenosis above the PV remnants (*red arrow*). The pulmonary trunk and the left pulmonary branch (*LPB*), including its intrapulmonary portion, are aneurysmal, the right pulmonary branch (*RPB*) is not dilated. The outlet septum (*asterisk*) is malaligned and deviated anteriorly, above the outlet VSD

Associated Lesions

Absent Pulmonary Valve

The leaflets of the pulmonary valve are either completely absent, or very hypoplastic, with very small nodular remnants (Fig. 3.2b). Because of the pulmonary regurgitation due to the absence of pulmonary valve leaflets, the pulmonary trunk and branches are often significantly dilated. The pulmonary annulus is small, the VSD and the subpulmonary stenosis are those encountered in classical TOF.

Complete Atrioventricular Canal

The association between tetralogy of Fallot and complete AV canal is encountered almost exclusively in the setting of Down syndrome. There are usually no attachments of the anterior bridging leaflet on the ventricular septal crest.

Anomalies of the Pulmonary Branches

The pulmonary branches can be stenotic and/or hypoplastic. They can be discontinuous, one of the branches being thus isolated, originating from the ductus arteriosus.

Right Aortic Arch

A right aortic arch is present in 28 % of TOF, especially in the setting of 22q11 microdeletion [8].

Coronary Abnormalities

In 5–7 % of cases of TOF, the left anterior descending coronary artery (LAD) connects to the right coronary artery, because of the more anterior location of the right coronary ostium [15]. The course of the LAD may cross the subpulmonary infundibulum with a high risk of injury during surgical repair.

Significant Systemic-to-Pulmonary Collateral Arteries

Major aortopulmonary collateral arteries (MAPCA) can occasionally be found in tetralogy of Fallot with pulmonary stenosis.

Aortic Coarctation

Tetralogy of Fallot and coarctation of the aorta is an exceptional association. Interestingly, two types of coarctation can be found in this context. In left aortic arch, coarctation is situated distal to the left subclavian artery. In right aortic arch, coarctation is distal to the right common carotid artery, mirror-image of interrupted left aortic arch type B, associated with anomalies of the branches of the aorta, and should be considered a complex anomaly of aortic arches in the setting of an outflow tract defect, due to abnormal migration of cardiac neural crest cells [16].

Tetralogy of Fallot with Pulmonary Atresia

This anatomic entity is considered to be an extreme form of tetralogy of Fallot, the development of the pulmonary valve having been impaired by the extreme anterior deviation of the outlet septum. We prefer the term "TOF with pulmonary atresia" to the term "pulmonary atresia with VSD" because of the lack of precision of this latter term, inferring that any congenital heart defect including both a VSD and an atretic pulmonary valve as part of its phenotype could be considered a pulmonary atresia with VSD, for example congenitally corrected TGA, VSD and pulmonary atresia, or DORV with complete AV canal in the setting of a heterotaxy syndrome and pulmonary atresia.

Intracardiac Anatomy

The intracardiac anatomy is the same than in TOF, except that the outlet septum is exaggeratedly deviated anteriorly, being fused with the anterior right ventricular wall in a significant number of cases (40 %) [12].

The pulmonary valve is atretic, and usually there is no remnant of the valve to be found (muscular atresia).

The VSD is, like in tetralogy of Fallot, an outlet malalignment VSD, located between the two limbs of the septal band. However, the presence of a fibrous postero-inferior rim (membranous extension) is less frequent in TOF-PA than in TOF (39 %) in our anatomic series [12].

The Pulmonary Arterial Supply

The current nomenclature describes three anatomic types of TOF-PA according to the type of arterial supply to the lungs [17].

In type A, the pulmonary branches are of relatively good size, often confluent, and supplied through the arterial duct (Fig. 3.3a). In type B, the pulmonary branches are present but hypoplastic, there is no arterial duct, and there are additional sources of blood for the lungs called MAPCA (major aortopulmonary collateral arteries, Fig. 3.3b). In type C, there are no central pulmonary branches and both lungs are supplied through MAPCA only (Fig. 3.3c).

The MAPCA can originate from the descending aorta (the majority, derived from the intersegmental arteries), from the subclavian arteries (derived themselves of the seventh intersegmental arteries), or rarely from the coronary arteries. MAPCA originating from the carotid arteries have been described but are exceptional.

Common Arterial Trunk

Common arterial trunk is defined by a single vessel arising from the base of the heart with a unique arterial valve, giving origin to the coronary arteries, at least one pulmonary artery, and systemic vessels, in that order [18, 19]. Typically the common trunk overrides a large outlet VSD due to total absence of development of the outlet septum.

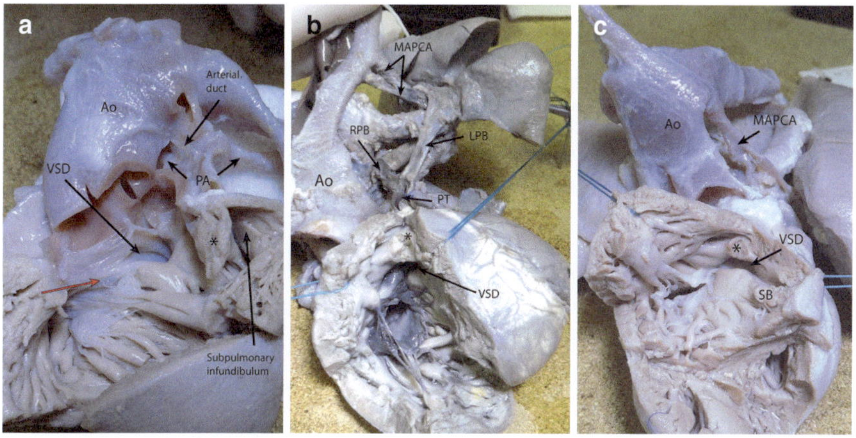

Fig. 3.3 Anatomy of the right ventricular outflow tract in tetralogy of Fallot with pulmonary atresia: the three major anatomic types. The outlet septum (*asterisk*) is exaggeratedly deviated anteriorly, obstructing completely the subpulmonary infundibulum. The ventricular septal defect (*VSD*) is always cradled between the two limbs of the septal band (*SB*). The aorta (*Ao*) is overriding the ventricular septum. (**a**) Type A of Barbero-Marcial. The pulmonary arteries (*PA*) are confluent and supplied through a widely patent arterial duct. (**b**) Type B of Barbero-Marcial. The pulmonary trunk (*PT*) and the left and right pulmonary branches (LPB and RPB) are confluent but hypoplastic. Two major aortopulmonary collateral arteries (*MAPCA*) originating from the descending aorta are supplying the left lung. (**c**) Type C of Barbero-Marcial. There are no central pulmonary arteries. The two lungs are supplied entirely through a major aortopulmonary collateral artery (*MAPCA*) originating from the descending aorta and dividing into two branches

Main Anatomic Types

The first classification of common arterial trunk was published by Collett and Edwards in 1949 [20]. Although still used by some, this classification is flawed by not incorporating CAT with interrupted aortic arch or with discontinuous pulmonary arteries, as well as by including its type IV, which represents TOF-PA with absence of central pulmonary arteries and blood supply to the lungs provided by MAPCA originating from the descending aorta. To remedy to this problem, Van Praagh introduced his classification in 1965 [21] and modified it in 1987 [18]. In the last version of this classification, type A1–2 has confluent or near confluent pulmonary arteries originating from the common arterial trunk (large aortic type of CAT, Fig. 3.4a), type A3 has one pulmonary artery branch originating from the common arterial trunk and the other from the arterial duct (large aortic type of CAT with discontinuous pulmonary arteries, Fig. 3.4b), and type A4 has interrupted aortic arch or severe coarctation (large pulmonary artery type of CAT, Fig. 3.4c). The concept of aortic or pulmonary dominance, introduced by Van Praagh in 1987, was recently reemphasized [22].

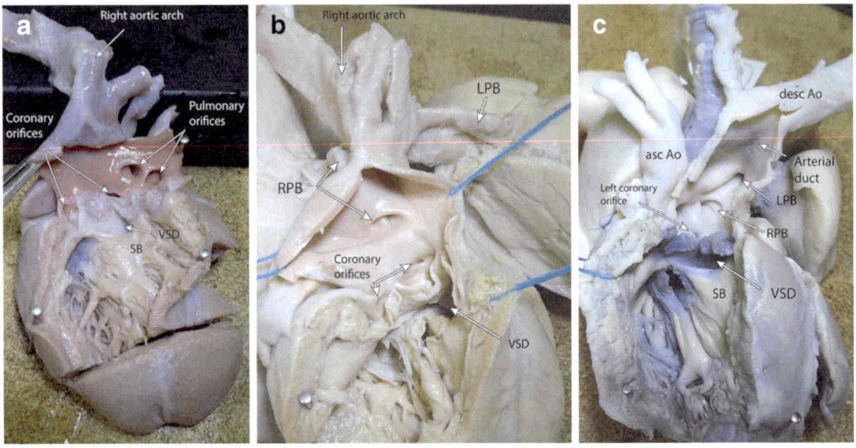

Fig. 3.4 Anatomy of the right ventricular outflow tract in common arterial trunk: the three major anatomic types. The ventricular septal defect (*VSD*) is an outlet VSD, located between the two limbs of the septal band (*SB*). (**a**) Type A1–2 of Van Praagh: the pulmonary orifices arise from the left side of the common trunk. The truncal valve has four leaflets and there is a right aortic arch. The left coronary orifice is posterior to the pulmonary orifices. (**b**) Type A3 of Van Praagh: the pulmonary branches are discontinuous, the right pulmonary branch (*RPB*) originates from the trunk, the left pulmonary branch (*LPB*) originates from the arterial duct. The truncal valve has three leaflets and there is a right aortic arch. (**c**) Type A4 of Van Praagh (pulmonary dominance): the aortic arch is interrupted between the left carotid artery and the left subclavian artery, the descending aorta (*desc Ao*) is supplied through the arterial duct. Note the dysplastic 3-leaflet truncal valve and the pinpoint left coronary orifice, located directly above a commissure. *Asc Ao* ascending aorta, *LPB* left pulmonary branch, *RPB* right pulmonary branch

The Ventricular Septal Defect

As in other cardiac neural crest defects, the VSD always lies between the two limbs of the septal band (outlet VSD), and is overhang by the truncal valve. Usually the truncal valve overrides both ventricles equally, but can be located almost entirely above the right ventricle, or more rarely above the left ventricle.

Among 54 heart specimens with CAT, we found a direct fibrous continuity between the truncal valve and the anterior leaflet of the tricuspid valve in only one case (1.8 %) [12]. This very low rate is probably due to the complete absence of rotation of the outflow tract in CAT, in addition to the absence of septation. The VSD has thus almost always entirely muscular borders.

Some exceptional cases without VSD have been described [23].

The Truncal Valve

The truncal valve has three leaflets in the majority of cases. It can also have four leaflets or more rarely two leaflets. Truncal leaflet dysplasia is frequent and can create valvar stenosis or insufficiency.

The Coronary Arteries

The pattern of the coronary orifices in CAT is unique among outflow tract defects. The left coronary ostium is displaced posteriorly with an anterior angle between the two coronary orifices significantly larger than in other outflow tract defects, in which this angle is constant. This may reflect the dual identity, aortic and pulmonary, of the common arterial trunk [15]. Anomalies of the coronary orifices are very frequent: anomalies of size and configuration of the coronary orifices (diminutive or pinpoint, tangential, intramural, slit-like, orificial ridge), of location relative to the commissures (paracommissural, supracommissural, intracommissural), of location relative to the sinotubular junction (too low or too high). We found at least one abnormal coronary orifice in 87 % of CAT. The left coronary orifice is more often abnormal that the right one regarding its shape or size, and is more often supracommissural [15].

Interrupted Aortic Arch

Interrupted aortic arch can result either from a complete obliteration of the aortic lumen with a fibrous continuity between the two segments of the arch (atretic aortic arch), or from a complete absence of development of one part of the arch (absent aortic arch).

Main Anatomic Types

The most widely used classification was developed by Celoria and Patton, who added to the types A and B described by Abbott in 1927 the exceptional type C [24, 25]. In type A, the interruption is located distal to the left subclavian artery, between this artery and the arterial duct; in type B, between the left carotid artery and the left subclavian artery; in type C, between the innominate artery and the left carotid artery (Fig. 3.5). Type A is considered an extreme form of aortic coarctation, while type B is caused by a lack of development of the fourth aortic arch [26]. Type C is extremely rare.

In IAA type A, the aortic arch can be atretic (with fibrous continuity between the two segments of the arch) or absent. In IAA type B, the aortic arch is almost always absent.

The Ventricular Septal Defect

The anatomy of the VSD is different according to the anatomic type of IAA. In an anatomic study about 28 heart specimens with isolated IAA (11 type A, 17 type B) and 19 with IAA associated with other congenital heart defects (7 type A, 12 type B), we found that the VSD in type B was always an outlet VSD, located between the two limbs of the septal band, while in type A the VSD could be of any type: membranous, muscular, of the outlet type, or of the inlet type in the setting of complete AV canal (personal data).

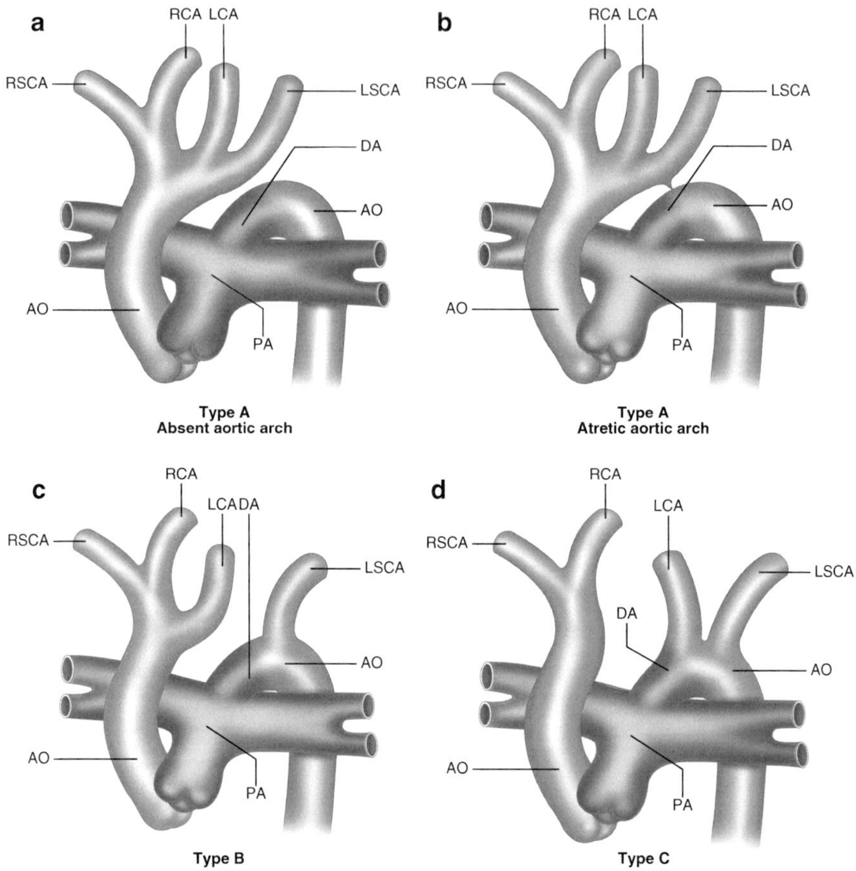

Fig. 3.5 The three anatomic types of interrupted aortic arch according to Celoria and Patton [24]. (a) Interrupted aortic arch type A with absent aortic arch. The aorta is interrupted after the left subclavian artery and there is no continuity between the two parts of the aorta. The descending aorta is supplied by the ductus arteriosus. (b) Interrupted aortic arch type A with absent aortic arch. The aorta is interrupted after the left subclavian artery and there a fibrous continuity between the two parts of the aorta. (c) Interrupted aortic arch type B. The aorta is interrupted between the left carotid artery and the left subclavian artery, the descending aorta (d) Interrupted aortic arch type C. The aorta is interrupted between the innominate artery and the left carotid artery. Ao, aorta; DA, ductus arteriosus; LCA, left carotid artery; LSCA, left subclavian artery; PA, pulmonary artery; RCA, right carotid artery; RSCA, right subclavian artery

When an outlet VSD is present, the outlet septum or its fibrous remnant is usually deviated posteriorly under the aortic valve, and the rims of the VSD are entirely muscular (100 % of the cases in our series, Fig. 3.6). However, other authors have reported a relatively high rate of posterior tricuspid-aortic continuity in this setting [27].

These differences regarding the type of VSD associated with the two anatomic types of IAA reinforces the hypothesis of different pathogenic mechanisms responsible for the two types of IAA, and the inclusion of IAA type B in the group of cardiac neural crest defects.

Very rarely, the VSD may be absent. This is usually the case when IAA is associated with aortopulmonary window, but it can happen in isolated IAA [28].

Associated Anomalies

Right Aortic Arch

A right aortic arch can be associated, as with all the neural crest defects, with IAA type B.

Bicuspid Aortic Valve

Bicuspid aortic valve is relatively frequent in association with IAA. In our anatomic series, we found eight bicuspid aortic valves, always associated with IAA type B. This underlines the recently described involvement of cardiac neural crest cells in the morphogenesis of bicuspid aortic valve [29].

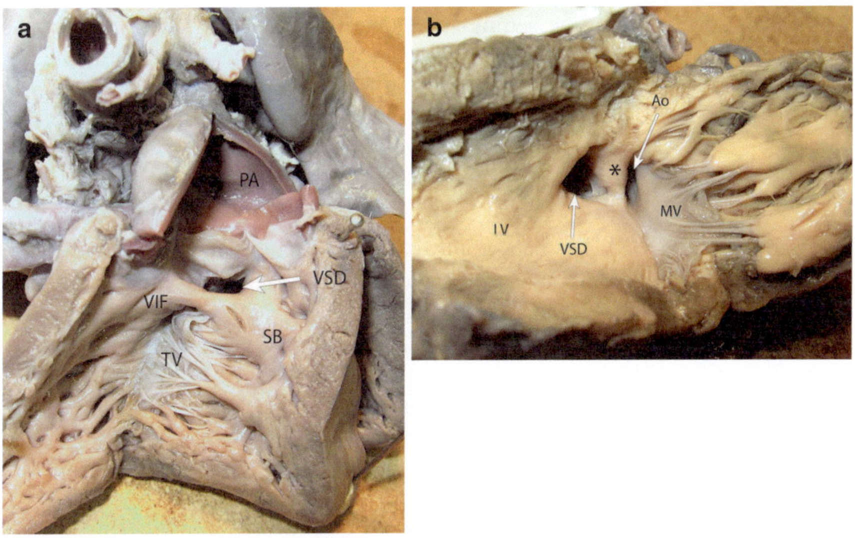

Fig. 3.6 Anatomy of the right ventricular outflow tract (**a**) and of the left ventricular outflow tract (**b**) in interrupted aortic arch type B. (**a**) The outlet ventricular septal defect (*VSD*) is cradled between the two limbs of the septal band (*SB*). The postero-inferior rim of the VSD is entirely muscular, due to the fusion of the posterior limb of the septal band with the ventriculo-infundibular fold (*VIF*), separating the leaflets of the pulmonary valve from the tricuspid valve (*TV*). The outlet septum is not visible from the right ventricle. *PA* pulmonary artery. (**b**) The outlet septum (*asterisk*) is deviated posteriorly, creating subaortic obstruction. There is a fibrous continuity between the leaflets of the aortic valve (*Ao*) and the mitral valve (*MV*). *LV* left ventricle, *VSD* ventricular septal defect

Aortopulmonary Window

Thirteen per cent of hearts with an aortopulmonary window have an associated IAA type A [30].

Common Arterial Trunk

The association of CAT and IAA represents the pulmonary dominance type, or type A4 of Van Praagh's classification [19, 22]. The most frequent site of interruption lies between the left subclavian artery and the left carotid artery (type B).

Other Outflow Tract Defects

Interrupted aortic arch has been described in association with double outlet right ventricle, tetralogy of Fallot and transposition of the great arteries.

Common AV Canal

Interrupted aortic arch in the setting of common AV canal is usually of type A, determined by a narrow left ventricular outflow tract with subaortic obstruction.

Double Outlet Right Ventricle

The definition of DORV has been controversial for a long time. A consensus has been achieved with the International Congenital Heart Surgery Nomenclature and Database Project in 2000: DORV is defined as a type of ventriculo-arterial connection (or alignment) in which both great vessels arise entirely of predominantly from the right ventricle [31].

This definition accounts for the great anatomic heterogeneity associated with this particular type of ventriculo-arterial relationship, which led to a number of classifications, focusing on one specific part of the cardiac phenotype:

- The location of the VSD relative to the great vessels (Lev): subaortic, subpulmonary, doubly committed, non committed [32]
- The associated lesions (Van Praagh): DORV with outflow tract anomalies only, DORV with anomalies of the atrioventricular valves and the ventricles, and DORV found in the setting of heterotaxy syndromes [33]
- The position of the great vessels relative to each other (De La Cruz) [34]

Of these, the Lev's classification remains the most significant, as the location of the VSD will be determinant for the surgical strategy.

The Ventricular Septal Defect

Like in tetralogy of Fallot, there is some controversy about the signification of the term "ventricular septal defect" in the setting of DORV with committed VSD, because of the different planes for deficient septation and the ventricular septum itself [14].

Committed VSDs

A VSD is dubbed "committed" when the blood coming from the left ventricle through the VSD goes directly into the aorta (subaortic VSD), the pulmonary artery (subpulmonary VSD), or both (doubly committed VSD). Committed VSD always open in the outlet of the right ventricle and are cradled within the limbs of the septal band (outlet VSD). They are due either to a lack of fusion of the outlet septum with the septal band (subaortic or subpulmonary VSD), or to a lack of formation of the outlet septum (doubly committed VSD). The three types of DORV corresponding to these three types of VSD are considered to be the result of an arrest in cardiac development during the process of wedging, preventing the aortic valve (in case of normal formation of the outflow tract with spiraling great arteries and establishment of aortic-to-mitral continuity), or the pulmonary valve (in case of abnormal formation of the outflow tract with parallel great arteries and establishment of pulmonary-to-mitral continuity) to achieve its connection, or alignment, with the left ventricle. In DORV with committed VSD, the outlet septum is malaligned with the ventricular septum, and the type of commitment of the VSD depends on the relationship of the outlet septum with the limbs of the septal band [35]: when the outlet septum is connected with the anterior limb of the septal band, the VSD is subaortic (Fig. 3.7a); when it is connected with the posterior limb of the septal band, the VSD is subpulmonary (Fig. 3.7b); when the outlet septum is fibrous or absent, the VSD is doubly committed (Fig. 3.7c).

Non-committed VSDs

The definition of non-committed VSD has been the subject of many controversies. Some authors have advocated an anatomic distinction between "truly non committed VSD" (inlet or muscular) and "not directly committed VSD" (VSD opening in the outlet of the right ventricle, located between the two limbs of the septal band, but "remote" from the aorta or the pulmonary artery [36, 37]). To solve these ambiguities, we propose, along with Anderson [38], to include in this category all VSD which are not located between the two limbs of the septal band, that is inlet, muscular, and also central membranous VSD, located below the posterior limb of the septal band, behind the septal leaflet of the tricuspid valve (Fig. 3.7d). The blood flow through a non-committed VSD is not directed towards the outflow tract, but directly towards the right ventricular cavity, running perpendicular to the ventricular septum. Double-outlet right ventricle with non committed VSD are due to a very early arrest in cardiac development, at the early looping stage, which accounts for the higher frequency

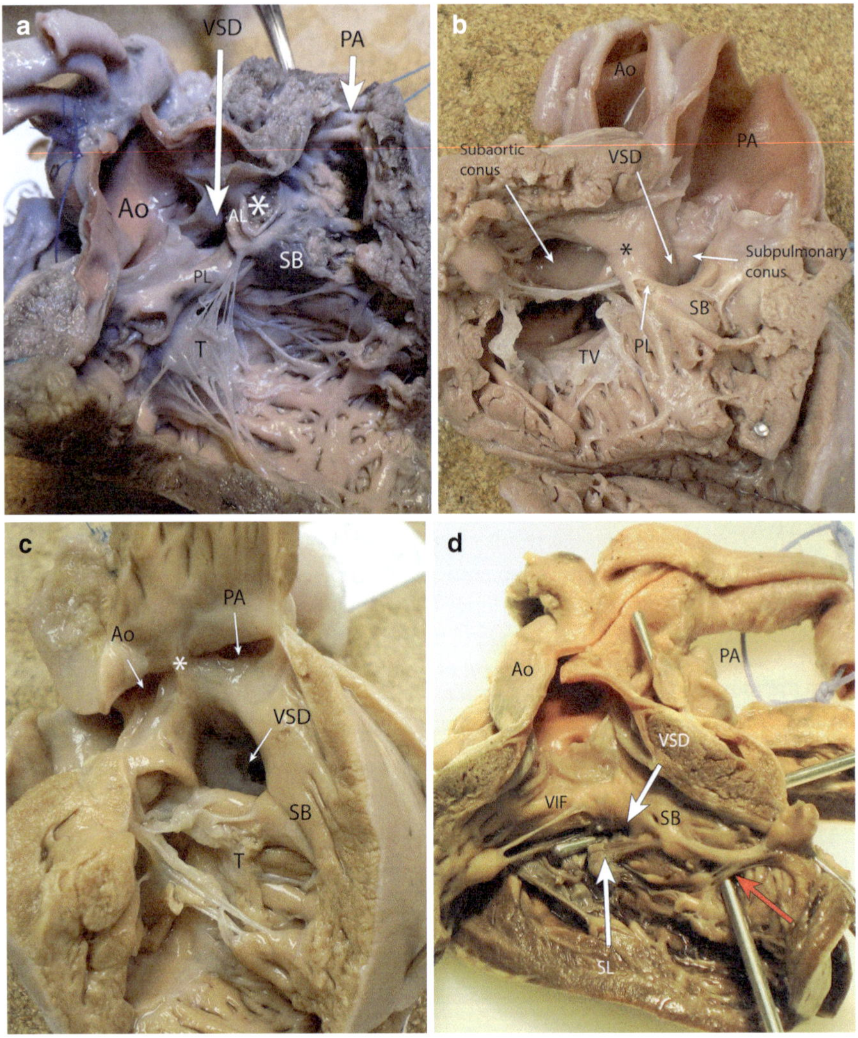

Fig. 3.7 Double outlet right ventricle (DORV): different anatomic forms according to the type and the location of the ventricular septal defect (*VSD*). (**a**) DORV with subaortic VSD. The ventricular septal defect (*VSD*) is cradled between the two limbs of the septal band (*SB*), and the outlet septum (*asterisk*) is in continuity with the anterior limb (*AL*) of the septal band (*SB*). The VSD is thus subaortic. There is a bilateral conus. *Ao* aorta, *PA* pulmonary artery, *PL* posterior limb of the septal band, *TV* tricuspid valve. (**b**) DORV with subpulmonary VSD. The ventricular septal defect (*VSD*) is cradled between the two limbs of the septal band (*SB*), and the outlet septum (*asterisk*) is in continuity with the posterior limb (*PL*) of the septal band (*SB*). The VSD is thus subpulmonary. There is a bilateral conus. *Ao* aorta, *PA* pulmonary artery, *TV* tricuspid valve. (**c**) DORV with doubly VSD. The outlet septum (*asterisk*) is extremely hypoplastic and fibrous, the LV blood flow goes through the VSD directly into both great vessels (*Ao* aorta, *PA* pulmonary artery). The VSD is cradled between the two limbs of the septal band (*SB*) and its postero-inferior rim is muscular. *T* tricuspid valve. (**d**) DORV with non committed central membranous VSD. The probe passes through a central membranous VSD, just beneath the ventriculo-infundibular fold (*VIF*), behind the septal leaflet of the tricuspid valve (*SL*). The blood flow coming from the left ventricle is perpendicular to the ventricular septum and is not directed towards either great vessel. There is a bilateral conus and a very severe stenosis of the ostium infundibuli (*red arrow*). *Ao* aorta, *PA* pulmonary artery, *SB* septal band

in this subgroup of hypoplasia of the AV valves and the ventricles [33]. If the left ventricle does not develop, then DORV is "obligatory" because the outflow tract is entirely supported by the right ventricle at this stage of development. In heterotaxy syndromes, which occur even earlier in development, DORV is very frequent and often associated with common AV junction, and/or double inlet right ventricle.

The Position of the Great Arteries

Double outlet right ventricle is a malposition of the great vessels, along with TGA, double outlet left ventricle (DOLV) and anatomically corrected malposition of the great arteries [33]. In fact, DORV is basically a malposition of the aorta. The relationships between the two great arteries are highly variable and represent a real spectrum, starting from an almost usual configuration (the aorta being posterior and to the right of the pulmonary trunk, with almost spiraling great vessels), to side-by side vessels with the aorta on the right, and finally to antero-posterior vessels, the aorta being to the right, anterior or to the left of the pulmonary artery, with parallel trunks. De la Cruz used the relationship between the two arterial trunks as an indicator for the location of the VSD [34]. However, there are so many exceptions to this rule that one should not any more infer the location of the VSD, and thus the type of surgical repair, from the position of the great vessels [38]. The position of the great vessels relative to each other should thus be described in addition to other features, of which the most important for determining the surgical management is the location of the VSD.

The Conal or Infundibular Morphology

Although this criterion is widely used by echocardiographists, the presence of a bilateral conus or infundibulum is not synonymous with double outlet right ventricle. Some hearts with the two great vessels entirely above the right ventricle have fibrous continuity between the mitral and either the aortic or the pulmonary valve, and some hearts with TGA, or even normal hearts, exhibit bilateral conus. However, bilateral conus is a frequent finding in DORV, especially in DORV with committed VSD [33].

The Taussig-Bing Anomaly

The cardiac anomaly described by Taussig and Bing in 1949 associates a double outlet right ventricular type of ventriculo-arterial connection, side-by-side great arteries, a bilateral conus, and a subpulmonary VSD [33, 39].

The VSD is always an outlet VSD, cradled between the two limbs of the septal band, and the outlet septum is connected to the posterior-inferior limb of the septal band, directing the blood from the left ventricle directly towards the pulmonary artery (Fig. 3.7b).

DORV with subpulmonary VSD might thus constitute the "bridge" between the two groups of outflow tract defects: cardiac neural crest defects and laterality defects. Mutations of some laterality genes like CFC1 and ZIC3 were identified in patients with TGA, DORV and heterotaxy, indicating that TGA and a subset of DORV share a common genetic basis with laterality defects [5, 40].

Several anatomic characteristics or associations are in favor of this hypothesis, and will be detailed further: the coronary arterial pattern, mitral anomalies, and juxtaposition of the atrial appendages. Moreover, the great arteries are not spiraled but parallel in DORV with subpulmonary VSD, like in TGA or ccTGA.

The Associated Anomalies

Obstruction of the Outflow Tracts

Because of the connection of the outlet septum to the anterior limb of the septal band, subpulmonary stenosis is relatively frequent in DORV with subaortic VSD, due to leftward deviation of the outlet septum (DORV, Fallot type), and in DORV with doubly committed VSD and fibrous outlet septum.

Similarly, subaortic stenosis (usually with aortic arch hypoplasia and coarctation as a consequence) is more frequent in DORV with subpulmonary stenosis, due to rightward deviation of the outlet septum.

Rarely however, subaortic stenosis can occur in DORV with subaortic VSD, due to muscular narrowing between the subaortic conus and the outlet septum, and subpulmonary stenosis can be found in DORV with subpulmonary VSD, due usually to abnormal attachments of a straddling mitral valve.

Severe obstruction of the outflow tracts can lead to pulmonary atresia (mostly in ventricular L-loop, and in heterotaxy syndromes) and more rarely to aortic atresia (especially in DORV with non-committed VSD).

Anomalies of the AV Valves

In the anatomic collection of the French Reference Center for Complex heart defects, anomalies of the AV valves were significantly more frequent in DORV than in TGA (Table 3.1). The mitral valve was more often concerned than the tricuspid

Table 3.1 Anomalies of the atrioventricular valves associated with DORV and TGA

Anomalies of the AV valves	DORV (n = 114)	TGA (n = 195)	p
Mitral valve anomalies	17.5 %	5.6 %	0.002
Cleft	25 %		
Straddling	40 %		
Subvalvar apparatus	35 %		
Tricuspid valve anomalies	3.6 %	4.4 %	ns
Complete AV canal	14 %	1 %	0.000

valve, and a complete AV canal was found in 14 % of all specimens with DORV (usually in the setting of heterotaxy).

The Mitral Valve

- Straddling mitral valve: the mitral valve always straddles through an outlet type of VSD (Fig. 3.8). In our anatomic series, this VSD was always subpulmonary, establishing a link between DORV with subpulmonary VSD and TGA, which could be the involvement of some laterality genes in these two types of malposition of the great arteries [39]. The mitral valve inserts within the right ventricular cavity, either on papillary muscles (Fig. 3.8a) or on the subpulmonary conus and/or the outlet septum, which can create subpulmonary obstruction.
- Cleft mitral valve: in three of five cases found in our series the cleft was isolated, splitting the anterior leaflet of the mitral valve in two equal parts, perpendicular to the ventricular septum but without any defect within the inlet septum. In two cases, the cleft was oriented towards the outflow tract, parallel to the ventricular septum (Fig. 3.9), contrarily to the so-called "cleft" in common AV junction which is perpendicular to the ventricular septum [41].
- Anomalies of the subvalvar apparatus (parachute mitral valve), mitral valvar hypoplasia and mitral atresia are found essentially in DORV with non committed VSD (DORV with mitral atresia usually have no VSD).

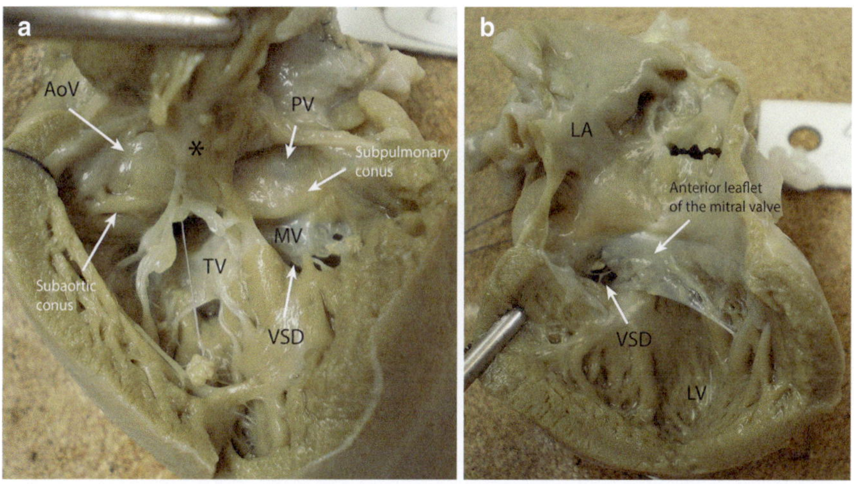

Fig. 3.8 Straddling mitral valve in a heart specimen with double outlet right ventricle, subpulmonary ventricular septal defect (*VSD*) and bilateral conus. (**a**) Right ventricular view: the aorta and the pulmonary artery originate from the right ventricle. There is a bilateral conus, the tricuspid valve (*TV*) has abnormal attachments on the outlet septum (*asterisk*). The mitral valve (*MV*) straddles through a subpulmonary VSD (outlet type), and has abnormal attachments on the right ventricular septal surface. *AoV* aortic valve, *PV* pulmonary valve. (**b**) Left ventricular view: the mitral valve straddles through an anterior, outlet type, VSD. *LA* left atrium, *LV* left ventricle

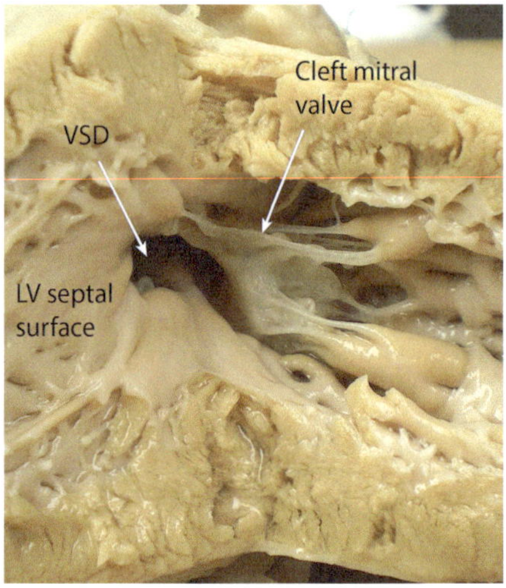

Fig. 3.9 Cleft mitral valve in a heart specimen with double outlet right ventricle and subpulmonary outlet ventricular septal defect (*VSD*), left ventricular (*LV*) view. The anterior leaflet is split in two asymmetric parts attached on the anterosuperior rim of the VSD. The cleft is directed towards the outflow tract, and not perpendicular to the ventricular septum

The Tricuspid Valve

- Abnormal insertions on the outlet septum are particularly frequent in DORV with subpulmonary VSD (Taussig-Bing anomaly) [42].
- Straddling tricuspid valve always occurs through an inlet VSD. Both mitral and tricuspid valves can straddle through a very large VSD extending from the inlet to the outlet.

Ventricular Hypoplasia

The left ventricle can be hypoplastic, especially in DORV with non-committed VSD. Hypoplasia of the right ventricle is less frequent and is found mostly in association with superior-inferior ventricles and/or criss-cross AV relations.

Coronary Arteries

DORV with Subaortic or Doubly Committed VSD

In all cardiac neural crest defects except for CAT, the left coronary orifice is displaced posteriorly and the right coronary orifice is displaced anteriorly, while the angle between the two orifices remains constant [15] (Fig. 3.10). The anterior displacement of the right coronary orifice is more important in DORV than in TOF and TOF-PA, which may indicate that the rotation of the outflow tract is less achieved in DORV than in TOF and TOF-PA [15].

No specific coronary anomalies are reported in DORV with subaortic VSD. However, in DORV with subaortic VSD and subpulmonary stenosis (Fallot type), anomalous connection of the LAD to the right coronary artery crossing anteriorly the subpulmonary infundibulum has been described.

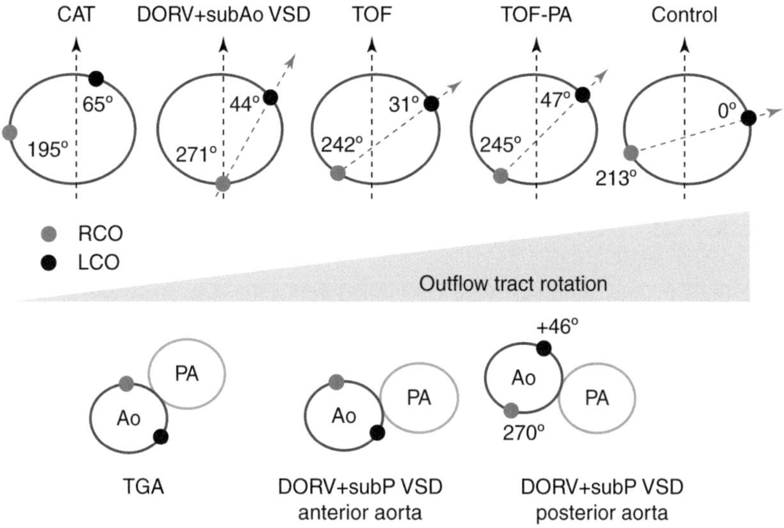

Fig. 3.10 The position of the coronary orifices on the aortic/truncal circumference in conotruncal defects varies according to the degree of rotation of the outflow tract. *CAT* common arterial trunk, *DORV* double-outlet right ventricle, *LCO* left coronary orifice, *RCO* right coronary orifice, *TOF* tetralogy of Fallot, *TOF-PA* tetralogy of Fallot with pulmonary atresia. In TGA and DORV with subpulmonary VSD and anterior aorta, the position of the coronary orifices is the same. In DORV with subpulmonary VSD and posterior aorta, the position of the coronary orifices is similar to that found in DORV with subaortic VSD (personal data)

DORV with Subpulmonary VSD

The pattern of the coronary orifices depends in this case not only on the rotation of the outflow tract, but also on the spatial relationships between the two great vessels. When the aorta is anterior, the left coronary orifice is anterior and to the left, and the right coronary orifice posterior and to the right, in the facing sinuses, like in TGA [33]. However, when the aorta is posterior, the position of the coronary orifices is similar to that observed in DORV with subaortic VSD. In side-by-side vessels (Taussig-Bing anomaly), these two patterns can be found, with often abnormal course of the coronary arteries [33].

Double Outlet Left Ventricle

Double outlet left ventricle (DOLV) is defined as a type of ventriculo-arterial connection (or alignment) in which both great vessels arise entirely of predominantly from the left ventricle [43]. This malformation is extremely rare and was considered for a long time an “embryologic impossibility”.

It is therefore not surprising that there is a great heterogeneity among the various anatomic forms of DOLV. Following the two largest series of patients with DOLV [44, 45], the current classification of DOLV is based, like in DORV, on the position of the VSD relative to the great vessels: subaortic, subpulmonary, doubly committed, non committed [43].

The VSD

Subaortic VSD

Among the 71 cases with two well-developed ventricles and atrioventricular concordance described by Van Praagh, the majority (75 %) had a subaortic VSD. This malformation is considered an anatomical continuum with TGA with VSD [43]. Van Praagh distinguishes four subtypes [45]:

- TOF type, the most frequent, with short subpulmonary conus and mitro-aortic fibrous continuity (Fig. 3.11)
- TGA type, with small subaortic conus and pulmonary to mitral fibrous continuity
- TGA with posterior aorta type, without pulmonary nor aortic stenosis
- Aortic stenosis type with preductal coarctation and absent conus

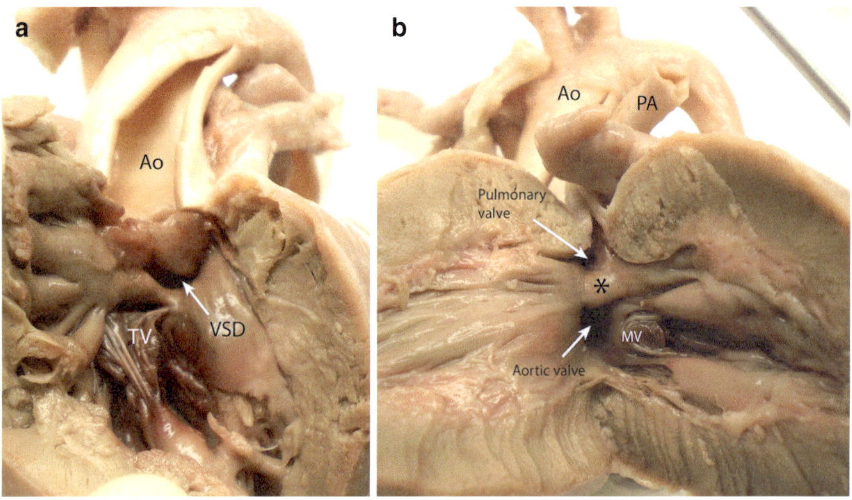

Fig. 3.11 Double-outlet left ventricle with mitro-aortic continuity, subpulmonary conus and subpulmonary stenosis. (**a**) Right ventricular view: the aorta (*Ao*) overrides the ventricular septal defect (*VSD*) but originates predominantly from the left ventricle. The VSD opens in the outlet of the right ventricle, its postero-inferior rim is entirely muscular, separating the anterior leaflet of the tricuspid valve (*TV*) from the aortic leaflets. (**b**) Left ventricular view: the outlet septum (*asterisk*) is an entirely left ventricular structure and is deviated anteriorly, creating subpulmonary obstruction. There is no subaortic conus but fibrous mitro-aortic continuity. The pulmonary artery (*PA*) lies anterior to the aorta (*Ao*). *MV* mitral valve

Subpulmonary VSD

In DOLV with subpulmonary VSD (15 % in the same series), the outlet septum tends to be very deficient, as in DOLV with doubly committed VSD.

Doubly Committed VSD

In the series of Van Praagh, doubly committed VSD, with fibrous or absent outlet septum, was found in 10 % of cases [45].

Non-committed VSD

DOLV with non-committed VSD is exceedingly rare [43].

The Great Vessels

The aorta can be posterior and to the right, side by side and to the right, anterior and to the right, or anterior and to the left.

The Conal or Infundibular Morphology

The conus can be absent, bilateral, subpulmonary or subaortic [43].

Associated Anomalies

Subpulmonary Stenosis

Subpulmonary stenosis is frequent, especially with subaortic VSD. It is usually due to a deviated outlet (conal) septum.

Subaortic Stenosis

Subaortic stenosis is associated with coarctation of the aorta and hypoplastic aortic arch.

Other Associated Anomalies

DOLV type of ventriculo-arterial connections have been reported in association with double inlet left ventricle, tricuspid or mitral atresia, heterotaxy syndrome, Ebstein anomaly. Cases with intact ventricular septum and hypoplastic right ventricle have also been reported and might be considered the complete form of DOLV [45].

Laterality Defects

Transposition of the Great Arteries

The first description of TGA was given by Baillie in 1797, but the term "transposition of the arteries" was coined by Farre in 1814 [46]. The definition of TGA is unequivocal: both great arteries are "placed across" ("trans-positioned") the ventricular septum, so that the aorta originates from the morphologically right ventricle and the pulmonary artery originates from the morphologically left ventricle (Fig. 3.12). Transposition is thus one particular type of relationships, or alignments, between the ventricles and the great vessels [47]. In other terms, there are discordant ventriculoarterial connections with concordant atrioventricular connections [48]. The aorta originates from the right ventricle above a subaortic conus, and the pulmonary valve is in continuity with the mitral valve, above the left ventricle. The great vessels run parallel to each other. Usually the aorta is slightly anterior and to the right of the pulmonary artery: TGA {S,D,D} according to the segmental approach developed by Van Praagh: situs solitus atria, D-loop (normal) ventricles, D-transposition of the great arteries [49]. In atrial situs inversus, the segmental set will thus be {I,L,L}: situs inversus atria, L-loop ventricles, and L-transposition of the great arteries with the aortic valve slightly anterior and to the left of the pulmonary valve.

The atria are normal, but the ventricular anatomy is slightly different from that in a normal heart. The infundibulum of the right ventricle is not deviated to the left as

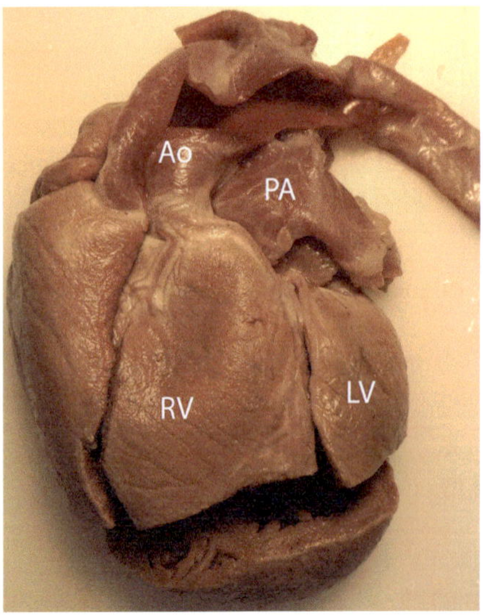

Fig. 3.12 Transposition of the great arteries {S,D,D}: the aorta (*Ao*) arises from the right ventricle (*RV*), anterior and to the right relatively to the pulmonary artery (*PA*), which arises from the left ventricle (*LV*), posterior and to the left. The great vessels are parallel

in the normal heart but stands straight under the aortic valve. The central fibrous body, the membranous septum and the atrioventricular septum are smaller than normal, with a straight ventricular septum, due to the absence of rotation of the outflow tract [50, 51]. The pulmonary valve is not as wedged between the mitral and tricuspid valve as the aortic valve in the normal heart [50].

Main Anatomic Features

Position of the Great Arteries

The aorta can be strictly anterior to the pulmonary artery: TGA {S,D,A}. Two other rare situations can be encountered:

- TGA {S,D,D} with posterior aorta was first reported by Van Praagh et al. in 1971 [47]. In the majority of the cases reported there is a subpulmonary conus, an relatively hypoplastic subaortic conus, and an outlet malalignment VSD due to hypodevelopment of the outlet septum. Like is classical TGA, arterial switch is the treatment of choice [52].
- TGA {S,D,L} or {I,L,D} represent exceptions to the "loop rule". TGA {S,D,L} is a rare variant (about 3 %) of TGA in situs solitus [53]. The aortic valve originates from the right-sided morphologically right ventricle, but is positioned to the left of the pulmonary artery, which originates from the left-sided left ventricle. This rare anomaly is never isolated, but may be regarded as an anatomic complex, because of the frequent abnormality of the ventricular segment, resulting in several related additional anomalies: VSD in 96 %, typically a malalignment outlet VSD, right ventricular hypoplasia in 50 %, pulmonary outflow tract stenosis in 27 %, ventricular malposition in 23 %, absent left coronary orifice in 23 % [53].

Conus

In the vast majority of cases the conus is subaortic, but it can be bilateral [47], or, even more rarely, subpulmonary. Exceptional cases of TGA {S,D,D} with bilaterally absent subarterial conus have been reported [54].

Coronary Artery Pattern

Anomalies of the epicardial course of the coronary arteries and of their connection to the aortic root are frequent in TGA. More than ten classifications have been proposed [55], the most well known being those of Yacoub and of the Leiden group [56, 57]. Serraf and Planché in Marie-Lannelongue Hospital in Paris proposed a classification based on the course of the coronary arteries: type I, usual pattern; type II, interarterial course; type III, anterior, posterior or bilateral loop; type IV, coronary arterial course not included in the above mentioned categories [58] (Fig. 3.13).

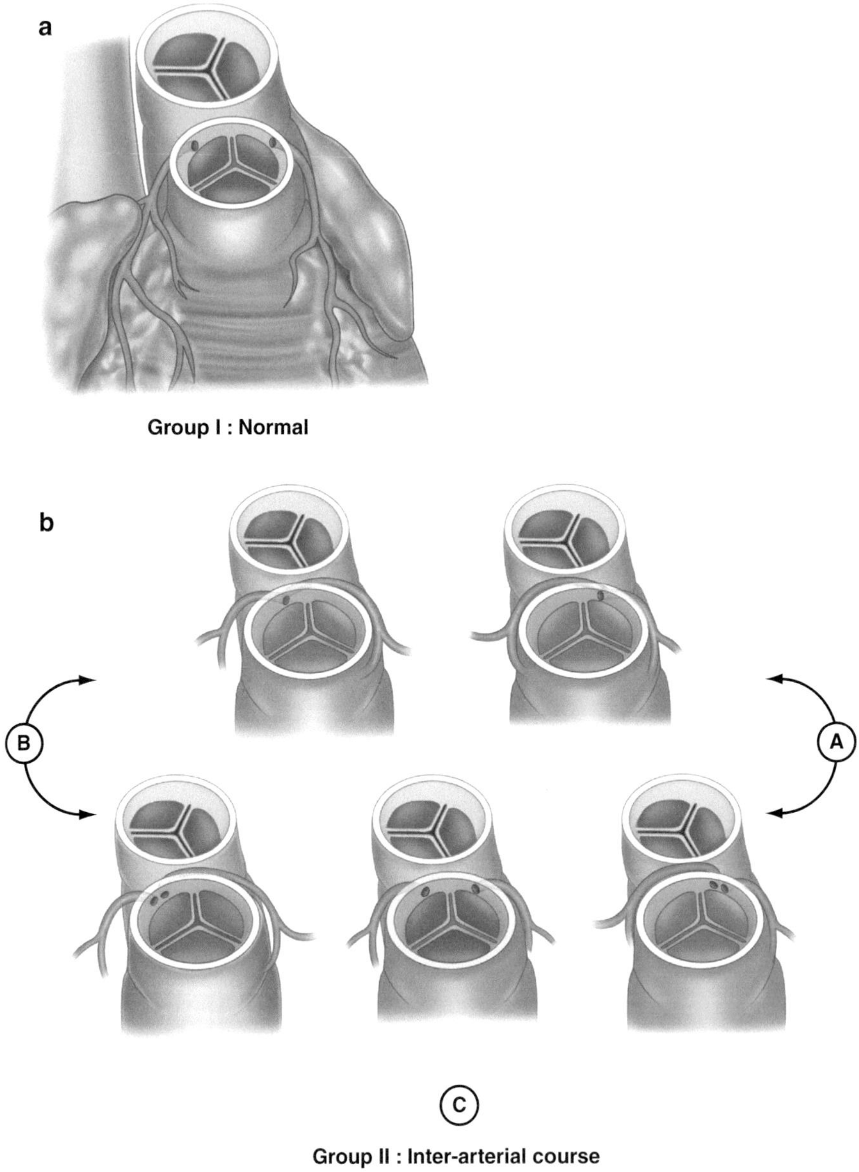

Fig. 3.13 Marie-Lannelongue's classification of coronary arteries pattern in transposition of the great arteries [58]. Group I: the left and right coronary artery orifices are located in the aortic sinus of Valsalva adjacent to the pulmonary artery root (usual pattern for TGA). Group II: abnormal interarterial course of one or two coronary arteries, whatever the number and the position of the orifices; this abnormal interarterial course is often associated with intramural course of one or two coronary arteries. Group III: abnormal course of one of two coronary arteries in front of or behind a great vessel; IIIa: abnormal anterior course of one coronary artery in front of the aorta (anterior loop); IIIb: abnormal posterior course of one of the coronary arteries behind the pulmonary artery (posterior loop); IIIc: abnormal anterior course of one coronary artery and abnormal posterior course of the other coronary artery (double loop). Group IV: any other anomaly of origin and/or course of the coronary arteries which is different from groups II and III or a combination of these two groups

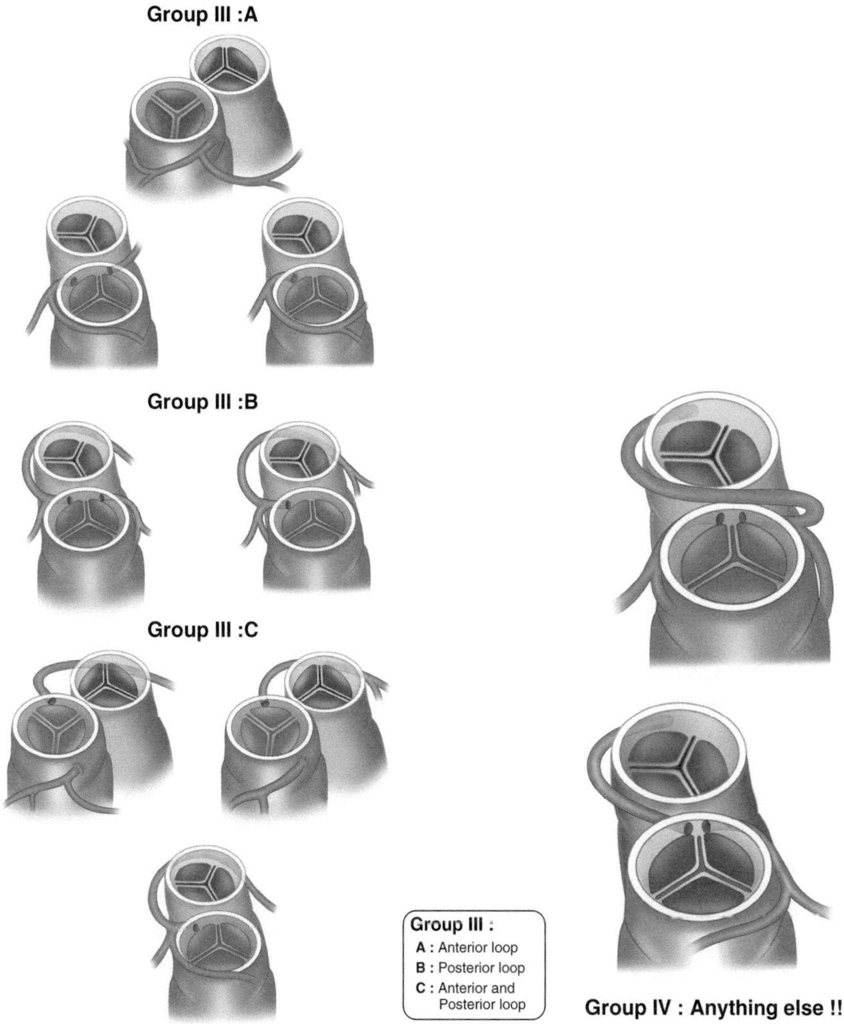

Fig. 3.13 (continued)

Associated Lesions

Ventricular Septal Defect

In an anatomic study based on the 1400 heart specimens of the anatomic collection of the French Reference Center for Complex Congenital Heart Defects, we have found a VSD in 54 % of the 195 hearts with TGA. Among these VSD, 40 % were of the outlet type, 25 % membranous, 25 % muscular, and 10 % opened into the inlet of the right ventricle (personal data). This underlines the different embryologic mechanisms involved in cardiac neural crest defects, in which the VSD is always of the outlet type, and TGA.

In clinical series, the incidence of VSD in TGA varies between 30 and 40 % [59], and their distribution is similar to our findings.

Obstruction of the Outflow Tracts

Left Ventricular Outflow Tract Obstruction (LVOTO)

The spectrum of lesions that can produce subpulmonary obstruction in TGA is exactly the same as in hearts with normally related great arteries [60]. The stenosis can be valvar, due to commissural fusion, often with a bicuspid pulmonary valve, or subvalvar, due to several mechanisms:

- Posterior deviation of the outlet septum
- Posterior and leftward deviation of the outlet septum associated with a malalignment VSD is the most common cause of LVOTO in the setting of discordant VA connections.
- Other muscular subpulmonary stenosis:
  A septal bulge, in the setting of TGA with intact ventricular septum, or a subpulmonary fibromuscular tunnel, can be associated with an anterolateral muscle bundle of the left ventricle [61]
- Discrete subpulmonary stenosis, caused by a fibrous diaphragm inserted on the septal surface, and/or on the anterior leaflet of the mitral valve (Fig. 3.14a).
- Tricuspid pouch, herniating through a membranous VSD, realizes a dynamic subpulmonary obstruction: the pouch will be pushed back to the right ventricle after the arterial switch procedure, due to the rise in left ventricular pressure (Fig. 3.14b).
- Abnormal attachments of the mitral valve on the septal surface, associated or not with a cleft of the mitral valve [60, 61]

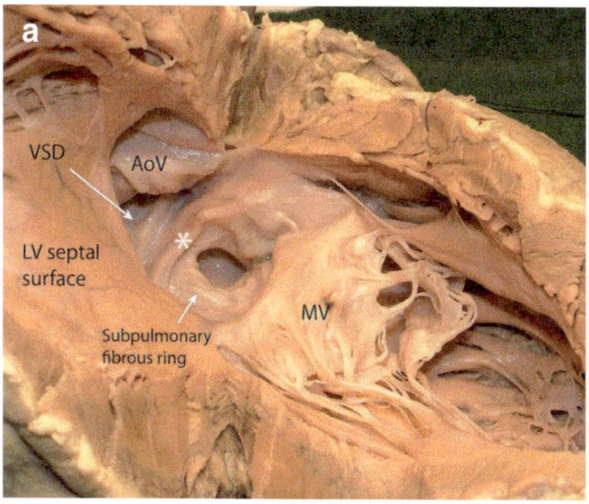

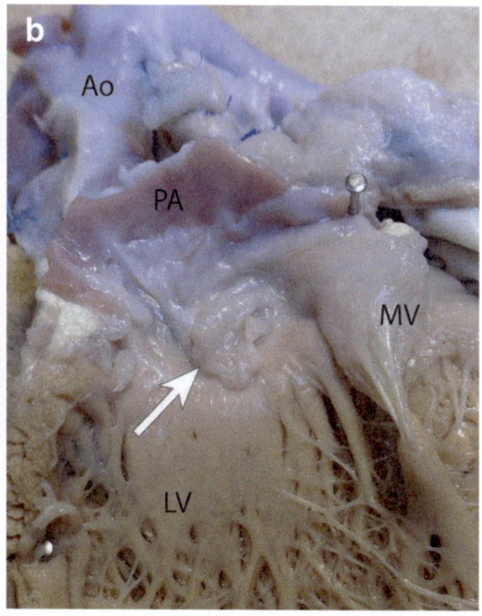

Fig. 3.14 Transposition of the great arteries, ventricular septal defect and subpulmonary stenosis. (**a**) Left ventricular view: discrete subpulmonary stenosis due to a fibrous diaphragm. This diaphragm is circular, inserted both on the anterior leaflet of the mitral valve (*MV*) and on the hypoplastic, fibrous, outlet septum (*asterisk*). The aortic valve (*AoV*) is visible through the large outlet ventricular septal defect (*VSD*). (**b**) Left ventricular view: a large membranous ventricular septal defect, centered under the commissure between the right anterior and posterior leaflets of the pulmonary artery (*PA*), is closed by a tricuspid pouch (*arrow*) developed from the septal leaflet of the tricuspid valve. This tricuspid pouch creates a dynamic left ventricular outflow tract obstruction. *Ao* aorta, *LV* left ventricle, *MV* mitral valve

Right Ventricular Outflow Tract Obstruction (RVOTO)

Like in hearts with concordant VA connections, the consequences of the reduced flow through the aortic valve will be aortic arch hypoplasia, coarctation or interrupted aortic arch (Fig. 3.15a).

Anterior and rightward deviation of the outlet septum, associated with an outlet malalignment VSD, is the most frequent cause of RVOTO in the setting of discordant VA connections (Fig. 3.15b).

The second most frequent cause is hypoplasia of the right ventricular sinus.

Juxtaposition of the Atrial Appendages

Juxtaposition of the atrial appendages (JAA) is present in 2–5 % of TGA. Both atrial appendages are located side by side, to the left (L-JAA) or rarely to the right (R-JAA) of the outflow tract. This anomaly is found predominantly in TGA and DORV with

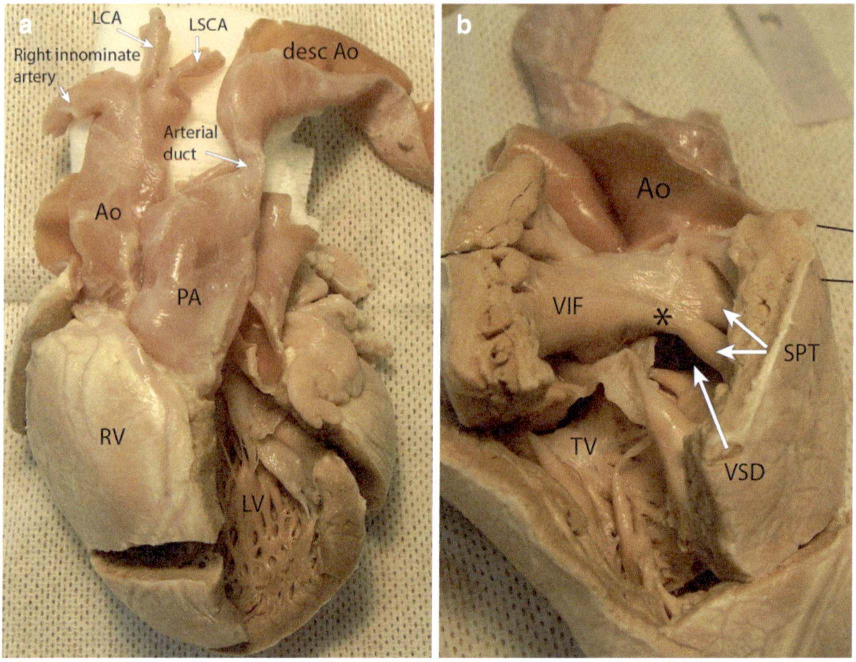

Fig. 3.15 Transposition of the great arteries {S,D,D} with ventricular septal defect and interrupted aortic arch. (**a**) The interruption is situated distal to the left subclavian artery (*LSCA*), on a left aortic arch. The descending aorta (*desc Ao*) is supplied through the arterial duct. *Ao* aorta, *LCA* left carotid artery, *LV* left ventricle, *PA* pulmonary artery, *RV* right ventricle. (**b**) right ventricular view of the same specimen. The ventricular septal defect (*VSD*) is an outlet VSD, cradled between the two limbs of the septal band, due to the malalignment of the outlet septum (*asterisk*). The outlet septum (*asterisk*) is deviated anteriorly, creating subaortic obstruction. *Ao* aorta, *SPT* septoparietal trabeculations (*arrow*), *TV* tricuspid valve, *VIF* ventriculo-infundibular fold

subpulmonary VSD, but also in double-inlet left ventricle and tricuspid atresia. In their anatomic study about 21 hearts with JAA, Meluish et al. found that in TGA with JAA, when compared with hearts with TGA and normal atrial appendages, there was a remarkably high incidence of bilateral conus, right ventricular hypoplasia, and tricuspid atresia or stenosis [62].

Anomalies of the Atrioventricular Valves

Mitral Valve

Mitral valve anomalies are mostly encountered in TGA with VSD. The main anomalies are straddling mitral valve through an outlet VSD, and cleft mitral valve, which can be of two types:

- Outlet type, directed towards the outlet: anomalous mitral attachments can cause subpulmonary obstruction
- AV canal type, directed perpendicular to the septum.

Tricuspid Valve

Like mitral valve anomalies, tricuspid valve anomalies are usually found in TGA with VSD. The main anomalies are:

- Straddling, through an inlet VSD, and annular overriding
- Abnormal attachments to the septal crest or the outlet septum
- Tricuspid pouch, which may create a dynamic subpulmonary obstruction, reversible after the arterial switch procedure (Fig. 3.14b).

Common Atrioventricular Canal

This association is extremely rare [63].

Anomalous Pulmonary Venous Connections

Although rare, this association is not exceptional and pulmonary venous drainage has to be carefully assessed during preoperative assessment [64].

Congenitally Corrected TGA

Congenitally corrected TGA (ccTGA), or "double discordance", is defined by the combination of discordant atrioventricular and ventriculo-arterial connections. Although it definitely involves a malformation of the outflow tract (TGA), the major determinant of this complex anomaly lies in the discordant atrioventricular connections. Atrioventricular discordance profoundly disturbs the internal architecture of the heart and determines the main associated anomalies that are sufficiently frequent to be considered part of the malformation, such as VSD and tricuspid valve anomalies, as well as the abnormal position of the atrioventricular conduction system [65, 66]. Developmentally, the first morphogenetic abnormality appears to be at the ventricular level, the transposition of the great arteries being probably secondary to this primitive malformation.

In the most common form of ccTGA, in atrial situs solitus, the right atrium is connected to the right-sided left ventricle, which ejects into the pulmonary artery. The mitral valve is oriented differently than in a left-sided LV, rotated anteriorly so that the mural leaflet is anterior and the pulmonary leaflet posterior, but it retains its fibrous continuity with the pulmonary valve. The left ventricle often possesses an antero-superior recess, characteristic of ccTGA (Fig. 3.16a). The left atrium is connected to the left-sided right ventricle, which ejects into the aorta above a subaortic conus (Fig. 3.16b). The tricuspid valve is abnormal in over 90 % of the cases [65, 66], which for Van Praagh et al. is associated with an abnormally small right ventricular sinus. The atrioventricular discordance leads to a malalignment between atrial and ventricular septa, creating

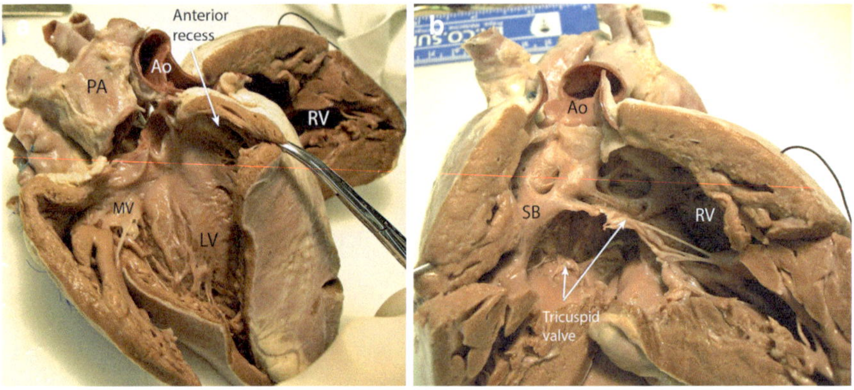

Fig. 3.16 Congenitally corrected transposition of the great arteries {S,L,L} with intact ventricular septum. (**a**) The right-sided left ventricle (*LV*) is opened. The LV possesses an anterior recess. The mitral valve (*MV*) is oriented anteriorly, there is a fibrous mitro-pulmonary continuity. The pulmonary artery (*PA*) arises from the left ventricle and is posterior and to the right. *Ao* aorta, *RV* left-sided right ventricle. (**b**) The left-sided right ventricle (*RV*) is opened. The aorta (*Ao*) arises from the RV above a subaortic conus and is anterior and to the left. The annulus of the tricuspid valve is verticalized with abnormal attachments of the septal and inferior leaflet, but without atrialization of the posterior wall of the RV. *SB* septal band

a gap that will be filled by an abnormally large membranous septum, which determines the abnormal position of the conduction tissues (Fig. 3.17). Like in isolated TGA, the great vessels arise from the ventricles parallel to each other. However, in the vast majority of cases of ccTGA in atrial situs solitus, the aorta lies anterior and to the left of the pulmonary artery (L-transposition). According to the segmental analysis developed by Van Praagh [48], this type of ccTGA is called ccTGA {S,L,L}.

Another consequence of the atrioventricular discordance is the high incidence of mesocardia and dextrocardia. In a series of 22 heart specimens with ccTGA among the anatomic collection of the French Reference Center for Complex Heart Defects, levocardia was present in only 12 % of cases (personal data).

The conduction system is always abnormal in ccTGA. This is due to the atrioventricular discordance, especially when there are L-looped ventricles, which produces malalignment of the atrial and ventricular septa. This malalignment and the resulting enlargement of the membranous septum prevent the regular posterior AV node to contact the ventricles and leads to the development of a second, anterior, AV node. This second AV node develops anteriorly beneath the entrance of the right atrial appendage, on the anterior margin of the right AV orifice. The penetrating AV bundle descends along the left side of the pulmonary annulus, to reach the expanded portion of the ventricular septum, anterior to the membranous septum. When there is a VSD, the penetrating AV bundle descends on the right ventricular surface, on the anterior margin of the VSD, before bifurcating into its branches (Fig. 3.18).

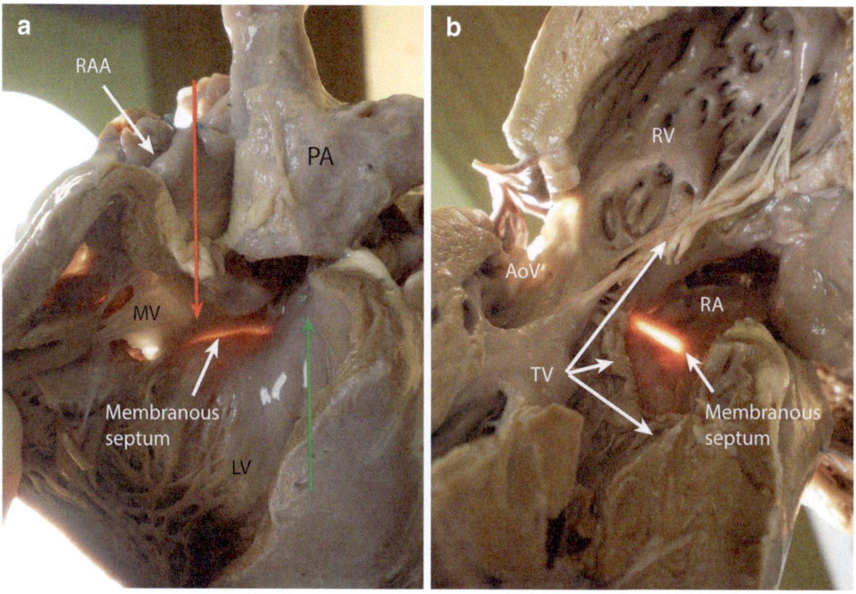

Fig. 3.17 Congenitally corrected transposition of the great arteries {S,L,L} with intact ventricular septum (same specimen than in Fig. 3.16): location of the membranous septum, viewed from the left ventricle (*LV*, **a**) and from the right ventricle (*RV*, **b**). Contrarily to the normal heart, the membranous septum is not an interventricular structure but separates the left ventricular chamber from the right atrial chamber (*RA*), filling the gap caused by the malalignment between the atrial septum (*red arrow*) and the ventricular septum (*green arrow*). *Ao* aorta, *MV* mitral valve, *PA* pulmonary artery, *RAA* right atrial appendage, *TV* tricuspid valve

Associated Anomalies

The Right Ventricle and the Tricuspid Valve

The right ventricle and the tricuspid valve are almost always malformed in ccTGA [65]. The apical part of the right ventricle (sinus) is often hypoplastic, especially if there is an Ebstein malformation of the tricuspid valve. The junction of inlet and outlet segment is constricted, and the anatomic landmarks of the right ventricle, such as the limbs of the septal band, tend to disappear. Tricuspid anomalies are extremely frequent (78 % in our anatomic series).

Ebstein anomaly occurs mainly in ccTGA with intact ventricular septum [65]. If there are similarities between Ebstein anomaly in ccTGA and in otherwise normal heart (defect of delamination of the septal and inferior leaflet, maximal displacement of the valve at the level of the septo-inferior commissure, verticalisation of the tricuspid orifice), there are also noticeable differences: the anterior leaflet usually has focal distal insertions on one or more papillary muscles, the annulus is usually not dilated, the right ventricle is small, and the inferior wall of the right ventricle, although somewhat thinner, remains muscular and not "atrialized".

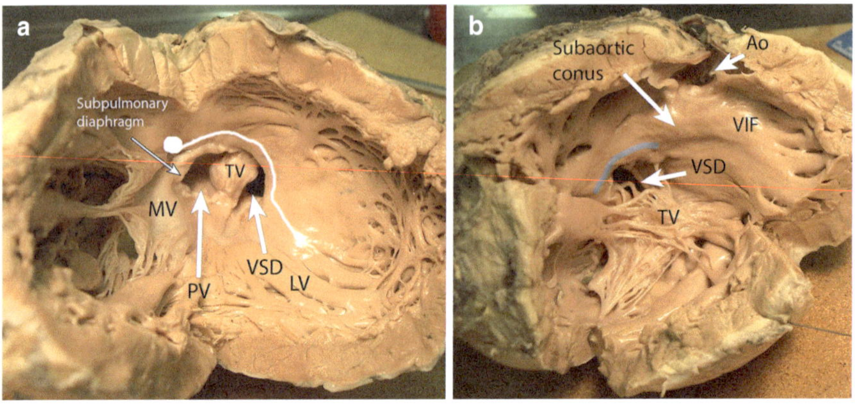

Fig. 3.18 Location of the atrioventricular (*AV*) node and of the bundle of His in a heart specimen with congenitally corrected transposition of the great arteries. (**a**) The right-sided left ventricle is opened. The anterior AV node is located on the anterior margin of the annulus of the mitral valve (*MV*). The penetrating His bundle (*in white*) circles anteriorly the pulmonary annulus, then descends on the anterior margin of the ventricular septal defect (*VSD*), before bifurcating into its branches. The left ventricular outflow tract is obstructed by a fibrous diaphragm under the pulmonary valve (*PV*). The tricuspid valve (*TV*) straddles through the VSD. (**b**) Right ventricular view: The His bundle (*light blue*) runs on the anterior margin of the VSD (outlet VSD with inlet extension). The aorta (*Ao*) is above a subaortic conus. *TV* tricuspid valve, *VIF* ventriculo-infundibular fold

Straddling tricuspid valve occurs through the inlet component of the VSD (38 % of ccTGA with VSD in our series). Other tricuspid anomalies include leaflet dysplasia, significant annular hypoplasia, and overriding.

The Ventricular Septal Defect

The VSD is extremely frequent (91 % of heart specimens in our series), especially in autopsy series. This VSD cannot be called perimembranous, as the "membranous" septum in ccTGA is not a septum any more: it is located between the left atrium and the left ventricle, filling the gap caused by the malalignment between the atrial and ventricular septa (Fig. 3.17). This particular type of VSD is located beneath the pulmonary valve, and opens then in the outlet of the LV, but almost always extends posteriorly and inferiorly, opening in the inlet of the left ventricle [66], this particular location being almost specific to ccTGA. Mitro-pulmonary fibrous continuity is the rule, except when there is pulmonary atresia. In this latter case, there is almost always a mitro-tricuspid continuity (75 % in our series). Fibrous continuity between the mitral, tricuspid and pulmonary valve can also occur. This "ccTGA type" of VSD (outlet with inlet extension) was found in all our specimens with associated VSD except in one heart with muscular inlet VSD. Two specimens had additional muscular VSDs.

Left Ventricular Outflow Tract Obstruction

Left ventricular outflow tract obstruction was found in 50 % of our specimens: pulmonary atresia in nine, all with a VSD, and pulmonary stenosis in two. The mechanism was anterior deviation of the outlet septum, and subpulmonary fibrous ring in one specimen (Fig. 3.18), but other mechanisms have been described.

The Left Ventricle and the Mitral Valve

Mitral anomalies are relatively rare (cleft, straddling, leaflet dysplasia). An anterolateral muscle bundle of the left ventricle was found in 11/23 specimens of our series (48 %), but was never obstructive.

Position of the Great Arteries

The great arteries run parallel to each other. The aorta is usually in L-malposition in atrial situs solitus (ccTGA {S,L,L}), but can occasionally be in D-malposition (ccTGA {S,L,D}), which constitutes an exception to the loop rule [65].

In atrial situs inversus, the aorta is usually in D-malposition (ccTGA {I,D,D}) but can rarely be in L-malposition (ccTGA {I,D,L}).

Conclusion

In this chapter we have provided the salient anatomic features of the different types of conotruncal defects, which share as a common characteristic to be due to an abnormal development of the outflow tract of the heart. The similarities and differences between these defects are reminiscent of their presumably different embryologic origin. All cardiac neural crest defects share as an essential part of their phenotype a VSD, which always opens in the outlet of the right ventricle and is cradled between the two limbs of the septal band. However, the differences observed regarding the postero-inferior and superior rims of the VSD suggest an anatomic continuum from tetralogy of Fallot to IAA-B rather than distinct physiological phenotypes, related to various degrees of abnormal rotation of the outflow tract during heart development, incomplete in TOF, TOF-PA and DORV, absent in CAT, excessive in IAA-B. On the contrary, the presence of a VSD is not constant in TGA and ccTGA, and when a VSD is present, it can be of any type in TGA (outlet, inlet, muscular, central membranous), and opens both in the outlet and in the inlet of the left ventricle in the majority of ccTGA. The anatomy of the coronary arteries and their orifices is also directly related with the rotation of the outflow tract during heart development, which explains the high frequency of coronary arterial anomalies in outflow tract defects. Finally, the anatomic particularities of ccTGA indicate that, although the ventriculo-arterial discordance (TGA) is part of its phenotype, the atrioventricular discordance is the major determinant of this complex malformation.

References

1. Digilio MC, Casey B, Toscano A, Calabro R, Pacileo G, Marasini M, Banaudi E, Giannotti A, Dallapiccola B, Marino B. Complete transposition of the great arteries. Patterns of congenital heart disease in familial precurrence. Circulation. 2001;104:2809–14.
2. Ferencz C, Loffredo CA, Correa-Villasenor A, et al. Genetic and environmental risk factors of major cardiovascular malformations: the Baltimore-Washington Infant Study, 1981–1989. Armonk: Futura Publishing Company; 1997.
3. Clark EB. Pathogenetic mechanisms of congenital cardiovascular malformations revisited. Semin Perinatol. 1996;20:465–72.
4. Hutson MR, Kirby ML. Seminars in cell and developmental biology model systems for the study of heart development and disease cardiac neural crest and conotruncal malformations. Semin Cell Dev Biol. 2007;18:101–10.
5. Goldmuntz E, Bamford R, Karkera JD, de la Cruz J, Roessler E, Muenke M. CFC1 mutations in patients with transposition of the great arteries and double outlet right ventricle. Am J Hum Genet. 2002;70:776–80.
6. De Luca A, Sarkozy A, Consoli F, Ferese R, Guida V, Dentici ML, Mingarelli R, Bellacchio E, Tuo G, Limongelli G, Diglio MC, Marino B, Dellapiccola B. Familial transposition of the great arteries caused by multiple mutations in laterality genes. Heart. 2010;96:673–7.
7. Unolt M, Putotto C, Silvestri LM, Marino D, Scarabotti A, Massaccesi V, Caiaro A, Versacci P, Marino B. Transposition of great arteries: new insights into the pathogenesis. Front Pediatr Cardiol. 2013;1:1–7.
8. Van Praagh R. The first Stella Van Praagh memorial lecture: the history and anatomy of tetralogy of Fallot. Semin Thorac Cardiovasc Surg Pediatr Card Surg Annu. 2009;12:19–38.
9. Fallot A. Contribution à l'anatomie pathologique de la maladie bleue (cyanose cardiaque). Mars Méd. 1888;25:77–93, 138–158, 207–223, 270–286, 341–354, 403–420.
10. Abbott ME, Dawson WT. The clinical classification of congenital cardiac disease, with remarks upon its pathological anatomy, diagnosis and treatment. Int Clin. 1924;4:156–88.
11. Anderson RH, Jacobs ML. The anatomy of tetralogy of Fallot with pulmonary stenosis. Cardiol Young. 2008;18 Suppl 3:12–21.
12. Mostefa-Kara M, Bonnet D, Belli E, Fadel E, Houyel L. Anatomy of the ventricular septal defect in outflow tract defects: similarities and differences. J Thorac Cardiovasc Surg. 2014;149(3):682–8.e1.
13. Dyer LA, Kirby ML. Sonic hedgehog maintains proliferation in secondary heart field progenitors and is required for normal arterial pole formation. Dev Biol. 2009;330:305–17.
14. Anderson RH, Spicer DE, Giroud JM, Mohun TJ. Tetralogy of Fallot: nosological, morphological, and morphogenetic considerations. Cardiol Young. 2013;23:858–66.
15. Houyel L, Bajolle F, Capderou A, Laux D, Parisot P, Bonnet D. The pattern of the coronary arterial orifices in hearts with congenital malformations of the outflow tracts: a marker of rotation of the outflow tract during cardiac development? J Anat. 2013;222:349–57.
16. Perdreau E, Houyel L, Baruteau AE. Tetralogy of Fallot with coarctation of the aorta: a newly recognized developmental and anatomic syndrome. Cardiol Young. 2014;24:714–20.
17. Barbero-Marcial M, Jatene AD. Surgical management of the anomalies of the pulmonary arteries in the tetralogy of Fallot with pulmonary atresia. Semin Thorac Cardiovasc Surg. 1990;2:93–107.
18. Van Praagh R. Truncus arteriosus: what is it really and how should it be classified? Eur J Cardiothorac Surg. 1987;1:65–70.

19. Jacobs ML. Congenital heart surgery nomenclature and database project: truncus arteriosus. Ann Thorac Surg. 2000;69:S50–5.
20. Collett RW, Edwards JE. Persistent truncus arteriosus: a classification according to anatomic subtypes. Surg Clin North Am. 1949;29:1245–70.
21. Van Praagh R, Van Praagh S. The anatomy of common aorticopulmonary trunk (truncus arteriosus communis) and its embryologic implications. A study of 57 necropsy cases. Am J Cardiol. 1965;16:406–25.
22. Russell HM, Jacobs ML, Anderson RH, et al. A simplified categorization for common arterial trunk. J Thorac Cardiovasc. 2011;141:645–53.
23. Murdison KA, McLean DA, Carpenter B, Duncan WJ. Truncus arteriosus communis associated with mitral valve and left ventricular hypoplasia without ventricular septal defect: unique combination. Pediatr Cardiol. 1996;17:322–6.
24. Celoria GC, Patton RB. Congenital absence of the aortic arch. Am Heart J. 1959;58:407–13.
25. Abbott M. Congenital heart disease. In: Osler's modern medicine, vol. 4. 3rd ed. Philadelphia: Lea and Febiger; 1927. p. 773–93.
26. Van Mierop LH, Kutsche LM. Interruption of the aortic arch and coarctation of the aorta: pathogenetic relations. Am J Cardiol. 1984;54:829–34.
27. Al-Marsawafy HM, Ho SY, Redington AN, Anderson RH. The relationship f the outlet septum to the aortic outflow tract in hearts with interruption of the aortic arch. J Thorac Cardiovasc Surg. 1995;109:1225–36.
28. Cazavet A, Seguela PE, Acar P, Leobon B. A new type of aortic arch interruption without significant patent ductus arteriosus and with no ventricular septal defect. J Thorac Cardiovasc Surg. 2012;143:237–9.
29. Phillips HM, Mahendran P, Singh E, Anderson RH, Chaudhry B, Henderson DJ. Neural crest cells are required for correct positioning of the developing outflow cushions and pattern the arterial valve leaflets. Cardiovasc Res. 2013;99:452–60.
30. Kutsche LM, Van Mierop LH. Anatomy and pathogenesis of aorticopulmonary septal defect. Am J Cardiol. 1987;59:443–7.
31. Walters HL, Mavroudis C, Tchervenkov CI, Jacobs JP, Lacour-Gayet F, Jacobs ML. Congenital heart surgery nomenclature and database project: double outlet right ventricle. Ann Thorac Surg. 2000;69:S249–63.
32. Lev M, Bharati S, Meng CC, Liberthson RR, Paul MH, Idriss F. A concept of double-outlet right ventricle. J Thorac Cardiovasc Surg. 1972;64:271–81.
33. Van Praagh S, Davidoff A, Chin A, Shiel FS, Reynolds J, Van Praagh R. Double outlet right ventricle: anatomic types and developmental implications based on a study of 101 autopsied cases. Coeur. 1982;13:389–439.
34. De la Cruz MV, Cayre R, Arista-Salado Martinez O, Sadowinski S, Serrano A. The infundibular interrelationships and the ventriculoarterial connection in double outlet right ventricle. Clinical and surgical implications. Int J Cardiol. 1992;35:153–64.
35. Peixoto LB, Leal SM, Silva CE, Moreira SM, Ortiz J. Double outlet right ventricle with anterior and left-sided aorta and subpulmonary ventricular septal defect. Arq Bras Cardiol. 1999;73:446–50.
36. Beekman RP, Bartelings MM, Hazekamp MG, Gittenberger-de Groot AC, Ottenkamp J. The morphologic nature of noncommitted ventricular septal defects in specimens with double-outlet right ventricle. J Thorac Cardiovasc Surg. 2002;124:984–90.
37. Belli E, Serraf A, Lacour-Gayet F, Hubler M, Zoghby J, Houyel L, Planche C. Double-outlet right ventricle with non-committed ventricular septal defect. Eur J Cardiothorac Surg. 1999;15:747–52.
38. Anderson RA, McCarthy K, Cook AC. Double outlet right ventricle. Cardiol Young. 2001;11:329–44.
39. Van Praagh R. What is the Taussig-Bing malformation? Circulation. 1968;38:445–9.
40. D'Alessandro LC, Latney BC, Paluru PC, Goldmuntz E. The phenotypic spectrum of *ZIC3* mutations includes isolated d-transposition of the great arteries and double outlet right ventricle. Am J Med Genet Part A. 2013;161A:792–802.

41. Van Praagh S, Porras D, Oppido G, Geva T, Van Praagh R. Cleft mitral valve without ostium primum defect: anatomic data and surgical considerations based on 41 cases. Ann Thorac Surg. 2003;75:1752–62.
42. Stellin G, Zuberbuhler JR, Anderson RH, Siewers RD. The surgical anatomy of the Taussig-Bing malformation. J Thorac Cardiovasc Surg. 1987;93:560–9.
43. Tchervenkov CI, Walters HL, Chu VF. Congenital heart surgery nomenclature and database project: double outlet left ventricle. Ann Thorac Surg. 2000;69:S264–9.
44. Bharati S, Lev M, Stewart R, McAllister HA, Kirklin JW. The morphologic spectrum of double outlet left ventricle and its surgical significance. Circulation. 1978;58:558–65.
45. Van Praagh R, Weinberg PM, Srebro JP. Double outlet left ventricle. In: Adams FH, Emmanouilides GC, Riemenschneider TA, editors. Moss' heart disease in infants, children, and adolescents. Baltimore: Williams and Wilkins.; 1989. p. 461–85.
46. Van Praagh R. Transposition of the great arteries: history, pathologic anatomy, embryology etiology, and surgical considerations. Card Surg State Art Rev. 1991;5:7–82.
47. Van Praagh R, Perez-Trevino C, Lopez-Cuellar M, Baker FW, Zuberbuhler JR, Quero M, Perez VM, Moreno F, Van Praagh S. Transposition of the great arteries with posterior aorta, anterior pulmonary artery, subpulmonary conus and fibrous continuity between aortic and atrioventricular valves. Am J Cardiol. 1971;28:621–31.
48. Anderson RH, Moorman AF, Webb S, Brown N. A system for describing congenital cardiac malformations and correlating them with abnormal cardiac development. In: Rosenthal N, Harvey RP, editors. Heart development and regeneration. Waltham: Academic Press; 2010. p. 255–77.
49. Van Praagh R. Nomenclature and classification: morphologic and segmental approach to diagnosis. In: Moller JH, Hoffman JIE, editors. Pediatric cardiovascular medicine. New York: Churchill Livingstone; 2000. p. 275–88.
50. Smith A, Wilkinson JL, Anderson RH, Arnold R, Dickinson DF. Architecture of the ventricular mass and atrioventricular valves in complete transposition with intact ventricular septum compared with the normal. I: the left ventricle, mitral valve, and interventricular septum. Pediatr Cardiol. 1986;6:253–7.
51. Smith A, Wilkinson JL, Anderson RH, Arnold R, Dickinson DF. Architecture of the ventricular mass and atrioventricular valves in complete transposition with intact ventricular septum compared with the normal. II: the right ventricle and tricuspid valve. Pediatr Cardiol. 1986;6:299–305.
52. Tam S, Murphy JD, Norwood WI. Transposition of the great arteries with posterior aorta: anatomic repair. J Thorac Cardiovasc Surg. 1990;100:441–4.
53. Houyel L, Van Praagh R, Lacour-Gayet F, Serraf A, Petit J, Bruniaux J, Planché C. Transposition of the great arteries {S, D, L}: pathologic anatomy, diagnosis, and surgical management of a newly recognized complex. J Thorac Cardiovasc Surg. 1995;110:613–24.
54. Pasquini L, Sanders SP, Parness IA, Colan SD, Van Praagh S, Mayer JE, Van Praagh R. Conal anatomy in 119 patients with d-loop transposition of the great arteries and ventricular septal defect: an echocardiographic and pathologic study. J Am Coll Cardiol. 1993;21:1712–21.
55. Amato JJ, Zelen J, Bushong J. Coronary arterial patterns in complete transposition – classification in relation to the arterial switch procedure. Cardiol Young. 1994;4:329–39.
56. Yacoub MH, Radley-Smith R. Anatomy of the coronary arteries in transposition of the great arteries and methods for their transfer in anatomical correction. Thorax. 1978;33:418–24.
57. Gittenberger-de Groot AC, Sauer U, Oppenheimer-Dekker A, Quaegebeur J. Coronary arterial anatomy in transposition of the great arteries: a morphologic study. Pediatr Cardiol. 1983;4(Suppl I):15–24.
58. Serraf A, Lacour-Gayet F, Bruniaux J, Touchot A, Losay J, Comas J, Sousa-Uva M, Planché C. Anatomic correction of transposition of the great arteries in neonates. J Am Coll Cardiol. 1993;22:193–200.
59. Paul MH. Complete transposition of the great arteries. In: Adams FH, Emmanouilides GC, Riemenschneider TA, editors. Moss' heart disease in infants, children, and adolescents. Baltimore: Williams and Wilkins; 1989. p. 371–420.

60. Martins P, Tran V, Price G, Tsang V, Cook AC. Extending the surgical boundaries in the management of the left ventricular outflow tract obstruction in discordant ventriculo-arterial connections: a surgical and morphological study. Cardiol Young. 2008;18:124–34.
61. Hazekamp M, Portela F, Bartelings M. The optimal procedure for the great arteries and left ventricular outflow tract obstruction. Eur J Cardiothorac Surg. 2007;31:879–87.
62. Melhuish BP, Van Praagh R. Juxtaposition of the atrial appendages: a sign of severe cyanotic congenital heart disease. Br Heart J. 1968;30:269–84.
63. Alfieri O, Plokker M. Repair of common atrioventricular canal associated with transposition of the great arteries and left ventricular outflow tract obstruction. J Thorac Cardiovasc Surg. 1982;84:872–5.
64. Gontijo B, Fantini F, Barbosa M, Gomes MV, Gutierrez C, Vrandecic M. Surgical repair of transposition of great arteries and total anomalous pulmonary venous return to the coronary sinus. Eur J Cardiothorac Surg. 1994;8:391–2.
65. Van Praagh R, Papagiannis J, Grünenfelder J, Bartram U, Martanovic P. Pathologic anatomy of corrected transposition of the great arteries: medical and surgical implications. Am Heart J. 1998;135:772–85.
66. Wallis GA, Debich-Spicer D, Anderson RH. Congenitally corrected transposition. Orphanet J Rare Dis. 2011;6:22.

Chapter 4
Outcomes Data of Surgery for Conotruncal Anomalies from the Congenital EACTS and STS Databases

Jeffrey P. Jacobs, Bohdan Maruszewski, and Francois Lacour-Gayet

Abstract Multi-institutional data can provide valuable information about outcomes. Rare lesions may not be seen enough in individual institutions to obtain a meaningful single institutional experience. Moreover, in comparison to data from individual institutions, data from a multi-institutional registry may provide a more realistic representation of overall global outcomes.

In this chapter, we provide multi-institutional data about the outcomes of patients undergoing surgery for Cono-Truncal Anomalies (CTA).

Keywords Outcomes • Quality of care • Pediatric cardiac surgery • Congenital cardiac surgery

Databases

STS and EACTS/ECHSA Congenital Heart Surgery Databases

The two largest clinical databases in the world containing data about patients undergoing surgery for congenital and pediatric cardiac disease are the Society of Thoracic Surgeons (STS) Congenital Heart Surgery Database (STS-CHSD) [1] and the European Association for Cardio-Thoracic Surgery/European Congenital Heart

J.P. Jacobs, MD (✉)
Division of Cardiovascular Surgery, Department of Surgery,
Johns Hopkins All Children's Heart Institute, 601 Fifth Street South, Suite 607,
Saint Petersburg, FL 33701, USA
e-mail: JeffJacobs@msn.com

B. Maruszewski, MD
Cardiothoracic Surgery, Children's Memorial Health Institute, Syta 108 AM 4, Warsaw
PL 02-987, Poland
e-mail: bmar@ecdb.pl.pl

F. Lacour-Gayet, MD
Department of Pediatric Cardiac Surgery, National Heart and Lung Institute,
Royal Brompton Hospital, Imperial College University, Sydney Street, London SW3 6NP, UK
e-mail: flacourgayet@mac.com

F. Lacour-Gayet et al. (eds.), *Surgery of Conotruncal Anomalies*,
DOI 10.1007/978-3-319-23057-3_4

Surgeons Association (EACTS/ECHSA) Congenital Heart Surgery Database (EACTS/ECHSA-CHSD) [2].

STS-CHSD is the largest database in North America dealing with congenital cardiac malformations. It has grown annually since its inception, both in terms of the number of participating centers submitting data, and the number of operations analyzed. The Report of the 2010 STS Congenital Heart Surgery Practice and Manpower Survey, undertaken by the STS Workforce on Congenital Heart Surgery, estimated that 125 hospitals in the United States of America and eight hospitals in Canada perform pediatric and congenital heart surgery. As of June, 2014, STS-CHSD contains data from 119 of the 125 hospitals (95.2 % penetrance by hospital) in the United States of America and three of the eight centers in Canada. With penetrance of over 95 % of the hospitals in the United States, the data in STS-CHSD is representative of pediatric and congenital heart surgery in the United States of America. As of June, 2014, the current number of cumulative total operations in the STS Congenital Heart Surgery Database was 314,674 (see Fig. 4.1).

EACTS/ECHSA-CHSD is the largest database in Europe dealing with congenital cardiac malformations. As of May 2013, EACTS/ECHSA-CHSD contained 157,772 operations performed in 130,534 patients, with 173 active Centers from 46 countries submitting data (see Fig. 4.2).

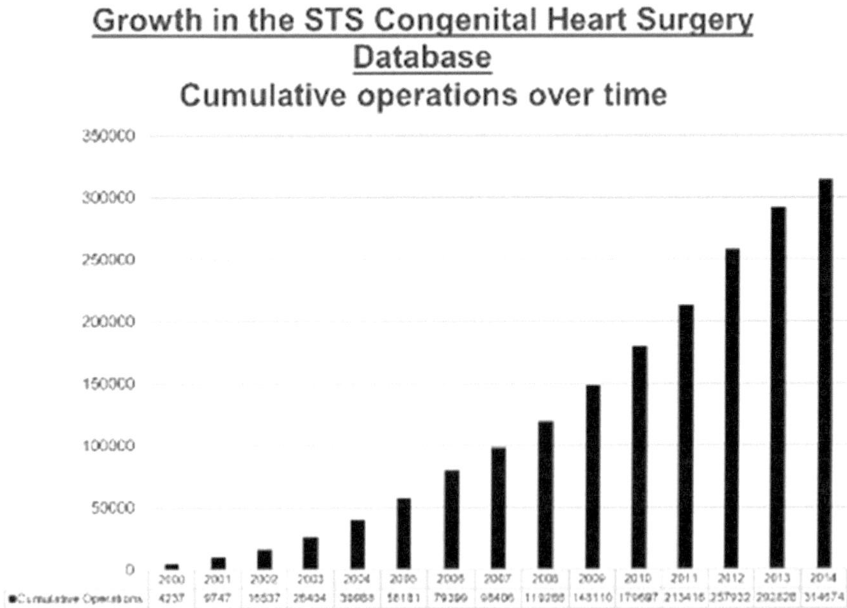

Fig. 4.1 Growth of procedures in the STS Congenital Heart Surgery Database (Data Source: Jacobs JP, Jacobs ML, Mavroudis C, Lacour-Gayet FG, Tchervenkov CI, Pasquali SK. Executive Summary: The Society of Thoracic Surgeons Congenital Heart Surgery Database – Twentieth Harvest – (January 1, 2009 – December 31, 2013))

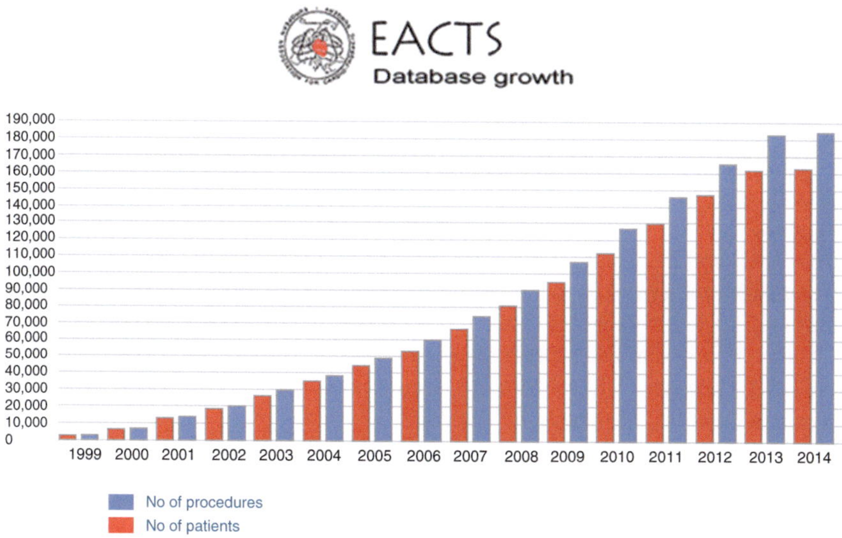

Fig. 4.2 Growth of patients and procedures in the EACTS/ECHSA Congenital Heart Surgery Database (Data Source: Bohdan Maruszewski et al. EACTS/ECHSA Congenital Heart Surgery Database [3])

Risk Adjustment Models in Congenital Heart Surgery

Five major multi-institutional tools for risk stratification of pediatric and congenital cardiac operations have been widely utilized:

- Risk Adjustment in Congenital Heart Surgery (RACHS-1) system [3]
- Aristotle Basic Complexity Score (ABC Score) [4]
- The Aristotle Comprehensive Complexity Score [5] (ACC Score)
- STAT Mortality Score and Categories (STS-EACTS Congenital Heart Surgery Mortality Score and Categories [6])
- STAT Morbidity Score and Categories (STS-EACTS Congenital Heart Surgery Morbidity Score and Categories [7])

Results from STS and EACTS/ECHSA Databases

The conotruncal anomalies are defined as abnormalities involving both the conus and the truncus (Chap. 1) and include:

- Tetralogy of Fallot
- Transposition of the great arteries
- Double outlet right ventricle (DORV)

- Double outlet left ventricle (DOLV)
- Congenitally corrected transposition (ccTGA)
- Truncus arteriosus
- Interrupted aortic arch (Type B)

The international nomenclature for congenital heart surgery [8] recognizes 25 different surgical procedures for the seven CTA diagnosis (Tables 4.1 and 4.2). The total number of CTA surgery procedures performed for the period 2010–2013 in the STS-CHSD and EACTS/ECHSA-CHSD are respectively: 85,302 and 65, 461. The Operative Mortality (30 days mortality and discharge mortality) for all CTA procedures are: 3.5 % for STS-CHSD and 3.7 % for EACTS/ECHSA-CHSD (Table 4.1).

The complexity of the procedures as evaluated by ABC Score, ABC Category, RACHS-1 Category, STAT Mortality Score and Category, and STAT Morbidity Score and Category, are shown on Table 4.2.

Mortality The overall mortality (Table 4.1) of this complex group of procedures is around 3.5 %, quite similar to the entire combined dataset of STS-CHSD and EACTS/ECHSA-CHSD. If Fallot is not considered, all the other procedures are quite complex and require an expert team.

The highest mortality is observed in Truncus-IAA and in ASO for TGA-VSD-CoA.

Some results should probably be double checked, such as 0 % mortality for Truncus-IAA in EACTS/ECHSA-CHSD.

Complexity Table 4.3 shows the ten most complex procedure. When examining the sum of the STAT Mortality and Morbidity Categories, we find ten procedures reaching eight and more, which corresponds to a rationale definition of complexity. The Aristotle Basic Complexity Score recognized nine of these ten complex procedures. However, although the Blalock–Taussig shunt is classified as a complex procedure by STAT Mortality and Morbidity Scores and Categories, the Blalock–Taussig shunt is "underscored" by Aristotle and RACHS-1. (Also, the Blalock–Taussig shunt is often performed for many complex lesions other than conotruncal anomalies.) (Chap. 12).

Table 4.1 Listing and operative mortality from procedures of Cono-Truncal anomalies, according to STS-CHSD and EACTS/ECHSA-CHSD.

		STS-CHSD 2010–2013		EACTS/ECHSA-CHSD 2010–2013	
	Cono-Truncal anomalies	N	Mortality (%)	N	Mortality (%)
Fallot	TOF repair, No ventriculotomy	967	0.8	646	0.8
	TOF repair, Ventriculotomy, Nontransanular patch	988	0.5	1000	1.2
	TOF repair, Ventriculotomy, Transanular patch	2105	1.4	2731	2.5
	TOF – AVC (AVSD) repair	160	5.6	123	10.6
	TOF absent pulmonary valve	158	9.5	124	12.9
	Pulmonary atresia – VSD (including TOF, PA) repair	192	4.7	356	3.7
	Pulmonary atresia – VSD – MAPCA (pseudotruncus) repair	222	6.8	141	5.7
	Conduit placement, RV to PA	849	2.6	1538	4.1
	Conduit reoperation	1614	0.9	823	2.3
	Shunt, Systemic to pulmonary, Modified Blalock–Taussig shunt (MBTS)	2051	6.6	2441	11.0
TGA	Arterial switch operation (ASO)	1724	2.6	1972	4.2
	Arterial switch operation (ASO) and VSD repair	784	5.0	815	7.7
	Arterial switch procedure and VSD repair + aortic arch repair	212	11.3	76	11.8
	Rastelli	324	3.1	134	4.5
	REV	13	15.4	89	4.5
	Aortic root translocation (Nikaidoh)	66	7.6	27	0.0
Cc TGA	Congenitally corrected TGA repair, Atrial switch and ASO (double switch)	70	4.3	65	6.2
	Congenitally corrected TGA repair, Atrial switch and Rastelli	44	9.1	34	5.9
	Congenitally corrected TGA repair, VSD closure	12	0.0	23	4.3
	Congenitally corrected TGA repair, VSD closure and LV to PA conduit	11	9.1	13	0.0
DORV	DORV, Intraventricular tunnel repair	687	4.7	649	4.9
DOLV	DOLV repair	9	0.0	12	8.3
Truncus	Truncus arteriosus repair	571	8.9	414	15.5
	Truncus + interrupted aortic arch (IAA) repair	58	20.7	21	0.0
IAA	Interrupted aortic arch repair	497	6.6	310	11.6
All patients		85,302	3.5	65,461	3.7

Table 4.2 Risk stratification of Cono-Truncal anomalies procedures, comparing: Aristotle Basic Score, RACHS1 score, STAT mortality score and category, STAT morbidity score and category

	Cono-truncal anomalies	Aristotle basic score 0.1–15	Aristotle basic category 1–4	RACHS-1 category 1–5/6	STAT mortality score 0.1–5	STAT mortality category 1–5	STAT morbidity score 0.1–5	STAT morbidity category 1–5
Fallot	TOF repair, No ventriculotomy	8	3	2	0.3	1	0.7	1
	TOF repair, Ventriculotomy, Nontransanular patch	7.5	2	2	0.3	1	0.7	1
	TOF repair, Ventriculotomy, Transanular patch	8	3	2	0.5	2	1.2	2
	TOF – AVC (AVSD) repair	11	4	4	1.6	4	2.3	3
	TOF absent pulmonary valve	9.3	3		1.5	4		
	Pulmonary atresia – VSD (including TOF, PA) repair	9	3	3	1.1	3	2.2	3
	Pulmonary atresia – VSD – MAPCA (pseudotruncus) repair	11	4	3	1.7	4	3.1	4
	Conduit placement, RV to PA	7.5	2	3	1.2	3	1.3	2
	Conduit reoperation	8	3		0.3	1	0.7	1
	Shunt, Systemic to pulmonary, Modified Blalock–Taussig shunt (MBTS)	6.3	2	3	1.5	4	2.5	4

TGA	Arterial switch operation (ASO)	10	4	3	0.8	3	1.7	3
	Arterial switch operation (ASO) and VSD repair	11	4	4	1.4	4	2.6	4
	Arterial switch procedure and VSD repair + aortic arch repair	13	4		2.4	4	4.1	5
	Rastelli	10	4	4	0.9	3	2.6	5
	REV	11	4		1.1	3	1.8	3
	Aortic root translocation (Nikaidoh)	12	4		2.4	4		
Cc TGA	Congenitally corrected TGA repair, Atrial switch and ASO (double switch)	13.8	4	4	3.4	5	2.5	4
	Congenitally corrected TGA repair, Atrial switch and Rastelli	11	4		3.2	5	1.7	3
	Congenitally corrected TGA repair, VSD closure	9	3		0.5	2		
	Congenitally corrected TGA repair, VSD closure and LV to PA conduit	11	4		1.7	4		
DORV	DORV, Intraventricular tunnel repair	10.3	4	3	1.4	4	2	3
DOLV	DOLV repair	11	4		1.4	4		
Truncus	Truncus arteriosus repair	11	4	4	2.4	4	3.4	4
	Truncus + interrupted aortic arch (IAA) repair	15	4	5	5	5	5	5
IAA	Interrupted aortic arch repair	10.8	4	4	2.1	4	3.5	4

Table 4.3 Ten most complex CTA procedures

	STAT mortality	STAT morbidity	Sum M+ m	Aristotle basic score	RACHS 1 score
Shunt, systemic to pulmonary, modified Blalock–Taussig shunt no CBP	4	4	**8**	2	3
Pulmonary atresia – VSD – MAPCA (pseudotruncus) repair	4	4	**8**	4	
Arterial switch operation (ASO) and VSD repair	4	4	**8**	4	4
Rastelli	3	5	**8**	4	4
Congenitally corrected TGA repair, Atrial switch and Rastelli	5	3	**8**	4	
Interrupted aortic arch repair	4	4	**8**	4	4
Truncus arteriosus repair	4	4	**8**	4	4
Arterial switch procedure and VSD repair + aortic arch repair	4	5	**9**	4	
Congenitally corrected TGA repair, Atrial switch and ASO (double switch)	5	4	**9**	4	
Truncus + interrupted aortic arch (IAA) repair	5	5	**10**	4	5

Conclusion

The raw data included in STS-CHSD and EACTS/ECHSA-CHSD show satisfactory results for the group of conotruncal anomalies, with a mean Operative Mortality at 3.6 %, despite a high complexity. Certainly, outcomes other than mortality are important to asses, and efforts are ongoing to use our multi-institutional databases to asses morbidity.

References

1. STS Congenital Heart Surgery Database. http://www.sts.org/sts-national-database/database-managers/congenital-heart-surgery-database.
2. EACTS Congenital Heart Surgery Database. Gold Standard public results on line. http://www.eactscongenitaldb.org/index.php?LANG=en&level=2&struct=14_1.
3. Jenkins KJ, Gauvreau K, Newburger JW, Spray TL, Moller JH, Iezzoni LI. Consensus-based method for risk adjustment for surgery for congenital heart disease. J Thorac Cardiovasc Surg. 2002;123(1):110–8.

4. Lacour-Gayet F, Clarke D, Jacobs J, Comas J, Daebritz S, Daenen W, Gaynor W, Hamilton L, Jacobs M, Maruszewski B, Pozzi M, Spray T, Stellin G, Tchervenkov C, Mavroudis C, Aristotle Committee. The Aristotle score: a complexity-adjusted method to evaluate surgical results. Eur J Cardiothorac Surg. 2004;25:911–24.
5. Comprehensive Aristotle Score. http://www.aristotleinstitute.org/aboutScore.asp.
6. O'Brien SM, Clarke DR, Jacobs JP, Jacobs ML, Lacour-Gayet FG, Pizarro C, Welke KF, Maruszewski B, Tobota Z, Miller WJ, Hamilton L, Peterson ED, Mavroudis C, Edwards FH. An empirically based tool for analyzing mortality associated with congenital heart surgery. J Thorac Cardiovasc Surg. 2009;138:1139–53.
7. Jacobs ML, O'Brien SM, Jacobs JP, Mavroudis C, Lacour-Gayet F, Pasquali SK, Welke K, Pizarro C, Tsai F, Clarke DR. An empirically based tool for analyzing morbidity associated with operations for congenital heart disease. J Thorac Cardiovasc Surg. 2013;145:1046–57.
8. International Pediatric and Congenital Cardiac Code. Available: at http://www.ipccc.net. Accessed December 30, 2013.

Chapter 5
Tetralogy of Fallot: Transventricular Repair, Including Pulmonary Atresia Without MAPCAs

David Kalfa, Paul J. Chai, and Emile Bacha

Abstract Timing and indications of surgical techniques in patients with Tetralogy of Fallot (TOF) remains controversial nowadays. The ideal timing for surgical repair of asymptomatic patients seems to be between 3 and 6–9 months. Severe persistent hypoxemia in neonates constitute an absolute indication to a surgical intervention, managed either by an aorto-pulmonary shunt or by a neonatal complete repair. The surgical techniques described in this chapter focus on all the techniques described to repair a TOF through the right ventricle, with a specific interest in the valve-sparing transventricular repair technique which can include pulmonary valve thinning, commissurotomy, intraoperative balloon dilation, or a patch augmentation of the pulmonary valve. The right ventricle-pulmonary artery connection using a transannular patch in patients with TOF with pulmonary atresia is also described. In contemporary practice, repair of TOF has become a safe procedure with excellent outcomes.

This chapter will focus on the surgical transventricular repair of Tetralogy of Fallot (TOF), including pulmonary atresia (PA) without MAPCAs. The transatrial repair, the palliation with a BT-shunt, the redo surgery and the repair of TOF-PA with main aortopulmonary collateral arteries (MAPCAs), TOF-AVSD and absent pulmonary valve syndrome are treated in other chapters. The valve-sparing transventricular repair technique will be emphasized.

Keywords Tetralogy of Fallot • Pulmonary atresia • Aorto • Pulmonary shunt • Neonatal repair • Transannular patch • Valve • Sparing transventricular repair • Balloon dilation • Pulmonary valve patch augmentation • Right ventricle • Pulmonary artery connection • Abnormal coronary artery

---

D. Kalfa, MD, PhD • P.J. Chai, MD • E. Bacha, MD, FACS (✉)
Division of Cardiac, Thoracic, and Vascular Surgery/Pediatric and Congenital Cardiac Surgery, New York Presbyterian-Columbia University Medical Center/Combined Morgan Stanley Children's Hospital of New York (CHONY) – Komansky Weill-Cornell Program, 3959 Broadway, CHN 274, New York, NY 10032, USA
e-mail: eb2709@columbia.edu

F. Lacour-Gayet et al. (eds.), *Surgery of Conotruncal Anomalies*,
DOI 10.1007/978-3-319-23057-3_5

Anatomy

Anatomy of TOF

The classic components of the Tetralogy of Fallot described by Arthur Fallot [28] in 1888 included: (1) ventricular septal defect (VSD), (2) aortic override, (3) right ventricular outflow tract obstruction (RVOTO) and (4) right ventricle (RV) hypertrophy. Actually, the condition results from a single anatomic abnormality: the anterior and left-ward displacement of the infundibular septum [1]. The borders of the VSD are (1) superiorly: the parietal extent of the infundibular septum, (2) anteriorly: the anterior limb of the septal band, (3) inferiorly: the posterior limb of the septal band, and (4) posteriorly: the anteroseptal leaflet of the tricuspid valve [2]. The VSD can also extend anteriorly under the pulmonary valve when the infundibulary septum is deficient. The course of the bundle of His is the same in TOF and perimembranous VSD: it penetrates at the posteroinferior edge of the VSD. The RVOT is most frequently obstructed at several levels: in the infundibulum in 70 %, at the valvar level in 75 % (annulus and cusps), main pulmonary artery (MPA) in 50 % and at the level of PA branches in 10 % [3]. Hypoplasia of the RV infundibulum directly results from the anterior and left-ward displacement of the infundibular septum. The infundibular obstruction is related to prominent muscle bands that extend from the septal extent of the infundibular septum to the RV free wall. The pulmonary valve often participates to the RVOT through two mechanisms: (1) the annulus is nearly always smaller than normal; (2) the valve leaflets are often thickened, with commissural fusion and tethering to the pulmonary artery wall. The pulmonary valve is bicuspid in 58–66 % of cases [4]. The MPA is often hypoplastic resulting from a long supravalvar stenosis. A hypoplastic MPA does not prejudge of the size of the PA branches that can be normal. The anatomy of PA branches is highly variable, varying from localized narrowing of the origins with post-stenotic dilation to diffuse hypoplasia. Pulmonary atresia is present in 7 % of TOF [5]. Associated anatomic lesions include: abnormal coronary arteries in 2–9 % [6], most often the left anterior descending artery coming from the right coronary artery; multiple VSD in 5 % of patients, most often in the muscular septum; diffusely hypoplastic PA branches; right aortic arch, left superior vena cava, atrial septal defect, patent ductus arteriosus, complete atrio-ventricular canal defect (see Chap. 20), absent pulmonary valve leaflets (see Chap. 20) and aberrant origin of the PA branches.

Anatomy of Pulmonary Atresia-TOF

Pulmonary atresia-TOF is characterized by the lack of luminal continuity between the right ventricle and the pulmonary artery, a marked anterior and leftward displacement of the infundibular septum, which is often fused with the anterior wall of the right ventricle, and a large outlet, malaligned VSD. The pulmonary arterial anatomy is extremely variable, from a vessel that is patent down to the heart, to a fibrous strand between the right ventricle and pulmonary arterial confluence. The anatomy of the PA branches is also variable. In pulmonary atresia-TOF without MAPCAs, the PA branches are usually well developped and supplied from a patent tortuous ductus arteriosus, There can be a stenosis at the origin of the left PA due to abnormal ductal tissue.

Diagnosis and Imaging

The severity of the cyanosis and the timing of presentation of patients with TOF depend on the severity and the predominant mechanism of the RVOTO: – early and constant cyanosis in patients with a fixed hypoplastic RVOTO, – late and variable cyanosis in those with a dynamic muscular infundibular stenosis. Besides gradually progressing cyanosis, cyanotic acute "spells" can occur and lead to profound desaturations. Cyanosis is associated to a characteristic systolic murmur resulting from the RVOTO and the VSD shunt. The EKG shows RV hypertrophy, right axis deviation. Chest x-ray shows a classic "boot-shaped" heart, resulting from elevation of the cardiac apex (RV hypertrophy) and a concave upper left heart border (narrow MPA). The main imaging modality establishing the diagnosis is echocardiography that describes the characteristics of the four components of the "tetrad". Usually, a detailed echocardiogram is all that is needed. Echocardiography can also help in the diagnosis of an abnormal coronary artery crossing the RVOT susceptible to injury from an incision in this area and in the detection of multiple VSDs. The anatomy of distal PA branches is poorly seen on echocardiography and constitutes one of the main indications for cardiac catheterization. Other indications for catheterization, which should not been done systematically, include the precise determination of the anatomy of MAPCAs and the measurement of PA pressure and pulmonary vascular resistance in older patients or those with pulmonary overcirculation related to MAPCAs. Low-radiation CT-scan, coro-scan and MRI are more and more useful to precise the anatomy of the coronary arteries and PA branches while avoiding the drawbacks of the catheterization.

Check List Prior to Surgery

- Detailed evaluation of the RVOT obstruction
  - diameter of the pulmonary valve annulus (z score)
  - morphology of the pulmonary valve leaflets
  - diameter of the pulmonary branches (z score)
- number and location of VSDs
- anatomy of coronary arteries
- presence of ASD
- presence of PDA
- presence of MAPCAs
- side of aortic arch

Surgery: Transventricular Repair of Tetralogy of Fallot

Indications

Timing and indications of surgical techniques in patients with TOF remain controversial nowadays. Most of patients with TOF have a satisfactory saturation at birth and do not require a surgery during the first month of life. Surgical repair is indicated when saturation progressively decreases down to low 80s, high 70s. The preferred timing for surgical repair seems to be between 3 and 6–9 months, according to a recent survey of the Society of Thoracic Surgeons Database [7] that included 3059 operations for TOF (patients with pulmonary atresia were excluded). This study also showed that a ventriculotomy with a transanular patch remains the most prevalent technique, both for primary repair and for repair following palliation, despite contemporary awareness of the late consequences of pulmonary insufficiency. Some groups prefer to favor the transatrial approach in order to avoid any incision of the right ventricle, hoping to limit the risk of long-term RV dysfunction and arrhythmias [8]. Other groups, including our institution, emphasis on sparing the pulmonary valve and the pulmonary annulus in the vast majority of patients, taking into account the deleterious consequences of pulmonary regurgitation on the long-term RV function and incidence of arrhythmias. In our institution, an elective valve-sparing surgical repair is performed typically at approximately 3–6 months of age in asymptomatic patients [9].

So-called “Tet Spells” or severe persistent hypoxemia in neonates constitute an absolute indication to a surgical intervention. The traditional management of these symptomatic patients has been palliation with an aortopulmonary shunt (Blalock–Taussig shunt) [10], but this continues to carry a significant mortality that has remained relatively constant even in the contemporary series [7, 11]. This has led to the promotion of neonatal complete repair [12, 13], as in our own center. Although some literature suggests that this primary neonatal repair strategy is also associated to a higher risk of mortality and morbidity when compared to patients operated after 3 months, especially in patients with low birth weight and small PAs [14], centers with experienced neonatal cardiac surgeons have very good results with neonatal TOF repair [15]. Patients with anomalous abnormal LAD coronary artery crossing the RVOT, significant extracardiac comorbidities, or contraindication to cardiopulmonary bypass still represent good indications to the BT-shunt.

The presence of PA branches hypoplasia is still currently traditionally managed in many centers by an aortopulmonary shunt (Chap. 12). More recently, the opening of the RVOT/connection of the RV to the PA through the creation of a transannular patch using the restrictive floor of the MPA or the left atrial appendage was adopted in many centers [16]. In cases with marked hypoplasia of the pulmonary trunk or atresia, the distal margin of the ventriculotomy can be approximated to the proximal end of the pulmonary arteriotomy. in order to enlarge the continuity of the RVPA connection. The anterior wall can then be reconstructed using a patch sized around a Hegar dilator depending on the patient’s body surface index. This strategy promotes symmetrical PA blood flow and decreases the risk of PA branch distortion by the shunt. Such a transannular patch can be associated to a BT-shunt if the pulmonary flow remains insufficient or to the VSD closure if the distal PA branch anatomy is judged suitable to a primary complete repair.

A new type of palliation based on percutaneous procedures such as PDA stenting [17], balloon dilatation of the pulmonary valve or RVOT stenting [18] may offer an alternative approach to neonatal repair in high-risk neonates and allow for PA growth and delay of repair.

Surgical Technique

Intraoperative transesophageal echocardiogram is systematically performed to assess the anatomy and adequacy of the repair. After median sternotomy or partial lower sternotomy, the heart is inspected from the outside: size of the PAs, abnormal coronary artery, and a “dimple” is often seen on the RVOT. The edges of the infundibulum are marked with 4–0 silk mattress stay sutures, placed several millimeters away from the LAD. A fine polypropylene suture can be placed to mark the exact middle of the PA bifurcation, to orientate the main PA incision. A patent ductus arteriosus, if present, is ligated or clipped.

Standard cardiopulmonary bypass techniques with bicaval cannulation, aortic cross clamping and mild hypothermia (32–34 °C) or normothermia (36–37 °C) are used. The branch PAs are controlled using Vessel Loops© or Heifetz mini-clamps, avoiding any deformation of the PA branches. After the right atriotomy is performed and a left ventricle vent is placed though the PFO, the intracardiac anatomy (borders of the VSD, RVOT muscle bundles) is inspected. Even if the surgeon chooses to do a transventricular repair of TOF and performs an infundibulotomy to treat the RVOTO, the VSD can be closed more easily through the right atrium in some patients, especially in those with a long conal septum.

The VSD will be closed using a patch with either 5–0 Tevdek mattressed pledgeted sutures, or a polypropylene running suture. The closure of the VSD though the RA is detailed in Chap. 7. The closure of the VSD through the RV usually starts at the nadir of the lower border of the VSD. Exposure can be improved by opening a forceps inside the VSD or placing a small retractor in the upper margin. Care must be taken to avoid the inferoposterior edge to avoid the conduction system and it is safer to place the sutures in the base of the tricuspid valve leaflet at that point (Fig. 5.1). Specific attention must be paid to the ventriculo- infundibular fold as this can be the site of troublesome intramural residual VSDs. Finally, the stitches on the upper border of the VSD can be placed transmurally from the outside of the infundibulum if there is little space between the edge of the ventriculotomy and the upper border of the VSD. A running suture can also be very satisfactory since the traction done on the running suture helps with the exposure.

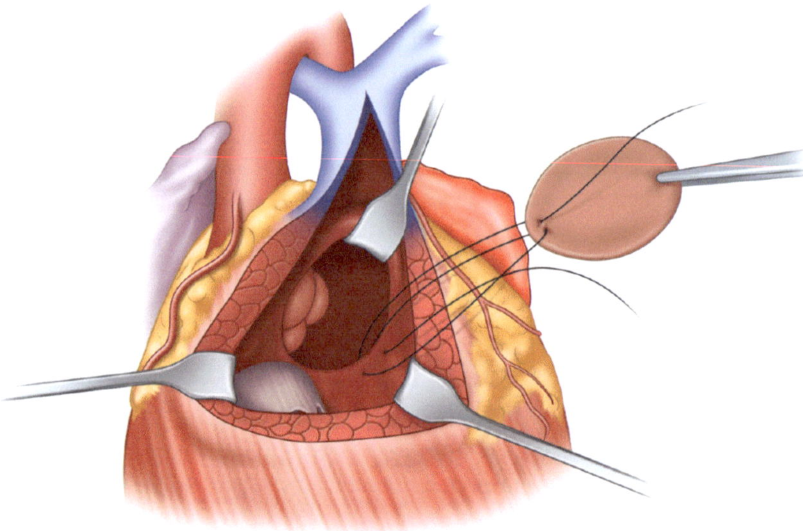

Fig. 5.1 The closure of the VSD through the RV usually starts at the nadir of the lower border of the VSD. Exposure can be improved by opening a forceps inside the VSD or placing a small retractor in the upper margin. Care must be taken to avoid the inferoposterior edge to avoid the conduction system and it is safer to place the sutures in the base of the tricuspid valve leaflet at that point (Reprinted from *Oper Tech Thorac Cardiovasc Surg*, 10(1), Monro, Transventricular repair of tetralogy of Fallot, 45–53, copyright (2005), with permission from Elsevier)

"Classic" Transannular Patch Repair of TOF Without Pulmonary Atresia

A longitudinal incision is made in the infundiblum (around 1.5 cm) stopping a few millimeters below the level of the pulmonary annlus. Obstructing muscle bundles in the RVOT are excised. Muscle trabeculations along the anterior limb of the septal band (trabecula septomarginalis) are divided down to the level of the moderator band. The parietal extent of the infundibular septum can also be excised. Muscle can also be removed from the edges of the infundibulotomy. The pulmonary valve can be inspected from below and some surgeons prefer to do valvar commissurotomy from below instead of opening the main PA. The annulus size is then measured using a Hegar dilator (Fig. 5.2). If the annulus diameter is close to the theoric diameter for the BSA or weight (Rowlatt table), the infundibulotomy is closed using a patch. If the annulus diameter is $<$z-score -2 (or if the RV/LV pressure ratio $>2/3$ after weaning the bypass), the incision is carried upwards through the pulmonary annulus until the bifurcation of the PAs, and a transannular patch is sewn. This transannular patch should not be excessively wide, in order to reduce the long-term deleterious effects of the pulmonary regurgitation. When opening the pulmonary annulus, care should be taken to try to cut the annulus between two cusps (along the anterior commissure) in order to spare the cusps and keep some degree of competency of the cusps. Some centers prefer to use a monocusp valved usually

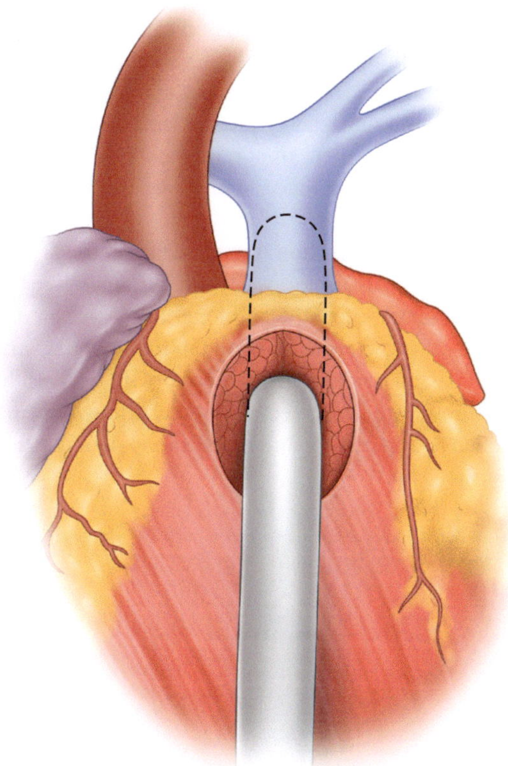

Fig. 5.2 A longitudinal incision is made in the infundiblum (around 1.5 cm) stopping a few millimeters below the level of the pulmonary annlus. The annulus size is then measured using a Hegar dilator (Reprinted from *Oper Tech Thorac Cardiovasc Surg*, 10(1), Monro, Transventricular repair of tetralogy of Fallot, 45–53, copyright (2005), with permission from Elsevier)

constructed of Gore-Tex in order to get a short-term competency of the valve and improve the postoperative course. This transannular patch technique is rarely used in our institution.

Valve-Sparing Repair of TOF Without Pulmonary Atresia

This is the preferred and most commonly used technique in our center. The main pulmonary artery (MPA) is almost always opened and later patched, as it is an easy approach to work on the pulmonary valve compared to the RVOT. It is incised longitudinally using the previously placed distal midpoint suture as a guide in order to avoid any distortion of the distal MPA and proximal LPA. A small infundibular incision (usually 1 cm) is performed at the point of greatest stenosis right below the level of the annulus. This "double-staged" approach allows to treat both supravalvar and infundibular stenoses (Fig. 5.3). The division of the obstructing muscle bundles can also been performed though the tricuspid valve and the pulmonary valve. A detailed analysis of the pulmonary valve anatomy and sinuses, noting the number of cusps, the number of commissures, and planes of the cusp, in particular the anterior cusp, is done. This inspection is more important than the preoperatively measured z score that only informs on the pulmonary annular size and not on valve morphology, repairability, or effective orifice.

Based on this information, a decision is made whether to (1) just perform pulmonary valve thinning and commissurotomy, (2) add intraoperative balloon dilation, or (3) perform a patch augmentation of the pulmonary valve. First, an Amato dilator is passed to measure the effective orifice rather than to dilate the valve. The cusps are thinned out gently, and each commissure is incised with a no. 15 blade down to the medial layers. Measure of the new effective orifice is now done again with Amato dilators. These maneuvers usually gain an additional 1–2 mm in effective orifice

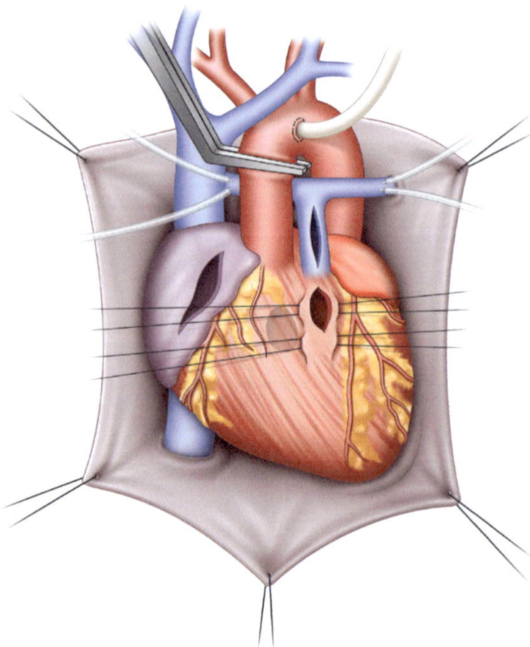

Fig. 5.3 The main pulmonary artery (MPA) is almost always opened and later patched, as it is an easy approach to work on the pulmonary valve compared to the RVOT. It is incised longitudinally using the previously placed distal midpoint suture as a guide in order to avoid any distortion of the distal MPA and proximal LPA. A small infundibular incision (usually 1 cm) is performed at the point of greatest stenosis right below the level of the annulus. These "double-staged" approach allows to treat both supravalvar and infundibular stenoses (Reprinted from *Oper Tech Thorac Cardiovasc Surg*, 18(4), Bacha E, Valve-sparing options in tetralogy of Fallot surgery, 316–27, copyright (2013), with permission from Elsevier)

diameter. Depending on the theoretical pulmonary annular size in relation to the body surface area, a decision is made about whether to stop or proceed with balloon dilation or pulmonary valve patch augmentation. A rough estimate is that if the effective orifice is within 1 mm of expected effective orifice for body surface area, nothing else is done. If the effective orifice is <2 mm from expected, slow and deliberate hand-controlled balloon dilation. Dilation occurs in static position, and the radial transmission of stress imparted by the balloon allows for splitting of commissures as well as dilation and stretching of the annulus (Fig. 5.4). The first balloon size should be the same size as the measured effective orifice after commissurotomy. One can then incrementally increase the balloon size by 1 mm.

If the orifice is still too small, the pulmonary annulus and anterior cusp are divided and a patch augmentation of the pulmonary valve is performed (Fig. 5.5). Such a patch is sutured starting at the edge of the divided anterior cusp on the distal part, and on the endothelial layers of the RVOT incision on the proximal part, to create a pseudo sinus of Valsalva. Another patch is then used to cover the entire RVOT.

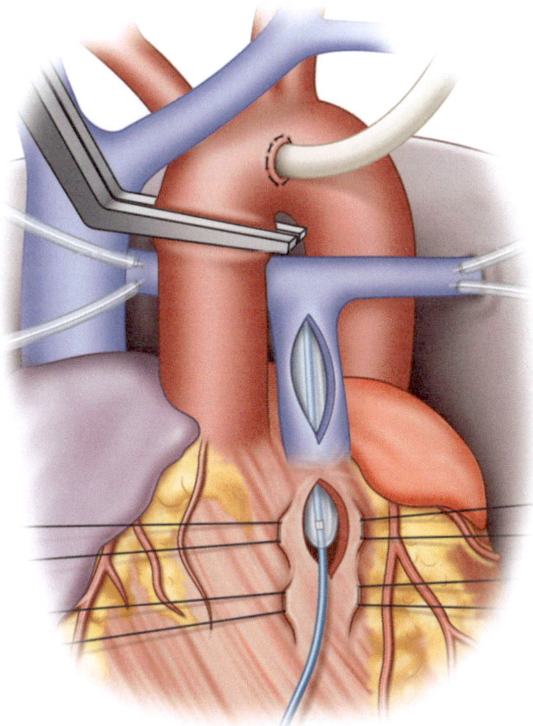

Fig. 5.4 If the effective orifice is <2 mm from expected, slow and deliberate hand-controlled balloon dilation. Dilation occurs in static position, and the radial transmission of stress imparted by the balloon allows for splitting of commissures as well as dilation and stretching of the annulus. The first balloon size should be the same size as the measured effective orifice after commissurotomy. One can then incrementally increase the balloon size by 1 mm (Reprinted from *Oper Tech Thorac Cardiovasc Surg*, 18(4), Bacha E, Valve-sparing options in tetralogy of Fallot surgery, 316–27, copyright (2013), with permission from Elsevier)

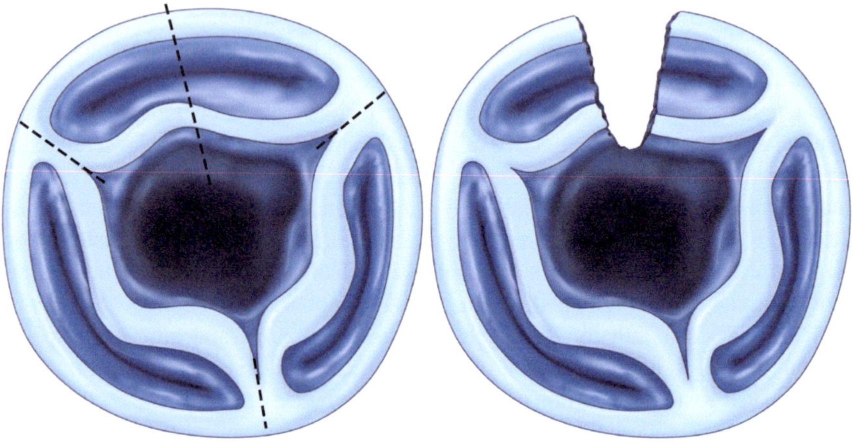

Fig. 5.5 If the orifice is still too small, the pulmonary annulus and anterior cusp are divided and a patch augmentation of the pulmonary valve is performed (Reprinted from *Oper Tech Thorac Cardiovasc Surg*, 18(4), Bacha E, Valve-sparing options in tetralogy of Fallot surgery, 316–27, copyright (2013), with permission from Elsevier)

Repair of TOF with Abnormal Coronary Arteries

The type of surgical technique for a given patient depended on the size of the pulmonary annulus and the exact location of the anomalous coronary artery in relation to the pulmonary annulus. Numerous techniques and surgical strategies were proposed, including the delay of the complete repair using a modified BT-shunt if the patient is symptomatic [19], a transatrial or transatrial-transpulmonary approach [10], a "tailored" right ventriculotomy and reconstruction by patch (below or above the coronary artery or below and above) [20], a RV-PA tube [21], dissection and mobilization of the coronary artery with a patch sewed underneath the coronary artery [22], an anterior translocation of the main pulmonary artery [23, 24], a "double outflow" technique [25],… The precise description of each technique cannot be made here. We would recommend to avoid the use of a conduit as often as possible and advocate the use of the transatrial approach if the size of the RVOT is adequate [6] or the anterior translocation of the main PA if the pulmonary annulus is excessively small.

Surgery: Transventricular Repair of Pulmonary Atresia-Tetralogy of Fallot without MAPCAS

Indications

Decision making largely revolves around whether to repair these patients with pulmonary atresia-TOF without MAPCAS with a one-stage neonatal repair or to stage the repair. The anatomy of the PA branches, evaluated by the Nakata index [29] (sum of the R and L PA cross-sectional areas divided by the BSA) or the McGoon ratio (diameter of the proximal extrapericardial R and L PAs divided by the diameter of the descending thoracic aorta at the diaphragm) can be useful in the decision making. The "traditional" staged repair is based on the confection of a modified BT-shunt (with or without bypass). New approaches of this staged repair can be based on (1) a transannular patch with reapproximation and augmentation of the posterior discontinuity between the RV and the atretic main PA or (2) a percutaneous PDA stenting. Such strategies provide a pulmonary flow in the neonatal period and aim at the growth of the PA branches, while defering the closure of the VSD and reconstruction of the RVOT until the patient is older. In a more recent era, more and more centers favor the one stage primary repair which can be performed with excellent outcomes, and decrease the risk of mortality related to the systemic-to-pulmonary artery shunt operation.

Surgical Technique

Conduit Repair of Tetralogy of Fallot with Pulmonary Atresia

The relief of the infundibular stenosis through a right ventriculotomy is the same as previously described. If the PA confluence is of good size, the vessel is transected horizontally, just cephalad to the atretic part. Different kinds of tubes can be used. We would recommend the use of a homograft if available or a Contegra conduit. The size of the conduit is adapted to the size of the child (often slightly oversized compared to the theoretical pulmonary valve diameter). Some groups also use a non-valved 5–6-mm polytetrafluoroethylene (PTFE) tube graft to connect the RV to the pulmonary bifurcation [16]. Try to place the conduit away from the back of the sternum is useful in order to avoid conduit compression or accidental entry during any future sternotomies, A hood can be needed to complete the RVOT (Fig. 5.6). Patients with moderately hypoplastic or nonconfluent pulmonary arteries can benefit from the enlargement of the central pulmonary artery confluence using a bifurcated pulmonary homograft. Some surgeons frequently patch the left PA branch in order to prevent stenosis at this level.

Transannular Patch for Tetralogy of Fallot with Pulmonary Atresia

Proximal branch pulmonary arteries together with the bifurcation need to be mobilized extensively. A vertical incision of the main PA is performed in continuity with an infundibular incision of 5–10 mm, taking care not to avoid any injury of the coronary arteries. Posterior continuity of the RVPA connection can be performed or augmented using interrupted sutures to approximate margins of the ventriculotomy

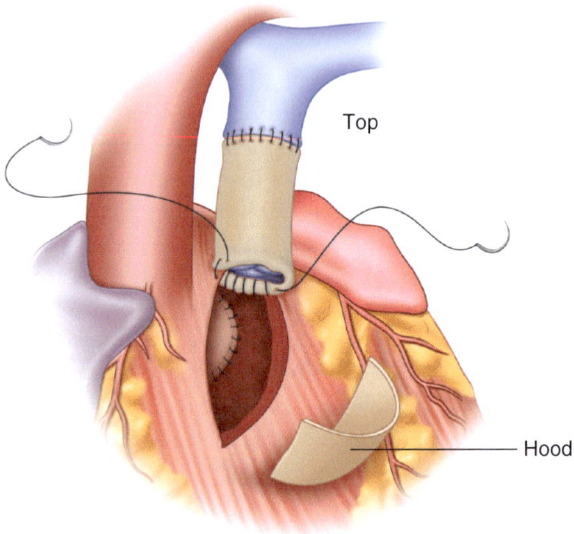

Fig. 5.6 A hood can be needed to complete the RVOT (Reprinted from *Oper Tech Thorac Cardiovasc Surg*, 8(3), van Dorrn C et al., Conduit repair of tetralogy of Fallot with pulmonary atresia, 131–145, copyright (2003), with permission from Elsevier)

and the pulmonary arteriotomy. The anterior wall of the RVOT is then reconstructed using a patch, sized on a Hegar dilator adapted to the theoretical diameter of the pulmonary valve. This technique can be used in TOF-PA with a main PA trunk. If there is no main PA trunk, the left atrial appendage can be used as the floor of the neo-RVOT, in order to avoid the use of a conduit.

Outcomes

In contemporary practice, repair of ToF has become a safe procedure with excellent outcomes. In North America, the STS database has recently published contemporary outcomes for over 3000 ToF repairs between 2002 and 2007 with excellent results of 1.9 % early mortality [7]. But the vast majority of repairs (>93 %) included in this series were performed in infants and older children—not in neonates. Moreover, these results did not include any mortality associated with BT shunts procedures carried out previously.

The results in symptomatic neonates requiring a procedure in the first month of life are not as good. The same STS database report found that during the study period of 2002–2007 there had been 178 neonatal repairs carried out with an early mortality of 7.8 % and that 154 neonates with ToF had undergone BT shunt in the same time period, with a mortality of 6.2 % [7]. The patient weight less than 3.0 kg was an important independent risk factor. Contemporary results in the United Kingdom are similar, with national statistics revealing a 7.5 % mortality from 2006 to 2009.

With increasing follow-up of patients after surgical repair of tetralogy of Fallot, the long-term complications of chronic pulmonary regurgitation, ventricular dilation and myocardial scarring are becoming apparent: exercise intolerance, right heart failure, arrhythmias,… The most common indications for late reoperation are the results of long-term complications of the RVOT, mainly severe pulmonary regurgitation, RVOTO or conduit failure. In addition to symptomatic patients, criteria for valve replacement in the asymptomatic patient continue to evolve and include increased RV size evaluated by magnetic resonance imaging (MRI), progressive or new tricuspid valve regurgitation, severity of pulmonary valve regurgitation, the development of ventricular arrhythmias and/or increased QRS >180 ms [26]. Indications for pulmonary valve replacement [27] will be discussed further in Chap. 20.

References

1. Van Praagh R, Van Praagh S, Nebesar RA, et al. Tetralogy of Fallot: underdevelopment of the pulmonary infundibulum and its sequelae. Am J Cardiol. 1970;26:25–33.
2. Suzuki A, Ho SY, Anderson RH, et al. Further morphologic studies on tetralogy of Fallot, with particular emphasis on the prevalence and structure of the membranous flap. J Thorac Cardiovasc Surg. 1990;99:528–35.
3. Howell CE, Ho SY, Anderson RH, et al. Variations within the fibrous skeleton and ventricular outflow tracts in tetralogy of Fallot. Ann Thorac Surg. 1990;50:450–7.
4. Shimazaki Y, Blackstone EH, Kirklin JW, et al. The dimensions of the right ventricular outflow tract and pulmonary arteries in tetralogy of Fallot and pulmonary stenosis. J Thorac Cardiovasc Surg. 1992;103:692–705.
5. Chiariello L, Meyer J, Wukasch DC, et al. Intracardiac repair of tetralogy of Fallot. Five year review of 403 patients. J Thorac Cardiovasc Surg. 1975;70:529–35.
6. Kalfa DM, Serraf AE, Ly M, et al. Tetralogy of Fallot with an abnormal coronary artery: surgical options and prognostic factors. Eur J Cardiothorac Surg. 2012;42:e34–9.
7. Al Habib HF, Jacobs JP, Mavroudis C, et al. Contemporary patterns of management of tetralogy of Fallot: data from the Society of Thoracic Surgeons Database. Ann Thorac Surg. 2010;90:813–9; discussion 819–20.
8. Luijten LW, van den Bosch E, Duppen N, et al. Long-term outcomes of transatrial-transpulmonary repair of tetralogy of Fallot. Eur J Cardiothorac Surg. 2014.
9. Bacha E. Valve-sparing options in tetralogy of Fallot surgery. Semin Thorac Cardiovasc Surg Pediatr Card Surg Annu. 2012;15:24–6.
10. Karl TR, Sano S, Pornviliwan S, et al. Tetralogy of Fallot: favorable outcome of nonneonatal transatrial, transpulmonary repair. Ann Thorac Surg. 1992;54:903–7.
11. Petrucci O, O'Brien SM, Jacobs ML, et al. Risk factors for mortality and morbidity after the neonatal Blalock-Taussig shunt procedure. Ann Thorac Surg. 2011;92:642–51; discussion 651–42.
12. Pigula FA, Khalil PN, Mayer JE, et al. Repair of tetralogy of Fallot in neonates and young infants. Circulation. 1999;100:II157–61.
13. Hirsch JC, Mosca RS, Bove EL. Complete repair of tetralogy of Fallot in the neonate: results in the modern era. Ann Surg. 2000;232:508–14.

14. Kanter KR, Kogon BE, Kirshbom PM, et al. Symptomatic neonatal tetralogy of Fallot: repair or shunt? Ann Thorac Surg. 2010;89:858–63.
15. Reddy VM, Liddicoat JR, McElhinney DB, et al. Routine primary repair of tetralogy of Fallot in neonates and infants less than three months of age. Ann Thorac Surg. 1995;60:S592–6.
16. Gerelli S, van Steenberghe M, Murtuza B, et al. Neonatal right ventricle to pulmonary connection as a palliative procedure for pulmonary atresia with ventricular septal defect or severe tetralogy of Fallot. Eur J Cardiothorac Surg. 2014;45:278–88; discussion 288.
17. Gibbs JL, Rothman MT, Rees MR, et al. Stenting of the arterial duct: a new approach to palliation for pulmonary atresia. Br Heart J. 1992;67:240–5.
18. Dohlen G, Chaturvedi RR, Benson LN, et al. Stenting of the right ventricular outflow tract in the symptomatic infant with tetralogy of Fallot. Heart. 2009;95:142–7.
19. Hallman GL, Cooley DA, Singer DB. Congenital anomalies of the coronary arteries: anatomy, pathology, and surgical treatment. Surgery. 1966;59:133–44.
20. Hekmat M, Rafieyian S, Foroughi M, et al. Associated coronary anomalies in 135 Iranian patients with tetralogy of Fallot. Asian Cardiovasc Thorac Ann. 2005;13:307–10.
21. Kyger 3rd ER, Chiariello L, Hallman GL, et al. Conduit reconstruction of right ventricular outflow tract. Experience with 17 patients. Ann Thorac Surg. 1975;19:277–88.
22. Bonchek LI. A method of outflow tract reconstruction in tetralogy of Fallot with anomalous anterior descending coronary artery. Ann Thorac Surg. 1976;21:451–3.
23. O'Blenes SB, Freedom RM, Coles JG. Tetralogy of Fallot with anomalous LAD: repair without conduit. Ann Thorac Surg. 1996;62:1186–8.
24. Tchervenkov CI, Pelletier MP, Shum-Tim D, et al. Primary repair minimizing the use of conduits in neonates and infants with tetralogy or double-outlet right ventricle and anomalous coronary arteries. J Thorac Cardiovasc Surg. 2000;119:314–23.
25. Dandolu BR, Baldwin HS, Norwood Jr WI, et al. Tetralogy of Fallot with anomalous coronary artery: double outflow technique. Ann Thorac Surg. 1999;67:1178–80.
26. Gatzoulis MA, Balaji S, Webber SA, et al. Risk factors for arrhythmia and sudden cardiac death late after repair of tetralogy of Fallot: a multicentre study. Lancet. 2000;356:975–81.
27. Geva T. Repaired tetralogy of Fallot: the roles of cardiovascular magnetic resonance in evaluating pathophysiology and for pulmonary valve replacement decision support. J Cardiovasc Magn Reson. 2011;13:9.
28. Fallot A. Contribution à l'anatomie pathologique de la maladie bleue (cyanose cardiaque). Mars Med. 1888;25:77–93.
29. Nakata S, Imai Y, Takanashi Y, Kurosawa H, Tezuka K, Nakazawa M, Ando M, Takao A. A new method for the quantitative standardization of cross-sectional area of the pulmonary arteries in congenital heart diseases with decreased pulmonary blood flow. J Thorac Cardiovasc Surg. 1984;88:610–9.

Chapter 6
Transatrial Repair of Tetralogy of Fallot

Jennifer C. Hirsch-Romano, Richard G. Ohye, Ming-Sing Si, and Edward L. Bove

Abstract Tetralogy of Fallot (TOF) is one of the most common congenital cardiac malformations and consists of: (1) ventricular septal defect (VSD), (2) right ventricular outflow tract obstruction (RVOTO), (3) aortic override, and (4) right ventricular hypertrophy (RVH). The initial presentation of the patient with TOF is variable and dependent on the degree of right ventricular outflow tract obstruction. In most children with TOF, elective complete repair is recommended preferably by 3–6 months of age. Single-stage complete repair is performed in most large centers with excellent results. The surgical repair of TOF can be performed via a transatrial or transventricular approach to the VSD and the RVOT. The transatrial repair allows excellent visualization of both the VSD and the obstructive muscle bundles within the RVOT while avoiding an incision on the right ventricle. For patients requiring a transannular patch to relieve pulmonary stenosis, the transatrial approach allows for minimal extension of the incision onto the infundibulum as the ventriculotomy is not used for the VSD closure. By avoiding a ventriculotomy, short and long-term impairment of ventricular function can be minimized.

Keywords Tetralogy of Fallot • Transatrial repair • Pulmonary stenosis • Right ventricular outflow tract obstruction • Malalignment ventricular septal defect • Aortic override • Infundibulum

Introduction

Tetralogy of Fallot (TOF) is the most common complex congenital heart defect, with an estimated incidence of 3.3 per 10,000 live births [1]. The first complete description of TOF was published in 1888 by the French physician Etienne Fallot [2]. It was not until 1945, however, that the first surgical treatment for TOF was performed by Alfred Blalock at Johns Hopkins University [3].

J.C. Hirsch-Romano, MD, MS (✉) • R.G. Ohye, MD • M.-S. Si, MD • E.L. Bove, MD
Department of Cardiac Surgery, Section of Pediatric Cardiovascular Surgery, C. S. Mott Children's Hospital and Michigan Congenital Heart Center, University of Michigan, Ann Arbor, MI 48109, USA
e-mail: jhirsch@med.umich.edu

F. Lacour-Gayet et al. (eds.), *Surgery of Conotruncal Anomalies*,
DOI 10.1007/978-3-319-23057-3_6

This landmark operation ushered in the era of surgery for congenital heart defects. A number of innovative systemic-to-pulmonary artery shunt procedures were soon described followed by the first successful intracardiac repair using human cross-circulation by Lillehei and Varco at the University of Minnesota in 1954 [4]. Numerous contributions have been made in the management of TOF since these initial pioneering efforts, which has led to a long-term survival rate approaching 90 % [5]. For the majority of patients, primary complete repair in infancy via a transatrial or transventricular approach is now the standard of care.

Anatomy

The classic components of the "tetrad" that comprise this defect are a ventricular septal defect (VSD), right ventricular outflow tract obstruction (RVOTO), aortic override, and right ventricular hypertrophy (RVH) (Fig. 6.1). All of these individual components result from one basic morphologic abnormality: anterior and leftward displacement of the infundibular, or conal, septum [6]. The VSD in

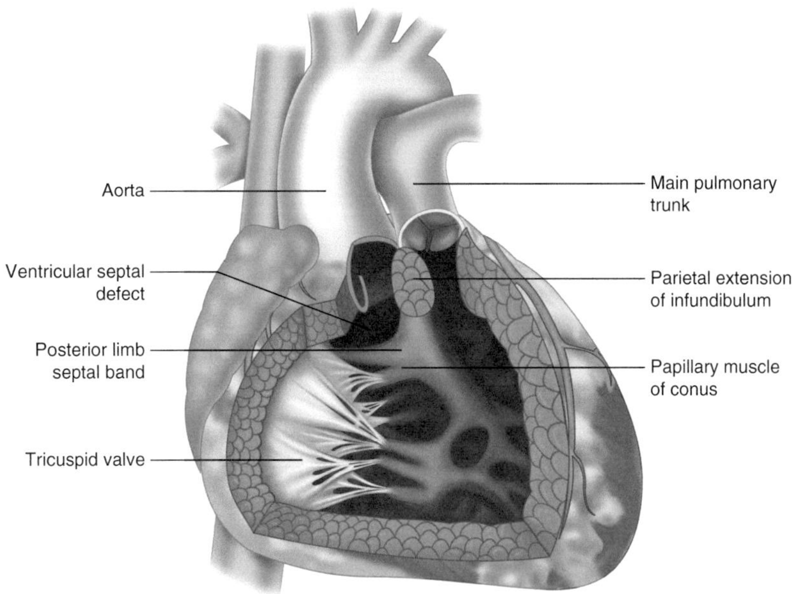

Fig. 6.1 Anatomy of TOF with a nonrestrictive VSD with aortic override, the papillary muscle of the conus along with the parietal and septal which result in RVOTO, and a hypoplastic pulmonary valve and main pulmonary artery trunk. *Ao* aorta, *TV* tricuspid valve, *VSD* ventricular septal defect, *MPT* main pulmonary trunk (Hirsch and Bove [22])

TOF is a large, nonrestrictive defect that results from malalignment of the leftward or septal extent of the infundibular septum with the septal band. The bundle of His penetrates at the posteroinferior edge of the defect. Although the VSD is generally subaortic in position, it may extend to the subpulmonary region when the infundibular septum is absent or deficient. Additional VSDs may exist in approximately 5 % of patients and generally occur in the muscular septum.

The anterior and leftward displacement of the infundibular septum also results in RVOTO from hypoplasia of the right ventricular infundibulum. The pulmonary valve (PV) is nearly always involved in the obstruction. The leaflets may be thickened and tethered to the pulmonary artery wall. The PV is bicuspid in approximately 2/3 of patients, but it is the narrowest part of the outflow tract in only a small minority of patients. The "annulus" of the PV, although not a true fibrous structure, is nearly always hypoplastic.

Important degrees of obstruction may also occur at the level of the right and left branch pulmonary arteries. Hypoplasia of one or both branches may be seen. Uncommonly, the left pulmonary artery may take origin from the ductus arteriosus and its intrapericardial portion may be completely absent. More commonly, localized narrowing of the origin of the right or left pulmonary arteries will be present. In extreme cases of anterior displacement of the infundibular septum, complete atresia of the distal right ventricular infundibulum and main pulmonary artery trunk may result. Pulmonary atresia is present in approximately 7 % of patients with TOF [7]. Multiple aortopulmonary collateral arteries (MAPCAs) are usually found in those patients with pulmonary atresia without an associated patent ductus arteriosus (PDA). These MAPCAs provide a variable degree of the pulmonary blood flow.

Aortic override is caused by dextroposition of the aortic root and results in a biventricular origin of the aorta. Continuity between the aortic and mitral valves is nearly always present even in extreme degrees of override. Double outlet right ventricle is considered to exist with TOF when the right ventricle supports 90 % or more of the aorta.

The origin of the left anterior descending (LAD) coronary artery from the right coronary artery (RCA) occurs in approximately 3–5 % of patients with TOF [8]. The LAD will cross the RVOT a short distance below the PV annulus to reach the anterior interventricular septum and is susceptible to injury from an incision in this area. Other important coronary artery patterns include a dual LAD distribution with the lower half of the septum supplied from the RCA and the upper half from the left coronary artery along with the presence of large right ventricular conal branches. Rarely, a single RCA gives rise to the left main coronary artery (LMCA), which then crosses the RVOT.

Major associated cardiac defects are relatively uncommon in TOF. The most frequently associated lesions are atrial septal defect (ASD), PDA, complete atrioventricular septal defect, and multiple VSDs. Other less common defects include persistent left superior vena cava, anomalous origin of the left anterior descending coronary artery, and aberrant origin of the right or left pulmonary artery.

Diagnosis and Imaging

Cyanosis is the main physical finding. The first heart sound is normal, but the second sound is often single due to an inaudible pulmonary component resulting from the low pulmonary artery pressure and the anterior location of the aorta that may obscure the soft pulmonary closure sound. The characteristic systolic murmur results from the RVOTO and is usually moderate in intensity. Typically the murmur disappears in the presence of a hypercyanotic "tet" spell.

The characteristic electrocardiographic finding is that of RVH from pressure overload of the right ventricle. Right axis deviation will also be found. On chest radiograph, the heart size is generally normal and the pulmonary artery segment may be small. The aortic arch is right-sided in approximately 25 % of patients. The characteristic "boot shaped" heart results from elevation of the cardiac apex from the hypertrophied right ventricle and a concave upper left heart border caused by a narrow main pulmonary artery.

The diagnosis is generally established by echocardiography (ECHO) [9]. The typical malalignment VSD with aortic override and RVOTO is well visualized. Often the location of the LAD can be visualized as well. If the anatomy of the peripheral pulmonary arteries is not well seen, cardiac MRI or catheterization can be useful for clarification. In the majority of patients, diagnostic cardiac catheterization is not necessary. Catheterization is more commonly used for interventional procedures before and after TOF repair to address branch pulmonary artery stenoses. In the rare instance when the coronary artery anatomy is not well delineated by ECHO, cardiac catheterization may be of benefit however visual inspection by the surgeon at the time of operation is usually sufficient.

Checklist for Surgical Repair

The surgical repair of tetralogy of Fallot is relatively straightforward in the majority of patients. Specific anatomic variations, however, can significantly impact the surgical repair as well as long-term surgical needs. Listed below are the necessary anatomic details that need to be considered prior to embarking on complete surgical repair.

1. Prior palliative operations: systemic to pulmonary artery shunt, branch pulmonary artery augmentation
2. Anatomy of the VSD, any additional VSDs
3. Degree and level of RVOTO
4. Nature and size of the pulmonary valve annulus size
5. Size and distribution of branch pulmonary arteries
6. Coronary artery distribution
7. Presence of an atrial level shunt
8. Any associated defects

Surgical Approach

Standard cardiac anesthesia with high dose narcotics and paralysis is employed during operation. Severe hypoxemic spells can be precipitated by the decrease in SVR caused by inhaled anesthetics. Therefore, care is taken to avoid significant changes in systemic as well as pulmonary vascular resistance that may increase the right-to-left (R–L) shunt. Should important hypoxemia occur, α-agonist drugs are recommended to increase SVR and minimize the R–L shunt. In the rare case of a refractory spell, emergent sternotomy and initiation of cardiopulmonary bypass (CPB) may be required. Standard bicaval cannulation is employed for all repairs with mild hypothermia (32–34 °C). The left ventricle is vented through the right superior pulmonary vein.

After initiation of CPB, all shunts are ligated and/or divided, the main pulmonary trunk and bifurcation (if branch stenoses are present) are mobilized, and the PDA is ligated if necessary. The coronary anatomy is evaluated by direct visual inspection in case a transannular patch is required. After the aortic cross-clamp is applied and the cardioplegic solution is administered, a right atriotomy is made to assess the anatomy. If an atrial septal defect or patent foramen ovale is present, it is closed at this time. In neonates with a patent foramen ovale only, it is left open to allow for a limited degree of right-to-left shunting helping to maintain the systemic output early after repair, although at the expense of mild systemic desaturation. The anatomy of the VSD and RVOTO is viewed from the tricuspid valve (Fig. 6.2). A retractor placed anteriorly through the tricuspid valve aids in the exposure of the distal outflow tract (Fig. 6.3). When the repair is accomplished entirely through the right atrial approach, as is preferred at the University of Michigan, the outflow tract obstruction is approached first. Traction sutures placed in the anterior and septal leaflets of the tricuspid valve facilitate exposure of the VSD and distal infundibulum. The position of the anterior margin of the VSD and the aortic valve leaflets are noted, and the parietal extent of the anterosuperiorly malpositioned infundibular septum is visualized. Invaginating the right ventricular free wall with a finger placed from outside the heart facilitates this exposure. Muscle trabeculations along the anterior limb of the septal band are divided down to the level of the moderator band if necessary (Figs. 6.4 and 6.5). When repair is performed in infancy, excision of the parietal extent of the infundibular septum is almost never necessary and simple division of the obstructing muscle bundles is all that is required.

Closure of the VSD is accomplished from the transatrial approach regardless of whether or not a transannular patch is needed, as that allows the ventricular extent of the incision to be minimized to the length necessary only for relief of obstruction, not for VSD exposure. Visualization of the VSD is generally adequate through the tricuspid valve and is facilitated by dividing the obstructing right ventricular muscle bundles first (Fig. 6.5). A patch of PTFE is cut to the appropriate size and sutured to the right side of the septum utilizing a continuous-suture technique (Fig. 6.6). Suturing is commenced at the angle between the anterior and posterior limbs of the septal band, directly opposite the perimembra-

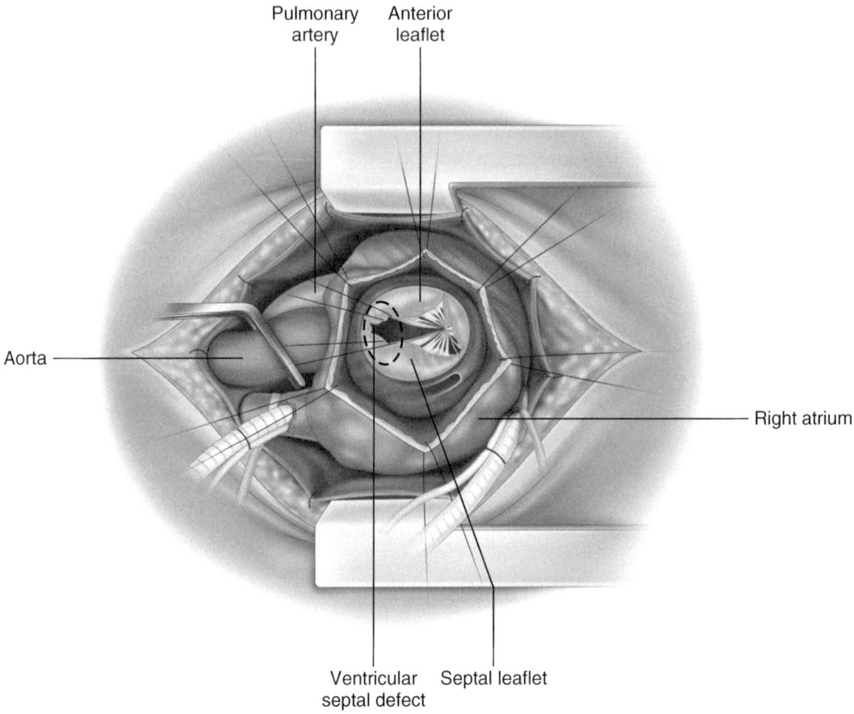

Fig. 6.2 The surgical anatomy as viewed through a right atriotomy with standard bicaval cannulation. The free edge of the atrial wall is retracted with sutures. The location of the VSD is denoted by the dashed line. Stay sutures are placed in the septal and anterior leaflets of the TV for retraction. *Ao* aorta, *PA* pulmonary artery, *RA* right atrium, *VSD* ventricular septal defect, *SL* septal leaflet, *AL* anterior leaflet (Hirsch and Bove [22])

nous rim, and begun superiorly over the infundibular septum and aortic valve. The sutures are kept close to the aortic valve annulus itself to avoid residual defects in muscle trabeculations. This initial arm of the suture is brought into the right atrium by passing the needle through the annulus of the tricuspid valve at its junction with the ventriculoinfundibular fold. The other needle is then brought inferiorly, past the medial papillary muscle and under any chordae tendinae from the septal leaflet, until the posteroinferior rim of the defect is reached. At this point suturing is done approximately 5 mm away from the crest of the VSD itself and only on the right ventricular side. This is done in order not to injure the A-V node or bundle of His which penetrate the floor of the atrial septum in the apex of the triangle of Koch and pass adjacent to this margin of the VSD. Attaching the patch to the base of the septal leaflet of the tricuspid valve over the penetrating bundle completes suturing.

A pulmonary valvotomy can now be performed through the right atrial approach. If exposure is not adequate, a vertical incision is made in the main pulmonary artery through which a pulmonary valvotomy may be performed. Valve

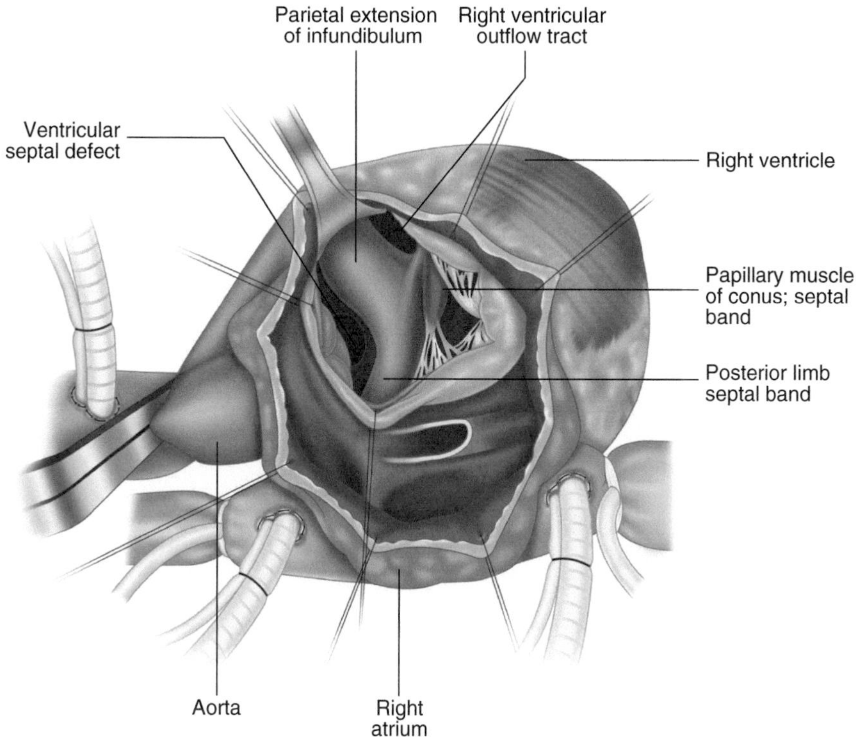

Fig. 6.3 The tricuspid valve leaflets have been retracted and a single valve retractor is placed to aid exposure. The inferior margin of the VSD can be seen superior to the posterior limb of the septal band. *Ao* aorta, *RA* right atrium, *VSD* ventricular septal defect, *RVOT* right ventricular outflow tract, *RV* right ventricle (Hirsch and Bove [22])

leaflets may be mobilized and fused commissures divided all the way to the pulmonary artery wall. At this time, an assessment of the diameter of the PV annulus is made by inserting calibrated dilators across the PV. In select patients (no unicusp valve, PV Z-score ≥ -3), a valve-preserving technique is an option. PV commissurotomy may be followed by high-pressure balloon dilation of the pulmonary valve annulus after complete relief of RVOTO. Early results of balloon dilation are encouraging [10].

The decision to place a transannular patch is made if the estimated post-repair RV/LV pressure is predicted to exceed 0.7. In this situation the main pulmonary artery incision is extended onto the RVOT across the PV annulus (Fig. 6.7). It can be kept quite short, extending only a few millimeters proximal to the annulus, as the infundibular obstruction has been adequately relieved transatrially. Whenever possible, this incision is placed directly through the anterior commissure of the valve to allow the pulmonary valve leaflets to remain functional and decrease the amount of pulmonary regurgitation. It is often possible to limit the incision such that it remains superior to an anomalous LAD when a transatrial repair is done.

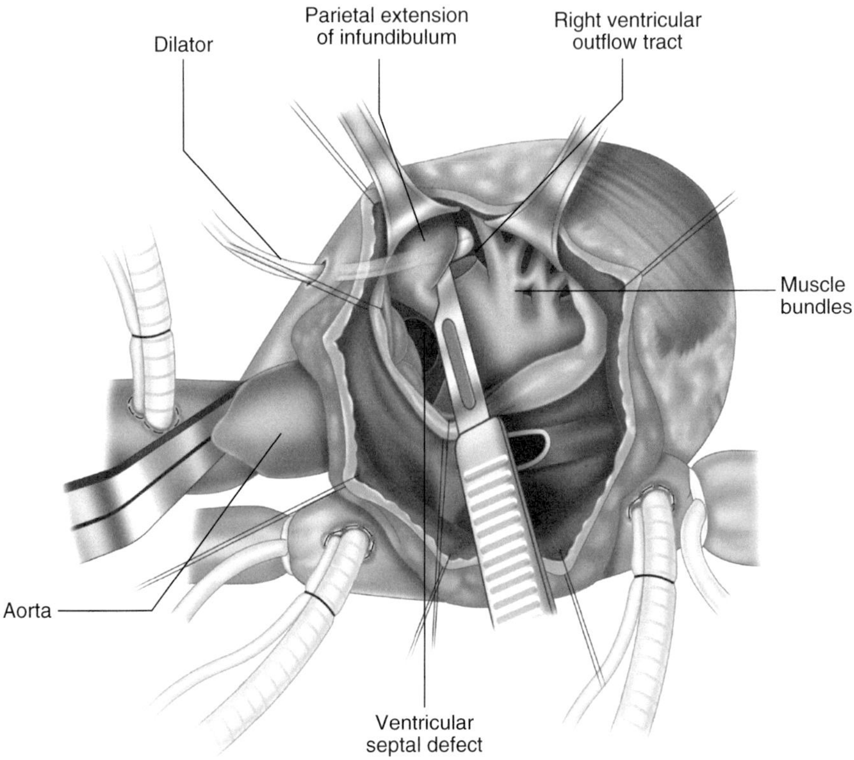

Fig. 6.4 A dilator placed through the pulmonary annulus delineates the course of the RVOT. The parietal extension of the infundibulum is visible at the tip of the dilator. The parietal extension is divided. *Ao* aorta, *VSD* ventricular septal defect, *RVOT* right ventricular outflow tract (Hirsch and Bove [22])

Upon completion of systemic rewarming, CBP is discontinued in the usual fashion and the hemodynamics are assessed for important residual lesions. The peak RV/LV pressure ratio is measured to ensure that significant residual RVOTO does not persist. If the post repair RV/LV pressure is in excess of 0.7 and a transannular patch has not been placed, bypass is resumed and a patch is inserted across the PV annulus. If a transannular patch has been placed, other causes of persistent elevation of right ventricular pressure must be considered, including branch pulmonary artery stenoses, hypoplastic peripheral pulmonary arteries, residual VSD, or residual infundibular obstruction. Often this elevation in right ventricular pressure can result from dynamic RVOTO, particularly when an outflow patch is avoided, as in the case of a transatrial repair. Administration of an ultra-short acting beta-blocking agent such as Esmolol can help to differentiate dynamic versus fixed residual right ventricular outflow tract obstruction intraoperatively.

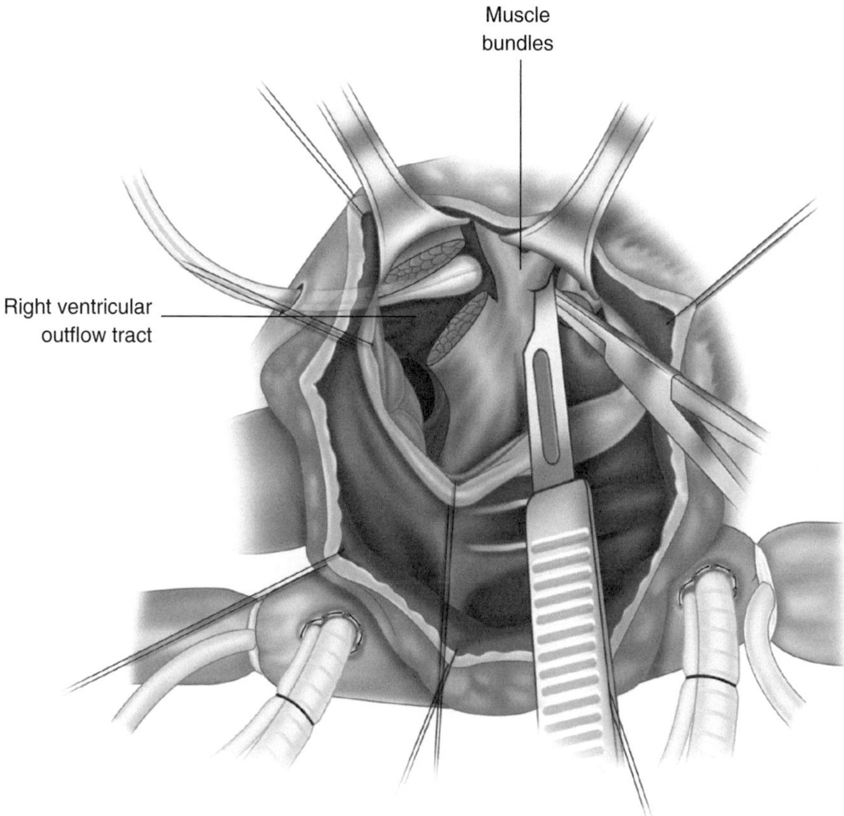

Fig. 6.5 Division of the obstructing muscle bundles along the anterior limb of the septal band. Division of these muscle bundles is usually sufficient to relieve the outflow tract obstruction. *RVOT* right ventricular outflow tract (Hirsch and Bove [22])

Results

The national 30-day mortality after repair of TOF is between 0.3 and 1 % depending on type of repair as reported in the Society of Thoracic Surgeons Congenital Heart Surgery Database [11]. Although most children undergoing TOF repair have a short ICU stay including early extubation, some patients will experience low cardiac output syndrome (LCOS) and may require prolonged inotropic support. Seen in approximately 25 % of infants with congenital heart disease who have any type of cardiac surgery, LCOS is characterized by signs of decreased systemic perfusion and is a risk factor for increased length of stay and post-operative morbidity and mortality [12]. Typically LCOS presents as tachycardia, oliguria, and metabolic acidosis. Among patients undergoing repair of TOF, approximately 1/3 will experience LCOS due to RV diastolic dysfunction, or "restrictive RV physiology" [13].

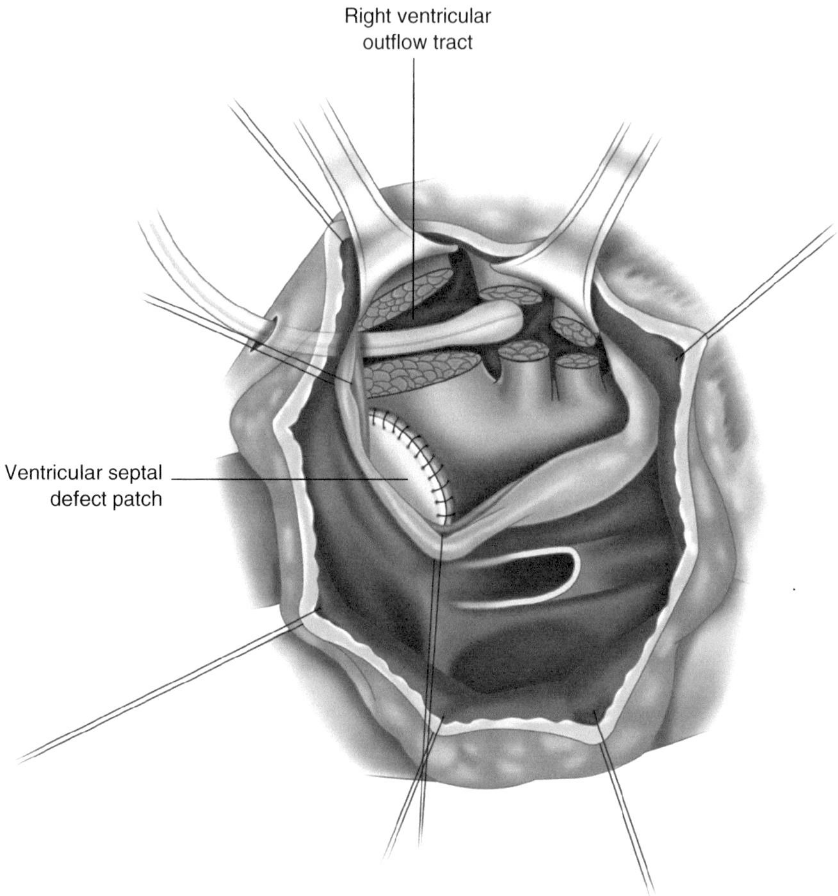

Fig. 6.6 View through the right atriotomy and TV following patch closure of the VSD. The ends of the divided muscle bundles can be visualized. *RVOT* right ventricular outflow tract, *VSD* ventricular septal defect (Hirsch and Bove [22])

Preoperative RVH, myocardial injury and edema after right ventriculotomy, arrhythmias, and residual anatomic lesions such as VSD, RVOTO, tricuspid regurgitation, and/or free pulmonary insufficiency (PI) may exacerbate the clinical presentation. Our preference for a transatrial repair reduces the potential for injury and subsequent impaired function of the RV in the post-operative period. In postoperative patients with LCOS, repeat bedside echocardiography is useful to rule out clinically significant residual anatomic lesions. Children with RV diastolic dysfunction require elevated RA pressures for adequate RV filling in diastole. Without an atrial-level communication, this situation leads to high central venous pressure, which can cause hepatic congestion, ascites, and pleural effusions [13]. Decreased RV filling leads to decreased LV preload and resultant low cardiac output. An atrial

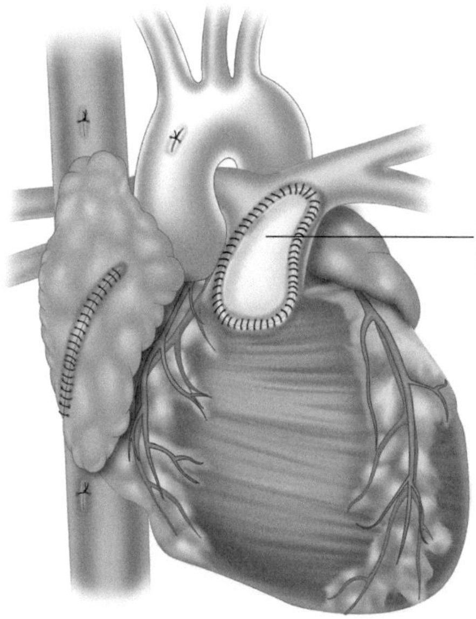

Fig. 6.7 The appearance of a transannular patch used to enlarge a hypoplastic PV annulus and main pulmonary trunk. The proximal extent of the patch on the RVOT should be kept as short as possible (Hirsch and Bove [22])

fenestration can decompress the right atrium via a R-L shunt that can help augment cardiac output, albeit at the expense of lower oxygen saturation.

Cullen et al. [13] showed that in patients with RV diastolic dysfunction, the non-compliant RV acts more like a passive conduit than a compliant chamber and results in antegrade diastolic flow into the pulmonary arteries during atrial systole. This flow pattern, though abnormal, is an important contributor to cardiac output in these patients. They also note that cardiac output is adversely affected by both the loss of sinus rhythm and the inspiratory phase of mechanical ventilation [13]. These findings have important implications for postoperative management. In particular, maintenance of low mean airway pressures and early (within 24 hours of ICU admission) extubation should be goals. Use of temporary pacing is recommended if there is a loss of AV synchrony. The incidence of complete heart block following tetralogy repair requiring permanent pacemaker is less than 1 %. The management of LCOS may also require inotropic support with dopamine, epinephrine, and milrinone infusions and sedation and neuromuscular blockade in refractory cases.

Junctional ectopic tachycardia (JET) is a rapid, catecholamine-sensitive, and self-limited arrhythmia that occurs in 4–22 % of patients following TOF repair [14]. The onset is typically within the first 24 hours postoperatively. At the University of Michigan, an algorithm for the management of JET includes correction of electrolyte derangements, sedation, decreasing catecholanergics, systemic cooling to 34–35° C, and amiodarone infusion with temporary epicardial pacing as necessary.

After repair of TOF, 6–10 % of patients will require reoperation [15]. A review of the University of Michigan TOF patients undergoing complete repair in the first month of life demonstrated 1-month, 1-year, and 5-year freedom from reoperation rates of 100 %, 89 %, and 58 %, respectively [16]. Most common indications for reoperation are: residual or recurrent VSD, recurrent RVOT obstruction or aneurysm formation, conduit failure, and severe PI or PS [15, 16].

The exact amount of residual RV outflow tract obstruction required for reoperation is controversial, but when RV pressure exceeds 2/3–3/4 systemic, relief of residual obstruction is generally indicated. An intraoperative pressure ratio between the right and left ventricles, at the time of initial repair, of 0.75 or greater is an independent risk factor for reoperation [17]. Overall survival and functional status following reoperation is very good with a 10 year actuarial survival of 92 % with 93 % of these patients in a New York Heart Association classification of I or II [18].

Long-standing PI, due to PV abnormalities or the need for a transannular patch, is associated with significant complications after the second postoperative decade. These include exercise intolerance, right heart failure, arrhythmia, and sudden death [19]. Two recent large studies of patients 30 years after TOF repair revealed that the annualized risk of death more than triples during the third postoperative decade (increasing from .27 to .95 %) [15, 20]. The observation that pulmonary valve replacement (PVR) in symptomatic patients late after TOF repair did not necessarily lead to functional recovery has supported replacement of the pulmonary valve before the onset of symptoms in many cases [21].

References

1. Eldadah ZA, Hamosh A, Biery NJ, Montgomery RA, Duke M, Elkins R, Dietz HC. Familial tetralogy of Fallot caused by mutation in the jagged1 gene. Hum Mol Genet. 2001;10:163–9.
2. Fallot ELA. Contribution a l'anatomie pathologique de la maladie bleue (cyanose cardiaque). Mars Med. 1888;25:77.
3. Blalock A, Taussig HB. The surgical treatment of malformation of the heart in which there is pulmonary stenosis or pulmonary atresia. JAMA. 1945;128:189.
4. Lillehei CW, Cohen M, Warden HE, Read RC, Aust JB, Dewall RA, Varco RL. Direct vision intracardiac surgical correction of the tetralogy of fallot, pentalogy of fallot, and pulmonary atresia defects; report of first ten cases. Ann Surg. 1955;142:418–42.
5. Lindberg HL, Saatvedt K, Seem E, Hoel T, Birkeland S. Single-center 50 years' experience with surgical management of tetralogy of fallot. Eur J Cardiothorac Surg. 2011;40:538–42.
6. Van Praagh R, Van Praagh S, Nebesar RA, Muster AJ, Sinha SN, Paul MH. Tetralogy of fallot: underdevelopment of the pulmonary infundibulum and its sequelae. Am J Cardiol. 1970;26:25–33.
7. Chiariello L, Meyer J, Wukasch DC, Hallman GL, Cooley DA. Intracardiac repair of tetralogy of fallot. Five-year review of 403 patients. J Thorac Cardiovasc Surg. 1975;70:529–35.
8. Humes RA, Driscoll DJ, Danielson GK, Puga FJ. Tetralogy of fallot with anomalous origin of left anterior descending coronary artery. Surgical options. J Thorac Cardiovasc Surg. 1987;94:784–7.
9. McConnell ME. Echocardiography in classical tetralogy of fallot. Semin Thorac Cardiovasc Surg. 1990;2:2–11.
10. Vida VL, Padalino MA, Maschietto N, Biffanti R, Anderson RH, Milanesi O, Stellin G. The balloon dilation of the pulmonary valve during early repair of tetralogy of fallot. Catheter Cardiovasc Interv. 2012;80:915–21.
11. Data Analyses of the Society of Thoracic Surgeons Congenital Heart Surgery Database. Period ending 6/30/2014:110.

12. Rajagopal SK, Thiagarajan RR. Perioperative care of children with tetralogy of Fallot. Curr Treat Options Cardiovasc Med. 2011;13:464–74.
13. Cullen S, Shore D, Redington A. Characterization of right ventricular diastolic performance after complete repair of tetralogy of fallot. Restrictive physiology predicts slow postoperative recovery. Circulation. 1995;91:1782–9.
14. Hoffman TM, Bush DM, Wernovsky G, Cohen MI, Wieand TS, Gaynor JW, Spray TL, Rhodes LA. Postoperative junctional ectopic tachycardia in children: incidence, risk factors, and treatment. Ann Thorac Surg. 2002;74:1607–11.
15. Nollert G, Fischlein T, Bouterwek S, Bohmer C, Klinner W, Reichart B. Long-term survival in patients with repair of tetralogy of fallot: 36-year follow-up of 490 survivors of the first year after surgical repair. J Am Coll Cardiol. 1997;30:1374–83.
16. Hirsch JC, Mosca RS, Bove EL. Complee repair of tetralogy of Fallot in the neonate: results in the modern era. Ann Surg. 2000;232:508–14.
17. Hennein HA, Mosca RS, Urcdlay G, Crowley DC, Bove EL. Intermediate results after complete repair of tetralogy of Fallot in neonates. J Thorac Cardiovasc Surg. 1995;109:332–42.
18. Oechslin EN, Harrison DA, Harris L, Downar E, Webb GD, Siu SS, Williams WG. Reoperation in adults with repair of tetralogy of fallot: indications and outcomes. J Thorac Cardiovasc Surg. 1999;118:245–51.
19. Burchill LJ, Wald RM, Harris L, Colman JM, Silversides CK. Pulmonary valve replacement in adults with repaired tetralogy of fallot. Semin Thorac Cardiovasc Surg Pediatr Card Surg Annu. 2011;14:92–7.
20. Murphy JG, Gersh BJ, Mair DD, Fuster V, McGoon MD, Ilstrup DM, McGoon DC, Kirklin JW, Danielson GK. Long-term outcome in patients undergoing surgical repair of tetralogy of fallot. N Engl J Med. 1993;329:593–9.
21. Therrien J, Siu SC, McLaughlin PR, Liu PP, Williams WG, Webb GD. Pulmonary valve replacement in adults late after repair of tetralogy of fallot: are we operating too late? J Am Coll Cardiol. 2000;36:1670–5.
22. Hirsch JC, Bove EL. Tetralogy of Fallot. In: Mavroudis C, Backer CL, editors. Pediatric cardiac surgery. 3rd ed. Philadelphia: Mosby; 2003.

Chapter 7
Tetralogy of Fallot: Management of the Pulmonary Valve

James A. Quintessenza

Abstract Repair of TOF can be accomplished with low mortality and excellent long-term survival. Event free survival however remains a significant problem. Long-term procedural risks related to right ventricular outflow tract obstruction or more importantly right ventricular dilatation, dysfunction and arrhythmia related to chronic pulmonary insufficiency, continue to affect our patients. Adequate relief of right ventricular outflow tract obstruction with emphasis on preserving a functional right ventricle as well as valve preservation strategies at the time of surgical repair, are recommended. A precise evaluation of the anatomy and technical readiness to perform valve-preserving procedures are essential for the surgeon. Inferences from long term data out to 50 years support these concepts.

Keywords Tetralogy of Fallot • Pulmonary valve morphology • Pulmonary valve sparing surgery • Pulmonary regurgitation

Introduction

The repair of the child with Tetralogy of Fallot (TOF), transforming the "blue baby" into a pink one, remains one of the most amazing accomplishments of modern medicine. As one of the most common forms of congenital heart disease, many advances have been made over the years, yet many challenges persist. One of the more central challenges to these patients is the management of the pulmonary valve and its effect on both the short and long-term lives of these patients. This chapter will attempt to explore some of these challenges and provide insights into options for therapy and their effect on surgical outcomes.

J.A. Quintessenza, MD
Division of Cardiac Surgery, Department of Cardiovascular Surgery, Johns Hopkins All Children's Heart Institute, All Children's Hospital, St. Petersburg, FL, USA
e-mail: JAQMD@mac.com

F. Lacour-Gayet et al. (eds.), *Surgery of Conotruncal Anomalies*,
DOI 10.1007/978-3-319-23057-3_7

History

The first anatomic description of the congenital malformation currently referred to as Tetralogy of Fallot is credited to Niels Stenson [1] in 1672. In 1888, Arthur Fallot [2] correlated the pathology and clinical course in his patients with these findings and described "la maladie bleue". Subsequently, Maude Adams [3] coined the term "Tetralogy of Fallot".

The initial surgical treatment was devised and performed by Alfred Blalock, Vivian Thomas and Helen Taussig [4], creating a systemic to pulmonary artery shunt for relief of cyanosis in 1945. Walton Lillehei is credited with the first successful open heart correction of Tetralogy of Fallot utilizing controlled cross circulation in 1956. Many other notable surgeons of the past and current era such as A. Castaneda, S. Barratt-Boyes, and J. Kirklin, to mention a few, are responsible for the approaches and today's outcomes.

Anatomy

There are many anatomical features that need to be clearly understood in order to successfully repair a child with Tetralogy of Fallot. The most surgically important are the atrial and ventricular septal defects, the degree of right ventricular obstruction, the pulmonary valve structure and function, the morphology of the main pulmonary artery and its branches and the coronary anatomy. This chapter will focus on specifics of the pulmonary valvar anatomy.

Pulmonary valve morphology in Tetralogy is complex and variable. Combining the reports by Winn et al. [5] and Rao [6] 120 patients with TOF were studied post mortem. Bicuspid pulmonary valves (Fig. 7.1) where present in 62 (63 %), unicuspid in 17 (14 %), tricuspid in 16 (13 %), and "domed" in 12 (10 %). They described shortened leaflets with limited mobility (tethering) and resultant stenosis as well as variable degrees of dysplasia or cauliflower like appearance, adding to flow obstruction. Thus, in addition to the information gained by the Z value of the pulmonary annulus, it is the combined effect of all these varied features that determine the functionality of the pulmonary valve.

Preoperative Evaluation and Assessment

The preoperative evaluation and assessment for successful repair of TOF includes the usual preoperative preparation of the patient and thorough knowledge of the important anatomic variables. Currently, echocardiography is the main imaging modality and usually provides the surgeon with the necessary information. On occasion however, cardiac catheterization, computed tomography (CT) or

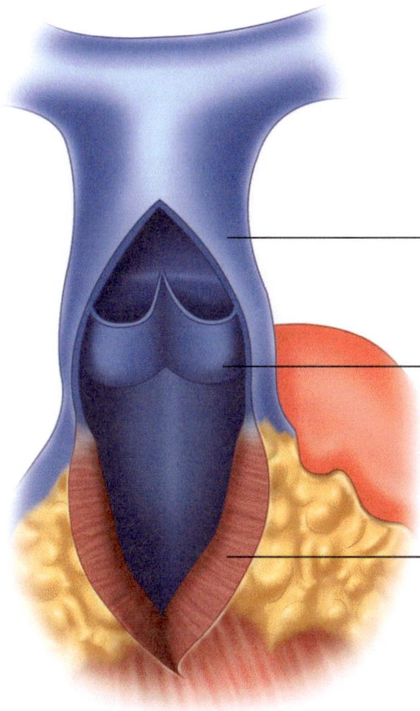

Fig. 7.1 Trans-annular incision divides the transversely oriented anterior leaflet of the bicuspid valve into hemi-leaflets. Incision extends onto anterior RV freewall as a limited ventriculotomy

magnetic resonance imaging (MRI) can be utilized to resolve a specific concern such as a rare MAPCA or coronary issue. A preoperative evaluation checklist (Table 7.1) can be used to ensure a thorough anatomical evaluation prior to surgery.

Surgical Strategy

The important goals for repair of Tetralogy include the closure of the ventricular septal defect(s), relief of right ventricular outflow tract obstruction, management of the pulmonary valve, and main and branch pulmonary arteries, and optional patency of a small atrial communication. Many aspects of surgical care vary from surgeon to surgeon and institution to institution. Some are fairly standard with minor variations amongst surgeons, such as the proposed cannulation strategy, cardiopulmonary bypass management, myocardial protection and overall plan for anatomic correction. On the other hand, there is no absolute consensus regarding specifics such as the optimal timing of repair, single versus two-stage approach, transatrial versus transventricular approach (see Chaps. 6 and 7) or preservation of pulmonary valve function.

Table 7.1 Preoperative check List

Anatomical component	Characteristics
Ventricular septal defect (s)	Location, size and any additional defects
Atrial septal defect	Size and flow pattern
Right ventricular outflow tract	Relative size and levels of flow disturbance
Pulmonary annulus	Diameter (Z value)
Pulmonary valve	Leaflet size, number, mobility, relative thickness
Main pulmonary artery	Diameter (Z value)
Pulmonary Branches	Diameter (Z value)
Patent ductus	Location and size
A-P collaterals (rare)	Number, size and location
Coronary arteries	Abnormal origin and course
Aortic valve	Structure and function
Left ventricle and mitral valve	Structure and function

In light of differing strategies and approaches resulting in reportedly good short and long-term outcomes [7, 8], it may be reasonable to focus on and ask, "what can we improve upon"? It is known that long-term survival is good but not normal [9]. There is a risk of earlier mortality as well as significant morbidity from residual right ventricular outflow tract obstruction or more importantly, severe pulmonary insufficiency, with subsequent right ventricular dilatation, dysfunction, arrhythmia and possible sudden death [10]. Therefore surgeons have the opportunity to refine their initial surgical approach in dealing with the right ventricular outflow tract and the pulmonary valve, in an attempt to improve upon the long-term issues that face our patients.

With regard to relief of right ventricular outflow tract obstruction, the ability to create a non-obstructive, normally functioning connection should be the goal. If the anatomy allows for a transatrial resection with adequate relief, this is generally deemed the optimal surgical technique. If severe infundibular hypoplasia exists, infundibular patch reconstruction is usually most effective. The specific technique may be less important than achieving the desired end goal of a non-obstructed and normally functioning right ventricular chamber.

More complex in many ways is the question of how best to deal with preservation of pulmonary valve function. These challenges relate to issues such as the poor quality of the anatomic substrate that the patient presents with, or the technical difficulty in creating an effective and durable repair of the pulmonary valve. There is convincing evidence that chronic pulmonary insufficiency is the most important variable that affects the lives of TOF patients [10]. There is also some early data to support the use of pulmonary valve preserving techniques at the initial surgery resulting in a decreased incidence of subsequent pulmonary valve replacement [11]. Additionally, recent data [12] suggests an improved immediate postoperative course with valve preservation. Therefore, it stands to reason that surgeons strive for a non-obstructive and competent pulmonary valve, given the limits of the anatomical substrate at hand.

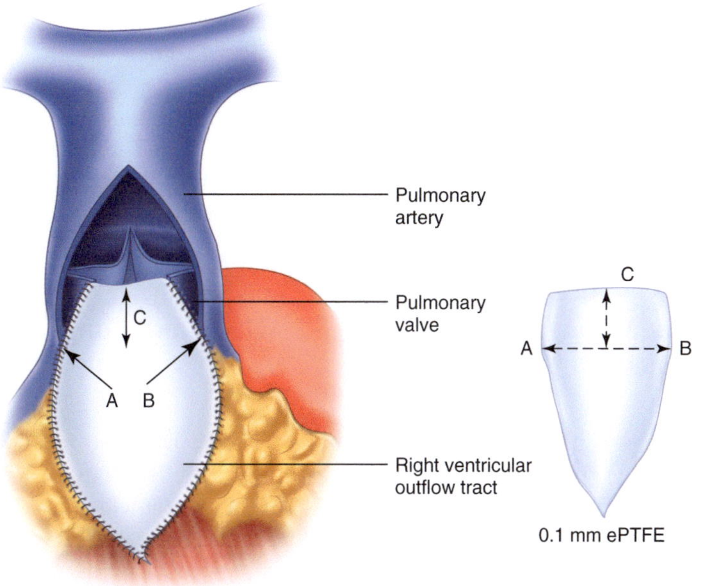

Fig. 7.2 Step 1. A triangular shaped patch of .1 mm ePTFE is sewn along the open ventriculotomy and onto the side edge of the divided pulmonary valve hemi-leaflets. It becomes part of the annulus and moves with the native valve hemi-leaflets. Line *A-B* is the length of the e PTFE patch needed to create an annular diameter of 1.5–2 Z value. The height of the patch (*C*), is the length of the native hemi-valve leaflet plus 1–2 mm

The intraoperative assessment should carefully evaluate the annular diameter, orifice size, and the number, length, mobility and quality (dysplasia) of the leaflets. Valve orifice sizes relating to a Z value $\geq -$ 1.5 and predicted post repair RV/LV pressure ratio $\leq$0.7 are usually acceptable for valve preservation. For the most favorable cases of a tri-leaflet or bi-leaflet valve with mild hypoplasia or leaflet abnormality, a precise, simple valvotomy may be all that is needed. As the valve abnormality increases, usually with progressive degrees of stenosis, additional maneuvers are necessary. One of the most versatile techniques incorporating a valve-preserving concept, is a transannular, leaflet-preserving technique, reported by Sung et al. [13] with modifications by others more recently [14–16]. Our current strategy is a modification of the "Sung" repair incorporating 0.1 mm ePTFE as the transannular, leaflet extension material (Fig. 7.2a–c). This type of repair can be used with a variety of valvular pathologies and small annular sizes, in patients as young as 3–4 weeks of age. For the extremely small annulus, preterm or small neonate, and if valve preservation is felt to be unlikely, we would recommend a systemic to pulmonary shunt and a two-stage approach.

There are a variety of other approaches used in the repair of Tetralogy of Fallot. Commonly, a transannular patch is used to create an unobstructed outflow tract.

This is actually the most commonly performed procedure in the STS database for Tetralogy repair [17]. Often a monocusp (pericardium or ePTFE) is used with a transannular patch achieving reasonable valve function in the immediate postoperative period [18]. Additional options such as intra-operative balloon dilatation have been reported with good initial results [19]. Interventionally based procedures such as stenting the RVOT have been reported, but these approaches are generally reserved for patients felt to be very high risk for surgery, such as those with recent intracranial hemorrhage or necrotizing enterocolitis.

Current Management Patterns (STS Data) and Long-Term Outcomes

The Society of Thoracic Surgeons Pediatric Cardiac Database report by Habib et al., 2010 [17] included 3059 patients with repair of Tetralogy of Fallot. They found out of 2534 primary repairs, 581 (23 %) had no ventriculotomy, 571 (23 %) had non-transannular patch, 1329 (52 %) had transannular patch, and 53 (2 %) had right ventricle to pulmonary artery conduits. Of patients who had repair following prior palliation (two stage approach, n = 217), 20 (9 %) had no ventriculotomy, 30 (14 %) had a non-transannular patch, 144 (66 %) had transannular patch, and 24 (11 %) had conduits. Discharge mortality was 7.5 % after initial palliation, 1.3 % for primary repair and 0.9 % for secondary repair. Neonatal mortality was 6.2 % for palliation and 7.8 % for primary neonatal repair. Primary repair, most commonly in the first year of life, is the most prevalent strategy, 2534 out of 3059 (82 %). Despite contemporary awareness of the late consequences of pulmonary insufficiency, ventriculotomy with transannular patch remains the most prevalent technique, both for primary repair and for repair following palliation. Also of note, the use of a transannular patch increased from 52 to 66 % following palliation. This report suggests prior palliation was not successful in preserving the pulmonary valve annulus in this real life data set.

Long-term outcome data for repair of Tetralogy of Fallot now includes patients operated over a half of a century ago. In 2011, Lindberg et al. [20] reported on 627 patients with follow-up extending 50 years, median follow-up 16 years, with an overall mortality of 7.9 %. They categorized five different surgical approaches consisting of: (1) Transatrial approach, with or without pulmonary artery (PA) patch, (2) Transventricular repair, with or without infundibular or PA patch, (3) Transventricular approach with transannular patch. (4) Transventricular approach with transannular patch and monocusp in PA. (5) Repair with conduit or valve. They found *no difference in survival* with any type of procedure. They did, however, report a significant difference with an increased need for reoperation in patients receiving a transannular patch (Fig. 7.3). These differences became more significant after 10 years and the authors state "conclusions drawn by others with limited follow up should be viewed with caution". In another long-term report, Cuypers et al.

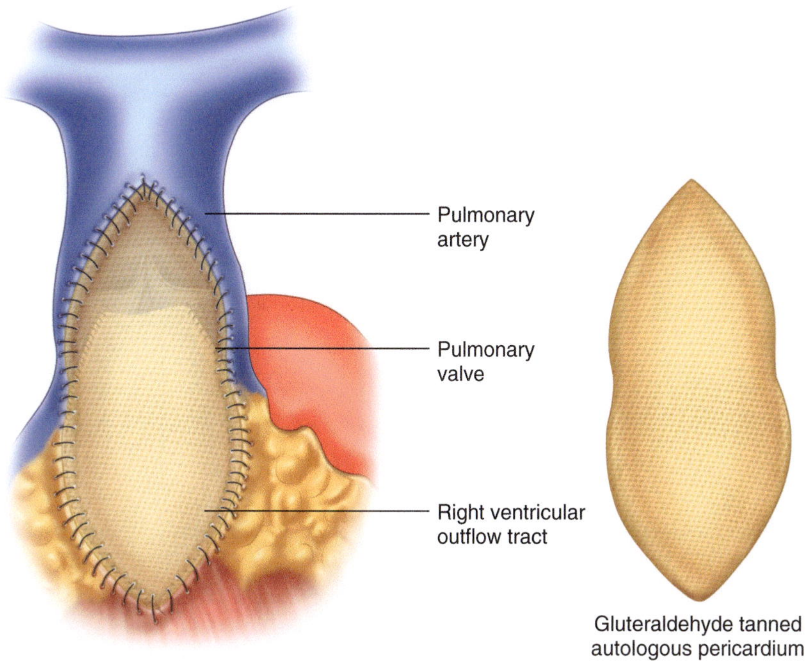

Fig. 7.3 Step 2. Next, a patch of glutaraldehyde treated autologous pericardium is used to cover the entire open defect creating a sinus between the ePTFE leaflet patch and the outflow tract pericardial patch

[9], reported on 144 patients followed more than 30 years following Tetralogy repair. They found an increased incidence of arrhythmias and need for pulmonary valvc rcplaccmcnt in paticnts rccciving a transannular patch, but no diffcrcncc in survival. Luijten et al. [21] reported on 453 Tetralogy patients using transatrial/transpulmonary approach. Transannular patches were used in 65 %. At 10 and 25 year follow-up there was no difference in survival but a significant difference in event-free survival (Figs. 7.4 and 7.5). Overall survival was 97.3 % and 91.8 % at 10 and 25 years, respectively. Event-free survival for transannular patch versus non-transannular patch patients was 80.2 % vs. 81.7 % at 10-year and 27.9 % vs. 78.5 % at 25-year follow-up ($P=0.016$).

In summary, it seems clear that long-term survival is quite good following Tetralogy repair. From these most recent long-term reports one may draw the inference that a transannular patch with creation of significant pulmonary insufficiency may be the most important operative variable determining the patient's long-term need for re-intervention. The relief of significant right ventricular outflow tract obstruction with the least traumatic derangement of the right ventricle would seem most beneficial. It would also follow from the available data that the initial surgical encounter should focus on preservation of pulmonary valve function utilizing conservative or reconstructive techniques where practicable.

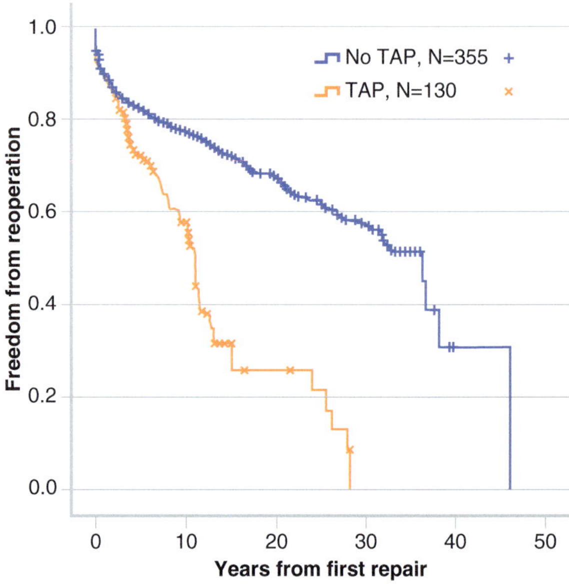

Fig. 7.4 The influence of trans-annular patch (*TAP*) upon freedom from reoperation in surgery of TOF (Reproduced from Lindberg et al. [20], with permission of Oxford University Press)

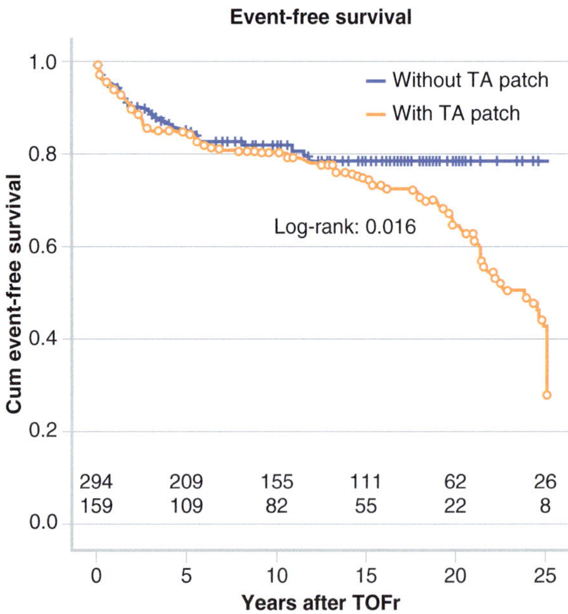

Fig. 7.5 Event-free survival at 25 years was 78.5% without TA patch and 27.9 % with trans-annular patch (*TAP*) (Reproduced from Luijten et al. [21], with permission of Oxford University Press)

References

1. Stensen N. Embryo monstro affins Parisiis dissectus. Acta Med Philos Hafniensa 1671–72;1:202–3.
2. Fallot A. Contribution à l'anatomie pathologique de la maladie bleue (cyanose cardiaque). Marseille Medicale. 1888;25:77–93.
3. Van Praagh R. The first Stella van Praagh memorial lecture: the history and anatomy of tetralogy of Fallot. Semin Thorac Cardiovasc Surg Pediatr Card Surg Annu. 2009;12:19–38.
4. Brogan TV, Alfieris GM. Has the time come to rename the Blalock-Taussig shunt? Pediatr Crit Care Med. 2003;4(4):450–3.
5. Winn KJ, Hutchins GM. The pathogenesis of tetralogy of Fallot. Am J Pathol. 1973;73(1):157–72.
6. Rao S. Anatomic variation in the tetralogy of fallot. Am Heart J. 1971;81(3):361–71.
7. Bacha EA, et al. Long-term results after early primary repair of tetralogy of Fallot. J Thorac Cardiovasc Surg. 2001;122(1):154–61.
8. Morales DL, et al. Right ventricular infundibulum sparing (RVIS) tetralogy of fallot repair: a review of over 300 patients. Ann Surg. 2009;250(4):611–7.
9. Cuypers JA, et al. Unnatural history of tetralogy of Fallot: prospective follow-up of 40 years after surgical correction. Circulation. 2014;130(22):1944–53.
10. Gatzoulis MA, et al. Risk factors for arrhythmia and sudden cardiac death late after repair of tetralogy of Fallot: a multicentre study. The Lancet. 2000;356(9234):975–81.
11. Kim GS, Han S, Yun TJ. Pulmonary annulus preservation lowers the risk of late postoperative pulmonary valve implantation after the repair of Tetralogy of Fallot. Pediatr Cardiol. 2015;36(2):402–8.
12. Sasson L, et al. Right ventricular outflow tract strategies for repair of tetralogy of Fallot: effect of monocusp valve reconstruction. Eur J Cardiothorac Surg. 2013;43(4):743–51.
13. Sung SC, et al. Pulmonic valve annular enlargement with valve repair in tetralogy of Fallot. Ann Thorac Surg. 2003;75(1):303–5.
14. Anagnostopoulos P, et al. Pulmonary valve cusp augmentation with autologous pericardium may improve early outcome for tetralogy of Fallot. J Thorac Cardiovasc Surg. 2007;133(3):640–7.
15. Yilmaz AT, et al. Simultaneous enlargement of the pulmonary annulus and the pulmonary cusp with a transannular patch. J Thorac Cardiovasc Surg. 2003;125(1):206–8.
16. Sasikumar N, et al. Prosthetic reconstruction of bicuspid pulmonary valve in tetralogy of Fallot. Asian Cardiovasc Thorac Ann. 2014;22(4):436–41.
17. Al Habib HF, et al. Contemporary patterns of management of tetralogy of Fallot: data from the Society of Thoracic Surgeons Database. Ann Thorac Surg. 2010;90(3):813–9; discussion 819–20.
18. Brown JW, et al. Right ventricular outflow tract reconstruction with a polytetrafluoroethylene monocusp valve: a twelve-year experience. J Thorac Cardiovasc Surg. 2007;133(5):1336–43.
19. Bacha E. Valve-sparing options in tetralogy of Fallot surgery. Semin Thorac Cardiovasc Surg Pediatr Card Surg Annu. 2012;15(1):24–6.
20. Lindberg HL, et al. Single-center 50 years' experience with surgical management of tetralogy of Fallot. Eur J Cardiothorac Surg. 2011;40(3):538–42.
21. Luijten LW, et al. Long-term outcomes of transatrial-transpulmonary repair of tetralogy of Fallot. Eur J Cardiothorac Surg. 2015;47(3):527–34.

Chapter 8
Pulmonary Atresia, Ventricular Septal Defect and Major Aorto-Pulmonary Collateral Arteries

Yves d'Udekem and Lucas Jon Eastaugh

Abstract The term pulmonary atresia and ventricular septal defect (VSD) covers a spectrum of conditions with various degrees of severity. The terminology of pulmonary atresia, VSD and major aortopulmonary collateral arteries (MAPCAs) is usually restricted to patients with diminutive central pulmonary arteries whose pulmonary circulation is dependent from systemic-pulmonary collateral arteries. It therefore excludes patients with ductus-dependent pulmonary circulation. The natural history of the condition is severe. In the 90s, only a fifth of the patients born with pulmonary atresia, VSD and MAPCAs survived to 30 years of age.

Significant progress has been made in the management of patients with pulmonary atresia, VSD and MAPCAs. Our understanding of the variations in pulmonary vasculature has evolved, although there remains debate about the best methods of classification. There is an ongoing debate on optimal surgical strategies between surgical rehabilitation of the native hypoplastic PA that our group favors and unifocalisation of MAPCAs early in infancy. There continues to be debate on the most effective strategy to provide long-term survival in this patient group.

Keywords Pulmonary atresia • Ventricular septal defect • Major aortopulmonary collaterals • Unifocalisation • Rehabilitation of pulmonary arteries • Congenital heart defect

Y. d'Udekem, MD, PhD, FRACS (✉)
Department of Cardiac Surgery, Royal Children's Hospital, Flemington Road, Parkville, Melbourne, VIC 3052, Australia
e-mail: yves.dudekem@rch.org.au

L.J. Eastaugh, MBBS, FRACP, FCSANZ
Department of Cardiology, Royal Children's Hospital, Flemington Road, Parkville, Melbourne, VIC 3052, Australia

F. Lacour-Gayet et al. (eds.), *Surgery of Conotruncal Anomalies*,
DOI 10.1007/978-3-319-23057-3_8

Background

In the 70s, attempts had been made to shunt the small native vessels of these patients with poor outcomes [1]. Subsequently, strategies of unifocalisation were developed whereby collateral vessels were joined to either native pulmonary vessels that were previously shunted to increase their size, or to centrally reconstructed vessels. Initially, unifocalisation was performed as a staged procedure with some via sternotomy to enlarge the size of the central native pulmonary arteries, and others performed by thoracotomy to anastomose collateral arteries to centrally reconstructed pulmonary vessels [2]. Later these unifocalisation procedures were completed in one stage via a sternotomy, even at an early age [3]. Doubt has been cast on the long-term benefits of the translocation of collateral arteries by unifocalisation procedures [4–6].

Today, treatment strategies are divided between two diverging approaches: rehabilitation of the native pulmonary vessels and unifocalisation [7–10]. Some have proposed the use of both approaches following the patients' own anatomic characteristics [11].

Rehabilitation Strategy

Supporters of this approach claim that central pulmonary arteries are present in the majority of neonates [12]. Before rehabilitation of these central vessels is attempted, the exact distribution of these vessels to lung fields should be evaluated. It is believed that these central pulmonary vessels have a better chance to grow if procedures are aimed at increasing flow in early life [9, 13]. The initial procedure is performed at 2–3 weeks of life, even if the patients are well saturated. In patients showing signs of heart failure related to pulmonary over-circulation, the procedure may be delayed if symptoms can be controlled with medical therapy. The rehabilitation approach requires multiple interventions upon the central pulmonary arteries. The second procedure usually consists of the insertion of a right ventricle (RV) to pulmonary artery (PA) conduit. The conduit is gradually increased in size during repeat procedures performed during the first years of life. Almost all patients necessitate one or more procedures involving patching of the central pulmonary arteries, generally from hilum to hilum. Complete repair, including the closure of the VSD and the insertion of a valved conduit between the right ventricle and the pulmonary arteries, is only performed when the clinicians have the subjective impression that the pulmonary vasculature is developed enough and the central vessels are connected to enough of the overall lung parenchyma. This type of repair may be performed as a second procedure or be delayed until the third, fourth or even fifth procedure.

Exception to this strategy includes patients who present with near normal native pulmonary vasculature in both hila. These patients tend to have one or two MAPCAs feeding these vessels. A single stage repair procedure in early life will connect the hilar vessels to either native central vessels enlarged with patches, pericardial tubes or Gore-Tex grafts. Additional procedures may be required in cases where native lobar branches fed by MAPCAs, are not in continuity with the central vessels. These near-normal lobar branches can then be connected to the rehabilitated central vessels either directly or via an interposition graft.

The benefit of the rehabilitation strategy is its relative safety. As long as the MAPCAs are left undisturbed, the pulmonary blood flow is maintained. We have observed in some instances the spontaneous regression of these collateral vessels while in others there is increased pulmonary blood flow resulting from the growth of the native vessels. This has necessitated surgical ligation of collateral vessels or occlusion by interventional catheterisation procedures.

Unifocalisation

In its early development, unifocalisation was performed in stages [2]. Procedures were performed with the aim to rehabilitate central pulmonary vessels via a sternotomy and to translocate collateral vessels to the central vessels via thoracotomy. This strategy has now been virtually abandoned. Today most teams would proceed with one-stage unifocalisation of all or most collateral arteries [10, 14]. The principles of this approach are seemingly clear but in most series, the unifocalisation strategy is applied with some variation between individual surgeons and patients within the one institution. Some patients have had previous procedures on the central pulmonary vessels in an attempt to develop these vessels prior to unifocalisation, while others were late referrals to a "unifocalising" team.

The collaterals are detached from their insertion, mainly the descending aorta and the subclavian vessels, and the most distal segment is reattached to the centrally rehabilitated or reconstructed vessels. Practices in unifocalisation procedures vary from the translocation of all identified collateral vessels, to the translocation of selected collaterals deemed to be the most important contributors to the pulmonary vasculature. The decision of the suitability for complete repair varies between teams. Most appear to base their decision on the subjective appreciation of the adequacy of the reconstructed pulmonary vessels and degree of peripheral arborization. It has been suggested to cannulate the reconstructed pulmonary circuit, and measure the pressure while maintaining a full cardiac output in the pulmonary arteries. This can be achieved by an independent bypass circuit and is thought to enable prediction of the pulmonary artery pressures post repair [8].

Anatomical Classification of the Pulmonary Arterial Supply

Brawn and Hanley, two pioneers of this field with the largest described experience, vary in their classification of the anatomy of the pulmonary vasculature. Brawn identifies patients as having "confluent intra-pericardial pulmonary arteries, confluent intra-pulmonary arteries and non-confluent intra-pulmonary arteries". While Hanley described four patient groups; "large caliber MAPCAs without significant segmental level stenoses, small-to-moderate caliber MAPCAs without segmental level stenoses, centrally confluent fully arborizing hypoplastic true pulmonary arteries with dual supply MAPCAs, and MAPCAs with extensive segmental level stenoses" [8, 15]. While there is no clear consensus on a single, specific classification, there is general agreement that pulmonary atresia, VSD and MAPCAs is spread across a spectrum of severity. In its most benign form, there are central pulmonary arteries which are small and connected to the majority of the lung fields. At the other extreme, there are no visible native central pulmonary vessels or they are severely hypoplastic, with the main source of pulmonary blood flow arising from multiple small collateral vessels which have no resemblance to normal intra-pulmonary vasculature. Pulmonary blood flow distribution may not be uniform across both lungs. In the extreme, one lung vasculature may be normal and dependent upon a ductus or a hemitruncus, while the other lung depends exclusively on diminutive collateral vessels.

In the absence of an agreed classification, we encourage clinicians to identify the characteristics that will be the most important to their individual management strategy.

Central Pulmonary Arteries

Central pulmonary arteries are incorporated in both the rehabilitation and unifocalisation strategies. This may be as a unique target of revascularization, or as a central point of reconstruction. The discrepancy in the appreciation of the proportion of patients with native central pulmonary arteries may be explained by the way they are managed. A strategy of early surgery is more likely to identify the native central pulmonary arteries while unifocalisation may not allow identification of these vessels especially if they are referred late [8, 12].

Near-Normal Intra-Pulmonary Pulmonary Arteries or Pulmonary Lobar Branches

MAPCAs may be connected to intra-pulmonary pulmonary vessels that appear to have a normal hilar distribution. They can also be directly connected to individual lobar branches with a normal appearing intra-pulmonary course. The goal is to identify these vessels and connect them to the central pulmonary circulation.

Multiple, Small Diminutive MAPCAs

Some collaterals do not connect to any vessels that bears resemblance to native pulmonary vasculature. They can be identified by their abnormal course (intimate contact with the bronchial tree), tortuous or tubular appearance, and their limited distribution to small lung segments with a lack of normal pulmonary arborization.

These vessels would be targeted in aggressive unifocalisation strategies and neglected in rehabilitation strategies. There is a general agreement that these patients are at the worst end of the spectrum of the condition [5, 16] and very often, have diminutive central pulmonary arteries.

Dual Pulmonary Blood Supply

Pulmonary segments or lobes may be vascularized by both native pulmonary vessels and MAPCAs. In rehabilitation strategies, dual blood supply can be the source of competitive flow. This has been identified to be a potential source of failure during rehabilitation of lobar branches. Dual blood supply can lead to pulmonary overcirculation and heart failure, precipitating the need for ligation or catheter occlusion. It is important to appreciate the presence of dual blood supply and consider preemptive MAPCA ligation at the time of surgical intervention. Those undertaking a unifocalisation strategy may decide to translocate these collateral vessels regardless of whether or not the territories have dual supply.

Diagnosis and Imaging

At birth, the intra-cardiac diagnosis is usually made by *transthoracic echocardiography*, but more accurate definition of the pulmonary blood supply is required pre-operatively.

Historically, all patients bearing this diagnosis underwent *cardiac catheterisation and selective angiographic examination.* Selective injection of contrast into collateral vessels allowed the most accurate demonstration of the sources of pulmonary blood supply to each lung segment. Today, this investigation is no longer performed at birth because of the need for vascular access, general anaesthesia and radiation exposure. Those opting for a rehabilitation strategy will attempt an early central shunt notwithstanding the quality of distal vessels. Those attempting aggressive unifocalisation will need to identify only the proximal portion of the collateral arteries and the timing of their procedure will be based on the clinical status of the patients rather than the morphology of their pulmonary circulation. Imaging of the distal vessels may be performed at an older age, before the planned unifocalisation.

Cardiac magnetic resonance imaging (cMRI) and Computerized Tomographic Angiography (CTA) are the more common, less invasive techniques employed for imaging the pulmonary vessels. While image quality may not be as accurate as selective catheter-based angiography, the anatomical definition provided is more than adequate for surgical planning. General anaesthesia is still required for cMRI due to the amount of time required to obtain the images and CTA exposes the patient to radiation but may not necessarily need general anaesthesia. Clinicians must weight up the risk-benefits in each individual patient and institution, but cMRI would be the preferred technique if available.

After the initial rehabilitation procedure, the progress in the growth of the central pulmonary arteries can usually be followed by echocardiography. More accurate measurements and extensive imaging of the distal vessels would be ideally be performed by cMRI or CTA, again depending on availability and institution preference.

Before repair or unifocalisation, cardiac catheterisation and extensive angiography is necessary. This allows for haemodynamic assessment of each pulmonary segment and accurate definition of the distribution of the central and collateral vessels, and their peripheral arborization. In particular, aortic root and ascending aorta angiography will demonstrate rare coronary collaterals and more proximal MAPCAs. The descending aorta should be injected with distal occlusion to allow back-filling of collaterals. Both subclavian vessels should be selectively injected because they are commonly a source of MAPCAs, especially on the right side. The superior portion of the abdominal aorta may similarly give rise to collateral vessels. Each identified MAPCA should be injected selectively.

Checklist Before Surgery

Mapping of PA and MAPCAs based on selective Angiogram and/or CTA-MRI

Nakata index or total neo-pulmonary artery index

Material to be ready:

- Gore-Tex shunts,
- Patch enlargement material: 0.4 mm Gore-Tex, autologuous pericardium (fresh and gluteraldehyde tanned)
- RV to PA valved conduit: pulmonary or aortic homografts, Bovine Jugular Vein conduit (Contegra)
- If perfusion of the main pulmonary artery is planned, the necessary circuit has to be prepared.
- Potential Intra-operative stenting

Surgical Techniques

Timing of Surgery

The timing of the surgery varies depending on the type of strategy employed. In a rehabilitation strategy, the first procedure is recommended to take place at 2–3 weeks of age [9]. Patients directed to a unifocalisation strategy are usually offered their first surgery from 3 to 9 months of age [7, 8]. As most patients with well-developed

MAPCAs are initially only moderately desaturated, there is no clinical need for the patients to be operated early. There appears to be a general consensus on clinical indications for early surgery: the rare cases of patients in heart failure despite medical treatment, and those with a ductus or a hemitruncus providing circulation to one lung.

The type of surgery depends of the anatomy of the patients. Patients with adequate intra-pulmonary branches should be offered a definitive repair. Those with a well-developed pulmonary circulation on one side and diminutive collateral arteries on the contralateral lung should undergo a connection between the right ventricle and the well-developed lung circulation and a rehabilitation procedure in the contralateral lung [17].

The decision to proceed with the definitive repair and ultimately the closure of the VSD depends of the appreciation of the development of the ultimate pulmonary circulation. Traditionally the measurements of the Nakata index of the reconstructed pulmonary circulation has been the predominant factor guiding this decision. An index superior to 150 mm/m^2 is usually considered as suitable to achieve a repair [18]. The total neopulmonary artery index, a calculation of the total surface of the pulmonary blood vessels supplying the lungs notwithstanding their origin has been quoted to equally be a good estimate of the postoperative pulmonary pressure with similar values being considerate adequate for repair [11, 19]. Others have suggested to base their decision on preoperative MRI estimates of the pulmonary blood flow calculated as the total pulmonary venous return or by subtracting superior vena cava and descending aortic flow from ascending aorta flow [19]. Apart for some rare teams, decision to proceed to repair is no longer based on the number of broncho-pulmonary segments perfused by the reconstructed or rehabilitated pulmonary vasculature [20]. In borderline cases of patients undergoing unifocalisation, intraoperative flow testing of the pressure achieved in the pulmonary circulation has been maintained by some teams who favours unifocalisation procedures [21, 22].

Rehabilitation of Native Pulmonary Arteries

Central shunt following Laks technique (Fig. 8.1) The creation of a shunt between the ascending aorta and the main pulmonary artery appears to be the best way to provide increased pulmonary blood flow to the small native central pulmonary arteries without distorting the branches. With this technique, the procedure can be performed without the need for cardio-pulmonary bypass. The branch pulmonary arteries are gently snared. A single 5/0 suture is passed at the base of the main pulmonary arteries. Traction on this suture and the two snugger's provide optimal exposure of the main pulmonary artery. A longitudinal incision is made on the main pulmonary artery. This incision is central and not directed towards either of the branches. The largest possible shunt is inserted at this level, but in the majority of patients (based on age/weight at the time of procedure), this is usually limited to a

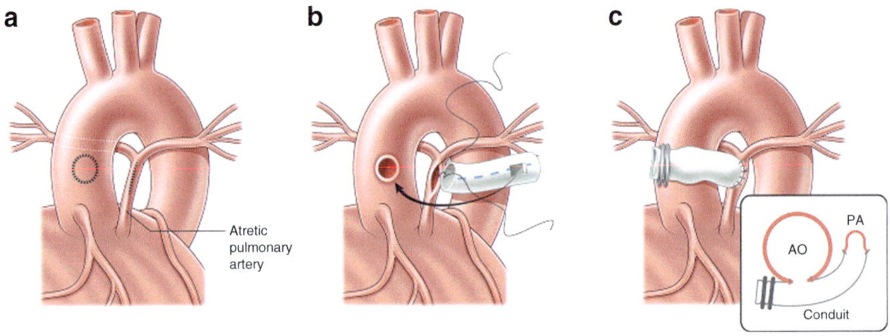

Fig. 8.1 (**a**, **b**, **c**) Central shunt following Laks technique

3.0 or 3.5 mm diameter shunt. Most of the time the extremity of the shunt does not need to be beveled as a transverse cut fits adequately to the vessel opening. After relieving traction on the suture, the length of the shunt is estimated. A slight upwards or transverse course gives the best curvature to the shunt. A rectangular slit incision is made on the shunt and a side-biting clamp is applied on the ascending aorta. The proximal orifice is best made with a punch of 2.8 or 3.5 mm diameter. After the completion of this side-to-side anastomosis, the shunt is de-aired and two clips are applied on the proximal end. Care should be taken to avoid positioning any chest drains across the path of the shunt.

Alternative techniques It has been recommended to divide the proximal end of the main pulmonary artery and re-implant the main pulmonary artery directly on the side of the aorta [16]. We have found this technique to be unreliable. In our review of this technique, close to half of the patients developed right pulmonary artery stenosis [4]. Invariably, these patients have a large aorta and we have found that after this technique, the right pulmonary artery may become adhered to the back of the aorta. Others have proposed to perform an opening and patching of the occluded right ventricular outflow tract [18]. This technique is more technically demanding and extensive patching may increase the risk of distortion of the proximal pulmonary arteries compared to performing a central shunt. Additionally, this procedure requires cardio-pulmonary bypass with cardioplegic arrest.

RV to PA conduit (Fig. 8.2) The second procedure of a rehabilitation strategy is commonly a definitive repair utilising an RV to PA conduit. This is performed as the infant outgrows the shunt and requires increased pulmonary blood flow to the central pulmonary vessels. The conduit is positioned between the right ventricle and main pulmonary artery. It provides a large amount of pulmonary blood flow in additional to giving the interventional cardiologist access to distal pulmonary arteries. At this stage, the central pulmonary vessels have increased to a size that decreases the risk of any distortion of the branch pulmonary arteries. We have found a 6 mm Gore-Tex conduit to be the ideal size around the age of 6 months. Later in life, we use the smallest size Contegra conduit of 12 mm diameter. By this stage, the central

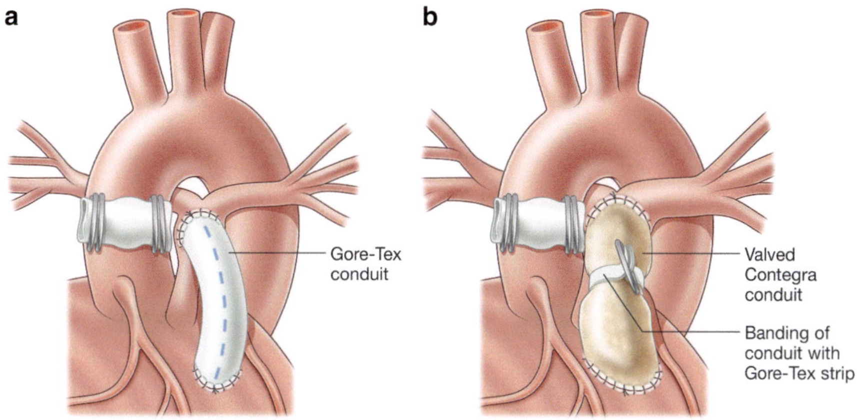

Fig. 8.2 Creation of a RV to PA conduit with (**a**) a Gore-Tex conduit and (**b**) with a Contegra conduit banded with a strip of Gore-Tex

pulmonary arteries have developed and patients are at risk of pulmonary overcirculation. Our strategy is to band all valved conduits while monitoring their pulmonary pressure. Banding of the conduit is performed with strips of Gore-Tex, secured with clips, to allow subsequent balloon dilatation of the conduit if required, which loosens the band and increases pulmonary blood flow.

Pulmonary artery patching (Fig. 8.3) During any of the procedures following the initial central shunt, it may be necessary to proceed with the patching of the central pulmonary arteries. Our preference has been to always enlarge both origins of the pulmonary arteries with an incision cephalad to the bifurcation. Patching is then extended to as far as necessary, sometimes crossing the origin of a pulmonary lobar branch. Patching of the pulmonary artery bifurcation results in the alteration of the shape of the bifurcation from a 'V' to a 'T' configuration.

Repair Repair is ultimately performed when there has been adequate growth of the pulmonary arterial branches and the central pulmonary vessels are connected to enough lung segments. In addition, lobar branches connected to MAPCAs, can be integrated into the native pulmonary circulation. It is very frequent to have to proceed with additional patching of the central pulmonary arteries concomitantly with the repair. Central pulmonary arteries which have been patched repeatedly have impaired long-term growth. In these circumstances, we favor the interposition of an adult size Gore-Tex graft conduit between both hila whenever possible (Fig. 8.4). We proceed with the repair of the central pulmonary arteries on bypass with the beating heart before proceeding to the VSD closure. The distal end of the RV to PA conduit is anastomosed to the pulmonary artery bifurcation before closing the VSD. In our experience, transection of the aorta is never necessary to access the pulmonary arteries. They can be accessed by gentle retraction of the aorta on both sides. After cardioplegia is administered the right ventriculotomy is performed. A

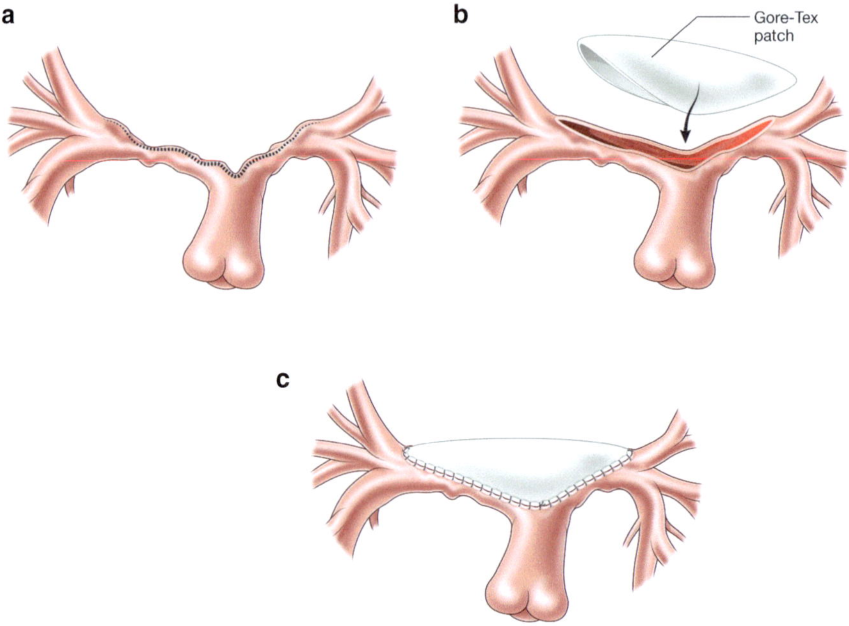

Fig. 8.3 (**a**, **b**, **c**) Patch reconstruction of the central pulmonary arteries

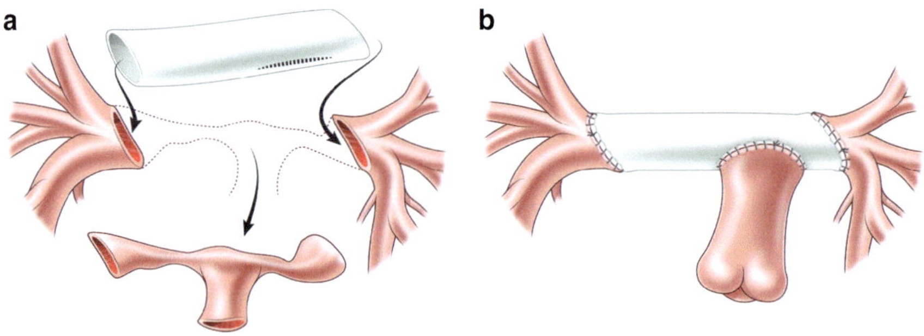

Fig. 8.4 (**a**, **b**) Replacement of the central pulmonary vessels with an interposition Gore-Tex graft

circumferential opening is made in the best identified location, usually below the level of infundibular obstruction. The area for the ventriculotomy is identified by examining the ventricular free wall from the outside and through the tricuspid valve, taking great care to stay away from the left anterior descending coronary artery and the aortic valve. After closure of the VSD, the proximal anastomosis of the conduit is completed. When there are concerns about the suitability of the pulmonary circulation, we have proceeded with closure of the VSD using a fenestrated flap patch or alternatively we have left a patent foramen ovale.

Additional procedures MAPCAs may need to be ligated if there is dual blood supply resulting in pulmonary over-circulation and heart failure, or because competitive flow results in a lack of growth of the rehabilitated pulmonary artery branches. The vascularization of the trachea and the bronchial tree is dependent upon some of these collateral vessels and tracheal necrosis has been described after the ligation [23]. We therefore avoid the systematic ligation of collaterals unless needed. Intra-pulmonary arterial branches may be reconnected to the centrally reconstructed circulation. There are two ways to access these branches. Whenever these branches are in continuity with a hypoplastic central vessel, dissection can proceed from this vessel and continue until the intra-pulmonary branch is adequately exposed. Alternatively, the dissection can proceed from the proximal segment of the MAPCA feeding the vessel, and be followed as distally as possible. These intra-pulmonary branches may then be connected to the pulmonary circulation directly, or by an interposition Gore-Tex graft.

Unifocalisation

Historically, unifocalisation procedures have been performed as staged procedures with multiple thoracotomies required at times. These techniques are now obsolete and most teams would proceed with a single-stage unifocalisation procedure. The most appropriate timing for the procedure will vary between teams and their preferred management strategy.

The procedure starts with an extensive time of dissection of the collaterals. It is possible at times to access these collaterals directly from the posterior mediastinum or directly in the hilum. At the best of times, these approaches are difficult and the identification of the vessels is not straightforward. It is therefore easier to identify the MAPCAs from their origin. Dissection proceeds from the transverse arch and is continued along the descending aorta. The dissection is made from an incision of the posterior mediastinum located on the left side of the SVC. The incision is extended caudally under the carina and may require the retraction of the roof of the left atrium. In rare circumstances, dissection requires the opening of the posterior mediastinum on the left side of the aorta, lifting up the heart to the right, while on cardio-pulmonary bypass. All attempts should be made to anastomoses these vessels as distally as possible as it is likely that the proximal segment of these collaterals will not allow adequate growth.

The team of Dr Hanley suggested proceeding with the isolated perfusion of the newly recreated pulmonary circulation with invasive pressure measurements in the central pulmonary vessels to identify whether the patients were suitable for the closure of the VSD. The cut-off of achieving a pulmonary flow of 3 l per minute per square meter and maintain a pulmonary to aortic pressure ratio of less than 0.4 has been suggested [16]. Others have proposed using the pre-operative cMRI evaluation of pulmonary blood flow [19].

Outcomes

To date, there have been no in-depth evaluations of the late functional capacity of patients born with pulmonary atresia, VSD, and MAPCAs. In reality the success of the various strategies can only be evaluated using three main outcome parameters: survival, number of patients palliated without complete repair, and right ventricular pressure after complete repair.

Survival

There is no data on the natural history of the disease. In a seminal manuscript of patients from the UK undergoing varied surgical strategies, survival to the age of 30 years was barely 20 % [24]. Following a strategy of staged procedures with unifocalisation, our team achieved a 30 year survival of 57 % [4]. More recently, groups performing unifocalisation have reported 3 year survival of 89 % and 5 year survival of 85 % [8, 20]. In a much smaller series of 25 patients using a rehabilitation strategy, we encountered only one unrelated death [12]. On the basis of these preliminary results, our institution believes higher survival may be achieved by pursuing a rehabilitation strategy. As long as the collateral arteries are not compromised and pulmonary blood flow is adequate, survival may be improved.

Palliation Without Complete Repair

Review of all strategies, demonstrates that some patients will not achieve a complete repair. In a historical series of staged palliation, 35 % of patients were palliated [4]. The team of Dr Hanley and Dr Brawn have reported this rate to be 10 and 44 % respectively [8, 20]. In our recent small series, 10 % of the patients were palliated after being deemed unsuitable for complete repair [12].

Right Ventricle Pressure After Complete Repair

This pressure is most often a reflection of the quality of the pulmonary circulation. While low physiological pressure is desirable, the minimum acceptable level of pressure for the right ventricle to provide adequate functional capacity over the course of an entire life-time is still unknown. It has been suggested that right ventricular systolic pressure should be less than 0.4 of the left ventricular systolic pressure. The Hanley team demonstrated that in their patients undergoing repeat conduit replacement, both early post-repair and late after replacement, the ratio between the right and left ventricular systemic pressures were below 0.4 [25]. In our small series describing the rehabilitation strategy, the ratio between the right and left to ventricular pressures was 0.57, and between the pulmonary artery and the left ventricle was 0.4 [12].

References

1. Sullivan ID, Wren C, Stark J, de Leval MR, Macartney FJ, Deanfield JE. Surgical unifocalization in pulmonary atresia and ventricular septal defect. A realistic goal? Circulation. 1988;78:III5–13.
2. Iyer KS, Mee RB. Staged repair of pulmonary atresia with ventricular septal defect and major systemic to pulmonary artery collaterals. Ann Thorac Surg. 1991;51:65–72.
3. Reddy VM, Liddicoat JR, Hanley FL. Midline one-stage complete unifocalization and repair of pulmonary atresia with ventricular septal defect and major aortopulmonary collaterals. J Thorac Cardiovasc Surg. 1995;109:832–44; discussion 844–5.
4. d'Udekem Y, Alphonso N, Nørgaard MA, Cochrane AD, Grigg LE, Wilkinson JL, Brizard CP. Pulmonary atresia with ventricular septal defects and major aortopulmonary collateral arteries: unifocalization brings no long-term benefits. J Thorac Cardiovasc Surg. 2005;130:1496–502.
5. Song S-W, Park HK, Park Y-H, Cho BK. Pulmonary atresia with ventricular septal defects and major aortopulmonary collateral arteries. Circ J. 2009;73:516–22.
6. Nørgaard MA, Alphonso N, Cochrane AD, Menahem S, Brizard CP, d'Udekem Y. Major aorto-pulmonary collateral arteries of patients with pulmonary atresia and ventricular septal defect are dilated bronchial arteries. Eur J Cardiothorac Surg. 2006;29:653–8.
7. Brawn WJ, Jones T, Davies B, Barron D. How we manage patients with major aorta pulmonary collaterals. Semin Thorac Cardiovasc Surg Pediatr Card Surg Annu. 2009;12:152–7.
8. Malhotra SP, Hanley FL. Surgical management of pulmonary atresia with ventricular septal defect and major aortopulmonary collaterals: a protocol-based approach. Semin Thorac Cardiovasc Surg Pediatr Card Surg Annu. 2009;12:145–51.
9. Brizard CP, Liava'a M, d'Udekem Y. Pulmonary atresia, VSD and MAPCAs: repair without unifocalization. Semin Thorac Cardiovasc Surg Pediatr Card Surg Annu. 2009;12:139–44.
10. Ishibashi N, Shin'oka T, Ishiyama M, Sakamoto T, Kurosawa H. Clinical results of staged repair with complete unifocalization for pulmonary atresia with ventricular septal defect and major aortopulmonary collateral arteries. Eur J Cardiothorac Surg. 2007;32:202–8.
11. Carotti A, Albanese SB, Filippelli S, Ravà L, Guccione P, Pongiglione G, Di Donato RM. Determinants of outcome after surgical treatment of pulmonary atresia with ventricular septal defect and major aortopulmonary collateral arteries. J Thorac Cardiovasc Surg. 2010;140:1092–103.
12. Liava'a M, Brizard CP, Konstantinov IE, Robertson T, Cheung MM, Weintraub R, d'Udekem Y. Pulmonary atresia, ventricular septal defect, and major aortopulmonary collaterals: neonatal pulmonary artery rehabilitation without unifocalization. ATS Elsevier Inc. 2012;93:185–91.
13. Metras D, Chetaille P, Kreitmann B, Fraisse A, Ghez O, Riberi A. Pulmonary atresia with ventricular septal defect, extremely hypoplastic pulmonary arteries, major aorto-pulmonary collaterals. Eur J Cardiothorac Surg. 2001;20:590–6; discussion 596–7.
14. Reddy VM, McElhinney DB, Amin Z, Moore P, Parry AJ, Teitel DF, Hanley FL. Early and intermediate outcomes after repair of pulmonary atresia with ventricular septal defect and major aortopulmonary collateral arteries: experience with 85 patients. Circulation. 2000;101:1826–32.
15. Griselli M, McGuirk SP, Winlaw DS, Stümper O, De Giovanni JV, Miller P, Dhillon R, Wright JG, Barron DJ, Brawn WJ. The influence of pulmonary artery morphology on the results of

operations for major aortopulmonary collateral arteries and complex congenital heart defects. J Thorac Cardiovasc Surg. 2004;127:251–8.
16. Mainwaring RD, Reddy VM, Perry SB, Peng L, Hanley FL. Late outcomes in patients undergoing aortopulmonary window for pulmonary atresia/stenosis and major aortopulmonary collaterals. Ann Thorac Surg. 2012;94:842–8.
17. Watanabe N, Mainwaring RD, Reddy VM, Palmon M, Hanley FL. Early complete repair of pulmonary atresia with ventricular septal defect and major aortopulmonary collaterals. Ann Thorac Surg. 2014;97:909–15; discussion 914–5.
18. Fouilloux V, Bonello B, Kammache I, Fraisse A, Macé L, Kreitmann B. Management of patients with pulmonary atresia, ventricular septal defect, hypoplastic pulmonary arteries and major aorto-pulmonary collaterals: Focus on the strategy of rehabilitation of the native pulmonary arteries. Arch Cardiovasc Dis. 2012;105:666–75.
19. Grosse-Wortmann L, Yoo S-J, van Arsdell G, Chetan D, MacDonald C, Benson L, Honjo O. Preoperative total pulmonary blood flow predicts right ventricular pressure in patients early after complete repair of tetralogy of Fallot and pulmonary atresia with major aortopulmonary collateral arteries. J Thorac Cardiovasc Surg. 2013;146:1185–90.
20. Ben D, Mussa S, Davies P, Stickley J, Jones TJ, Barron DJ, Brawn WJ. Unifocalization of major aortopulmonary collateral arteries in pulmonary atresia with ventricular septal defect is essential to achieve excellent outcomes irrespective of native pulmonary artery morphology. J Thorac Cardiovasc Surg. 2009;138:1269–75.
21. Reddy VM, Petrossian E, McElhinney DB, Moore P, Teitel DF, Hanley FL. One-stage complete unifocalization in infants: when should the ventricular septal defect be closed? J Thorac Cardiovasc Surg. 1997;113:858–66; discussion 866-8.
22. Honjo O, Al-Radi OO, MacDonald C, Tran K-CD, Sapra P, Davey LD, Chaturvedi RR, Caldarone CA, Van Arsdell GS. The functional intraoperative pulmonary blood flow study is a more sensitive predictor than preoperative anatomy for right ventricular pressure and physiologic tolerance of ventricular septal defect closure after complete unifocalization in patients with pulmonary atresia, ventricular septal defect, and major aortopulmonary collaterals. Circulation. 2009;120:S46–52.
23. Schulze-Neick I, Ho SY, Bush A, Rosenthal M, Franklin RC, Redington AN, Penny DJ. Severe airflow limitation after the unifocalization procedure: clinical and morphological correlates. Circulation. 2000;102:III142–7.
24. Bull K, Somerville J, Ty E, Spiegelhalter D. Presentation and attrition in complex pulmonary atresia. J Am Chem Soc. 1995;25:491–9.
25. Mainwaring RD, Reddy VM, Peng L, Kuan C, Palmon M, Hanley FL. Hemodynamic assessment after complete repair of pulmonary atresia with major aortopulmonary collaterals. Ann Thorac Surg. 2013;95:1397–402. 24.

Chapter 9
Tetralogy of Fallot with Complete Atrioventricular Canal

Thomas L. Spray and Michael Lewis

Abstract Tetralogy of Fallot associated with complete atrioventricular canal (TC) is a relatively rare form of conotruncal anomaly. The indications for a systemico-pulmonary shunt are few today. We favor a two patch technique. Most of the time, the VSD patch closure is performed through the right atrium only; however a ventriculotomy is used when needed.

The early mortality is contemporarily between 0 and 10 %. Risk factors for morbidity and mortality include: persistent or residual left AVV insufficiency, residual shunting at the ventricular level, residual RVOT obstruction particularly in association with TV regurgitation, and LVOT obstruction. Long-term actuarial survival in recent series show: 86 % survival at 1-year, 82 % at 5 years, 77 % at 7 years, and 72 % at 15 years.

Modern management of patients with Tetralogy of Fallot and Complete AVSD has proven that surgical intervention does not confer mortality, morbidity, or long-term functional status significantly outside the range of what could be expected for isolated TOF or CAVC patients.

Keywords Tetralogy of Fallot • Complete AVSD • Congenital heart diseases • Cardiac surgery • Cyanotic heart disease

T.L. Spray, MD • M. Lewis, MD
Division of Cardiothoracic Surgery, Department of Cardiothoracic Surgery,
The Children's Hospital of Philadelphia, 34th Street and Civic Center Blvd., Suite 8527,
Philadelphia, PA 19104, USA
e-mail: spray@email.chop.edu

F. Lacour-Gayet et al. (eds.), *Surgery of Conotruncal Anomalies*,
DOI 10.1007/978-3-319-23057-3_9

Introduction

Tetralogy of Fallot associated with complete atrioventricular canal (TC) is a relatively rare form of conotruncal anomaly, consisting of 6–16 % complete common atrioventricular canal [1–9] and 1–5 % of cases of tetralogy of Fallot (TOF) [10, 11].

Complete surgical correction of TC is the ultimate goal. A fundamental knowledge of both TOF and CAVC is essential to understanding TC. Furthermore, subtypes of both TOF and CAVC can exist that are not TC. In particular, we will not be discussing cases of double outlet right ventricle (DORV) with CAVC (Chap. 26) which have historically been grouped with cases of TC. As TOF and DORV have been recognized to be, while similar, unique pathologic entities, grouping DORV with complete common atrioventricular canal (DC) with TC would run contrary to the efforts of modern classification schemes of congenital heart disease (Chaps. 25 and 26).

Routine shunting with eventual complete repair had been the predominant surgical strategy in the 1960–1970s. This has been supplanted by initial complete repair as the dominant modern surgical paradigm, and mortality rates for surgical treatment of TC have dropped from near 35 % to less than 5 %. As this strategy has evolved, many issues have been debated and will be addressed in this chapter: appropriate age at repair, number of patches used in repair, and management of the RVOTO.

History

The first reported description of TC has been attributed to Bull [12], who described a patient in France in 1885 [13]. The patient was a 9 year old girl with cleft palate who presented with an upper respiratory infection. She was noted to have stigmata of chronic cyanotic as well as congestive heart disease. She died, and was found on autopsy to have situs inversus with an enlarged heart. While the intracardiac anatomy certainly describes what appears to be a CAVSD with right ventricular infundibular obstruction, it also seems that the right ventricle was hypoplastic.

The first described complete repair of TC was reported by Al Pacifico in 1980 [4].

The surgical series (Table 9.1) are small in number and mostly retrospective with a few prospective trials.

Anatomo-Pathology

Embryology

As we view TC as a net result of two distinct pathologic anomalies, so must we view the genesis of TC through the processes that result in both TOF and CAVSD.

Table. 9.1 Published series of TOF-AVC repair

Authors	Reference	Center	N	30 D mortality (%)	Study period
Kotani et al. [14]	JTCVS 2013	Toronto, Canada	41	7.3	1990–2010
Shuhaiber et al. [15]	JTCVS 2012	Boston, MA, USA	61	7.0	1979–2008
Hoohenkerk et al. [16]	ATS 2008	Leiden. Netherlands	20	0.0	1979–2007
Prifti et al. [13]	J Card Surg 2004	Massa, Italy	17	17.6	1990–2002
Okada et al. [11]	Jpn Circ J 1999	Tokyo, Japan	9	1.1	1986–1996
Najm et al. [17]	JTCVS 1998	Toronto, Canada	38	6.4	1981–1997
O'Blenes et al. [18]	ATS 1998	Halifax, Canada	11	9.1	1988–1996
Delius et al. [19]	EJCTS 1997	London, UK	14	10.3	1980–1995
Gatzoulis et al. [20]	BHJ 1994	London, UK	10	10.0	1987–1992
Malm et al. [21]	J Card Surg. 1993	Melbourne, Australia	13	0.0	1981–1992
Alonso et al. [9]	EJCTS 1990	Madrid, Spain	9	0.0	1982–1999
Pacifico et al. [22]	ATS 1988	Birmingham, AL, USA	12	8.3	1982–1986
Vouhe et al. [23]	ATS 1986	Paris, France	9	11.1	1975–1985
Uretzky et al. [5]	JTCVS 1984	Rochester, MN, USA	14	29	1962–1979
Pacifico et al. [4]	ATS 1980	Birmingham, AL, USA	5	40.0	1967–1978

The chief embryologic defect in TOF [2] is the anterior and leftward displacement of the infundibular septum, leading to a "malaligned" VSD, with malalignment of the infundibular septum and the muscular interventricular septum. Both ventricles consequently open up into the aorta (the left solely, the right less than 50 %) giving rise to the term "overriding aorta". Possible etiologies proposed have been faulty septation of the bulbis cordis resulting in unequal-sized great vessels (i.e., a large aorta and small pulmonary trunk) or underdevelopment of the subpulmonary conus with consequent rightward and superior shift of the aortic valve.

The chief embryologic defect in CAVC [2] is the failure of contribution of the AV cushion towards formation of the atrial and ventricular septae. These have been shown to be neural crest-derived structures (Chap. 39), and their failure to form normal cardiac structures is either an error in their own genesis, migration, or development.

Morphology

The great arteries are normally-related (aorta posterior and to the right), and there exists fibrous continuity between the leaflets of the aortic and common atrioventricular valves. The infundibular (muscular outlet) septum is deviated in an antero-superior fashion.

The mechanism of RVOTO in TC is valvar or subvalvar, like in TOF. The degree of preoperative RVOT peak pressure gradient has been shown to be less in TC patients as compared to TOF patients (3–6). The septo-parietal trabeculations can have an abnormal location.

The presence of thoracic visceral situs inversus should prompt concern that the patient is not TC, but DORV-AVSD [4, 5]. The common AV valve in most cases (>90 %) of TC is classified as Rastelli type C [2, 4, 5, 8], with a "free floating anterior" bridging leaflet. The VSD is an inlet-type with a large anterior and superior extension. The rightward and anterior deviation of the ventricular septum causes an increased risk of subaortic narrowing after VSD closure and reattachment of the LAVV components to the ventricular septum. This can further increase the degree of aortic dextroposition, predisposing the patient to LVOTO.

The aorta in TC patients is "unwedged" and the aortic valve sits anterior to and above the base of the anterior bridging leaflet, resulting in the classic "gooseneck" deformity of the elongated LVOT. The striking difference between the hearts with TC and isolated CAVC is the ventricular and AVV dimensions. Due to the presence of concomitant RVOTO, the size of both the ventricles and the AVV's in those with TC is considerably smaller than those in isolated CAVC patients. No difference is noted in the degree of AVV regurgitation between those two groups.

The conduction system is similar to that in CAVC. The AV node is not in the triangle of Koch and the conduction bundle lies in contact with the annulus of the posterior bridging leaflet. Commonly-associated cardiovascular anomalies include right-sided aortic arch, PDA, secundum ASD, LSVC, bicuspid pulmonic valve, aberrant LAD, anomalous RSCA, and multiple VSD's.

Diagnosis and Imaging

Presentation

The symptomatology of patients is a net result of the degree of RVOTO and of the severity of AVV regurgitation [24]. By and large, the symptomatology is governed by the degree of obstruction of the RVOT.

The majority of the TC patients present with trisomy 21 and cyanosis. *Prenatal diagnosis* of TC is today accurate. The frequent associated trisomy 21 can be detected early in pregnancy [25].

The gender of TC patients is essentially evenly-split. Down's syndrome is associated in 90 %, compared to DORV-AVSD where T21 is very rare [26]. In fact, the presence of trisomy 21 in TOF should arouse suspicion for a diagnosis of TC [5]. The severity of cyanosis depends on the age at presentation.

Imaging

Echocardiography is the methodology by which TC should be thoroughly investigated, and generally obviates the need for further investigation. All the salient morphologic characteristics can be well-delineated, and AVV function and gradients across the RVOT can be assessed. Furthermore, TEE is invaluable for post-operative evaluation of surgical repair.

CT scan and MRI are becoming quite popular and provide accurate information.

Catheterization is rarely necessary but could be useful to evaluate PA branch narrowing following a BT shunt.

Surgery

Palliation by Modified BT Shunt

The indications for a systemic-PA shunt are few today. Palliation remains indicated when the saturation is less than 75 % in the first month of life. The operation is performed by sternotomy using a 3.5 or 4 mm Goretex shunt (see Chap. 12)

Surgical Repair

We use routine aortic and bicaval cannulation with single cross-clamping of the aorta and single dose of cardioplegia for arrest at normothermia. After right atriotomy, the AV canal anatomy is evaluated.. The anterior free floating leaflet is gently retracted and the antero-superior component of the VSD is observed. Saline is injected into the ventricles to float the AV valves and assess the areas of coaptation. The PA trunk is opened longitudinally and the pulmonary valve explored as well as the subpulmonary area. We favor a two patch technique using Dacron or Goretex patch for the VSD and autologous pericardium for the ostium primum, as previously described [24].

VSD Patch Closure (Fig. 9.1)

Most of the time, the VSD patch closure is performed through the right atrium only. The septoparietal trabeculation (parietal band) is resected. Depending on the surgeon preferences, the anterior bridging leaflet is incised or respected. A

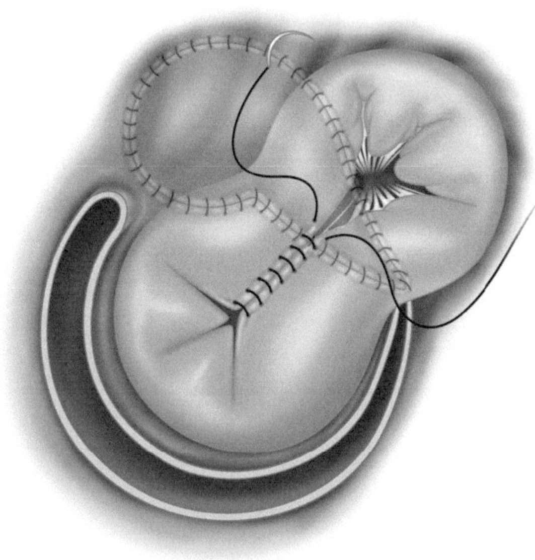

Fig. 9.1 The left AV valve "cleft" is totally closed. The tricuspid valve is carefully repaired, because combined residual pulmonary and tricuspid regurgitation is poorly tolerated

patch with a large superior coma shape is tailored and sutured on the RV side. The superior component of the patch is sutured around the aortic annulus. The anterior component of the patch should be large enough to avoid subaortic obstruction. We have rarely required the use of an incision in the RVOT for enhanced exposure of the antero-superior portion of the VSD. We would perform an incision in the RVOT at this time for improved exposure of the subaortic region of the VSD. The right and left components of the common AV valve leaflets are implanted on the VSD patch.

Common AV Valve Management

The "cleft" of the left AV valve is completely closed, up to the tip of the leaflets. A Hegar dilator of appropriate diameter, normalized for patient weight, ensures the absence of left AV valve stenosis. The valve is evaluated by saline installation and additional commissuroplasty is performed as needed, should the valve continue to be regurgitant.

The right AV valve orifice is inspected and likewise tested for insufficiency via instillation of saline. Commissuroplasty sutures may be needed. The tricuspid valve should have minimal or no residual regurgitation because a combined regurgitation of the tricuspid and pulmonary valves is poorly tolerated.

Ostium Primum Closure

The ostium primum defect is closed with autologous pericardium (Fig. 9.2). In the area of the conduction system, shallow bites are taken in the mouth of the coronary sinus, leaving it to drain to the right atrium. On occasion, however, it has appeared necessary to avoid the conduction system by taking bites laterally around the coronary sinus, and letting it drain into the left atrium.

RVOT Reconstruction

We prefer to do the least amount of intervention on the RVOT that is necessary. If we make an incision in the RVOT, it is to ensure the VSD patch implantation. The RVOT obstruction in TC is either valvar and/or subvalvar. Obstructing muscle bundles can usually be completely resected from the RA approach. If the pulmonary valve is amenable to dilation, we approach this via the RA incision. It not reachable, we would then perform a pulmonary arteriotomy, using a dilator 2 mm larger than the normal PV annulus size for weight. If the Z-score of the PV annulus is smaller than – 2 Z score, we tend to perform a transannular patch. If there is significant coronary arterial supply crossing the obstructed RVOT, we would perform an RV-PA conduit with valved pulmonary homograft.

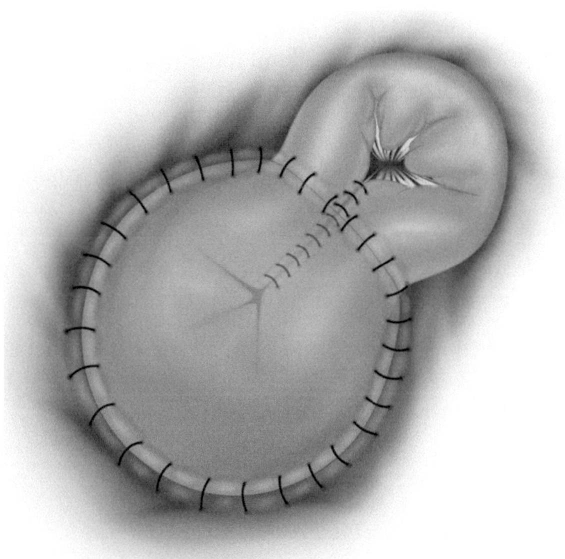

Fig. 9.2 The ostium primum is closed using autologous pericardium. The coronary sinus is frequently left in the left atrium

Post-repair Evaluation

After separation from bypass and a period of modified ultrafiltration, we perform routine TEE to evaluate for residual VSD or ASD, AVV insufficiency, RVOTO, and ventricular function. Results prompting a reinstitution of CPB and revision include a RV/LV pressure ratio >0.7, residual atrial or ventricular shunts, and more then moderate left- or right-sided AV valve regurgitation.

Outcomes

The 30-day mortality has dropped from rates of around 20–38 % from the 1960s to about 0–10 % contemporarily [24–26] Factors associated with both increased morbidity and mortality include persistent or residual left AVV insufficiency, residual shunting at the ventricular level, residual RVOTO particularly in association with TV regurgitation, or LVOTO [27].

Reoperations include both catheter-based and surgical interventions. Around 40 % of repaired TC patients will require surgical reintervention, with a mean time to reoperation of about 2 years [27], with longer times to reoperation noted in those patients that had been initially definitively repaired versus those who had undergone initial palliation [27]. The most common causes of surgical reintervention [19, 28] include RVOT reconstruction (5 %), left AVV regurgitation (15–20 %), or residual VSD (5–25 %).

Catheter-based reinterventions largely include those focused on relieving residual problems with the RVOT (41 %) or with PA obstruction [25]. Freedom from reintervention at 10 years [26] was higher in those patients who had their PV preserved (95 %) versus those who did not (70 %).

Long-Term survival Contemporary studies show that the long-term survival for patients who have undergone complete repair for TC (whether initially palliated or not) to be 86 % at 1-year, and 82 % at 5 years, and 77 % at 7 years, and 72 % at 15 years [29]. As studies have evolved over the last few decades, it has been shown that patients who were treated with initial complete anatomical correction have a better survival than those who had been initially palliated with a systemic-PA shunt [27]

Functional Status The long-term outcome for patients with completely repaired TC, whether initially shunted or not, is quite good, with the vast majority of patients in NYHA class I or II assessed years after definitive repair [21, 22, 29].

Conclusion

Thoughtful management of patients with Tetralogy of Fallot and Complete AVSD has proven that surgical intervention does not confer mortality, morbidity, or long-term functional status significantly outside the range of what could be expected for isolated TOF or CAVC patients.

References

1. Arciniegas E, Hakimi M, Farooki ZQ, Green EW. Results of total correction of tetralogy of Fallot with complete atrioventricular canal. J Thorac Cardiovasc Surg. 1981;81(5):768–73.
2. Bharati S, Kirklin JW, McAllister HA, Lev M. The surgical anatomy of common atrioventricular orifice associated with tetralogy of Fallot, double-outlet right ventricle and complete regular transposition. Circulation. 1980;61:142–9.
3. Bertolini A, Dalmonte P, Bava GL, Calza G, Lerzo F, Zannini L, Pongiglione G, Moretti R. Surgical management of complete atrioventricular canal associated with tetralogy of Fallot. Cardiovasc Surg. 1996;4(3):299–302.
4. Pacifico AD, Kirklin JW, Bargeron Jr LM. Repair of complete atrioventricular canal associated with tetralogy of Fallot or double-outlet right ventricle: report of 10 patients. Ann Thorac Surg. 1980;29(4):351–6.
5. Uretzky G, Puga FJ, Danielson GK, Feldt RH, Julsrud PR, Seward JB, Edwards WD, McGoon DC. Complete atrioventricular canal associated with tetralogy of Fallot. Morphologic and surgical considerations. J Thorac Cardiovasc Surg. 1984;87(5):756–66.
6. Karl TR. Atrioventricular septal defect with tetralogy of Fallot or double-outlet right ventricle: surgical considerations. Semin Thorac Cardiovasc Surg. 1997;9:26–34.
7. Schmid FX, Kampmann C, Hake U, Choi YH, Wipperman F, Oelert H. Complete atrioventricular septal defect associated with tetralogy of Fallot. Favourable outcome of transarterial transpulmonary repair. J Cardiovasc Surg (Torino). 2000;41:17–21.
8. He GW, Mee RB. Complete atrioventricular canal associated with tetralogy of Fallot or double-outlet right ventricle and right ventricular outflow tract obstruction: a report of successful surgical treatment. Ann Thorac Surg. 1986;41(6):612–5.
9. Alonso J, Núñez P, de LJ P, Sánchez PA, Villagrá F, Gómez R, López Checa S, Vellibre D, Brito JM. Complete atrioventricular canal and tetralogy of Fallot: surgical management. Eur J Cardiothorac Surg. 1990;4(6):297–9.
10. Berger TJ, Kirklin JW, Blackstone EH, Pacifico AD, Kouchoukos NT. Primary repair of complete atrioventricular canal in patients less than 2 years old. Am J Cardiol. 1978;41:906–13.
11. Okada Y, Tatsuno K, Kikuchi T, Takahashi Y, Shimokawa T. Complete atrioventricular septal defect associated with tetralogy of fallot: surgical indications and results. Jpn Circ J. 1999;63(11):889–92.
12. Bull C. Anomalie congénitale du coeur avec transposition des viscères. Semaine Med. 1885;5:318.
13. Prifti E, Crucean A, Bonacchi M, Bernabei M, Luisi VS, Murzi B, et al. Total correction of complete atrioventricular septal defect with tetralogy of Fallot. J Heart Valve Dis. 2003;12:640–8.
14. Kotani Y, Chetan D, Ono N, Mertens LL, Caldarone CA, Van Arsdell GS, Honjo O. Late functional outcomes after repair of tetralogy of Fallot with atrioventricular septal defect: a double case-match control study. J Thorac Cardiovasc Surg. 2013;145(6):1477–84, 1484.
15. Shuhaiber JH, Ho SY, Rigby M, Sethia B. Current options and outcomes for the management of atrioventricular septal defect. Eur J Cardiothorac Surg. 2009;35:891–900.
16. Hoohenkerk GJ, Schoof PH, Bruggemans EF, Rijlaarsdam M, Hazekamp MG. 28 years' experience with transatrial-transpulmonary repair of atrioventricular septal defect with tetralogy of Fallot. Ann Thorac Surg. 2008;85(5):1686–9.
17. Najm HK, Van Arsdell GS, Watzka S, Hornberger L, Coles JG, Williams WG. Primary repair is superior to initial palliation in children with atrioventricular septal defect and tetralogy of Fallot. J Thorac Cardiovasc Surg. 1998;116:905–13.
18. O'Blenes SB, Ross DB, Nanton MA, Murphy DA. Atrioventricular septal defect with tetralogy of Fallot: results of surgical correction. Ann Thorac Surg. 1998;66(6):2078–82.
19. Delius RE, Kumar RV, Elliott MJ, et al. Atrioventricular septal defect and tetralogy of Fallot: a 15-year experience. Eur J Cardiothorac Surg. 1997;12:171–6.

20. Gatzoulis MA, Shore D, Yacoub M, Shinebourne EA. Complete atrioventricular septal defect with tetralogy of Fallot: diagnosis and management. Br Heart J. 1994;71(6):579–83.
21. Malm T, Karl TR, Mee RB. Transatrial-transpulmonary repair of atrioventricular septal defect with right ventricular outflow tract obstruction. J Card Surg. 1993;8:622–7.
22. Pacifico AD, Ricchi A, Bargeron Jr LM, Colvin EC, Kirklin JW, Kirklin JK. Corrective repair of complete atrioventricular canal defects and major associated cardiac anomalies. Ann Thorac Surg. 1988;46(6):645–51.
23. Vouhe PR, Neveux JY. Surgical repair of tetralogy of Fallot with complete atrioventricular canal. Ann Thorac Surg. 1986;41:342–4.
24. Spray TJ. Operative cardiac surgery. In: Gardner T, Spray T, editors. Atrioventricular septal defects. 5th ed. London: Arnold publisher; 2004. p. 605–13.
25. Mansfield C, Hopfer S, Marteau T. Termination rates after prenatal diagnosis of down syndrome, spina bifida, anencephaly, and Turner and Klinefelter syndromes: a systematic literature review. Prenat Diagn. 1999;19:808–12.
26. Lacour-Gayet F. Biventricular repair of double outlet right ventricle with noncommitted ventricular septal defect. Semin Thorac Cardiovasc Surg Pediatr Card Surg Annu. 2002;5:163–9.
27. Hanley FL, Fenton KN, Jonas RA, et al. Surgical repair of complete atrioventricular canal defects in infancy. J Thorac Cardiovasc Surg. 1993;106:387–97.
28. Prifiti E, Bonacchi M, Bernabei M, et al. Repair of complete atrioventricular septal defect with Tetralogy of Fallot: our experience and literature review. J Card Surg. 2004;19:175–83.
29. Shuhaiber JH, Robinson B, Gauvreau K, Breitbart R, Mayer JE, Del Nido PJ, Pigula F. Outcome after repair of atrioventricular septal defect with tetralogy of Fallot. J Thorac Cardiovasc Surg. 2012;143(2):338–43.

Chapter 10
Tetralogy of Fallot with Absent Pulmonary Valve Syndrome

Viktor Hraška

Abstract The absent pulmonary valve syndrome occurs in 3–6 % of patients with tetralogy of Fallot. This syndrome is physiologically distinctive from other forms of tetralogy of Fallot, due to tracheobronchial compression resulting from massive dilatation of the main pulmonary artery and its first and second-order branches, and from the abnormal branching of segmental arteries. Symptomatic newborns and infants, in particular, have a poor prognosis because of severe central pulmonary artery dilatation and bronchial compression. Here, one-stage early primary repair is the method of choice. Apart from the correction of tetralogy of Fallot, surgery must address the dilated pulmonary arteries in order to minimize the incidence of postoperative and long-term bronchial compression and peripheral lung damage. The traditional approach has focused on plication and reduction of the anterior and/or posterior wall of the normally positioned pulmonary arteries. An alternative approach advocated by some groups involves translocation of the pulmonary artery anterior to the aorta away from the trachea and bronchial tree, which may reduce or eliminate bronchial compression by the pulmonary artery. Insertion of a valved homograft or other suitable conduit should be considered particularly in symptomatic newborns and infants. Failure of treatment may be expected in symptomatic patients, in whom the pathology of the airways extends beyond the proximal pulmonary arteries.

Keywords Tetralogy of Fallot • Absent pulmonary valve syndrome • Airway compression • Respiratory distress • Surgical repair • Bronchoscopy

---

V. Hraška, MD, PhD
Department of Pediatric Cardiac Surgery, German Pediatric Heart Center,
Asklepios Clinic Sankt Augustin, Arnold Jansen Str. 29,
Sankt Augustin 53757, Germany
e-mail: v.hraska@asklepios.com

F. Lacour-Gayet et al. (eds.), *Surgery of Conotruncal Anomalies*,
DOI 10.1007/978-3-319-23057-3_10

Introduction

The absent pulmonary valve syndrome (APVS) occurs in 3–6 % of patients with tetralogy of Fallot (TOF). APVS can also occur in isolation, with an intact ventricular septum (IVS), or it may occur in conjunction with other cardiac anomalies such as major aortopulmonary collateral arteries (MAPCAs), atrioventricular septal defect, double outlet right ventricle, transposition of the great arteries, or atrial septal defect [1, 2]. This syndrome is physiologically distinctive from other forms of TOF due to tracheobronchial compression, resulting from massive dilatation of the main pulmonary arteries (PAs). Consequential tracheomalacia and bronchomalacia determine the timing and severity of respiratory compromise, as well as the morbidity and mortality of these patients. Mortality still remains considerable, predominantly in symptomatic newborns and infants.

Anatomy

TOF/APVS is associated with massive enlargement of the central PA's, a malalignment-type of ventricular septal defect (VSD) due to anterior and leftward displacement of the infundibular septum, and the absence, or extremely vestigial development, of the pulmonary valve leaflets in association with varying degrees of hypoplasia of the pulmonary annulus. This is almost always associated with absence of the ductus arteriosus. The aneurysmal development of the central PA's is attributed to the combination of the absence of the ductus arteriosus, the orientation of the infundibulum, the degree of valvar stenosis and free pulmonary regurgitation during fetal development [3]. The main and other branches of the PA's may be markedly enlarged in utero. Depending on the degree of external compression from the central PAs and its first and second-order branches, as well as from the abnormal branching of segmental PA's, secondary tracheomalacia and bronchomalacia may develop. Abnormalities of arborization, with tufts of arteries encircling and compressing the intrapulmonary bronchi, and dysplasia and/or absence of bronchial cartilages, have also been described [1]. The incidence of genetic mutations and associated defects is the same as for other conotruncal lesions.

Diagnostic – Imaging

Clinical Presentation

Because right ventricular outflow tract obstruction is generally mild at birth, clinical presentation reflects the degree of respiratory distress secondary to airway obstruction, infections, and heart failure as a result of the left to right shunt. The spectrum of clinical presentation is generally bimodal. In the most extreme forms, neonates and infants present with severe respiratory distress due to compression of the central airways by the aneurysmal central PA's. At the other end of the spectrum are patients whose course and development are most similar to those with simple TOF. Approximately 40–50 % of patients present as newborns or infants with respiratory syndromes ranging from inspiratory and expiratory stridor to severe respiratory compromise, caused by lobar collapse or lobar emphysema and subsequent infection. Some patients require mechanical ventilation or even extracorporeal membrane oxygenation (ECMO) support for stabilization before surgery. The rest of the patients, who do not suffer from respiratory compromise, follow the course of the typical TOF, presenting with cyanosis, cyanotic spells caused by dynamic infundibular stenosis, and cardiac failure, depending on the degree of pulmonary stenosis [4].

Chest X-ray

Chest radiography may reveal varying degrees of pulmonary over-inflation caused by air-trapping; otherwise, the heart does not resemble the typical "boot-shaped" heart found in TOF, due to the dilated PAs.

Echocardiography

Echocardiography is the mainstay for anatomic evaluation of patients with TOF in general, providing comprehensive diagnostic and hemodynamic information. Many patients are even diagnosed by prenatal fetal echocardiogram. The distal PAs and airways are not well visualized by echocardiography. A sequential approach is preferable. The details of the VSD should be clarified. The defect is usually perimembranous – conoventicular with a postero-inferior rim. If there is a short or absent subpulmonary infundibulum, which is rarely seen, the VSD can extend to the outflow to become a doubly committed defect. Multiple VSD's should be ruled out.

The degree of aortic overriding and narrowed subpulmonary outflow tract, with malalignment of the anteriorly displaced muscular outlet septum, and the size of pulmonary annulus should be evaluated. The diameter of the pulmonary annulus and the valve function in TOF/APVS have no impact on the way the RVOT is reconstructed. The dilated main and proximal branches of the PA's should be shown. The size of the PA's at the level of their first bifurcation can be determined. The more distal pattern of branching cannot be visualized.

The origins of the right and left coronary arteries from the aorta and their branching should be determined. Anomalous arteries crossing the RVOT and their origin can be identified.

An absent or non-confluent left pulmonary artery should be ruled out. Additional sources of pulmonary blood flow (aorto-pulmonary collaterals, ductus arteriosus) should be ruled out.

Straddling or overriding of the tricuspid valve should be ruled out. The systemic and pulmonary venous connections should be determined. A left superior vena cava (SVC) should be ruled out and the innominate vein should be visualized.

The side of the aortic arch should be determined. In the right-sided arch, the first branch from the arch itself divides into the left carotid and subclavian arteries; it then can be inferred that this vessel is the brachiocephalic artery, and that the arch itself is right-sided.

Cardiac Catherization

Cardiac catheterization is rarely indicated. In late presenters with pulmonary overcirculation, evaluation of pulmonary resistance may be helpful. Cardiac catheterization may be considered if additional anatomic information regarding the coronary artery anatomy, architecture of the distal PA's, and aorto-pulmonary collaterals is needed.

Bronchoscopy

It is selectively performed to delineate the cause and the site of the airway obstruction and to rule out intrabronchial pathology which could cause collapse. It may be useful for demonstrating airway obstruction during or after surgery.

CT Scan, MRI

In order to evaluate the extent and severity of airway compression, particularly in patients with significant respiratory compromise, computer tomography (CT), magnetic resonance imaging (MRI) have proved to be helpful. A helical CT with 3-dimensional reconstruction is used to delineate the anatomy of the PA's and the degree of airway obstruction. As acquisition time is short, it is useful in the case of compromised newborns and infants. A cardiac MRI provides precise information on the RVOT and on aneurysmal enlargement of the PA's and their relationship to the airways. Obtaining a cardiac MRI in newborns and infants may require intubation, or at least sedation, which limits the applicability of this method.

Check List

- Overinflation of the lungs, with lobar emphysema and/or infection
- Diameter of PA branches and first proximal branches
- Bronchial obstruction at bronchoscopy
- Non confluent or absent PA branches
- MAPCAs
- VSD anatomy, degree of aortic overriding
- Multiple VSD
- Aortic arch side
- Abnormal coronary artery
- Left SVC
- AV valve straddling and/or overriding
- Lung resistances in late presenters

Decision Making & Management Strategy

Decision-Making

In the current era, early primary repair should always be considered. Palliative surgical approaches are suboptimal unless there is a contraindication to cardiopulmonary bypass. Symptomatic newborns and infants need to proceed directly to surgery, regardless of their age and size. Early repair in asymptomatic patients can eliminate the potentially harmful effects of the dilated PA's on the tracheobronchial tree and persistent bronchopulmonary infections requiring repeated hospital admissions often with failure to thrive. These patients are operated on an elective basis at between 3 and 6 months of age [4–9].

Medical Management

The medical management of a symptomatic child is devoted principally to preparation for surgery [4, 6]. Severely ill newborns or infants are placed in the prone position and noninvasive positive pressure ventilation is utilized to obtain respiratory stability. Intubation with mechanical ventilation with a high positive end-expiratory pressure (10 cm H_2O) is initiated as required. If these measures fail, the only alternative is respiratory ECMO and subsequent high-risk surgery. Patients who do not present in infancy with respiratory compromise are generally managed similar to standard TOF patients.

Surgical Management

Apart from the standard TOF repair (see Chaps. 6 and 7), the specific goal of surgical management is decompression of the airways.

Traditional Approach to Decompression of the Airways

The traditional approach incorporates plication or resection of the anterior or posterior wall of the normally positioned PA's [4, 5, 9–11]. The downsized pulmonary arteries may decrease compression of the adjacent airways. Suspension of the left pulmonary artery to the retrosternal fascia might be also useful [6]. In rare cases, excision of nearly all the aneurysmal mediastinal pulmonary arteries and replacement by a pulmonary homograft might be considered [12]. The specific steps of the operation are as followed.

- Standard cardiopulmonary bypass is instituted with direct bicaval cannulation. The aorta is cannulated as high as possible. A left atrial vent is inserted through the right pulmonary veins. Myocardial protection is provided by crystalloid antegrade cardioplegia.
- First, the TOF is repaired (see Chaps. 6 and 7) preferentially using trans – atrial approach
- Downsizing of the PA by plication or resection of the anterior and/or posterior wall of the normally positioned PAs is performed. Transection of the aorta is useful (Fig. 10.1) to improve the approach to the dilated PAs,
- Alternatively, the PA trunk is transected, the PAs are downsized and a valve conduit is inserted (Fig. 10.2).

Alternative Approach of Decompression of the Airways

An alternative approach incorporates translocation of the PA anterior to the aorta (Lecompte maneuver) and away from the airways. Plication of the pulmonary arteries may or may not be necessary [7, 13, 14]. The specific steps of the operation are as followed.

- First, the TOF is repaired first, preferentially using trans-trial approach. After TOF repair, the aorta is divided. At this point, one should consider shortening the aorta by resecting the appropriate tubular segment to facilitate anterior translocation of the PA (Fig. 10.3).
- The PA is transected above the annulus (Fig. 10.4).
- The transected PA is brought anterior to the aorta and an end-to-end anastomosis of the ascending aorta is performed (Fig. 10.5)
- If needed, downsizing of the PA is performed to decrease wall tension and prevent later development of aneurysmal dilatation of the PA (Fig. 10.6).

- The right ventricular outflow tract is reconstructed (Figs. 10.7, 10.8, 10.9, and 10.10). Particulary in symptomatic newborns and infants valve conduit should be considered.

There are several technical pitfalls to keep in mind during the performance of this procedure. It is essential to gain adequate space between the SVC and ascending aorta for the translocated right PA. In addition to SVC mobilization, appropriate shortening of the ascending aorta, if necessary, allows the aorta to ultimately reside posteriorly and to the left of its usual location. This maneuver calls for a thorough mobilization of the aortic arch and brachiocephalic vessels. Shortening of the ascending aorta and mobilization of the PA beyond the pericardial reflection avoids the potential compression of the right coronary artery and the SVC [13]. On the other hand, it is not always necessary to make the aorta shorter and to risk too close a relationship of the ascending aorta to the trachea [2, 7, 14]. The relationship of the posteriorly located aorta and tracheobroncheal tree should be evaluated to rule out compression of the airways. Another relevant detail is shortening of the left PA (which is always too long), by oblique transection of the PA trunk with the

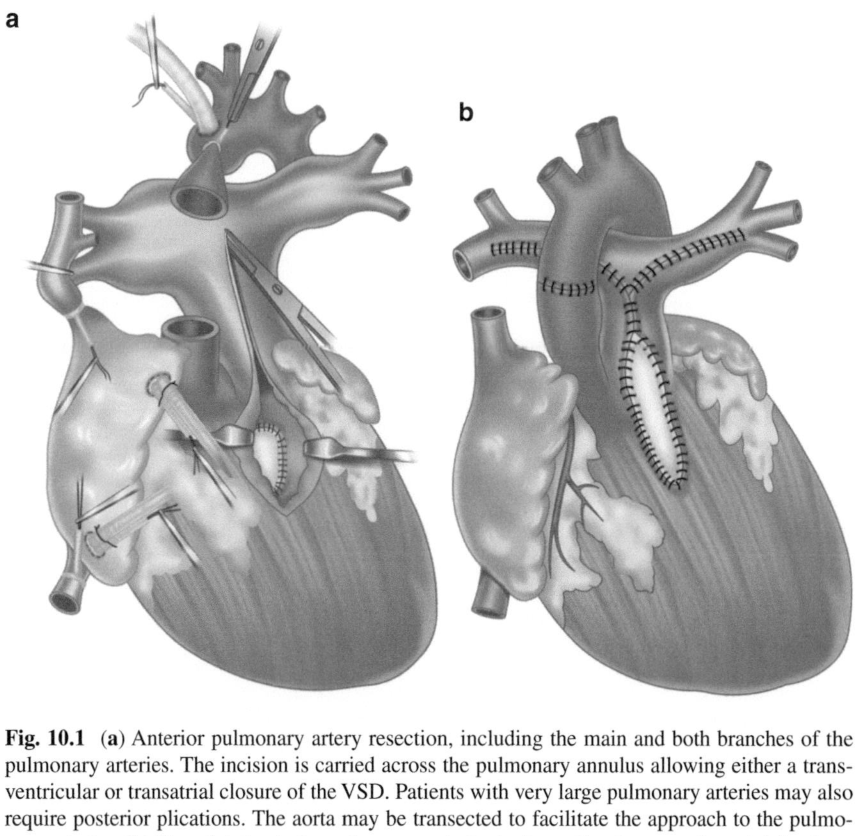

Fig. 10.1 (**a**) Anterior pulmonary artery resection, including the main and both branches of the pulmonary arteries. The incision is carried across the pulmonary annulus allowing either a transventricular or transatrial closure of the VSD. Patients with very large pulmonary arteries may also require posterior plications. The aorta may be transected to facilitate the approach to the pulmonary arteries. (**b**) Completed anterior pulmonary arterioplasties with a transannular patch in place

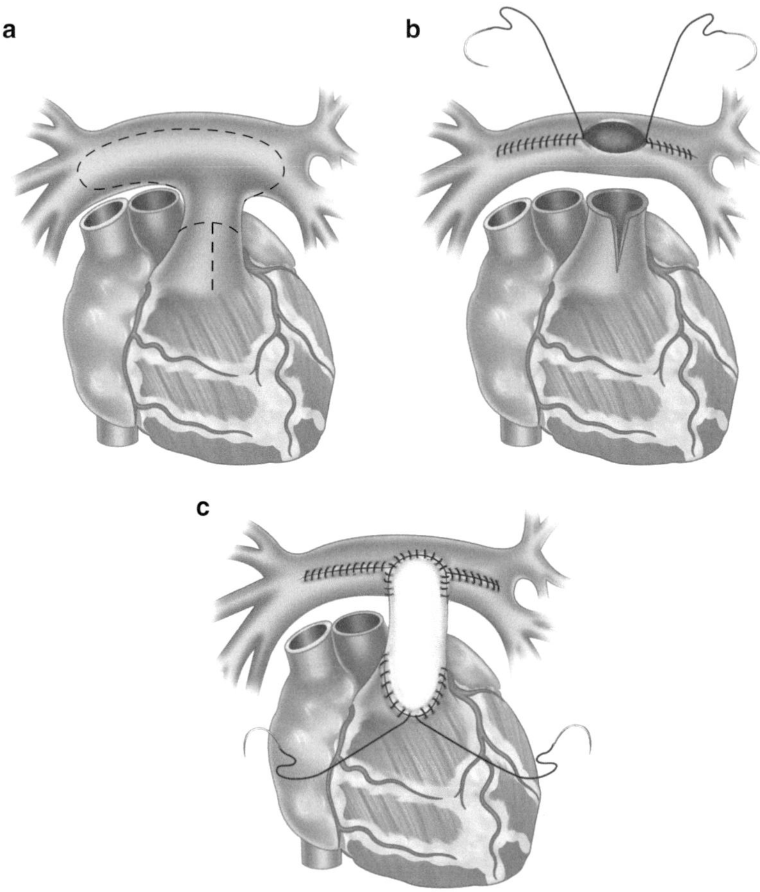

Fig. 10.2 (**a**) Line of resection of the main pulmonary artery and anterior portion of the main branches. The pulmonary artery is transected at the annulus and an incision is made into the right ventricular outflow tract. (**b**) Arterioplasty of the right and left pulmonary artery branches reduces their caliber. (**c**) Completed repair using a bovine jugular vein conduit

connection to the RVOT [7, 15]. A crossing left anterior descending coronary artery is a contraindication for translocation of the PA anterior to the aorta.

Outcomes

Airway morbidity determines the prognosis of patients with TOF/APVS. Older patients with no respiratory compromise follow the outcomes of standard TOF patients. At the other end of the clinical spectrum are symptomatic newborns and infants, in whom mortality and morbidity still remains considerable, despite improvements in surgical techniques and critical care. In this group, complete repair

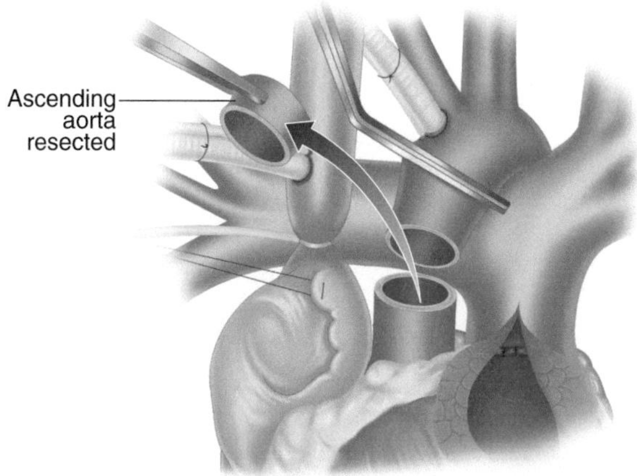

Fig. 10.3 The aorta is divided above the aortic valve commissures. A short tubular segment of the aorta is resected. This maneuver brings the future ascending aorta more posterior and to the left. Resection of the aorta, especially in newborns, may be omitted to avoid too close a relationship between the aorta and the trachea and left bronchus

with the placement of a valved conduit and decompression of the airways at the onset of symptoms should be considered. With this approach the patient outcome is determined by the status and management of their airways. These infants may require multiple postoperative hospitalizations for recurrent respiratory infections secondary to their tracheobronchomalacia.

The surgical approach to dilated PAs, especially in symptomatic newborns and infants remains controversial. The traditional approach focuses on plication and reduction of the anterior or posterior wall of the normally positioned PA, with or without pulmonary valve replacement. Nørgaard et al. (2006) [11] analyzed a group of 36 patients with a high prevalence of airway obstruction symptoms before surgery. PA plication was performed in 86 % of the patients. The majority of patients underwent transannular patching only. The survival benefit was 79 % at 15 years of follow-up. Postoperative survival was strongly associated with preoperative ventilator dependency, due to disease of the airways. In this group of patients, survival was less than 50 % at 10-year follow-up. Freedom from reoperation 10 years after repair was 55 %. A group in Toronto reviewed 61 patients who had undergone complete repair. Thirty-three patients (54 %) had undergone PA plication or reduction, and RVOT reconstruction with a valved conduit or bioprosthetic valve was performed in 80 % of the patients. The 10-year survival benefit was 87.5 %. Time-related survival stratified by age groups (infants vs. others), showed a significantly worse outcome for infants, with only 34.5 % survival at 12 years of follow-up. Freedom from RVOT reoperation was 60 % at 10 years. There were no significant risk factors for time-related survival or RVOT reoperation on multivariable analysis [6]. McDonnell et al. (1999) [9] analyzed 28 patients. Thirteen patients were ventilated for respiratory failure preoperatively and ECMO was used in three patients. Twenty-six

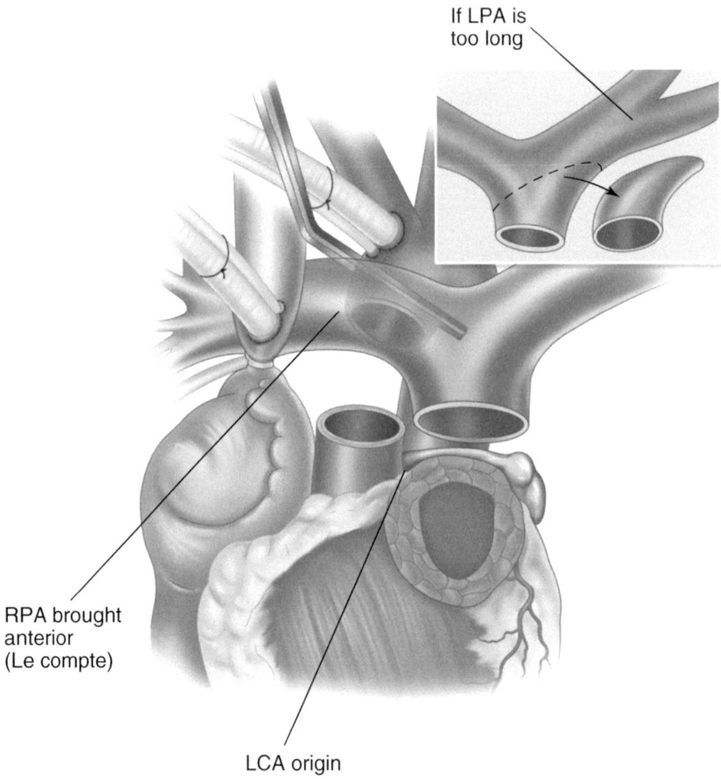

Fig. 10.4 The pulmonary artery is transected above the annulus. Care is taken to stay away from the left coronary artery. If the left pulmonary artery is too long, the pulmonary trunk is obliquely cut toward the left pulmonary artery. *LCA* left coronary artery, *LPA* left pulmonary artery, *RPA* right pulmonary artery

patients (93 %) had undergone pulmonary artery plication, and the right ventricular outflow tract was reconstructed with a valved conduit in 18 % of the patients. Survival was 72 % at 10 years. The need for preoperative intubation was associated with a worse outcome. Freedom from death or reoperation was 52 % at 10 years. The prognosis of patients requiring preoperative ventilation was significantly worse, with freedom from death or reoperation less than 30 % at 5 years. Brown et al. (2006) [5] reported an 85 % survival benefit at 15 years in 20 patients operated on using a valved conduit for reconstruction of the RVOT (45 %), or a transannular patch and/or transannular patch with monocusp valve with PA reduction arterioplasty. Preoperative ventilator dependency was associated with a worse outcome. Six patients (33 %) underwent reoperation for pulmonary valve incompetence and right ventricular dysfunction. Freedom from reoperation was 66 % at 15 years.

Another approach is the removal of the entire main pulmonary artery and placement of a bifurcated pulmonary homograft. This technique effectively decreases the size of the pulmonary vessels, minimizing potential compression of the bronchi.

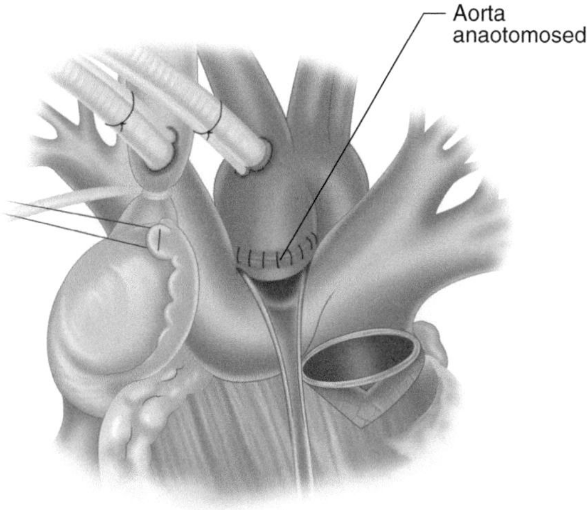

Fig. 10.5 If necessary, the transected pulmonary artery is mobilized, and brought anterior to the aorta. At this point, end-to-end anastomosis of the ascending aorta is performed. Care is taken to avoid compression of the right coronary artery by the translocated pulmonary artery. In particular, the right pulmonary artery must be mobilized adequately to avoid undue tension on the right coronary artery

Hew et al. (2002) [12] reported the experience of the Boston Children's Hospital with 54 patients. Overall, the 10-year survival rate was 78 %. Respiratory distress, younger age, and lower weight at surgery were important prognostic risk factors for early mortality. Replacement of the central PA's by a valved pulmonary homograft has been associated with improved survival in comparison with other techniques, especially in neonates with severe respiratory distress.

The combination of a pulmonary reduction arterioplasty and anterior displacement of the pulmonary artery by the use of the Lecompte maneuver seems to achieve better results by combining the various techniques. Hraska et al. (2009) [8] have used this novel technique in eight infants, including three newborns with persistent tracheobronchial compression and severe respiratory distress. Six patients (75 %) were ventilator-dependant before surgery. The RVOT was reconstructed using a valved homograft in two newborns; a monocusp valve was utilized in one infant. Combined anterior and posterior plication of the PA was performed in four patients. There were no deaths, with a mean follow-up of 4 years. Freedom from reoperation due to conduit failure was 78 % at 5 years of follow-up. Respiratory symptoms disappeared or were significantly reduced in all patients. No patient was ventilator-dependent or had a tracheostomy after surgery. Based on positive experiences with primary correction of TOF/APVS, this concept was applied to five other patients as a secondary procedure, after primary correction of the truncus arteriosus communis, double outlet right ventricle, TOF, and traditional correction of the TOF/APVS had failed, the patients thus requiring tracheostomy and ventilatory support. These patients presented with severe respiratory distress and persistent

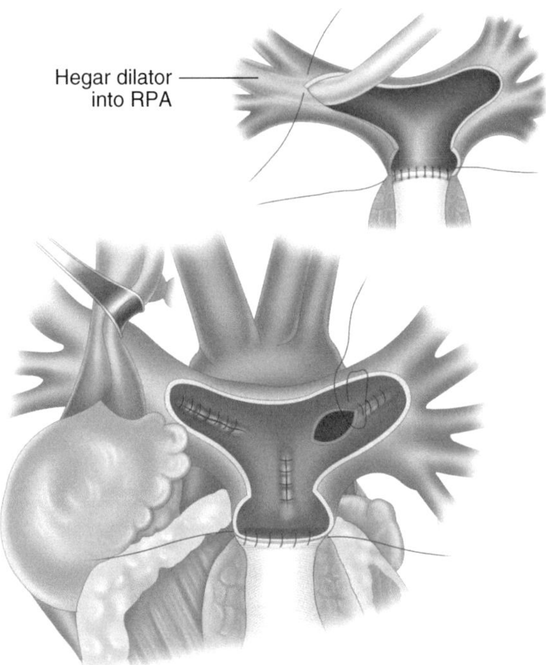

Fig. 10.6 Especially in symptomatic patients, anterior plication of the pulmonary artery is performed to decrease wall tension and prevent later development of aneurysmal dilation of the pulmonary artery. Triangular segments of the anterior wall of each branch of the pulmonary artery and part of the anterior wall of the pulmonary artery trunk are excised. An appropriately chosen Hegar dilator is used to guide the extent of the resection of the pulmonary artery and the magnitude of plication. An anterior wall resection may be combined with posterior wall plications of the main and both pulmonary arteries. *RPA* right pulmonary artery

tracheobronchomalacia, based on the altered relationship of the tracheobronchial tree and the PA's. The intermediate-term functional outcomes have been encouraging, with zero mortality and with the disappearance of respiratory symptoms in the majority of patients. The effectiveness of the Lecompte maneuver to relieve airway compression in severe symptomatic patients has also been confirmed by other studies [2], but long-term data are not yet available.

Severely symptomatic neonates and infants, with the risk of elevated pulmonary artery resistance due to grossly abnormal intra-parenchymal pulmonary arteries, reactive pulmonary artery pressure, or pulmonary artery branch stenosis, are sensitive to significant pulmonary insufficiency, and may benefit from placement of a competent pulmonary valve in the RVOT. In the intermediate term, pulmonary valve insertion may improve the early postoperative hemodynamics and diminish the incidence of persistent pulmonary artery dilatation and bronchial compression through elimination of pulmonary artery pulsatility, due to the larger pulmonary regurgitant fraction and the increased total pulmonary blood

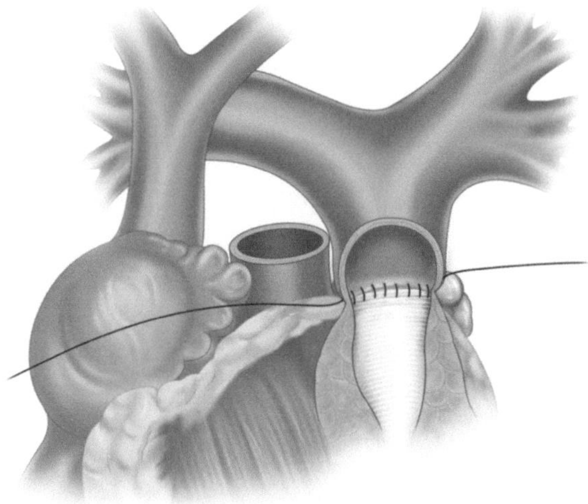

Fig. 10.7 A direct connection between the pulmonary artery and the RVOT is accomplished using a continuous suture technique (the aorta is cut off for clarity)

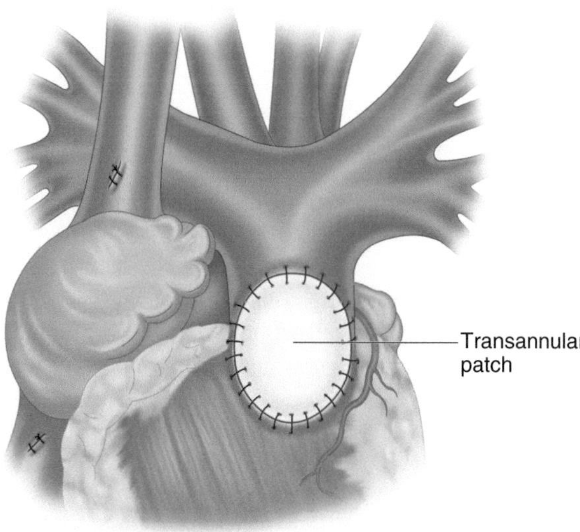

Fig. 10.8 The right ventricular outflow tract is enlarged and reconstructed by use of a transannular pericardial patch treated with glutaraldehyde, with the aim of achieving a normal Z-value for the annulus. The newly created right ventricular outflow tract should have growth potential

flow. In the long term, a competent valve in the RVOT reduces the risk of arrhythmias and late right ventricular dysfunction. A younger age at the time of the implantation of a valved conduit is a factor for earlier reoperation, but the advantage of maintaining valve competency and the low operative risk for conduit/

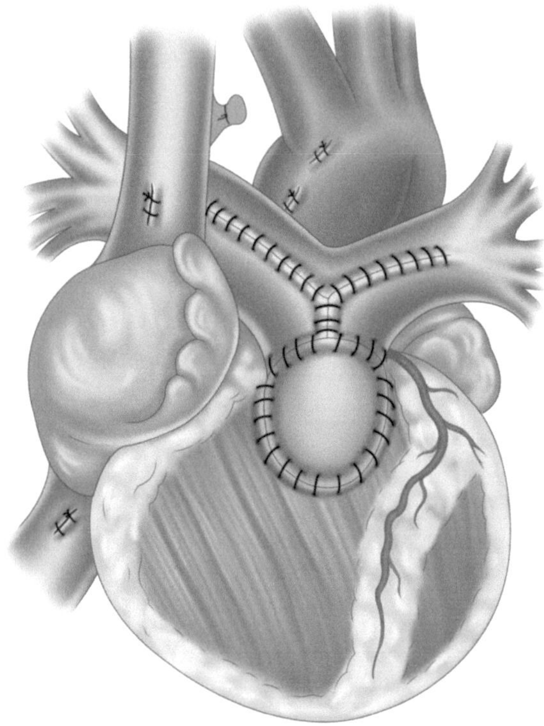

Fig. 10.9 The final outcome of translocation of the pulmonary artery, with direct connection to the right ventricle, patch reconstruction of the right ventricular outflow tract, and anterior plication of the pulmonary arteries. If a homograft is not used, the reconstruction has growth potential. The usual monitoring lines and temporary atrial and ventricular pacing wires are always placed

pulmonary valve replacement outweighs this drawback. Older patients without respiratory symptoms typically do well without placement of a pulmonary valve, and a limited transannular patch is a reasonable alternative for reconstruction of the RVOT [2, 8, 9].

Pulmonary arteriopexy for the relief of distal left bronchial collapse may be useful [6], however an arteriopexy operation alone is usually not sufficient to relieve the airway compression in TOF/APVS [2].

In patients with abnormalities of bronchial arborization, with tufts of arteries encircling and compressing the intrapulmonary bronchi that cannot be addressed during primary surgery, and which may contribute to air entrapment in emphysematous lobes and subsequent compression of the remaining lung, a lobectomy might be successful in relieving airway compression [6].

Endobronchial stents may represent another potential tool for the treatment of patients with a long segment of tracheobronchomalacia. However, the results are disappointing and the deployment of stents is generally not recommended [2].

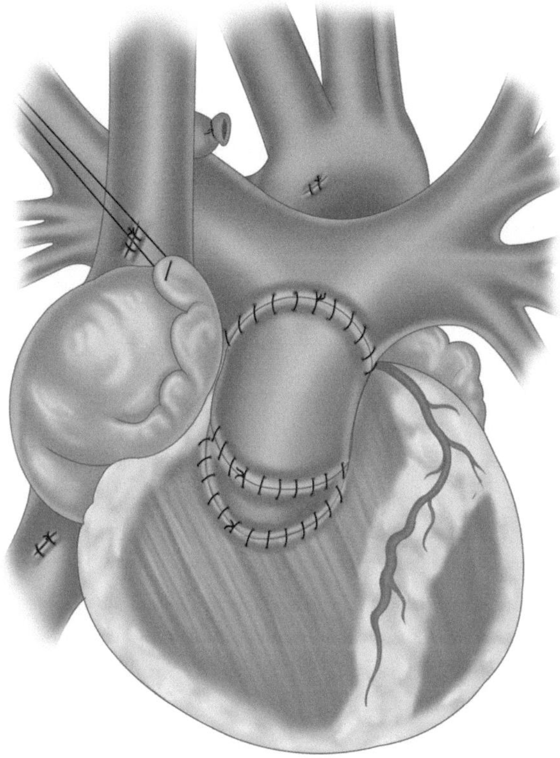

Fig. 10.10 If necessary, homograft insertion (recommended in symptomatic newborns) or monocusp valve placement is performed. A short pulmonary homograft is orthotopically placed the proximal anastomosis is supplemented with a roof of autologous pericardium treated with glutaraldehyde

Summary

1. Overall survival is closely related to airway pathology. The need for preoperative intubation and ventilation are risk factors predictive of poor outcome.
2. The treatment of patients should be individualized on the basis of the patient's age and clinical symptoms.
3. Asymptomatic patients with no respiratory compromise should undergo elective repair between 3 and 6 months of age. Placement of a pulmonary valve is not needed, and a limited transannular patch is a reasonable alternative for reconstruction of the RVOT.
4. In symptomatic newborns and infants, mortality and morbidity still remain considerable. Complete repair, with the placement of a valved conduit in the right ventricular outflow tract and decompression of the airways at the time of symptom onset, should be considered.
5. Symptomatic patients may require multiple postoperative hospitalizations for recurrent respiratory infections secondary to tracheobronchomalacia. Understanding the mechanism of airway compression is of paramount importance.

Under these circumstances, additional reinterventions for airway decompression may be helpful.

6. Long-term survival beyond the perioperative period is satisfactory, but patients are likely to present later for reoperation of the RVOT.
7. Future improvement in the management of symptomatic patients will require better evaluation of the long-term outcomes of different surgical approaches, including evaluation of exercise capacity and pulmonary function testing.

References

1. Rabinovitch M, Grady S, David I, et al. Compression of intrapulmonary bronchi by abnormally branching pulmonary arteries associated with absent pulmonary valves. Am J Cardiol. 1982;50:804–13.
2. Nolke L, Azakie A, Anagnostopoulos PV, et al. The Lecompte maneuver for relief of airway compression in absent pulmonary valve syndrome. Ann Thorac Surg. 2006;81:1802–7.
3. Jacobs ML. Congenital heart surgery nomenclature and database project: tetralogy of Fallot. Ann Thorac Surg. 2000;69:S77–82.
4. Kirshbom PM, Kogon BE. Tetralogy of Fallot with absent pulmonary valve syndrome. Semin Thorac Cardiovasc Surg Pediatr Card Surg Annu. 2004;7:65–71.
5. Brown JW, Ruzmetov M, Vijay P, et al. Surgical treatment of absent pulmonary valve syndrome associated with bronchial obstruction. Ann Thorac Surg. 2006;82:2221–6.
6. Alsoufi B, Williams WG, Hua Z, et al. Surgical outcomes in the treatment of patients with tetralogy of Fallot and absent pulmonary valve. Eur J Cardiothorac Surg. 2007;31:354–9.
7. Hraska V. Tetralogy of Fallot with absent pulmonary valve syndrome using a new approach. Semin Thorac Cardiovasc Surg Pediatr Card Surg Annu. 2005;8:132–5.
8. Hraska V, Photiadis J, Schindler E, et al. A novel approach to the repair of tetralogy of Fallot with absent pulmonary valve and the reduction of airway compression by the pulmonary artery. Semin Thorac Cardiovasc Surg Pediatr Card Surg Annu. 2009;12:59–62.
9. McDonnell BE, Raff GW, Gaynor JW, et al. Outcome after repair of tetralogy of Fallot with absent pulmonary valve. Ann Thorac Surg. 1999;67:1391–5.
10. Conte S, Serraf A, Godart F, et al. Technique to repair tetralogy of Fallot with absent pulmonary valve. Ann Thorac Surg. 1997;63:1489–91.
11. Norgaard MA, Alphonso N, Newcomb AE, et al. Absent pulmonary valve syndrome. Surgical and clinical outcome with long-term follow-up. Eur J Cardiothorac Surg. 2006;29:682–7.
12. Hew CC, Daebritz SH, Zurakowski D, et al. Valved homograft replacement of aneurysmal pulmonary arteries for severely symptomatic absent pulmonary valve syndrome. Ann Thorac Surg. 2002;73:1778–85.
13. Hraska V. A new approach to correction of tetralogy of Fallot with absent pulmonary valve. Ann Thorac Surg. 2000;69:1601–3.
14. Hraska V, Murin P. Surgical management of congenital heart disease I: complex transposition of great arteries right and left ventricular outflow tract obstruction, Ebstein's anomaly. A video manual. Heidelberg: Springer; 2012.
15. Hraska V. Absent pulmonary valve repair. Op Tech Thorac Cardiovasc Surg. 2007;12:36–46.

Chapter 11
Fallot: Palliation with BT Shunt

Pirooz Eghtesady and Mohammed Said Ghanamah

Abstract Tetralogy of Fallot (TOF) is a constellation of conotruncal anomalies involving anterior malalignment of the conal septum and right ventricular outflow tract obstruction. When symptomatic in the neonatal period or early infancy, it can be treated either by complete surgical repair or by initial palliation with a systemic to pulmonary shunt, most commonly in the form of a modified Blalock-Taussig shunt. This chapter describes the details of the surgical technique used to perform a BT shunt. The procedure continues to carry a relatively high mortality rate close to 4 %. The chapter also discusses perioperative management including preoperative evaluation, decision making and important aspects of postoperative anticoagulation.

Keywords Tetralogy of Fallot • Blalock-Taussig shunt • Systemic to pulmonary shunt • Congenital heart surgery

Introduction

Tetralogy of Fallot (ToF) is a constellation of conotruncal anomalies that can really be ascribed to the abnormal development of the conal septum resulting in what has been described as a "Monology" of Fallot by Van Praagh [1]. Specifically, the anterior malalignment of the conal septum and subsequent overriding of the aorta with protrusion of the conal septum toward the right ventricular outflow tract lead to the various associated pathologic changes observed. A number of different approaches have been described. Complete repair, which is our typical approach to the

P. Eghtesady, MD, PhD (✉)
Section of Pediatric Cardiothoracic Surgery, Department of Cardiothoracic Surgery, St. Louis Children's Hospital, Suite 5 S, One Children's Place,, St. Louis, MO 63110, USA
e-mail: eghtesadyp@wudosis.wustl.edu

M.S. Ghanamah, MD
Department of Cardiothoracic Surgery, St. Louis Children's Hospital, St. Louis, MO, USA

F. Lacour-Gayet et al. (eds.), *Surgery of Conotruncal Anomalies*,
DOI 10.1007/978-3-319-23057-3_11

symptomatic neonate or infant, is discussed in Chaps. 6 and 7. The purpose of this chapter is to describe the application of systemic to pulmonary artery shunting, often in the form of the Blalock-Taussig (BT) shunt, as an alternative palliation for management of the patient with ToF.

From a historical perspective, the BT shunt or more appropriately the Blalock-Taussig-Thomas shunt, giving credit to the late technician Vivien Thomas responsible for developing the operation while working in Dr. Blalock's laboratory at Johns Hopkins, marks an important landmark step in the history of congenital heart surgery [2]. Classically, that operation involved the sacrifice of the right subclavian artery by diverting the blood from that vessel to the right pulmonary artery, through a thoracotomy approach. Today, this author still on occasion uses the classic BT, particularly for very small infants who are less than two kilograms at the time of the operation.

In general, our approach for management of the asymptomatic Tetralogy of Fallot is to perform complete repair electively around 4–6 months of age. Symptomatic neonates are treated also with complete repair pending other confounding factors with the clinical scenario. Part of this bias stems from the fact that overall risks of complete repair are not substantially different from palliative systemic to pulmonary artery shunting. A relatively "simple" procedure, ironically, the BT shunt is associated with approximately 7 % mortality overall in the Society of Thoracic Surgery (STS) database [3]. However, for two ventricle physiology, the mortality rate is around 4 %. Neonatal repair of ToF is associated with ~4 % mortality in the STS database. The BT shunt mortality has been constant over the last decade, despite advances and improves in many other areas (e.g., NIRS monitoring, etc.>). As well, most single institution series have not shown any distinctly better outcomes and recent analysis of the individual institutions within STS, did not reveal significant outliers, highlighting the overall challenge to the pediatric cardiothoracic surgery community for this "simple" operation. A few factors more recently have been shown to be important in these outcomes; these are discussed later.

Diagnosis and Imaging

The preoperative evaluation includes patients' clinical symptoms, SaO_2, chest radiograph, and mainly 2D echocardiography. The echo findings include: the morphology of the VSD, the pulmonary valve annulus diameter and Z- score, the diameter of the PA branches and Z score, abnormal coronary artery pattern and the arch and neck vessel anatomy. In ToF presenting in infancy, the diameter of the pulmonary branches can be underestimated with diminished antegrade flow and presence of a patent ductus arteriosus (PDA). Association with MAPCAs should be suspected in presence of a relatively good SaO_2 despite a tight RVOT obstruction. Multiple VSD's are also assessed carefully, though quite rare in this condition. Abnormal presence of an LAD (or accessory LAD) arising from the RCA and crossing the infundibulum can be suspected by echocardiography. It will be confirmed by catheterism-angiogram or by CT angiogram, which allows assessing the distance between the abnormal coronary and the PA annulus. Others rely on intra-operative evaluation during sternotomy. Catheterization is rarely used in infancy. However, it is needed in severe forms presenting late. CT scan and MRI are becoming quite popular, particularly for more complex subtypes of Tetralogy of Fallot, such as association with complete AV canal (Chap. 10) or DORV-Fallot type (Chap. 26).

Check List Prior to BT Shunt

- Weight, SaO_2
- PA annulus diameter and Z score
- PA branch diameter and Z score
- PDA location, size
- Abnormal coronary pattern
- Additional VSD
- Aortic arch side
- Neck vessels morphology
- Prematurity, extra cardiac damage
- Complex cardiac association
- Coagulation disorder

Surgery

Below 3 months of age, there is some debate between BT shunt and one stage repair, while the later is becoming the rule. However, there are still some indications for palliation in Tetralogy of Fallot.

Indications for BT Shunt

ToF with pulmonary atresia are treated in Chaps. 6 and 9 and are excluded from this chapter.

In infancy, the indications for Blalock-Taussig shunt in ToF are limited to infants with: hemodynamic instability, multiple organ failure as a result of late unrecognized presentation, abnormal coronaries that could limit the feasibility of the right ventricular outflow tract patch if that is indicated, – and any contra-indication to cardiopulmonary bypass. Neonatal patent ductus stenting is an alternative used by some centers [4–6]. We have had limited experience with this modality which can be complicated with entrapment of the branch PA. Lastly, medical therapy with continued prostaglandins may have a place in the management of premature babies with SGA <34 weeks and birth weight <2.0 kg.

Although rare in the US, *late presentation of ToF* may alter the indication. Severe forms of ToF could be seen in emergency with SaO_2 <70 % and high hematocrit and hemoglobin. A BT shunt is usually preferred in an emergency as a saving procedure. Other ToF, seen late, present with hypoplasia of the PA branches and require a BT shunt as it is unlikely that the hypoplastic PA branches accept a full circulation after 6 months of age. Other ToF have significant MAPCAs with good SaO_2 and severe RVOT obstruction. The MAPCAs should be obturated by surgery or interventional cardiology at the time of ToF repair.

Surgical Technique

For the conduct of the operation, our bias is to give a quarter dose of baby aspirin the morning of surgery for reasons elaborated on later. Intraoperatively, our approach involves a median sternotomy. Others have described performing the shunt through a thoracotomy on the side opposite to the aortic arch. Our preference with regard to use of median sternotomy relates to the fact that it provides easy access for alteration of the plan, as well as ease with ligation of the PDA which we do routinely.

A Genesee retractor with a superior extension that retracts the superior skin edge northward toward patient's head (or other equivalent maneuvers that enhance exposure in the superior aspect of the wound) are worthwhile for conduct of the procedures to allow ample exposure. To that end, advance conversation with anesthesia colleagues to explain lack of access to the infant head during the procedure (due to limited real-estate after draping) is important. No manipulations can be done easily without hitting the elbow of the surgeon or assistant during the critical time that the clamps are on and the vessels are incised. Thymic tissue is resected (either both lobes or at least the right sided one) to allow exposure of the great vessels. Limited dissection of the innominate vein as well as the innominate arteries is carried out prior to opening up the pericardium. In babies that are slightly on the unstable side the pericardium is proactively opened and purse string sutures are placed in the right atrium and the ascending aorta in case there would be a need for urgent use of cardiopulmonary bypass. Otherwise the pericardium is left intact to reduce the chances of dysrhythmias which can occur with manipulation.

Once the innominate artery has been dissected up to the level of the bifurcation and the anatomy has been clearly delineated, the pericardium is incised and the right pulmonary artery is dissected and a vessel is isolated with a vessel loop and occluded temporarily to ensure the patient tolerates single lung ventilation. Of note, the morning of surgery a chest radiograph is always obtained, and intraoperatively there is confirmation that the right lung and left lung are being ventilated adequately, to ensure that the endotracheal tube position is appropriate and avoid an intraoperative mishap from single lung ventilation, (e.g., right lung intubation).

The underbelly of the innominate artery is identified and marked; as well, a PTFE graft is measured and marked. For nearly vast majority of our cases we use a 3.5 mm, non-stretch graft. Rarely, if the infant is over 4 kg (and this is not due to hydrops or other fluid retention), will we use a 4 mm graft. Typically the length of graft is about one and half centimeters long. While some have used heparin bonded PTFE grafts, we have used the standard PTFE and are not aware of any particular data showing improved outcomes with use of the heparin bonded PTFE. Of note, manufacturer of the heparin bonded grafts (which were developed for hemodialysis patients) reports that the heparin bonding dissolves within approximately 48 h.

It is essential that the underside of the innominate artery is *cleaned off of any adventitial tissue* (adventitial tissue, in contrast to intima, is highly thrombogenic) and clearly marked. Placement of the graft more anteriorly can lead to inappropriate angulation that can then lead to thrombosis of the shunt. It is the author's practice to mark the underbelly of the innominate artery to ensure the correct orientation is maintained during clamping. One hundred fifty units of heparin per kilogram is administered prior to clamping the innominate artery. While some clamp the vessel without the application of heparin, it is the author's bias to avoid any potential clot build up during clamping, specially since the clamp is maintained during the pulmonary artery end anastomosis. The heparin is allowed to circulate for a couple of minutes before clamping. Clamp is applied for approximately a minute before an arteriotomy is performed. This is to ensure the patient has hemodynamic stability. Of note, it is important if possible that the arterial line placed preoperatively or in the operating room, is not in the right wrist, allowing for continued accurate hemodynamics monitoring during the procedure.

A beaver blade is used to make an arteriotomy that approximately corresponds to the opening in the PTFE shunt. It is better to err on the side of making the arteriotomy smaller than the graft, since the vessel can stretch. The PTFE shunt is flushed with heparinized saline and cut in a beveled fashion. A 6–0 Prolene tack up suture is used to maintain opening of the upper lip of the arteriotomy. This is attached to the subcutaneous tissue in the upper aspect of the wound (Fig. 11.1). 7–0 Prolene® (Everpoint needle) is then used to sew the PTFE to the arteriotomy. One limb of the suture is first passed through the upper lip of the anastomosis on the assistant side and shodded. The lower aspect of the anastomosis is then carried out toward the surgeon using a running 7–0 Prolene suture (Fig. 11.2). At the heal and the toe of the anastomoses, using the standard principles of vascular surgery, the sutures are passed in two steps bringing up the suture in between each pass through the graft or the vessel. This is to ensure a tight opposition of the graft around the corners, preventing the potential for bleeding at those sites. Once the running suture line comes around the toe of the anastomosis, it is shodded (Fig. 11.3). The upper anastomosis (relative the innominate artery arteriotomy) is then completed by bringing the first limb of suture initially shodded, toward the surgeon (Fig. 11.4). Heparin containing saline solution is then introduced into the graft to assess for suture line tightness and any leakage. Tisseel glue® is then applied to the anastomosis, and then the graft is cut to appropriate length, corresponding to the upper border of the right pulmonary artery (RPA).

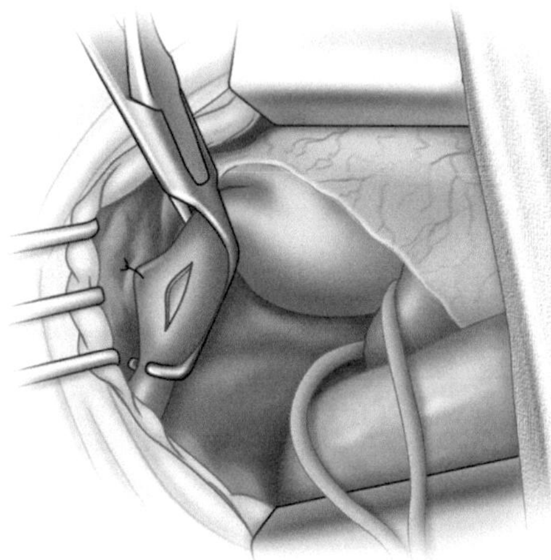

Fig. 11.1 Innominate artery open and tack up stitch in place

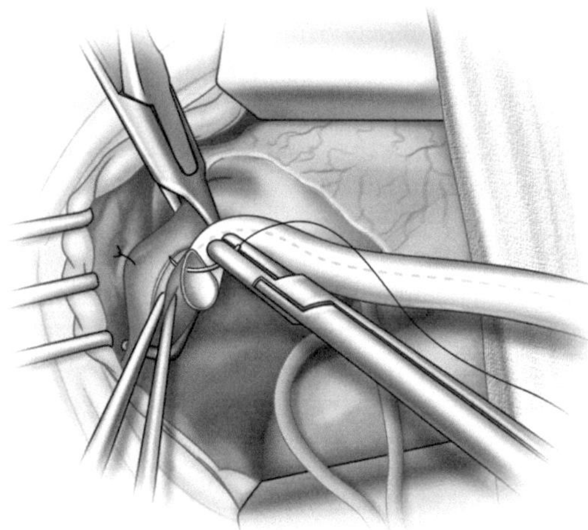

Fig. 11.2 The initiation of the anastomosis at the heel

In the same fashion as described previously, the upper aspect of the RPA is marked prior to clamping. Typically the pulmonary artery dissection is carried out unto the branch bifurcation to allow mobilization; however, the anasomtomis is kept off of the upper lobe branch. At times, in a patient who is dependent on the ductal flow, placing the clamp too proximally (toward the MPA) can lead to distortion or alteration of flow through the PDA into LPA. This can lead to desaturation, specially as the assistant may move the RPA clamp to assist the surgeon with the anastomosis. Therefore, it is prudent to take some time and ensure the patient can tolerate the clamping of the RPA prior to proceeding with the RPA arteriotomy. It's the author's

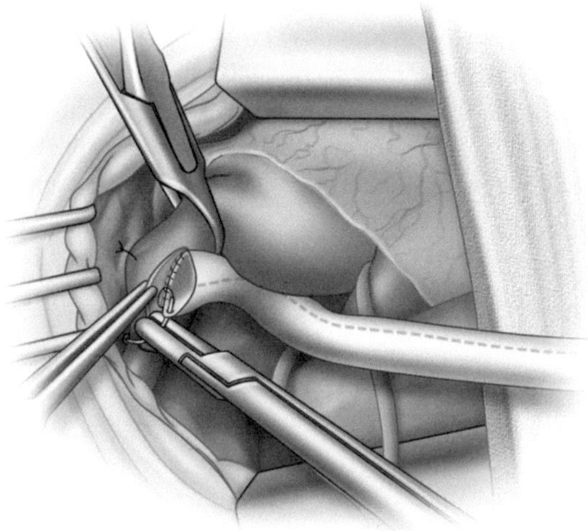

Fig. 11.3 The conduct of the toe anastomosis

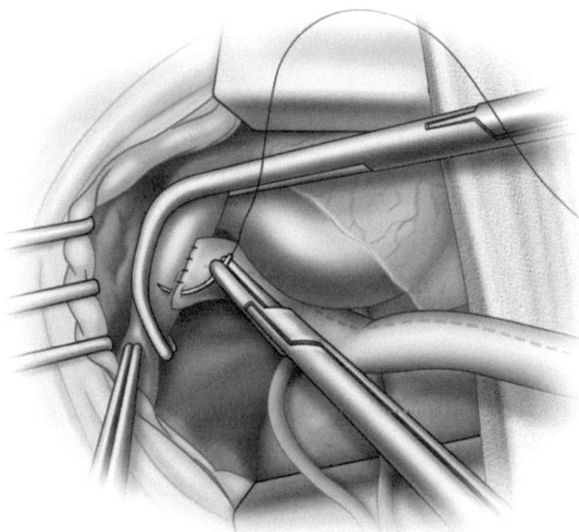

Fig. 11.4 The completion of the anastomosis

approach to use a side biting clamp to apply to the right pulmonary artery; other techniques involving two clamps or vessels loops have been described. The authors preference to use a single clamp for the RPA is because it typically pulls the aorta out of the way as well as eliminating the need for any additional hands by anyone else beyond the assistant to enhance the exposure.

A beaver blade is used once again to open up the upper aspect of the right pulmonary artery (Fig. 11.5) and a 6–0 Prolene® is placed onto the inferior lip of RPA with downward traction (toward patient feet) to enhance the exposure. As well, a previously placed purse-string suture on the right atrial appendage can be placed on traction to enhance exposure and limit the impingement of that structure in the operative field. A running 7–0 Prolene® (Everpoint) is then used for the anastomosis of RPA to the PTFE graft, again starting in the midpoint of the graft toward the assistant side (i.e., starting at the heel) (Fig. 11.6) sweing to the lower lip toward the surgeon (Fig. 11.7) and ultimately finishing on the upper lip as described previously (Fig. 11.8). Once again Tisseel® glue is applied and left in place for a few minutes

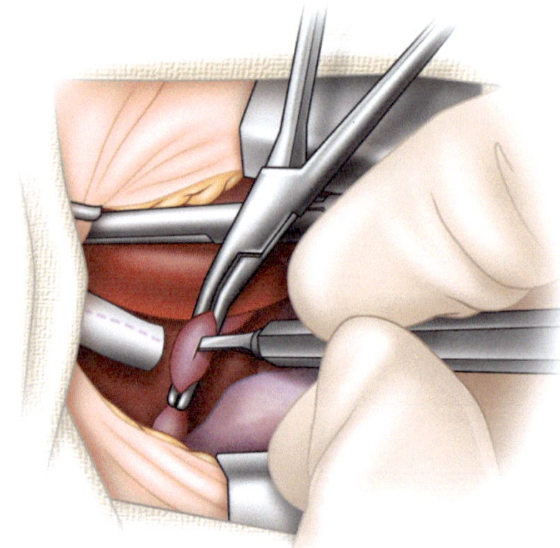

Fig. 11.5 RPA clamped and open

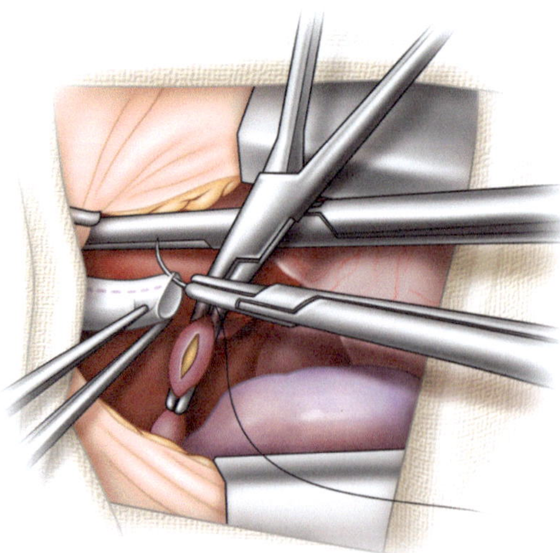

Fig. 11.6 Initiation of the anastomosis between PTFE and RPA (toward assistant side)

before the clamps are removed. The RPA clamp is removed first, and then subsequently the innominate artery clamp is removed to establish flow into the shunt. At this point then, attention is directed to the ductus arteriosus.

While some prefer to leave the ductus [7], it is author's preference to remove this to eliminate any potential for overcirculation immediately after the procedure as well as reduce competitive flow that can disadvantage the BT shunt. Of note,

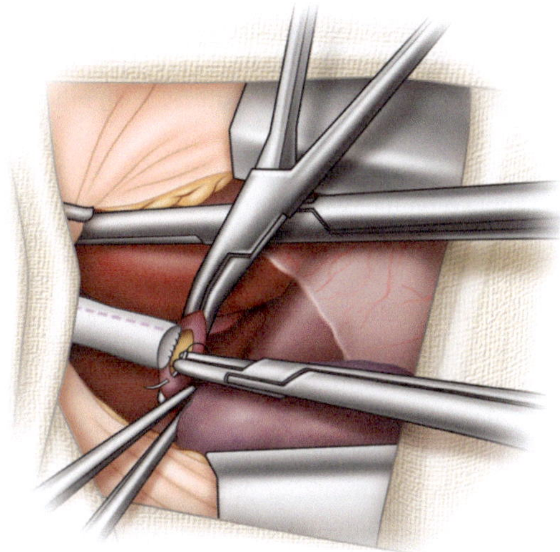

Fig. 11.7 Coming around the opposite end of the anastomosis (surgeon's side)

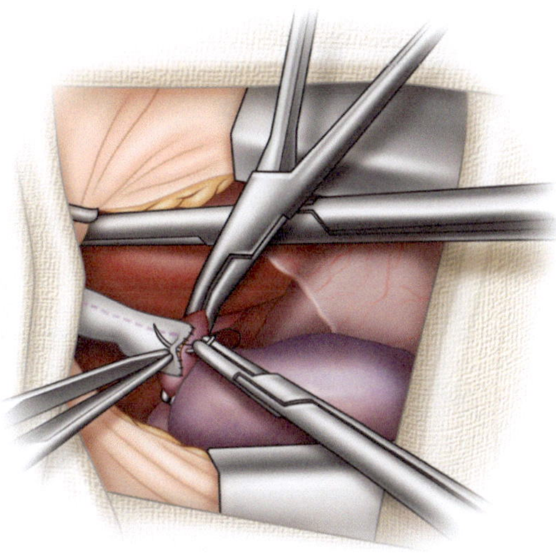

Fig. 11.8 Completion of the anastomosis on the lower lip

however, no data to date has clearly shown (recognizing the limitations of prior studies) whether ligation of PDA is critical or not. Typically limited dissection of ductus has been carried out earlier on after opening up the pericardium, although we avoid complete dissection to avoid ductal spasm that which would complicate the conduct of the operation. Once again, it is important that the PA end of the ductus is defined clearly so that with ductal ligation there is no question of potentially distorting the junction with the main pulmonary artery/LPA. This is critical specially for babies who have pretty minimal antegrade flow (i.e., almost all of the pulmonary atresia variants) because the potential distortion can lead to LPA stenosis or unexplained hypoxia post-operatively. This dissection (Fig. 11.9) will also give a "poor-man's" gauge for the potential future LPA stenosis (if there is significant difference in caliber of vessel at that junction). For the ligation of ductus arteriosus, a single 2–0 silk is passed around the ductus and a hem clip is applied in a downward fashion, while upward pressure is applied on the two ends of the silk ligature surrounding the ductus (Fig. 11.10). The reason this technique is used as opposed to tying off the ductus is that in case of inadequate pulmonary blood flow and or decompensation post-ligation, an immediate intervention to re-establish flow through the ductus can be achieved by removing the clip/pulling apart the two ends of the suture.

At completion of the BT shunt, the heparin is not reversed and following hemostasis closure is carried out in the standard fashion leaving the pericardium open and leaving behind a single chest tube. Typically pacing wires or intracardiac lines are not placed for this procedure minimizing potential risk of bleeding subsequently. Heparin infusion is then started upon return to the intensive care unit.

Preoperative seagull appearance of the branch pulmonary arteries with particular tenting toward the ductus can be a potential tell tale sign of subsequent LPA stenosis. However, to be able to discern ductal tissue from actual native PA can be

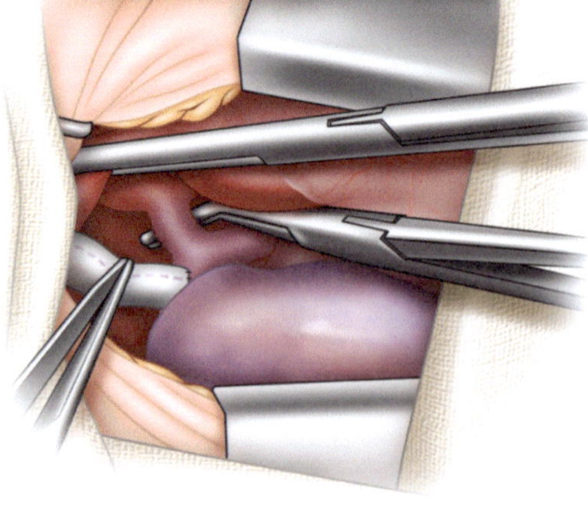

Fig. 11.9 PDA dissection

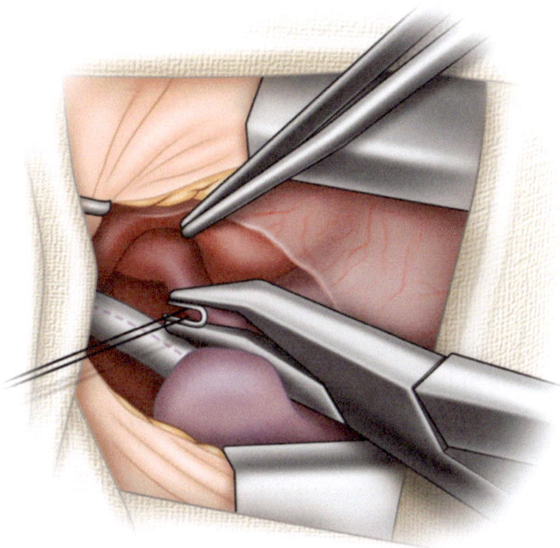

Fig. 11.10 PDA ligation with sutures pulling up and clip going down

difficult, and for that reason it is important that postoperatively close monitoring of the patient's pulmonary blood flow is carried out by looking at both chest radiographs and possibly a perfusion scan if routine echocardiographic findings are of concern. This would obviously be of greater concern in single ventricle patient as opposed to patients with Tetralogy of Fallot.

Outcomes

As noted before, remarkably the mortality of systemic pulmonary artery shunting is relatively high for a closed heart procedure. Nevertheless, some centers have routinely used this palliative approach for the first step management of ToF patients that require intervention within the first year of life. Their rationale is to minimize the use of transannular patch, avoid use of cardiopulmonary bypass (and attendant complications), and reduce hospital costs, among others. Risk factors that have been identified for the Blalock Taussig shunt are patient weight, gestational age, presence of extracardiac anomalies, chromosomal anomalies, and in some single institutions series the size of the shunt. The most consistent risk factor however has been weight, with nearly an exponential increase in risk with weight below 3 kg [8, 9]. Most centers use a 3.5 mm PTFE graft. Some surgeons have used 3.0 mm shunt for the smaller infants; typically the shunt size is correlated to the size of the infant. It is the author's practice to use a 3.5 mm shunt for infants in the 2.5–2.0 kg, mainly because unpublished observations has shown that often the size of the innominate artery (or size of the branch PAs) is a rate-limiting step in these babies and therefore, a bigger shunt rarely translates into significant overcirculation. Of note, the author has noted through echo and angiographic measurements of PDA (unpublished observations) that often the size of this structure is around 3.0–3.5 mm, but longer and often tortuous. An alternative approach in particularly small babies is use of the classic BT shunt with sacrifice of the right subclavian artery. Unfortunately, in author's experience reestablishing continuity of flow into the subclavian artery subsequently is not feasible and there is some tenting of the RPA subsequently, but the patency rate is remarkably good likely because of the native to native anastomosis. The author has used this for the very small babies (<2.0 kg). There is an increased risk of right recurrent laryngeal nerve injury during this procedure. This nerve passes around the more distal subclavian artery.

Our group has done extensive analyses of the outcomes of systemic pulmonary artery shunting looking at both practices at institutions who have the best outcomes, as well as the collective experience across the Society of Thoracic Surgeons and that reported by nearly 43 pediatric institutions in the Pediatric Health Information Systems database. One of the most profound findings from these studies has been the importance of aspirin anticoagulation (superior to heparin alone management) [10]. Early initiation of aspirin, particularly on the day of surgery, shows remarkable impact on mortality and complications as defined by need for return to the operating room, a trip to the cardiac catheterization lab, or need for ECMO. While direct data is lacking, there is evidence that there is significant activation of platelets during flow through the PTFE (often with significant shear stress from the acute angulations); it is the authors' hypothesis that this leads to release of vasogenic substances from the platelets that can impact pulmonary and systemic vasculature, often giving rise to the picture of presumed shunt thrombosis or occlusion (when in reality it is diminished flow from spasm).

Dual therapy with heparin and aspirin within the first 48–72 h appears to give some marginal additional benefit in the outcomes. Author's practice as noted before involves aspirin initiation either immediately prior to surgery or within the operating room and then continuing that postoperatively. In addition, a heparin infusion is started at 15 units per kilogram per hour starting upon return from the operating room to the Intensive Care Unit as long as there is no significant bleeding from the chest tube (i.e., <1 cc/kg/hr). The heparin is then continued for approximately 48–72 h and then discontinued. At that point aspirin administration continues at the same dose as started initially (20.25 mg or ¼ dose of baby aspirin). As well, small amounts of inotropic support are initiated in the operating room and continued in the post-operative period to ensure adequate cardiac output; again, though not proven, it is the authors suspicion that cardiac output is typically impacted following the conduct of this simple procedure (not too dissimilar to perhaps results seen following the hybrid palliation) and therefore, focusing beyond saturations and hemodynamics (i.e., NIRS or mixed venous monitoring) is important in the immediate post-operative period. Typical hospital stay is approximately a week (assuming early extubation) and most patients tend to do well, with hospital stay being impacted either by perioperative complications or development of low cardiac output following the conduct of the procedure. We employ home surveillance [11–13] in our program though it appears that since initiation of early aspirin initiation there have been less problems with interstage events. Lastly, the aspirin is continued until next operative intervention and not discontinued prior to any cardiac catheterizations or surgical procedures.

As noted earlier, some centers have explored the potential application of ductal stenting in this or other settings to which systemic-pulmonary artery shunting has been applied. Still few others have employed RVOT stenting. This is an evolving field and likely with increasing experience and data, this modality will impact the frequency of BT shunting done in the setting of ToF or other ductal dependent pulmonary blood flow settings.

References

1. Van Praagh R, Van Praagh S, Nebesar RA, AJ. M, Sinha SN, Paul MH. Tetralogy of Fallot: underdevelopment of the pulmonary in fundibulum and its sequela. Am J Cardiol. 1970;26:25–33.
2. Blalock A, Taussig HB. The surgical treatment of malformations of the heart in which there is pulmonary stenosis or pulmonary atresia. JAMA. 1945;128:189–202.
3. Society of Thoracic Surgeons (STS) 2010 congenital report executive summary. STS congenital heart surgery database, Spring 2010 harvest (2006–2009). Available at: http://www.sts.org/sites/default/files/documents/pdf/ndb2010/STSCONG-NeonatesSummary_spring2010.pdf.
4. Gibbs JL. Stenting of the arterial duct: a new approach to palliation for pulmonary atresia. Br Heart J. 1992;67(3):240–5.
5. Gwelling M, Boshoff DE, DensJ ML, Benson LN. Stenting of the neonatal arterial duct in duct-dependent pulmonary circulation: new techniques, better results. J Am Coll Cardiol. 2004;43:107–12.
6. McMullan DM, Permut LC, Jones TK, Johnston TA, Rubio AE. Modified Blalock-Taussig shunt versus stenting for palliation of cardiac lesions with inadequate pulmonary blood flow. J Thorc Cardiovasc Surg. 2014;147(1):397–401.
7. Zahorec M, et al. A comparison of Blalock-Taussig shunts with and without closure of the ductus arteriosus in neonates with pulmonary atresia. Ann Thorac Surg. 2011;92(2):653–8.
8. Petrucci O, O'Brien SM, Jacobs ML, Jacobs JP, Manning PB, Eghtesady P. Risk factors for mortality and morbidity after the neonatal Blalock-Taussig shunt procedure. Ann Thorac Surg. 2011;92(2):642–51.
9. Curzon CL, Milford-Beland S, Li JS, et al. Cardiac Surgery in infants with low birth weight is associated with increased mortality: analysis of the Society of Thoracic Surgeons Congenital Heart Database. J Thorac Cardiovasc Surg. 2008;135:546–51.
10. Li JS, Yow E, Berezny KY. Clinical outcomes of palliative surgery including a systemic to pulmonary shunt in infants with cyanotic congenital heart disease: does aspirin make a difference? Circulation. 2007;116:293–7.
11. Ghanayem NS, Hoffman GM, Mussatto KA, et al. Home surveillance program prevents interstage mortality after the Norwood procedure. J Thorac Cardiovasc Surg. 2003;126(5):1367–77.
12. Dobrolet NC, Nieves JA, Welch EM, Khan D, Rossi AF, Burke RP, Zahn EM. New approach to interstage care for palliated high-risk patients with congenital heart disease. J Thorac Cardiovasc Surg. 2011;142(4):855–60.
13. Stephanie LS, Jana KN, et al. Nome monitoring program reduces interstage mortality after the modified Norwood procedure. J Thorac Cardiovasc Surg. 2014;147(2):718–23.

Chapter 12
Redo Fallot: Surgery for Pulmonary Valve Implantation

Ed Peng, Neil Wilson, Robert A. Hanfland, and David Neil Campbell

Abstract Since tetralogy of Fallot was first successfully repaired in 1954, an encouraging long-term survival has been reported. However, an increasing number of adult survivors will present late after repair for re-intervention, and pulmonary regurgitation has been the most common indication. The timing and indications for pulmonary valve replacement continue to evolve but the trend has now moved towards earlier intervention before irreversible changes in right ventricular function occur. Late survivors are also at an increased risk of developing arrhythmias due to right ventricular scarring related to corrective surgery and sudden death remains the commonest cause of late death. The need to restore pulmonary valve competency to preserve right ventricular function and reduce the arrhythmia burden have therefore become the important indications for late intervention in this disease. In addition to traditional surgical approaches, the role of percutaneous valve intervention is also emerging. It is anticipated that this strategy will improve the long-term mortality and morbidity and will be the focus of this chapter.

Keywords Tetralogy of Fallot • Redo-operation • Pulmonary regurgitation • Valve surgery • Arrhythmia surgery

E. Peng, MD, FRCS(CTh)(UK)
Department of Pediatric Cardiac Surgery, Children's Hospital of Colorado, Aurora, CO, USA

N. Wilson, MD
Department of Pediatric Cardiology, Children's Hospital Colorado, Denver, CO, USA

R.A. Hanfland, MD
Department of Pediatric Cardiothoracic Surgery, Children's Hospital of Colorado, Aurora, CO, USA

D.N. Campbell, MD (✉)
Department of Pediatric Cardiovascular Surgery, The Children's Hospital Colorado Heart Institute, University of Colorado Denver Health Sciences Center, Aurora, CO, USA
e-mail: david.campbell@childrenscolorado.org

F. Lacour-Gayet et al. (eds.), *Surgery of Conotruncal Anomalies*,
DOI 10.1007/978-3-319-23057-3_12

Introduction

Since tetralogy of Fallot was first successfully repaired by Lillihei and Varco in 1954 at the University of Minnesota [1], long-term survival of 85 % at 36 years has been reported [2]. The need to relieve the right ventricular outflow tract obstruction (RVOTO) is often accompanied by residual pulmonary regurgitation (PR). Surgical techniques to relieve RVOTO by means of infundibular resection and patch enlargement of the outflow tract and pulmonary annulus often render the pulmonary valve incompetent. Pulmonary regurgitation is the commonest residual lesion following complete repair in infancy.

Although pulmonary regurgitation is well tolerated early after surgery, it results in ventricular dilatation and, ultimately, right ventricular dysfunction in the long term. Late survivors also have an increased risk of developing ventricular arrhythmias as a result of scarring of the right ventricle related to corrective surgery. Arrhythmias requiring intervention has been reported in more than 40 % of survivors late after repair [3]. Sudden death remains the commonest cause of late death, and is most likely arrhythmogenic in etiology. Therefore, the need to restore pulmonary valve competence and reduce the arrhythmia burden have become the most important indications for late interventions in this disease.

Diagnosis and Imaging

Transthoracic echocardiography (TTE) is the first line imaging to assess the degree of pulmonary regurgitation, RV volume overloading, and any residual lesion such as RV outflow tract stenosis, pulmonary artery stenoses and ventricular septal defect. Echocardiography can also be used to assess tricuspid regurgitation, and thus estimate right ventricular and pulmonary artery pressure. Competence of the aortic valve, aortic root dilatation and ventricular function can also be assessed semi-quantitatively. We routinely perform a bubble contrast study to look for shunting at atrial or ventricular level using trans-esophageal echocardiography prior to cardiopulmonary bypass as this may alter our cannulation strategy.

Cardiac MRI (CMR) has emerged as the most important imaging for accurate quantification of pulmonary regurgitation, right ventricular volume and function. Branch PA anatomy can also be shown clearly and differential flow to each lung can be calculated to assess the functional effect of any branch stenosis visualized. Currently, CMR is performed routinely for each of our patients referred for pulmonary valve replacement. Gadolinium enhancement can demonstrate myocardial fibrosis, and provide useful information on the extent of myocardial scarring. There is some evidence to suggest that this information can be used as risk stratification for tachydysrhythmia and sudden cardiac death. Besides precise volumetric and hemodynamic evaluation, the proximity of cardiac structures/conduit to the sternum can also be assessed and is relevant to the planning of sternal reentry. MRI is not universally applicable of course in the context of patients with a pacemaker.

Cardiac catheterization may not be required unless percutaneous intervention is planned such as a percutaneous pulmonary valve implantation or stenting of the branch pulmonary arteries. Angiography may also be considered to exclude coronary artery disease in older patients. In the latest guideline for ACHD (ESC 2010), pre-operative coronary angiography is recommended for men older than 40 years, post-menopausal women, and in patients with risk factors or sign of ischemic heart disease [4]. CT-angiography of the coronary anatomy is efficient in excluding significant CAD with high negative predictive value and can be used as a reliable alternative to coronary angiography in non-high risk patients without risk factors or symptoms of CAD [5, 6]. However, CT can overestimate the degree of any atherosclerotic obstruction, and before any decision making regarding revascularisation, coronary angiography is advised and fractional flow reserve quantification may be required in this setting [6].

Other useful investigations, which are sometimes performed in our practice include Holter monitoring, electrophysiology laboratory study and cardiopulmonary exercise testing. A formal cardiopulmonary exercise test provides objective exercise capacity (time, maximum oxygen uptake, peak oxygen consumption - peak VO_2) and can provide useful prognostic information, particularly regarding the timing of intervention [7]. Formal and serial exercise testing may also be useful to assess symptomatology particularly in the context of sedentary patients, which make up a large proportion of this group of patients.

Pre-operative Checklist

- Patency of peripheral vessels e.g., femoral vessels for peripheral cannulation if required
- The proximity of RV or any valved conduit behind the sternum to predict risk of cardiac injury on sternal re-entry.
- Electrophysiologic study may be needed if there is any history of arrhythmia.
- Intracardiac shunt: PFO/ASD, VSD to plan cannulation strategy and the need to arrest the heart.
- The anatomical relation between the aorta and pulmonary artery. A main pulmonary artery, which is rotated more posteriorly will require more extensive dissection to mobilize the heart.
- Aberrant coronary artery crossing the RV outflow tract
- Branch PA stenosis needing concomitant patch enlargement or stent insertion
- Tricuspid valve regurgitation – severity of regurgitation, degree of annular dilatation, any leaflet prolapse

Indications and Timing for Pulmonary Valve Replacement (Table 12.1)

The indications for replacing the pulmonary valve continue to evolve and the tendency has moved towards earlier intervention before irreversible myocardial damage has occurred. Pulmonary regurgitation (PR) remains the most common

Table 12.1 Indications for pulmonary valve implantation

PVR is indicated in the presence of criteria from I + II *OR* I + III
(I) Severe pulmonary regurgitation and/or stenosis
PR grading based on CMR: mild (regurgitation fraction, RF < 20 %), moderate (RF 20–40 %), and severe (RF > 40 %); Echo: broad regurgitant jet and diastolic retrograde flow seen at branch PA in the parasternal short axis RVOT view indicates severe PR
PS: severe stenosis as indicated by RV systolic pressure >60 mmHg, TR velocity >3.5 m/s
(II) Symptom(s): Dyspnea, reduced exercise capacity, heart failure, or arrhythmia
(III) In the absence of symptom:
Decrease in objective exercise capacity, VO_2 max <70 % of gender-age predicted or a decline >20 % on serial testing
Sustained atrial/ventricular arrhythmias
ECG CRITERIA: QRS duration 180 ms, QRS prolongation >3.5 ms/year
MRI CRITERIA: RVEF <40 %, RVESV > 80 mL/m^2, RVEDV >150 mL/m^2 (Z-score >4),
Progressive RV dysfunction or dilation on serial imaging
RVOT aneurysm
Tricuspid regurgitation: at least moderate or progressive TR
Residual RVOTO: RVSP > 2/3 systemic, RV systolic pressure >80 mmHg (TR velocity >4.3 m/s), branch PA stenosis
Coexisting cardiac lesions requiring surgery: Significant residual shunt (Qp:Qs > 1.5:1) or with LV volume overloading, severe aortic regurgitation (with symptoms or LV dysfunction) and/or aortic root dilatation

indication for pulmonary valve replacement (PVR) but it may also be indicated for residual RVOTO or mixed disease. Magnetic resonance imaging (MRI) has enabled precise quantification of RV volumes and reports have suggested that once the indexed right ventricular end-diastolic volume (RVEDV) exceeds 170 ml/m^2 or the end-systolic volume (RVESV) is greater than 85 ml/m^2 remodeling of the ventricle is unlikely even when the pulmonary valve competency is restored [8]. Therefore, PVR should be undertaken before these thresholds were reached to increase the likelihood that the RV volume will normalize after PV replacement and indexed RVEDV of 150 ml/m^2 has been recommended as a practical cut-off for intervention [8–10].

The reason why some patients appear more symptomatic with lesser degree of PR, and some with severe PR remain asymptomatic is not well understood. This paradox continues to confound decision-making but attempts to objectify exercise tolerance with cardiopulmonary exercise testing maybe helpful looking longitudinally in individual patients. The presence of severe PR alone does not necessarily indicate the need for pulmonary valve replacement, and, notwithstanding the potential subjectivity of symptoms mentioned above, the presence of symptoms or other clinical and imaging criteria need to be taken into account in decision making. Both the American (AHA 2008) and European (ESC 2010) guidelines for grown-up congenital heart patients advocated pulmonary valve implantation only in severe PR in symptomatic patients (Class 1 recommendation) [11, 12]. In the absence of symptoms, AHA and ESC recommend surgery when there is evidence of moderate to severe progressive RV dilatation, RV dysfunction or sustained arrhythmia (Class IIa). The presence of less than severe PR is not addressed by current guidelines and the indications for valve replacement requires individualized decision-making.

Surgical Techniques for Pulmonary Valve Replacement

Pulmonary valve replacement is performed under cardiopulmonary bypass. In the absence of an intracardiac shunt, it can be accomplished on a beating heart using a single right atrial cannulation with a two-stage venous cannula. Otherwise, bicaval cannulation and cardioplegic arrest are required to close any intracardiac shunt. The residual VSD or ASD/PFO is closed first following cardioplegic arrest and the subsequent pulmonary valve replacement can be performed on a beating heart.

Following redo sternotomy, dissection is undertaken first to expose the cannulation sites, and to free the areas around the aorta, pulmonary artery, right atrium and the anterior right ventricle. If bicaval cannulation is planned, then the area around the IVC will also need to be exposed. The temperature of the patient on cardiopulmonary bypass should not be lower than 32 °C (Figs. 12.1, 12.2, 12.3, 12.4 and 12.5).

Sizing and Choice of Prostheses for PVR

The options for pulmonary valve replacement include mechanical, bioprosthetic or homograft (aortic or pulmonary). The ideal valve choice does not exist. In adolescents and adult patients, we prefer the use of a bioprosthetic valve over homografts due to their easy availability, preparation, and durability in the adult population. Additionally, the use of a bioprosthesis has the potential to limit further redo surgery by allowing transcatheter valve implantation (Medtronic Melody™ or Edwards SAPIEN™ Pulmonic Transcatheter Heart Valve) when this becomes necessary in the future. The use of a transannular patch to enlarge the pulmonary valve annulus allows a larger prosthesis to be implanted. Typically, in adult patients, the largest available aortic bioprosthesis is chosen, but consideration is also given to the valve size, which will allow the largest transcatheter valve to be implanted if required in the future (Fig. 12.6 and Table 12.2).

Studies suggest better durability of a bioprosthetic valve over a homograft when a larger size (>19 mm) can be implanted [13]. Although a bioprosthetic valve has a shorter durability compared to mechanical valve, it allows future transcatheter valve-in-valve implantation [14, 15]. Bioprostheses have an excellent 5-year durability with over 94 % freedom from valve replacement. This decreases to 36–51 % at 10-year follow-up [14, 16]. In a contemporary analysis, younger age appears to be the primary determinant of the durability of bioprosthetic valves in the pulmonary position [16]. In this study, all the structural valve

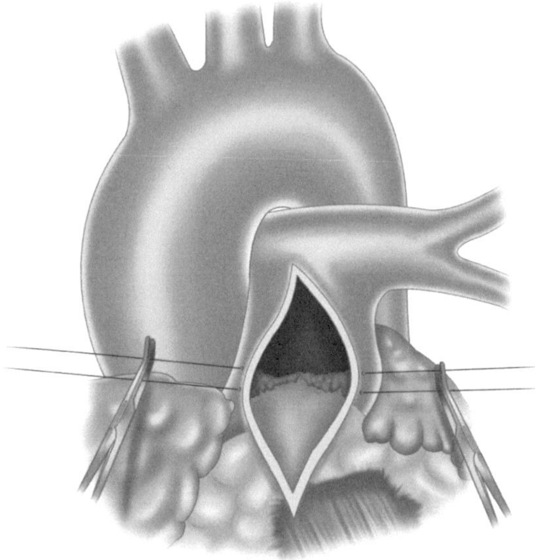

Fig. 12.1 An incision is made into the previous transannular patch, or in the absence of one, a transannular incision is created. The size of the incision should be adequate and starts at or just below the bifurcation of the main pulmonary artery. This technique augments the annulus and the right ventricular outflow tract to facilitate the implantation of a larger prosthesis

failure was observed in patients younger than 15 years, and re-intervention was only required in one patient older than 15 years due to endocarditis. There is no apparent advantage of using a pericardial valve over porcine valve, and both seem to be comparable [16]. Mechanical prostheses are more durable but large studies and long-term follow-up of their use in the pulmonary position is lacking. Besides anticoagulant related bleeding, thrombogenic complications have been the major concern associated with mechanical prostheses. In contemporary studies, valve thrombosis was not reported with adequate anticoagulation, but severe right ventricular dysfunction has been linked to a higher thrombogenic risk [15, 17]. Mechanical prostheses are also not immune from dysfunction, which can be due to thrombosis, fibrosis, or pannus formation and mandatory replacement with redo surgery is required. A percutaneous option is not possible in this context. Nevertheless, use of a mechanical valve may be justified in patients who are already on anticoagulation for other reasons such as a coexisting mechanical heart valve, compliant to anticoagulation medications, and those who have previously demonstrated accelerated degeneration of a bioprosthesis [15–18]. A generation of mechanical valves that are less thrombogenic and require lower levels of anti-coagulation, and the use of newer generation anticoagulants such as dabigatran may encourage the wider use of mechanical valves in the pulmonary position.

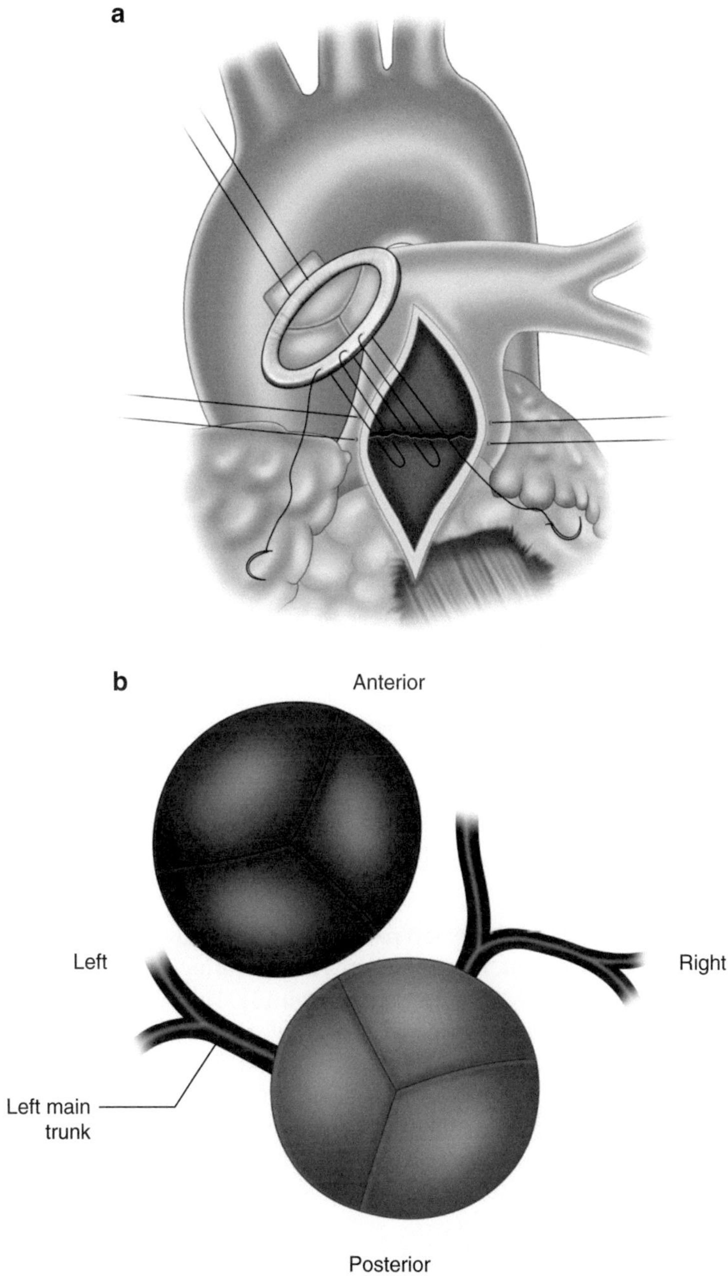

Fig. 12.2 PV leaflets are not routinely excised and can be used as tissues to anchor valve sutures during implantation. The prosthesis is first sutured on the posterior annulus starting with 4/0 Prolene™ using a continuous suture. We prefer to start closer to Y and suture towards X before parachuting the prosthesis down after several stitches. Deep bites on the posterior annulus are avoided to prevent any inadvertent injury to the left common coronary trunk which courses behind the main pulmonary artery. (**a**) Suturing valve in place (**b**) Relationship of pulmonary valve to left main coronary artery

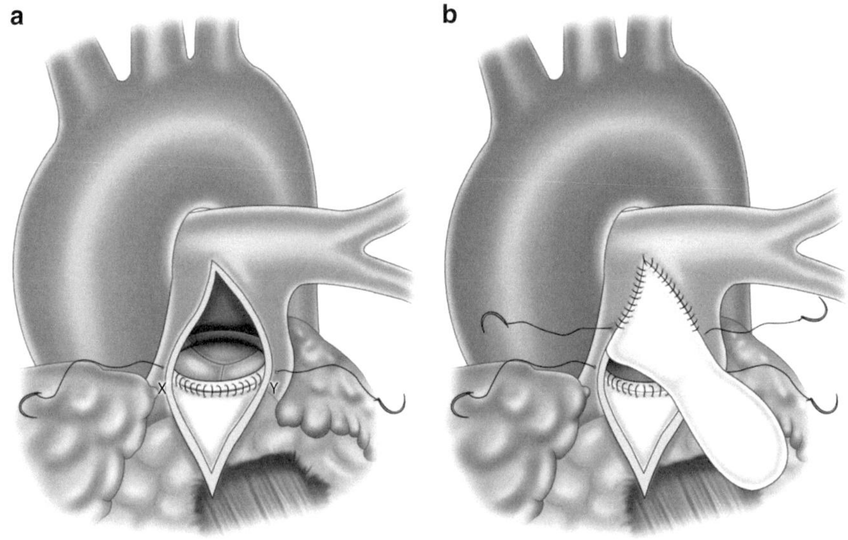

Fig. 12.3 A bovine pericardial patch (Peri-Guard®, Synovis, Deerfield, IL, USA) is measured to fit the size of the augmented RVOT. The patch is first sutured at the apex adjacent to the pulmonary artery bifurcation using double-armed 4/0 Prolene™ and brought on each side towards the prosthesis. At points X and Y, the needle is brought out from the edge of ventriculotomy and tied to the previous stitch. (**a**) Running 4/0 ProleneTM sutures anchoring the valve in place brought to outside the opened pulmonary artery (**b**) Pericardial patch being sewn in place

Surgical Ablation for Ventricular Tachycardia during Redo Surgery for Tetralogy of Fallot

In a multi-institutional study of 556 patients, 43 % of those older than 18 years of age had a documented sustained arrhythmia during adulthood and/or an arrhythmia needing intervention late after repair [3]. This may occur as a supraventricular and/or ventricular tachyarrhythmia with a prevalence of 20.1 % and 14.6 % respectively [3]. In several other studies, the incidence of late sustained ventricular tachycardia (VT) is 3–14 % and the risk of sudden death is 3–6 % amongst survivors at 25–30 years after corrective surgery [2, 19–21]. Due to a significant incidence of tachyarrhythmia among late survivors, cryoablation of the RVOT pathway is sometimes required concomitantly with the pulmonary valve replacement. The presence of ventricular fibrosis was shown to be the major predisposing factor for inducible monomorphic ventricular tachycardia in non-ischemic cardiomyopathy patients [22]. Based on intra-operative mapping studies, the mechanism for inducible VT in post repair patients is most commonly secondary to monomorphic and macro-reentrant circuits around the ventriculotomy scars or surgical patches [23].

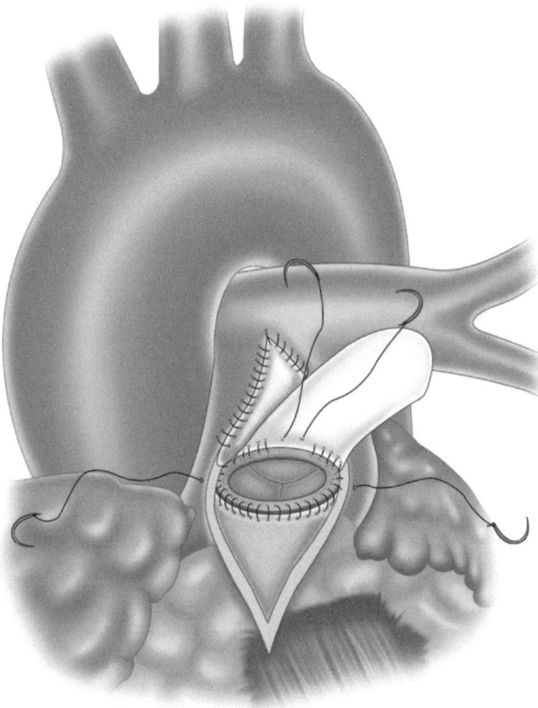

Fig. 12.4 The prosthesis is adjusted so that it is seated in a desirable position before it is fixed anteriorly. One of the needles at junction X/Y will be used to suture the prosthesis anteriorly and the other needle to suture the pericardial patch to the infundibulum. The needle is passed from outside to inside through the pericardial patch and the prosthesis. Once the prosthesis is secured anteriorly, the bottom half of the pericardial patch is sutured to the edge of the ventriculotomy. Before the patch is fixed on its lower half, the prosthetic valve leaflets are checked to ensure that they are not caught by any suture

Supraventricular arrhythmias can occur in the form of intra-atrial reentrant tachycardia or atrial fibrillation [3]. Typical atrial flutter is the most common form of intra-atrial reentrant tachycardia and usually originates from the isthmus between the tricuspid valve and inferior vena cava [24]. The occurrence of sustained ventricular tachyarrhythmia is the most concerning and carries the highest risk of sudden cardiac death, a leading cause of mortality among late survivors after repair of tetralogy of Fallot. In the most recent multi-centers study (N=873), RV hypertrophy, ventricular dysfunction and atrial tacharrhythmia are predictive of sustained ventricular tachycardia and sudden death in adults with repaired Fallot [25]. These high-risk patients should not be managed with anti-dysrhythmia agents alone. More definitive therapy in the form of catheter or surgical ablation and an implantable cardiac defibrillator is warranted [4, 12].

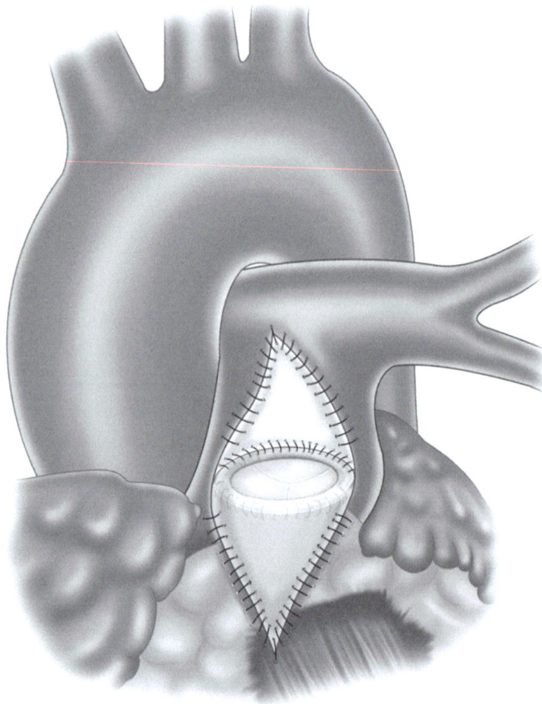

Fig. 12.5 When the pericardial patch is sutured down, a closer bite is taken on the pulmonary artery and ventriculotomy edges as opposed to a larger bite on the patch itself. This technique allows the pericardial patch to billow when the heart is full and ejecting

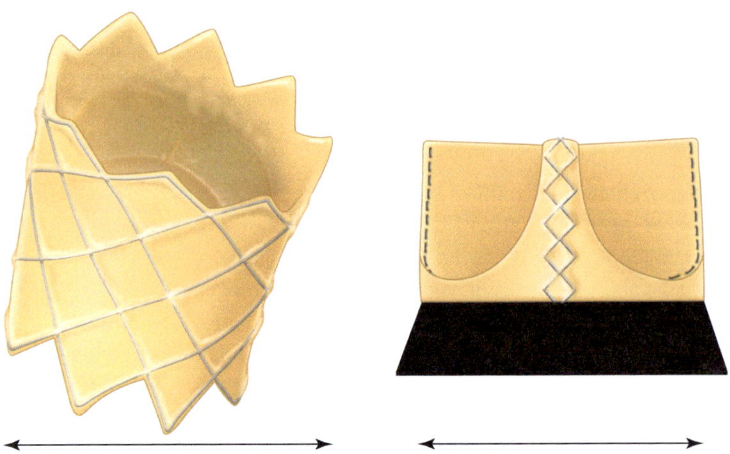

Fig. 12.6 The inner diameter of an aortic bioprosthesis should accommodate the outer diameter of a Melody™ valve. A size 27 mm Sorin Aortic Mitroflow™ (*right*) (outer diameter of 27.3 mm, inner diameter 22.9 mm) will facilitate the largest available Melody™ valve (*left*) (a Melody™ valve deployed with a 22 mm balloon diameter has an outer diameter of approximately 22–24 mm

Table 12.2 The dimensions of the Melody™ valve system and available aortic bioprostheses (the sizes which accommodate the largest Melody™ valve 22 mm are highlighted)

Melody® transcatheter pulmonary valve, Medtronic Inc	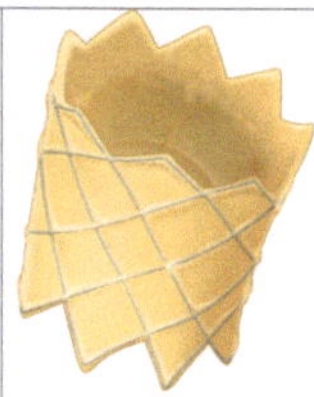	Valve size	Outer ballon pressure-outer diameter
		18 mm (smallest)	1 atm – 17.93 mm
			4 atm – 20.06 mm
		20 mm	1 atm – 19.65 mm
			4 atm – 22.42 mm
		22 mm (largest)	1 atm – 21.80 mm
			2 atm – 22.79 mm
			3 atm – 24.06 mm
Carpentier-Edwards PERIMOUNT aortic heart value	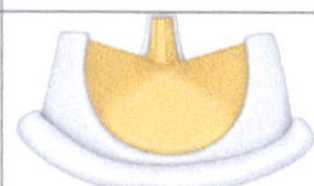	Valve size	Inner diameter
		19 mm (smallest)	18 mm
		21 mm	20 mm
		23 mm	22 mm
		25 mm	24 mm
		27 mm	26 mm
		29 mm (largest)	28 mm
Sorin aortic mitroflow	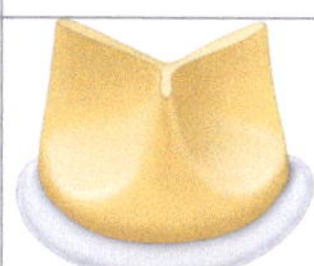	Valve size	Inner diameter
		19 mm (smallest)	15.4 mm
		21 mm	17.3 mm
		23 mm	19.0 mm
		25 mm	21.0 mm
		27 mm (largest)	22.9 mm
Medtronic Hancock II aortic bioprosthesis	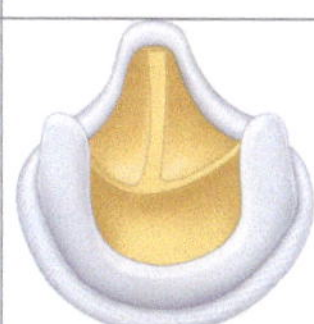	Valve size	Inner diameter
		21 mm (smallest)	18.5 mm
		23 mm	20.5 mm
		25 mm	22.5 mm
		27 mm	24.0 mm
		29 mm (largest)	26.0 mm

Indications for Electrophysiologic (EP) Study and Ablation

The American and European Guidelines (AHA 2008, ESC 2010) recommend electrophysiologic study and/or ablation for symptomatic patients with suspected or documented clinical arrhythmia (atrial or ventricular) [4]. Unexplained syncope is alarming and symptoms such as palpitations and dizziness should raise suspicion for serious arrhythmias and prompt assessment including cardiac catheterization and electrophysiology studies. A catheter ablation of the ventricular tachycardia circuit may be performed if stable monomorphic ventricular tachycardia can be induced and sustained sufficiently to permit mapping in the electrophysiology laboratory [12]. If unsuccessful, surgical ablation with or without intraoperative mapping can be performed as part of the pulmonary valve replacement surgery [12]. A concomitant Cox-Maze procedure during surgery should also be considered in the presence of atrial flutter or fibrillation. A more aggressive approach to perform electrophysiologic studies in all patients undergoing surgical pulmonary valve replacement is adopted in some centers, but whether this aggressive protocol will influence late outcome remains to be seen.

Surgical Techniques for Cryoablation of RVOT pathway

Cryoablation of RVOT pathways to ablate macro re-entrant circuits is usually undertaken with pulmonary valve replacement under cardiopulmonary bypass. The cryo-ablation is performed after the RVOT is opened and prior to implanting a prosthetic valve. Several ventricular isthmuses have been identified as critical in the pathogenesis of re-entrant monomorphic VT and ablation lines are performed in these critical regions (Fig. 12.7) [22, 26, 27]. A cryoablation probe is applied at each ablation line for 60 s, with caution to avoid collateral damage to adjacent structures. The cryothermy (Cardioblate® CryoFlex™ Argon-powered Surgical Ablation System, Medtronic, Inc) consists of a metal probe, which can be rapidly cooled using Argos gas to reach −150 °C. The metal probe is flexible with an adjustable insulation sheath, which is malleable and conforms to the endocardial

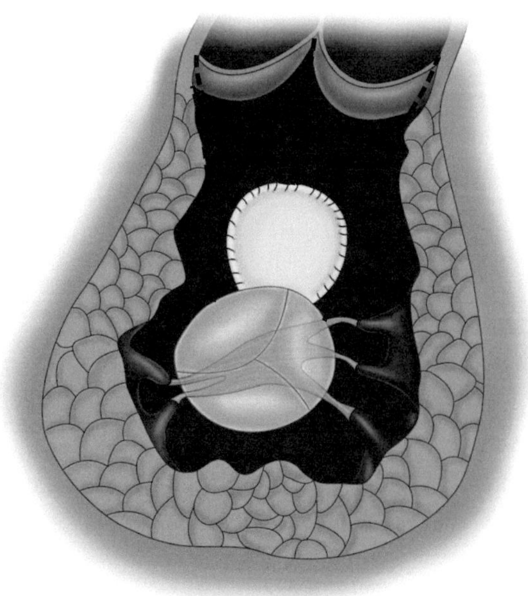

Fig. 12.7 Ablation lines in ventricular isthmuses which serve as critical substrate for VT: (i) from the posterior pulmonary annulus to the VSD patch (ii) from both edges of the ventriculotomy to the VSD patch (iii) from the edges of ventriculotomy on each side towards tricuspid annulus

surface to achieve good contact. The ideal application time is unknown, but in our experience we have observed complete heart block with a longer contact time, hence each ablation is reserved to 60 s. After completion of each ablation line, warm saline is used to rinse the probe, which allows easy removal from the endocardial surface.

Tetralogy of Fallot with Pulmonary Atresia

At the severe end of the spectrum of tetralogy of Fallot the pulmonary valve is completely atretic in approximately 20 % of patients [28]. This group represents a complex spectrum of malformation in itself and the use of a conduit to restore right ventricle to pulmonary artery continuity when confluent pulmonary arteries are present or to grow the pulmonary arteries is an important part of the surgical management.

An ideal conduit does not exist and patients require repeated intervention throughout life. The homograft conduits are used in countries where they are readily available [29, 30]. The early experience of using aortic homograft in pulmonary position was off set by rapid calcification especially in the very young patients and also lack of reliable preservation technique [30]. However, the durability of homograft has improved with cryopreservation technology and introduction of pulmonary homograft. A pulmonary homograft is thinner with less transvalvular gradient, is easier to work with, begets less calcification, and clinical studies suggest that it is more durable than an aortic homograft [30, 31]. More recently, decellularized homografts have been introduced to reduce immunogenicity and potentially attenuate the host–graft response and may improve homograft longevity [32].

Homograft conduits are not universally available and in some countries homograft availability is scarce thus alternatives are required. Xenograft and synthetic material have been used with satisfactory results in clinical series, either implanted as an extracardiac conduit or in an orthotopic position such as in the Ross procedure [33]. These various alternatives include stented (e.g., Hancock, Carpentier Edwards), or stentless xenografts (e.g., Medtronic Freestyle, RVOT élan, Contegra valved bovine jugular vein) [33]. Non-valved conduits have also been used but are associated with the deleterious long-term effects of free pulmonary regurgitation.

Each conduit has a finite life span. Whilst there is no single conduit that has been shown to be consistently superior compared to the others, younger age (under 1-year old), smaller conduit size, lower weight, and extra-anatomical conduit implantation had emerged as important risk factors across studies [34–36]. A truly ideal conduit that grows and does not degenerate will not exist in the foreseeable future. Currently, an acceptable conduit to restore RV to PA continuity should be one that will provide durable competent valve function without obstruction, be resistant to calcification, easy to handle, and is hemostatic when implanted.

Redo Surgery in Patients with Right Ventricle to Pulmonary Artery Conduit

RV to PA conduit may need replacement, either because it became stenotic, incompetent, or both. The criteria for PV replacement as outlined above can be used to decide timing of intervention. Redo surgery is not always necessary, as the availability of percutaneous transcatheter pulmonary valve has reduced the need of resternotomy to replace an old conduit in the current era. When the percutaneous option is deemed not suitable (common reason for this is the conduit size is too big for the largest available Melody™ valve), a redo surgery will then become necessary.

In the presence of an old, calcified conduit, sternal re-entry needs to be approached with an extreme caution due to high risk of the conduit being adherent to the back of sternum. We routinely placed a Goretex patch overlying the conduit in the first surgery to reduce risk of complication during resternotomy. Pre-operative imaging provides information of the risk of conduit injury and pre-emptive measures may be required, including preparation of femoral or iliac vessel to go on bypass immediately in any event of conduit injury or alternatively, peripheral cardiopulmonary bypass can be instituted prior to sternal re-entry.

The old conduit does not necessarily need to be explanted and replaced with a new one. Instead, the surgeon can simply lay open the previous conduit and implant a stented bioprosthetic valve in-situ with or without an overlying patch to fit in an appropriate size valve (Fig. 12.8). In our experience, this is achievable even in young children and this

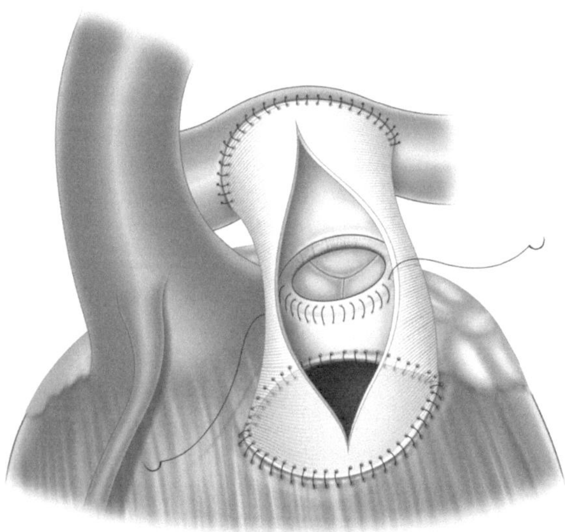

Fig. 12.8 The old conduit is opened anteriorly and the prosthesis is sutured in-situ. This can be achieved providing that the old conduit was not too calcified for implantation of the prosthesis. A patch can be used to accommodate larger prosthesis is needed

strategy will also allow replacement with a percutaneous valve in the future. Occasionally, the whole conduit may need to be explanted and replaced in the setting of endocarditis, when it is excessively aneurysmal or when it is too calcified to implant a prosthesis or achieve a hemostatic suture closure. When conduit replacement is required, it's important to ensure that the stent of the valve does not impinge on the left coronary artery posteriorly ("S" in Fig. 12.9). The conduit is trimmed as such that the valve within the conduit sits close to the central PA bifurcation (Fig. 12.9). The surgery can be usually completed on a beating heart when there is no intra-cardiac shunt present.

The Role of Percutaneous Pulmonary Valve Replacement

Since the first report of percutaneous pulmonary valve replacement in 2000, Melody^{TM} valve, Medtronic Inc (previously by VenPro Corp) has been used widely as an alternative to surgical replacement of RV-PA conduit [37]. The available

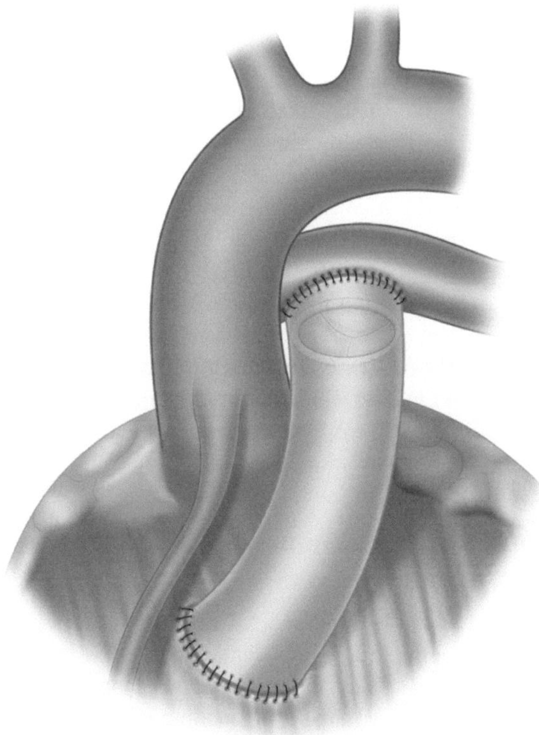

Fig. 12.9 RV to PA conduit implantation: the conduit is trimmed so that the valve sits close to the bifurcation. The LCA can be potentially compressed by stent (S) of the valve and sometimes, removal of the stent may be required to allow a stentless implantation

technology has been augmented with comparable results by the more recent use of the Edwards SAPIEN™ valve [38]. Transcatheter valve implantation has been shown to improve hemodynamics by reducing obstruction and abolishing regurgitation resulting in mechanical and electrical 'remodeling' of the right ventricle [39–42]. The topic of transcatheter pulmonary valve replacement is comprehensively covered in another chapter of this book. We would like to briefly state its role in the context of surgical pulmonary valve replacement in our practice.

It is acknowledged that any type of valve replacement in any position will have finite longevity before failure with stenosis or regurgitation or both intervene. The longevity and hemodynamic efficiency of a valve in the pulmonary position may be constrained by the younger age of the patient, the effects of somatic growth, the existing ventricular substrate, the relationship of the great arteries, the branch pulmonary artery anatomy, proximity of the implant to the posterior aspect of the sternum and the more imponderable chronic effects of inflammation and its accompanying results of neo-intima and calcification. The inevitability of repeated surgery in this group of patients and the prospect of procrastinating reoperation using a technique, which in practical terms did not make subsequent surgery more hazardous supported the inception of catheter based technology. This has been incorporated into the clinical problem of conduit dysfunction of predominant stenosis, predominant regurgitation or, more commonly, combined stenosis and regurgitation.

At our institution, we support an active transcatheter pulmonary valve replacement service and see our roles as complementary. We have therefore tailored our approach such that when our surgically implanted valve fails as a consequence of the factors above, we have effectively left a legacy of a 'landing site' for the implantation of a transcatheter valve. A Sorin Aortic Mitroflow™ in the pulmonary position has an outer diameter of 27 mm and inner diameter of 22.9 facilitates the interventional deployment of the Melody™ using the largest (22 mm inner diameter) delivery system (Ensemble Medtronic) ensuring maximal gradient reduction when present and greatest available competent valve area (Fig. 12.6, Table 12.2). Arguably, with the recently available Edwards SAPIEN™ valve for transcatheter deployment in the pulmonary position one could justify, where substrate permits, to use even larger bioprostheses, as the SAPIEN™ valve is available in 23 and 26 mm diameters.

Surgical Outcomes after Pulmonary Valve Replacement with or without Ablation Surgery

Despite the perceived benefits of PVR, current evidence has not shown a survival benefit. Nonetheless, a meta-analysis of 3118 patients demonstrated: (1) Remodeling of the RV with improvement in volume and function; (2) Improvement in left ventricular function; (3) Decreased QRS duration and (4) Improvement in functional status. Surgery can be performed with low mortality and the pooled 30-day mortality from this meta-analysis was 0.87 % (47 studies; 27 of 3100 patients). At mid-term follow-up, the pooled 5-year mortality was 2.2 % (24 studies; 49 of 2231 patients) and the pooled 5-year re-intervention rate was 4.9 % (15 studies; 88 of 1798 patients) [43].

Unlike studies in atrial fibrillation following the Cox-Maze procedure, available outcome data following ablation for VT are from small series, largely non-surgical, with mixed cohorts of structural and non-structural heart disease [44, 45]. Early results following ablation are satisfactory but long-term success may be seen in only 60 % of patients [45]. Ablation therapy should not be considered as sole therapy to prevent sudden cardiac death in high-risk patients and an implantable defibrillator (ICD) should be considered [46]. Those patients with documented sustained VT or cardiac arrest are at high risk and should receive an ICD regardless of the early success of ablation therapy as the late outcome of ablation is too uncertain [12]. In others, a repeat EP assessment and implantation of an ICD only in the presence of inducible VT seems to be a reasonable approach.

Tricuspid Regurgitation in Late Survivors

Tricuspid regurgitation can be seen in late survivors who present for pulmonary valve replacement. Moderate to severe regurgitation has been reported in one-fifth to one-third of survivors of Fallot surgery [47, 48]. Despite these observations, in our experience, the need of concomitant tricuspid valve surgery has been very rare. Tricuspid regurgitation is usually secondary to annular dilatation consequent on right ventricular enlargement from severe pulmonary regurgitation, and pulmonary valve replacement alone is usually all that is required to reverse this process. Studies have suggested that RV remodeling occurs with PV replacement, and improvement in TR is usually observed as a consequence of this [49]. Much less commonly, TR can occur as a result of injury to the valve and supporting apparatus during the initial reparative surgery. Tricuspid leaflet injury can occur during a trans-atrial approach to close the VSD and to relieve RV outflow tract obstruction. Injury of the chordae tendinae can also occur during the resection of obstructive muscle bundles, leading to TR.

We reserve surgery for TR only when it is severe and we will strive to avoid prosthetic valve replacement in this position. Our philosophy is to reduce the severity of TR and to allow any lesser degree of residual TR to improve with RV remodeling, which we believe is always better than achieving perfect tricuspid competency with a prosthetic valve replacement. A repair is tailored according to the underlying mechanism of the TR. An annuloplasty ring (e.g., Edwards MC3) sparing the AV node region is usually adequate to address annular dilatation. When compared with the De Vega technique without a ring, the placement of an annuloplasty ring has been associated with better long-term survival and freedom from recurrent TR [50]. Less frequently, leaflet repair, or neo-chordae may be needed when tricuspid valve leaflets or subvalvar apparatus have been injured.

Acknowledgement Dr. N Wilson MD illustrated the figures in this chapter.

References

1. Lillehei CW, Cohen M, Warden HE, Read RC, Aust JB, Dewall RA, Varco RL. Direct vision intracardiac surgical correction of the tetralogy of Fallot, pentalogy of Fallot, and pulmonary atresia defects; report of first ten cases. Ann Surg. 1955;142:418–42.
2. Nollert G, Fischlein T, Bouterwek S, Böhmer C, Klinner W, Reichart B. Long-term survival in patients with repair of tetralogy of fallot: 36-year follow-up of 490 survivors of the first year after surgical repair. J Am Coll Cardiol. 1997;30:1374–83.
3. Khairy P, Aboulhosn J, Gurvitz MZ, Opotowsky AR, Mongeon FP, Kay J, Valente AM, Earing MG, Lui G, Gersony DR, Cook S, Ting JG, Nickolaus MJ, Webb G, Landzberg MJ, Broberg CS, for the Alliance for Adult Research in Congenital Cardiology (AARCC). Arrhythmia burden in adults with surgically repaired tetralogy of Fallot: a multi-institutional study. Circulation. 2010;122:868–75.
4. Baumgartner H, Bonhoeffer P, De Groot NMS, de Haan F, Deanfield JE, Galie N, Gatzoulis MA, Gohlke-Baerwolf C, Kaemmerer H, Kilner P, Meijboom F, Mulder BJM, Oechslin E, Oliver JM, Serraf A, Szatmari A, Thaulow E, Vouhe PR, Walma E, Task Force on the Management of Grown-up Congenital Heart Disease of the European Society of Cardiology (ESC), Association for European Paediatric Cardiology (AEPC), ESC Committee for Practice Guidelines (CPG). ESC Guidelines for the management of grown-up congenital heart disease (new version 2010). Eur Heart J. 2010;31:2915–57.
5. Task Force Members, Montalescot G, Sechtem U, Achenbach S, Andreotti F, Arden C, Budaj A, Bugiardini R, Crea F, Cuisset T, Di Mario C, Ferreira JR, Gersh BJ, Gitt AK, Hulot J-S, Marx N, Opie LH, Pfisterer M, Prescott E, Ruschitzka F, Sabate M, Senior R, Taggart DP, van der Wall EE, Vrints CJM, ESC Committee for Practice Guidelines, Zamorano JL, Baumgartner H, Bax JJ, Bueno H, Dean V, Deaton C, Erol C, Fagard R, Ferrari R, Hasdai D, Hoes AW, Kirchhof P, Knuuti J, Kolh P, Lancellotti P, Linhart A, Nihoyannopoulos P, Piepoli MF, Ponikowski P, Sirnes PA, Tamargo JL, Tendera M, Torbicki A, Wijns W, Windecker S, Document Reviewers, Valgimigli M, Claeys MJ, Donner-Banzhoff N, Frank H, Funck-Brentano C, Gaemperli O, Gonzalez-Juanatey JR, Hamilos M, Husted S, James SK, Kervinen K, Kristensen SD, Maggioni AP, Pries AR, Romeo F, Rydén L, Simoons ML, Steg PG, Timmis A, Yildirir A. 2013 ESC guidelines on the management of stable coronary artery disease: the Task Force on the management of stable coronary artery disease of the European Society of Cardiology. Eur Heart J. 2013;34:2949–3003.
6. Task Force on Myocardial Revascularization of the European Society of Cardiology (ESC) and the European Association for Cardio-Thoracic Surgery (EACTS), European Association for Percutaneous Cardiovascular Interventions (EAPCI), Kolh P, Wijns W, Danchin N, Di Mario C, Falk V, Folliguet T, Garg S, Huber K, James S, Knuuti J, Lopez-Sendon J, Marco J, Menicanti L, Ostojic M, Piepoli MF, Pirlet C, Pomar JL, Reifart N, Ribichini FL, Schalij MJ, Sergeant P, Serruys PW, Silber S, Sousa Uva M, Taggart D. Guidelines on myocardial revascularization. Eur J Cardiothorac Surg. 2010;38 Suppl:S1–52.
7. Diller G-P, Dimopoulos K, Okonko D, Li W, Babu-Narayan SV, Broberg CS, Johansson B, Bouzas B, Mullen MJ, Poole-Wilson PA, Francis DP, Gatzoulis MA. Exercise intolerance in adult congenital heart disease: comparative severity, correlates, and prognostic implication. Circulation. 2005;112:828–35.
8. Therrien J, Provost Y, Merchant N, Williams W, Colman J, Webb G. Optimal timing for pulmonary valve replacement in adults after tetralogy of Fallot repair. Am J Cardiol. 2005;95:779–82.
9. Dave HH, Buechel ERV, Dodge-Khatami A, Kadner A, Rousson V, Bauersfeld U, Prêtre R. Early insertion of a pulmonary valve for chronic regurgitation helps restoration of ventricular dimensions. Ann Thorac Surg. 2005;80:1615–20; discussion 1620–1.
10. Buechel ERV. Remodelling of the right ventricle after early pulmonary valve replacement in children with repaired tetralogy of Fallot: assessment by cardiovascular magnetic resonance. Eur Heart J. 2005;26:2721–7.

11. McDonagh T. ESC guidelines for the management of grown-up congenital heart disease (new version 2010). Eur Heart J. 2010;31:2915–57.
12. Warnes CA, Williams RG, Bashore TM, Child JS, Connolly HM, Dearani JA, Del Nido P, Fasules JW, Graham Jr TP, Hijazi ZM, Hunt SA, King ME, Landzberg MJ, Miner PD, Radford MJ, Walsh EP, Webb GD. ACC/AHA 2008 guidelines for the management of adults with congenital heart disease: executive summary: a report of the American College of Cardiology/American Heart Association Task Force on Practice Guidelines (writing committee to develop guidelines for the management of adults with congenital heart disease). Circulation. 2008;118:2395–451.
13. Dearani JA, Danielson GK, Puga FJ, Schaff HV, Warnes CW, Driscoll DJ, Schleck CD, Ilstrup DM. Late follow-up of 1095 patients undergoing operation for complex congenital heart disease utilizing pulmonary ventricle to pulmonary artery conduits. Ann Thorac Surg. 2003;75:399–411.
14. Lee C, Park CS, Lee CH, Kwak JG, Kim SJ. Durability of bioprosthetic valves in the pulmonary position: long-term follow-up of 181 implants in patients with congenital heart disease. J Thorac Cardiovasc Surg. 2011;142:351–8.
15. Stulak JM, Dearani JA, Burkhart HM, Connolly HM, Warnes CA, Suri RM, Schaff HV. The increasing use of mechanical pulmonary valve replacement over a 40-year period. Ann Thorac Surg. 2010;90:2009–15.
16. Chen X-J, Smith PB, Jaggers J, Lodge AJ. Bioprosthetic pulmonary valve replacement: contemporary analysis of a large, single-center series of 170 cases. J Thorac Cardiovasc Surg. 2013;146:1461–6.
17. Dos L, Muñoz-Guijosa C, Mendez AB, Ginel A, Montiel J, Padro JM, Subirana MT. Long term outcome of mechanical valve prosthesis in the pulmonary position. Int J Cardiol. 2011;150:173–6.
18. Stulak JM, Dearani JA. Technique of mechanical pulmonary valve replacement. Oper Tech Thorac Cardiovasc Surg. 2006;11:200–6.
19. Gatzoulis MA, Balaji S, Webber SA, Siu SC. Risk factors for arrhythmia and sudden cardiac death late after repair of tetralogy of Fallot: a multicentre study. Lancet. 2000;356:975–81.
20. Murphy JG, Gersh BJ, Mair DD, Fuster V. Long-term outcome in patients undergoing surgical repair of tetralogy of Fallot. N Engl J Med. 1993;329:593–9.
21. Aliot EM, Stevenson WG, Almendral-Garrote JM, Bogun F, Delacretaz E, Bella Della P, Hindricks G, Jaïs PJ. EHRA/HRS Expert Consensus on Catheter Ablation of Ventricular Arrhythmias: developed in a partnership with the European Heart Rhythm Association (EHRA), a Registered Branch of the European Society of Cardiology (ESC), and the Heart Rhythm Society (HRS); in collaboration with the American College of Cardiology (ACC) and the American Heart Association (AHA). Heart Rhythm, Oxford University Press; 2009. p. 771–817.
22. Misaki T, Tsubota M, Watanabe G, Watanabe Y, Matumoto Y, Ishida K, Iwa T, Okada R. Surgical treatment of ventricular tachycardia after surgical repair of tetralogy of Fallot. Relation between intraoperative mapping and histological findings. Circulation. 1994;90:264–71.
23. Kurzidim K, Schneider H-J, Kuniss M, Sperzel J, Greiss H, Berkowitsch A, Pitschner HF. Cryocatheter ablation of right ventricular outflow tract tachycardia. J Cardiovasc Electrophysiol. 2005;16:366–9.
24. Khairy P, Stevenson WG. Catheter ablation in tetralogy of Fallot. Heart Rhythm. 2009;6:1069–74.
25. Valente AM, Gauvreau K, Assenza GE, Babu-Narayan SV, Schreier J, Gatzoulis MA, Groenink M, Inuzuka R, Kilner PJ, Koyak Z, Landzberg MJ, Mulder B, Powell AJ, Wald R, Geva T. Contemporary predictors of death and sustained ventricular tachycardia in patients with repaired tetralogy of Fallot enrolled in the INDICATOR cohort. Heart. 2014;100:247–53.
26. Zeppenfeld K, Schalij MJ, Bartelings MM, Tedrow UB, Koplan BA, Soejima K, Stevenson WG. Catheter ablation of ventricular tachycardia after repair of congenital heart disease: electroanatomic identification of the critical right ventricular isthmus. Circulation. 2007;116:2241–52.

27. Moore JP, Seki A, Shannon KM, Mandapati R, Tung R, Fishbein MC. Characterization of anatomic ventricular tachycardia isthmus pathology after surgical repair of tetralogy of fallot. Circ Arrhythm Electrophysiol. 2013;6:905–11.
28. Ferencz C, Rubin JD, Mccarter RJ, Brenner JI, Neill CA, Perry LW, Hepner SI, Downing JW. Congenital heart disease: prevalence at livebirth. The Baltimore-Washington Infant Study. Am J Epidemiol. 1985;121:31–6.
29. Ross DN. Homograft replacement of the aortic valve. Lancet. 1962;2:487.
30. Campbell DN, Clark DR. Use of the allograft aortic valved conduit. Ann Thorac Surg. 1990;50:320–2.
31. Livi U, Kay P, Ross DN. The pulmonary homograft: an improved conduit for RVOT reconstruction. Circulation. 1986;74(Supplement 2):250.
32. Ruzmetov M, Shah JJ, Geiss DM, Fortuna RS. Decellularized versus standard cryopreserved valve allografts for right ventricular outflow tract reconstruction: a single-institution comparison. J Thorac Cardiovasc Surg. 2012;143:543–9.
33. Caldarone CA, McCrindle BW, Van Arsdell GS, Coles JG, Webb G, Freedom RM, Williams WG. Independent factors associated with longevity of prosthetic pulmonary valves and valved conduits. J Thorac Cardiovasc Surg. 2000;120:1022–30; discussion 1031.
34. Vitanova K, Cleuziou J, Hörer J, Kasnar-Samprec J, Vogt M, Schreiber C, Lange R. Which type of conduit to choose for right ventricular outflow tract reconstruction in patients below 1 year of age? Eur J Cardiothorac Surg. 2014;46:961–6.
35. Forbess JM, Shah AS, St Louis JD, Jaggers JJ, Ungerleider RM. Cryopreserved homografts in the pulmonary position: determinants of durability. Ann Thorac Surg. 2001;71:54–9.
36. Sierra J, Christenson JT, Lahlaidi NH. Right ventricular outflow tract reconstruction: what conduit to use? Homograft or Contegra? Ann Thorac Surg. 2007;84:606–10.
37. Bonhoeffer P, Boudjemline Y, Saliba Z, Merckx J, Aggoun Y, Bonnet D, Acar P, Le Bidois J, Sidi D, Kachaner J. Percutaneous replacement of pulmonary valve in a right-ventricle to pulmonary-artery prosthetic conduit with valve dysfunction. Lancet. 2000;356:1403–5.
38. Faza N, Kenny D, Kavinsky C, Amin Z, Heitschmidt M, Hijazi ZM. Single-center comparative outcomes of the Edwards SAPIEN and Medtronic Melody transcatheter heart valves in the pulmonary position. Catheter Cardiovasc Interv. 2013;82:E535–41.
39. Chowdhury SM, Hijazi ZM, Rhodes J, Kar S, Makkar R, Mullen M, Cao Q-L, King L, Akin J, Shirali G. Early echocardiographic changes after percutaneous implantation of the Edwards SAPIEN transcatheter heart valve in the pulmonary position. Echocardiography. 2013;30:786–93.
40. Hasan BS, McElhinney DB, Brown DW. Short-term performance of the transcatheter Melody valve in high-pressure hemodynamic environments in the pulmonary and systemic circulations. Circ Cardiovasc Interv. 2011;4:615–20.
41. Harrild DM, Marcus E, Hasan B. Impact of transcatheter pulmonary valve replacement on biventricular strain and synchrony assessed by cardiac magnetic resonance feature tracking. Circ Cardiovasc Interv. 2013;6:680–7.
42. Plymen CM, Bolger AP, Lurz P, Nordmeyer J. Electrical remodeling following percutaneous pulmonary valve implantation. Am J Cardiol. 2011;107:309–14.
43. Ferraz Cavalcanti PE, Sá MP, Santos CA, Esmeraldo IM, de Escobar RR, de Menezes AM, de Azevedo Jr OM, de Vasconcelos Silva FP, Lins RF, Lima Rde C. Pulmonary valve replacement after operative repair of tetralogy of fallot: meta-analysis and meta-regression of 3,118 patients from 48 studies. J Am Coll Cardiol. 2013;62:2227–43.
44. Furushima H, Chinushi M, Sugiura H, Komura S, Tanabe Y, Watanabe H, Washizuka T, Aizawa Y. Ventricular tachycardia late after repair of congenital heart disease: efficacy of combination therapy with radiofrequency catheter ablation and class III antiarrhythmic agents and long-term outcome. J Electrocardiol. 2006;39:219–24.
45. Morwood JG, Triedman JK, Berul CI, Khairy P, Alexander ME, Cecchin F, Walsh EP. Radiofrequency catheter ablation of ventricular tachycardia in children and young adults with congenital heart disease. Heart Rhythm. 2004;1:301–8.

46. Le Gloan L, Khairy P. Management of arrhythmias in patients with tetralogy of Fallot. Curr Opin Cardiol. 2011;26:60–5.
47. Mahle WT, Parks WJ, Fyfe DA, Sallee D. Tricuspid regurgitation in patients with repaired tetralogy of fallot and its relation to right ventricular dilatation. Am J Cardiol. 2003;92:643–5.
48. Kobayashi J, Kawashima Y, Matsuda H, Nakano S, Miura T, Tokuan Y, Arisawa J. Prevalence and risk factors of tricuspid regurgitation after correction of tetralogy of Fallot. J Thorac Cardiovasc Surg. 1991;102:611–6.
49. Kogon B, Patel M, Leong T, McConnell M, Book W. Management of moderate functional tricuspid valve regurgitation at the time of pulmonary valve replacement: is concomitant tricuspid valve repair necessary? Pediatr Cardiol. 2010;31:843–8.
50. Tang GHL, David TE, Singh SK, Maganti MD, Armstrong S, Borger MA. Tricuspid valve repair with an annuloplasty ring results in improved long-term outcomes. Circulation. 2006;114:I577–81.

Chapter 13
Transcatheter Pulmonary Valvulation

Kalyani R. Trivedi, Nilesh Oswal, and Alain Fraisse

Abstract Transcatheter Pulmonary Valve Implantation (TPVI) has emerged as an attractive therapeutic option for the treatment of right ventricular outflow tract dysfunction. By 2015, more than 7000 transcatheter pulmonary valve implantation have been performed. Two valves are currently used for TPVI. The Melody Valve (MeV) (Medtronic Inc., Minneapolis, Minnesota), which can be expanded to 22 mm diameter. The Edward Sapien Valve (ESV) (Edwards Lifesciences LLC, Irvine, California), which can be expanded to 26 mm diameter. This chapter summarizes the concept, its evolution in clinical practice, current applications, and the devices in current use. Early and mid-term outcomes are presented as well as projected long term results and future developments.

Keywords Tetralogy of Fallot • RVOT obstruction • Pulmonary valve • Interventional cardiology • Transcatheter pulmonary valve implantation • Melody valve • Sapien valve • Stent

K.R. Trivedi, MD, FSCAI
Pediatric Interventional Cardiology, University of Chicago Medical Center, Comer Children's Hospital, Chicago, IL, USA

Biological Sciences Division, Department of Pediatrics, The University of Chicago, Chicago, IL, USA
e-mail: kalyani_trivedi@msn.com

N. Oswal, MD • A. Fraisse, MD, PhD (✉)
Paediatric Cardiology Services, Royal Brompton and Harefield Hospitals Trust, London, UK
e-mail: a.fraisse@rbht.nhs.uk

F. Lacour-Gayet et al. (eds.), *Surgery of Conotruncal Anomalies*,
DOI 10.1007/978-3-319-23057-3_13

Introduction

Transcatheter pulmonary valvulation implantation (TPVI) was proposed at the turn of the century in the year 2000 [1]. It is a major innovation in the treatment of congenital heart disease (CHD). It has widened the scope of transcatheter therapeutics in the management of CHD. Over the course of a decade, it has become widely used in clinical practice [2–10].

TPVI has been in permanent technical evolution since the introduction of the first transcatheter procedure of the right ventricular outflow tract (RVOT). Balloon pulmonary valvuloplasty in 1953 [11] followed by stent implantation in the RVOT in the 1990s [11–16], were essential technical precursors to transcatheter deployment of a valved stent in the year 2000 [1] for the management of dysfunctional RVOT. The Melody Valve (MeV) (Medtronic Inc., Minneapolis, Minnesota), a device designed specifically for the RVOT, underwent design modifications to reach its current state of clinical application [17]. The Edward SAPIEN Valve (ESV) (Edwards Lifesciences LLC, Irvine, California) was used for RVOT reconstruction after a period of application to the left ventricular outflow tract (LVOT) [18].

One fifth of children born with CHD have defects involving the RVOT. These defects are tetralogy of Fallot and its variants, transposition of the great arteries with ventricular septal defect and pulmonary stenosis, and common arterial trunk. These children undergo RVOT reconstruction in infancy either by patch augmentation of the RVOT or insertion of a right ventricle (RV) to the pulmonary artery (PA) conduit. TPVI is also performed for conduit failure following the Ross operation. Progressive conduit dysfunction occurs in a large majority of patients with RV to PA conduits due to patient growth and/or conduit degeneration. There may be conduit obstruction, regurgitation or both. Consequently the majority of these patients require 2–4 operations before reaching adulthood. The pulmonary regurgitation (PR) created by a trans-annular patch compromises in the long term the RV function. TPVII offers a non surgical option for pulmonary valvulation. This strategy has had a major impact in the lifetime management of patients with CHD as the number of surgical procedures undergone by the patient is considerably reduced.

Devices

The Melody Valve (Me V) (Fig. 13.1)

The MeV is a bovine jugular vein valve set within a balloon expandable stent for transcatheter pulmonary valvulation [17]. This valve is produced by Medtronic Inc©. It is the same valve than the Contegra© jugular valved conduit (Medtronic Inc, Minneapolis, Minnesota, USA). The valved segment of bovine jugular vein is first fixed in glutaraldehyde and then sutured inside a closed cell CP stent (NuMed Inc, Canada). The length of the valve is quite long, from 28 mm to 23.6 on full

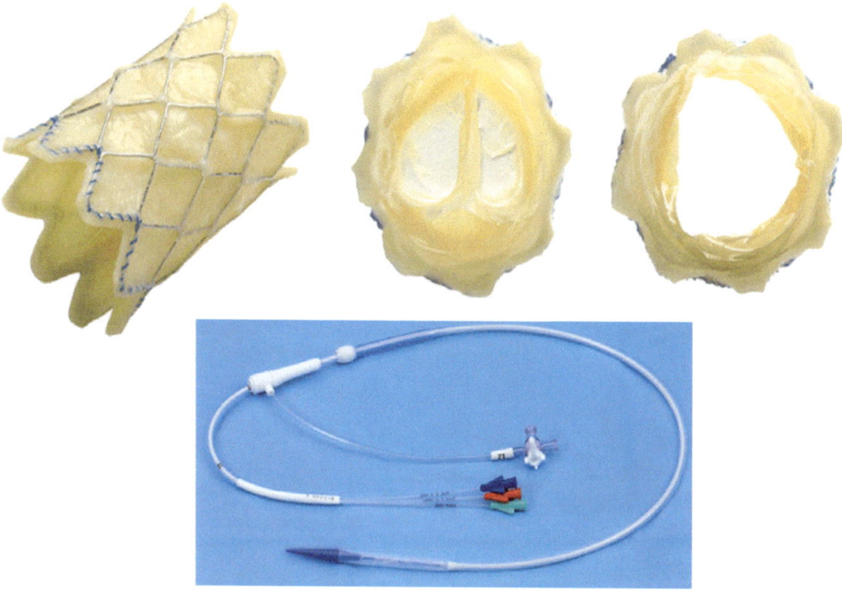

Fig. 13.1 Melody valve & Ensemble delivery system

expansion. A specially designed delivery system, the Ensemble delivery system is used for deployment of the MeV. The MeV can be implanted with 3 diameters through the Ensemble delivery system: 18, 20 and 22 mm. The maximum scope for the expanded MeV is set at 22 mm. There is an extended application to achieve a deployed diameter of up to 23–24 mm [19]. The MeV received approval for clinical use in Europe and Canada in 2006. It was approved by the US Food and Drug Administration in January 2010 under the humanitarian device exemption protocol.

The Edward Sapien Valve (ESV) (Fig. 13.2)

The ESV is a bovine pericardial tissue valve, with three leaflets [20]. The valve tissue is mounted from three equal sections of bovine pericardium preserved in low-concentration solutions of buffered glutaraldehyde. The valve is available in two sizes: 23 mm (14 mm height) and 26 mm (16 mm height); the size denoting the outer diameter of the valve. A 29 mm valve, already used for TAVI, is under progress for TPVI through the XT version. There is a large body of experience with the ESV in the aortic position. In the United States, at the time of writing this chapter, the ESV is an investigational device for use in the pulmonic position through the COMPASSION trial. Active recruitment for primary endpoint was concluded in January 2014. In Europe the ESV reached CE mark in 2010 and early experience with the device was published in 2013 [9]. A prospective multicenter trial (PREMIER Registry) is underway.

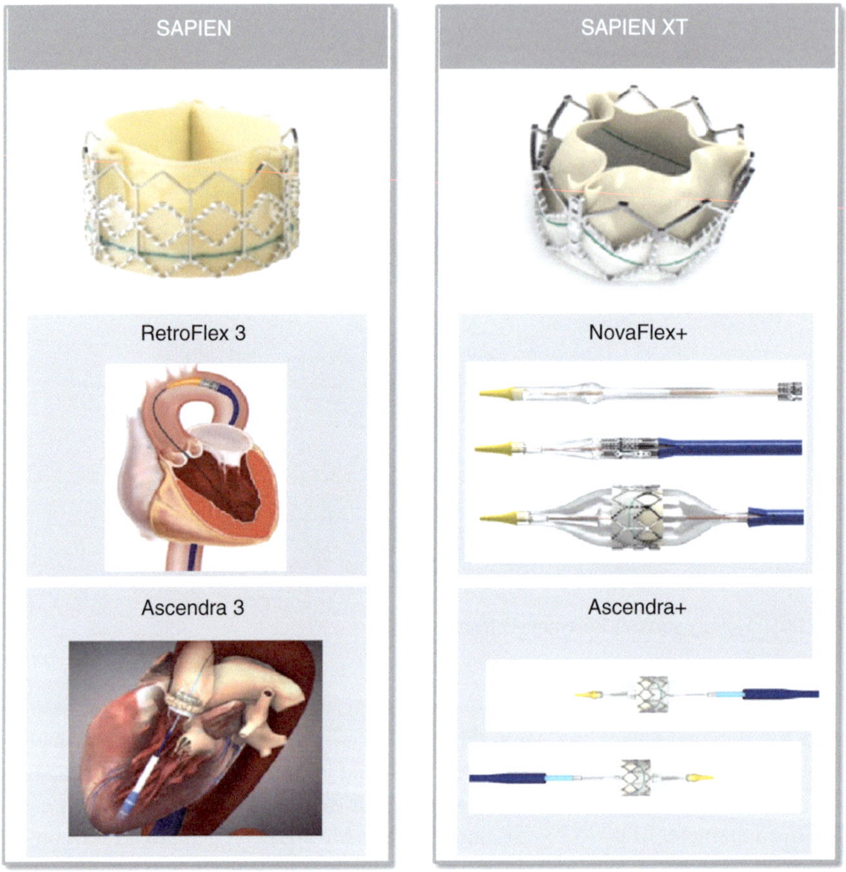

Fig. 13.2 Edward SAPIEN valve with the retroflex delivery system (*left*) and the XT version with new NovaFlex+ delivery system (*right*)

Indications for TPVI

Indications for TPVI are identical to those for surgical PV replacement. AHA-ACC practice recommendations statement lists TPVI with the MeV as a class IIa [21]. Primarily RVOT dysfunction of a specified severity secondary to obstruction, regurgitation or a combination of both and deterioration of cardiopulmonary exercise capacity and cardiac conduction of specified severity together constitute indications for TPVI. These can be summarized as follows:

(a) In symptomatic patients RVOT Doppler mean gradient ≥35 mmHg and/or pulmonary regurgitation (PR) quantified as ≥ moderate.
(b) In asymptomatic patients RVOT Doppler mean gradient ≥40 mmHg or PR quantified as severe with tricuspid annulus dilation (Z-score > 2).
(c) Any degree of RVOT obstruction in the presence of right ventricular systolic dysfunction.

Supportive Data:

(d) Impaired exercise capacity: peak oxygen consumption (VO_2) <65 % predicted on bicycle ramp protocol
(e) Arrhythmias on 24 h Holter.
(f) Prolonged QRS duration ≥150 ms on surface EKG
(g) PR fraction >40 % by cardiac Magnetic Resonance Imaging (MRI)
(h) Right ventricular end diastolic volume (RVEDV) ≥150 ml/m^2 and RV to LV end diastolic ratio >1.7 by MRI

Severity of RVOT dysfunction is further verified by cardiac catheterization. An RVOT peak-to peak gradient greater than 25-mmHg and RV pressure greater than or equal to 2/3 systemic pressure is an indication for TPVI.

Suitability for TPVI

Morphological features and technical aspects of the individual patient determine whether the patient is suitable for TPVI.

RVOT Substrate

The largest experience of TPVI with both the MeV and the ESV is in patients with RVOT conduit [2–10], including valved conduit with bioprosthesis [22]. Such patients are considered to be the most optimal candidates for TPVI. Selected patients with native RVOT dysfunction, occurring on solely or predominant native tissue, may be eligible for TPVI [23, 24].

RVOT Size

With specific techniques referred to as pre-dilation that enlarges the RVOT and pre-stenting which strengthens the RVOT as well as reduces its internal dimension, MeV can be applied to a wide range of RVOT conduits sizes [19]. It can be deployed within a 25-mm bioprosthetic valves as the internal dimension of a 25 mm bioprosthesis is≈23 mm [22]. MeV tolerates deformation from its size and its circular cross section well without loss of function. The ESV is applicable in RVOT of 23–26 mm diameter and soon will be applicable in 29 mm diameter RVOT. It functions best when the RVOT closely matches its nominal size and shape. Marked deviations from native size and shape are not well tolerated by the ESV, although this may be improve with the future generation of transcatheter ESV. TPVI can be offered in RVOT conduits which are as small as 12 mm in diameter at the time of initial surgical placement [25]. More TPVI of larger RVOT is pending definition although it has been shown to be feasible [22, 24].

RVOT Shape

TPVI relies on a device being held in situ by a comparable length of RVOT with a uniformly circular or oval cross section. Such a segment of RVOT is referred to as the landing zone. The landing zone offers a scaffold where the valved stent is embedded. RVOT morphology is heterogeneous [22]. It is shaped by many factors such as the initial surgical reconstruction of RVOT, the patient's hemodynamic status and the individual tissue response. The net result of these various factors is that the RVOT can be of myriad shapes. The funnel shaped RVOT that tapers distally to the PA bifurcation presents a challenge for TPVI and usually requires surgical PV placement. It is estimated that more than >50 % of RVOT morphologies may be suitable for TPVI [26]. This is expected to increase over time as operator experience increases and newer deployment strategies emerge [27, 28].

Patient Body Weight

TPVI with MeV is currently FDA approved in the US for application in patients ≥30 kg in weight. This is expected to change in the near future. There is data supporting application in children less than 30 kg with good technical and short to medium-term clinical outcomes. Of a group of 25 patients with median age 8 years, median weight 21.4 kg and a 17 mm for a median conduit diameter at surgical implant, 23 could undergo TPVI with MeV with good procedural results and early hemodynamic outcomes [25]. In Europe, there is application of TPVI in patient weighing 20 kg and more [29]. ESV is routinely offered to patient ≥35 kg [9].

Impact of RVOT Expansion on Coronary Flow

Up to 5–6 % of patients with RVOT dysfunction who meet the criteria for TPVI do not proceed to TPVI due to identification of direct or indirect coronary compression with expansion of RVOT [29, 30]. The techniques for identification of coronary compression resulting in clinically significant impairment of coronary perfusion are well described [29].

Techniques for TPVI (Fig. 13.3)

Right and left heart catheterization is performed under sedation or general anesthesia with acquisition of hemodynamic data. Angiogram of the dysfunctional conduit is performed (Fig. 13.3a). Indication and feasibility for TPVI is ascertained. Aortic root or selective coronary angiograms are obtained to evaluate coronary artery anatomy and proximity to RVOT [29].

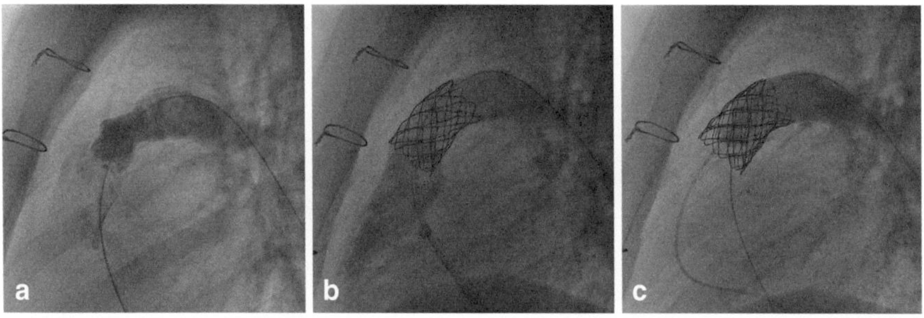

Fig. 13.3 Frontal right ventricular outflow tract angiogram showing a purely stenotic lesion (**a**) that is successfully pre stented (**b**) with relief of the stenosis. Free regurgitation is evident. A 22 mm Melody valve has been implanted with no residual regurgitation on the control angiogram (**c**)

Pre-dilation refers to the technique of RVOT balloon dilation prior to TPVI. It serves to enlarge the RVOT to the intended final dimension in patients with RVOT obstruction and to demonstrate RVOT behavior during placement of the valve when PR is the dominant dysfunction. A variety of high pressure, low compliance balloons are suitable for pre-dilation. Angiography and hemodynamic data are obtained following each pre-dilation to verify integrity of the conduit and efficacy of RVOT balloon angioplasty. Pre-dilation also unmasks the risk of coronary compression. Aortic root and/or selective coronary angiograms are obtained at the height of balloon inflation with the largest balloon used for pre-dilation.

Pre-stenting (Fig. 13.3b) refers to the technique of establishing a rigid zone called the landing zone within which the PV is deployed. Pre-stenting ensures that the valve is safely anchored within the RVOT. Pre-stenting has been shown to reduce the risk of MeV stent fractures [6, 8, 31–34]. Pre-stenting with multiple stents until the RVOT recoil is eliminated has become a standard procedure. Following ascertainment that TPVI is indicated, RVOT morphology is suitable and no risk exists for coronary compression, TPVI is accomplished by advancing the PV mounted on the delivery system. Femoral (or internal jugular) venotomy (femoral or internal jugular vein) is enlarged by sequential dilations for insertion of the delivery system. Hemodynamics and angiography are repeated after deployment to confirm adequate valve placement, competency and continued integrity of RVOT (Fig. 13.3c).

Procedural Complications

Contained and Non-contained Conduit Rupture

Contained tears of the RV to PA conduits are generally limited to the calcified wall and surrounding scar tissue. They can occur during pre-dilation, pre-stenting and valve implantation (Fig. 13.4). TPVI usually isolates the tear and contains hemorrhage. Extensive conduit rupture or dissection is a major adverse event that may require emergent management of acute hemothorax, implantation of covered stents to isolate the rupture and/or rescue surgery. Appropriate surgical backup is

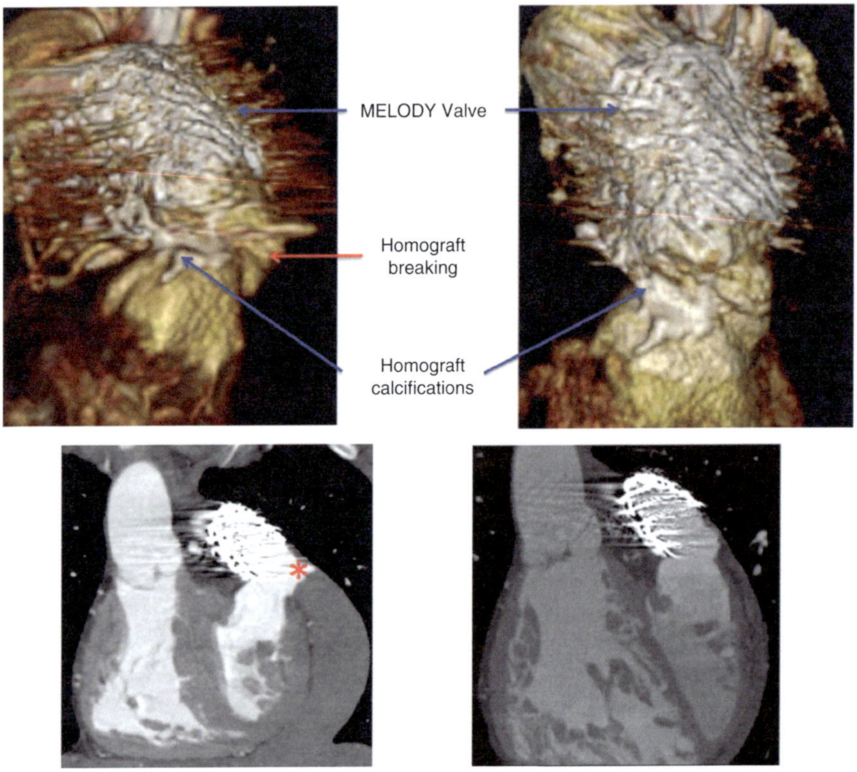

Fig. 13.4 3D reconstruction CT image (*up*) and CT scan of the right ventricular outflow in a patient following transcatheter valvulation with a 22 mm Melody Valve showing a tear with extravasation that is confined (*). A moderate pericardial effusion resolved over 5 days. No further intervention was required. Ultimately the result of transpulmonary valvulation was satisfactory

mandatory during TPVI. The incidence of extensive conduit rupture is between 1.5 and 1.9 % [5, 9].

Pulmonary Artery Dissection

PA dissection occurs during manipulation of stiff guide wires that are required to advance long sheaths as well as the delivery system for PV implantation. These are large rather stiff systems that are advanced across dysfunctional RV and RVOT. The potential for injury remains with dissection and hemorrhage of the proximal and distal PAs. This complication was noted in up to 1.3–1.5 % [3, 9] of MeV implants and 6 % of ESV implants although none of the patients with ESV implants required transfusion therapy. The hemorrhage was not deemed to be clinically significant [9]. Interventional techniques applied to treat PA dissection include device occlusion of the perforation, temporary balloon tamponade proximal to the dissected artery and definitive treatment with deployment of a covered stent across the dissection.

Valve Embolization and Malposition

In the US multicenter MeV trial, no cases of valve embolization were reported but embolization was described in 2 of the 155 initial patients undergoing TPVI with MeV [3]. Valve malposition can result in partial or complete obstruction of a branch PA [3]. During the feasibility phase of the COMPASSION trial, ESV embolization occurred in 3/33 implants. This trial included larger conduits than the conduits in the MeV trial. The shorter valve length may also have contributed.

Coronary Artery Compression

Coronary artery compression (Fig. 13.5) is a potentially fatal adverse event that is well known to occur during surgical RV to PA conduit interventions [31]. Coronary artery compression is also known to occur with transcatheter RVOT interventions including balloon angioplasty and stent implantation. It was noted to occur with TPVI early in the experience with MeV [3]. The procedural protocol was modified subsequently to include coronary imaging prior to TPVI. The most common reason for exclusion from TPVI in the US MeV trial was the risk of coronary compression [5]. Later report identified coronary compression by simultaneous RVOT angioplasty and coronary angiography in 5 % of the 404 patients who underwent cardiac catheterization for potential TPVI at four centers [30]. Risk of coronary compression was identified in 6 % of the 100 consecutive patients who underwent transcatheter RVOT evaluation in France. It was further demonstrated that pre-procedural non invasive imaging (CT-scan and/or CMR) are not fully accurate in identifying the potential for coronary compression [29]. Coronary compression is a major adverse event that is preventable by meticulous biplane angiographic evaluation of the coronary arteries [29]. The left main coronary artery was the most frequent coronary artery involved. Patients with abnormal left anterior descending (LAD) coronary coming off the right coronary artery (RCA) and crossing the infundibulum are likely to experience LAD compression from RVOT expanding interventions [29, 30]. Dense homograft calcification can contribute to coronary compression even when the internal conduit appears well separated from the coronary artery wall [5].

Hammock Effect

This complication is of historical interest. In 7 of the first 21 implants RVOT obstruction was noted following MeV implant due to prolapse of the valve tissue within the lumen [2]. This complication has not been observed following a design modification that included insertion of sutures anchoring the bovine vein wall to the entire length of the stent.

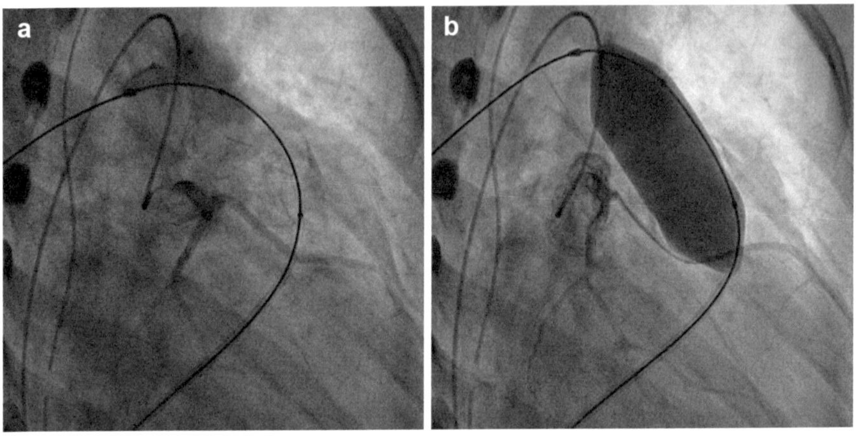

Fig. 13.5 Selective left coronary angiogram in right anterior oblique projection showing normal distribution of the left main and left anterior descending coronary artery (**a**). Another selective angiogram during balloon inflation of a high pressure 22 mm balloon (Atlas) shows compression of the left main and anterior descending coronary artery contraindicating stent and/or pulmonary valve implantation in this patient (**b**)

Early and Mid-term Results

TPVI can be accomplished with relatively low risk, and provides immediate and effective restoration of valve competence, resolution of right and left heart hemodynamic dysfunction and improvement of exercise capacity. This has been demonstrated consistently for both the transcatheter valves currently available for clinical use [2, 4, 10].

MeV Implants

In a study [2] of 58 patients who underwent TPVI with MeV for RVOT dysfunction, RV pressure, RVOT gradient and Pulmonary Regurgitation (PR) decreased significantly after MeV implant. Significant reduction in PR fraction, RV end-diastolic volume (EDV), a significant increase in left ventricular EDV and effective RV stroke volume was demonstrated by CMR in a subset of 28 patients in this study. On metabolic exercise testing performed in 16 patients, significant improvement in peak oxygen consumption (VO_2) was demonstrated. This was accomplished without procedural mortality.

The preliminary results from the US multi center trial confirmed the feasibility, safety and success with restoration of RVOT function in the short term following TPVI with MeV in 2009 [4]. Updated data from the trial was published in 2010 confirming ongoing high procedural success rate and encouraging immediate rehabilitation of valve dysfunction [5]. Of the 124 patients undergoing TPVI with MeV,

PR was the indication in 65 and mixed dysfunction (both regurgitation and obstruction) or obstruction in 59. In both groups of patients significant resolution of hemodynamic dysfunction was reported. Complications of a severe category occurred in 6 % (n =8) including 1 death at 7 days following the procedure from sequela of an acute procedural complication (dissection of coronary artery). Thus procedural mortality was 0.8 %. Freedom from stent fracture was 77.8 (±4.3) % at 14 months. Freedom from MeV dysfunction or reintervention was 93.5 (±2.4) % at 1 year and 85.7 (±4.7) % at 2 years. A higher RVOT gradient at discharge and younger age were associated with shorter freedom from dysfunction. Recurrent obstruction, usually associated with stent fracture, resulted in RVOT reintervention in 10 patients, 9 of whom received a second Melody valve. Although significant change in ventricular function was not shown in this series, it has been shown in other cohorts that RV pressure and/or volume unloading following TPVI is associated with improved RV and septal strain and improved biventricular function [32].

In the 102 patients undergoing TPVI with MeV for RVOT dysfunction reported from 2 large centers in Germany [6], it was demonstrated that the conduit diameter enlarged significantly from 13 mm (median, 11–15 mm) to 20 mm (median, 19–22 mm). Median peak systolic RVOT gradient, ratio of RV/aortic pressure, median CMR RV end-diastolic volume index and CMR PR fraction decreased significantly following TPVI The median follow-up time was 357 days (99–388 days). At the latest follow-up examination the median Doppler RVOT gradient was significantly lower as compared to the gradient before TPVI.

ESV Implants

The body of experience with the ESV is smaller than with the MeV however comparable acute results have been were demonstrated with the ESV implant indicating effective and safe resolution of dysfunctional RVOT in 2011. Of the 36 patients from 4 centers, 34 were offered TPVI. It was accomplished in 33 patients. Thus the success rate was 97 %. RVOT gradient and right ventricular/aortic pressure ratio decreased significantly. RV systolic pressure, RV diastolic pressure and PA mean and diastolic pressure changed significantly toward normalization. There were no deaths but a rather high (20.5 %, n=7) adverse event rate including 3 patients with valve migration 2 of whom requiring surgical retrieval. At 6-month follow-up, all patients were alive. There was improvement in exercise capacity with number of patients in New York Heart Association functional class I. PR was <2+ in 97 % of patients. Freedom from reintervention was 97 %. Elective placement of a second valve was undertaken in 1 patient due to conduit-induced distortion of the initial implant [9].

The European experience with the ESV was reported in 2013. TPVI with ESV was performed using a standardized procedure in 22 patients with a variety of RVOT substrate (transannular patch, bioprosthesis, homograft and Contegra conduit). RVOT dysfunction consisted of stenosis (n=2), regurgitation (n=11) and a combination lesion (n=9). TPVI was performed successfully with placement of 23 mm device in

10 and 26 mm device in 11 patients. RV-systolic pressure, RV to PA gradient and PR decreased and the PA systolic and diastolic pressure increased substantially [10]. Complication rate was 6 %, in contrast of the 20.5 % adverse event rate in the COMPASSION trial [9]. None of the complications in the European study were related to the ESV per se. At the time of writing this chapter, Premier Registry of the ESV has 131 enrolled patients from 16 centers in 9 countries and thus far there is no mortality and a 91 % success rate after 1 year.

In summary, ESV can be applied safely in a wide range of patients with various underlying RVOT substrate and dysfunction and offers restoration to an adult-size RVOT and reinstatement of valvar function. The immediate and short-term results are promising. The long-term effects and safety are pending assessment in further clinical follow-up studies.

Specific Applications: TPVI in Native RVOT

Following pioneering experimental work [27], there is increasing clinical application of TPVI for dysfunctional native PV and native repaired RVOTs (Fig. 13.6) [23, 24, 28, 33, 34]. TPVI in a native large regurgitant RVOT was first performed in 2010 with the "Atlas pulmonary valve" [33]. Applications of the MeV in native RVOT was reported in 2012 with preparatory techniques such as the Russian dolls technique and/or the PA jailing technique [28]. The first case series of patients with significant PR following RVOT patch repair demonstrated that ESV can be offered to patients with larger outflow tracts and can be treated with sustained relief of PR and significant decrease of RV end-diastolic pressure [35]. More recently, 5 patients with large native severely regurgitant RVOT successfully underwent TPVI with a new transcatheter self-expanding valve called the Venus P Valve [34]. The

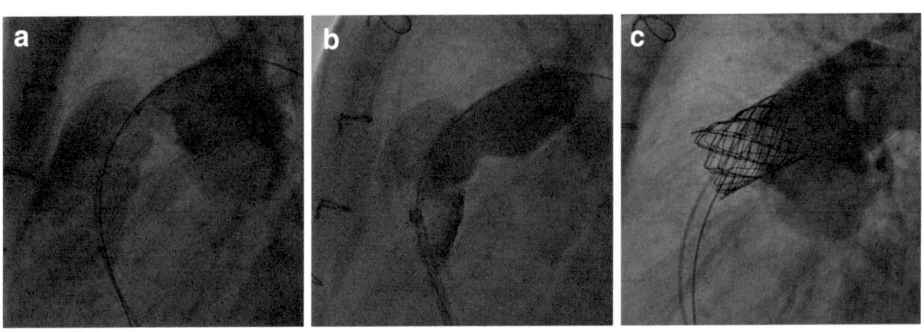

Fig. 13.6 Frontal right ventricular outflow tract angiogram (RVOT) in a patient with tetralogy of Fallot and absent pulmonary valve, status-post complete repair with pericardial patch RVOT reconstruction. A discrete stenosis is seen (**a**). In (**b**), a 25 mm diameter, 4 cm long Tyshak balloon is inflated while contrast injection is performed through the long sheath with tip in the proximal RVOT. The presence of a residual waist without distal passage of the contrast indicates feasibility of transcatheter pulmonary valvulation in a native RVOT. After pre stenting, a 22 mm Melody valve is successfully implanted. Frontal angiogram shows no regurgitation (**c**)

applicability of TPVI over a large range of anatomical variations of the RVOT is very much the current quest as the potential to provide transcatheter options for patients with large native regurgitant RVOT is there. We expect a device to receive approval for clinical application from the regulatory agencies within the following years. A multi center US trial is launched in the near future with a "native transcatheter PV" for implantation in large native regurgitant RVOT.

Adverse Events During Follow Up

Stent Fractures

The early studies of TPVI with the MeV reported an incidence of stent fractures of 25–28 % (Fig. 13.7) [3–5, 36]. Stent fractures presents early in the majority of patients — 26 of the 39 presented within the first 6 months in the US MeV trial [37]. New stent fractures were seen up to 3 years post valve implantation. Not all stent fractures were significant clinically but up to 35 % eventually progress to be of clinical significance with onset of significant outflow tract obstruction and/or fragmentation with embolization [36, 37]. However pre-stenting has resulted in significant reduction of stent fractures to 5–18 % [6, 38, 39].

Nordmeyer et al. reported results of TPVI with the MeV in 108 patients. Pre-stenting was performed in 50 %. The overall incidence of stent fracture was 22 % for the entire group. However, the incidence was only 18 % in the group with

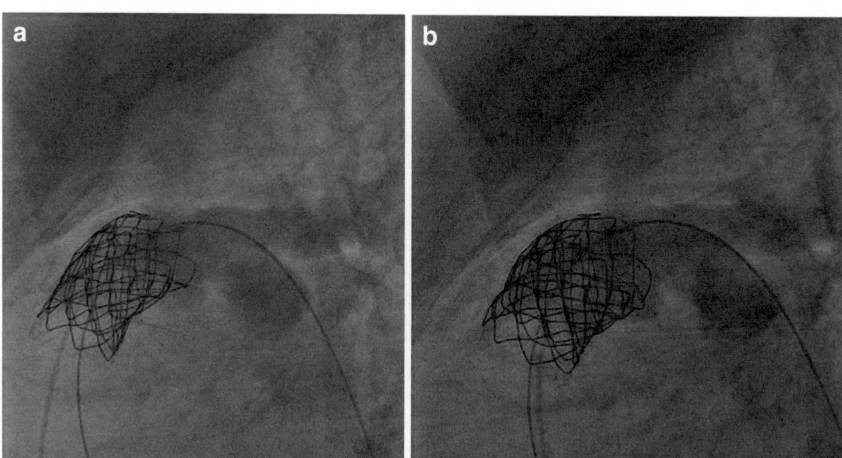

Fig. 13.7 Frontal right ventricular outflow tract (RVOT) angiogram shows recurrent stenosis, 2 years after a 22 mm Melody valve implant for conduit dysfunction status post repair of pulmonary atresia-ventricular septal defect (**a**). Notice the narrowing at the proximal part of the stent (*arrow*) and a distal stent fracture (*). RVOT angiogram performed following dilatation of the RVOT with a 22 mm Atlas balloon showing relief of the stenosis (**b**)

pre-stenting as compared to 31 % in those not pre-stented. The data implied protective effect of pre-stenting [38].

Eicken et al. reported 102 patients with TPVI with MeV. Majority of the patients underwent pre-stenting prior to MeV implantation. At a median follow-up of 357 days, there were only 5 patients (5 %) with stent fractures [6]. This is lower than reported by other investigators. While these could be secondary to the relatively short follow-up period, the data are supportive that pre-stenting likely is effective in preventing stent fractures.

Pre-stenting of RV to PA conduits is recommended prior to TPVI for stenotic conduits, conduits in the retrosternal area, in the absence of RVOT calcification and for persistent stent recoil following implantation. These have been identified as risk factors for stent fracture [36]. Multiple stents implants are recommended until there is no recoil of the stent during deflation of the implanting balloon. Additionally a substernal location of the valve and asymmetry of the valve following implantation are also identified to be associated with higher risk of stent fracture while pre-stenting and implant within a bioprosthesis were associated with protection and longer freedom from stent fractures [39].

Stent fractures have not been reported thus far in the patients enrolled in the COMPASSION trial for placement of the ESV in the pulmonic position [9]. The stainless steel frame- work and shorter length of the ESV may afford protection. Besides that the deployment of the ESV has always been following pre-stenting. Also fractures are less likely in the larger conduits which are typically where the ESV has been used. Positioning of the ESV in the RVOT is however very different from the placement in the LVOT. It is possible that dense adhesions in the post surgical RVOT patient and proximity to the sternum may contribute to stent fatigue over time.

Recurrent Stenosis

This is commonly due to stent fracture. An RVOT substrate such as a small conduit and external compressive constraints from a retrosternal conduit also cause recurrent stenosis. TPVI within the previous implant with MeV called the valve in valve therapy is an effective treatment for recurrent stenosis [5, 6, 8, 39, 40]. This was initially performed in a patient with acute severe stenosis due to hammocking of the MeV. This demonstration of concept and its effectiveness, resulted in valve in valve therapy being electively offered in all patients with recurrent RVOT stenosis. TPVI was feasible in all of the 20 patients who underwent repeat TPVI with MeV for recurrent stenosis related to device failure [40]. Balloon redilation of a stenotic MeV can also be performed successfully as an alternative to valve-in-valve implantation (Fig. 13.7), especially in cases where the MeV stenosis is associated with non longitudinal stent fractures [5, 6, 37]. In a recent study, up to 50 % of the patients could be successfully treated with balloon dilation of the MeV alone [6].

Infective Endocarditis

IE was first described following TPVI with MeV in 2008 [3]. Subsequent to this there have been several reports of IE following TPVI with MeV [3, 6–8, 22, 41–47]. A prospective North American and European study sponsored by the manufacturer reported an annualized rate of 0.88 % per patient-year for first episode of IE. This was derived from 16 cases of IE from among the 311 patients who underwent TPVI with MeV [46].

Common pathogens identified thus far are the various species of Staphylococcus (Aureus, Epidermidis) and Streptococcus (Sanguis, Mitis, Viridans, Aurelius). IE due to Aspergillus, Candida Albicans, Corynebacterium, Moraxella Catarrhalis and Hemophilus have also been reported [47]. Culture-negative endocarditis due to Bartonella Henselae has also been reported 5 years after MeV implant [41].

Temporal relationship between the implant and onset of IE are not in favor of infective seeding at the time of the implant procedure. The earliest case of IE occurred 50 days after TPVI with MeV and 13 of the 16 were diagnosed 6 months following the implant procedure in the manufacturer sponsored study [46]. Risk factors identified thus far are male gender [45], previous IE [3, 45, 46], dental treatment [3, 45], tattooing, previous fungal infection [3], septic wound [3, 45], incomplete opening of RVOT during TPVI resulting in residual gradient [46], multiple stents, stent fracture, altered anatomy of the RVOT [45], and history of abrupt withdrawal of aspirin [42]. It has been speculated if the irregular geometry of the implanted valve and long valve coaptation surface predisposes to IE [46]. Also, intrinsic characteristics of the bovine jugular vein, the valve apparatus for the MeV as well as the Contegra conduit may play a role; higher rates of IE following the Contegra conduit are known raising the possibility of risk stemming from the bovine valve tissue [48–53]. Immunological characteristics of the bovine tissue may predispose to idiosyncratic reactions with formation of non bacterial thrombotic endocarditis, disrupted laminar flow, and turbulence. Such endocardial injury is known to predispose to IE [53, 54].

It has been suggested that an increase in RVOT gradient in the presence of positive blood cultures should be considered diagnostic of IE [42, 55, 56].

It has been proposed that MeV replacement is not necessary when there is no involvement of the valve system [45]. However surgery should be offered early and promptly for acute RVOT obstruction related to valvar involvement in IE. It should also be considered when there is failure of clinical improvement with medical therapy. Almost half of all published cases received medical therapy alone including 1 of the 4 patients in the report by Villanave et al. [47]. In patients with history of IE, TPVI with MeV may be pursued after a period of clinical and bacteriological cure. Explantation of MeV may be indicated in as many as 50 % of cases [42, 47]. All patients should follow the recommendations for lifelong IE prophylaxis [45, 47].

Thus far there are no reports of IE following TPVI with ESV. This may be a reflection of the more recent application of ESV for TPVI. IE is known to occur following transcatheter implantation of the ESV in the LVOT.

When comparing TPVI strategy with the conventional surgical management strategy for RVOT dysfunction it is well worth acknowledging that IE is known to occur following RVOT conduits or bioprosthetic valves [53, 54, 57]. A higher incidence has been observed in bovine conduits such as the Contegra® conduits (Medtronic Inc, Minneapolis, Minnesota, USA) [48–53].

Long Term Prospects

Long term adverse effects of RVOT dysfunction are exercise intolerance, arrhythmia, and death [58, 59]. Pending the test of time, the impact of TPVI on long-term outcomes can be assessed through its impact on electrical and mechanical remodeling of ventricular synchrony, volume and function.

Sudden Cardiac Death and TPVI

The effects of TPVI on surface electrocardiogram were studied in 99 patients (43 % stenosis, 27 % regurgitation and 29 % mixed lesion) undergoing TPVI with the MeV before, after, and 1 year subsequent to TPVI [60]. QRS duration decreased significantly in patients with regurgitation following TPVI as has been reported for equivalent surgical cohorts [61]. RV end-diastolic volume correlation with QRS duration was not maintained 1 year following TPVI. Corrected QT interval and QRS, QT, and JT dispersions decreased significantly at 1 year in the entire group suggesting increased homogeneity of repolarization and improved conduction following TPVI. These data suggests favorable electrical remodeling following TPVI. A decrease in arrhythmic events and improved longevity can therefore be expected in patients undergoing TPVI.

Right Ventricular Function and TPVI

Persistent impairment of RV contractility after TPVI is reported [62]. However, ventricular strain and strain-derived synchrony are more sensitive indicators than ventricular ejection fraction for long term outcomes [63, 64]. MRI and EKG data in 31 patients (18 with stenosis and 13 with regurgitation) from one of the centers participating in the US Melody TPVI trial were analyzed for biventricular strain and mechanical synchrony [65]. TPVI was associated with improved global longitudinal and circumferential left ventricular strain; patients with RVOT stenosis had improved RV circumferential strain and patient with dominant regurgitant dysfunction had more synchronous left ventricular longitudinal contraction. These findings suggest a potential long-term beneficial impact of TPVI because of the known association of strain and synchrony with clinical outcomes.

Exercise Performance and TPVI

Exercise performance in patients with RVOT dysfunction is known to improve following surgical relief of RVOT dysfunction [66]. There is sophisticated information on the impact of TPVI on exercise performance. Briefly, exercise capacity improves with adequate relief of obstructive RVOT dysfunction but not with relief of regurgitant RVOT dysfunction [62, 67]. Improvement in VO_2, a surrogate for exercise performance, was highest among patients with the lowest baseline peak VO_2. Additionally baseline VO_2 is the only variable identified on multivariate analysis to predict significant change of peak oxygen consumption following TPVI [68].

Quality of Life and TPVI

Self-estimated quality of life increases following TPVI. Significant improvements were reported in "physical function", "general health perception" and "health transition" in patients treated for obstructive and regurgitant RVOT while improvement of "physical role functioning", "vitality" and "mental health" was reported in patients treated for obstructive RVOT [67].

Future Perspectives

An ideal pulmonary valve would be universally applicable to all morphological types of RVOT. The first steps in the search of such a valve have been taken as new lower profile devices undergo evaluation [34]. A living autologous valve similar to the native valve with the capacity of growth, repair and remodeling is the utopia in transcatheter valve therapy and may not be too far from reach [69, 70]. Application to native pulmonary valve and the native repaired RVOT [23, 24] has been accomplished with equivalent acute and medium terms results. TPVI will receive recognition as the standard of care for RVOT dysfunction. Surgical management of CHD will be impacted by the wide and easy availability of TPVI strategy such that an RVOT substrate will be selectively offered that is best suited to future TPVI. It may be the standard of care to offer expandable RV-to-PA conduits of 18–22 mm diameter as the preferred RVOT substrate. Non expandable conduits like the bioprothesis will fall out of favor. To prepare prospectively for conduit failure and its early management by application of TPVI is prevention of RVOT dysfunction disease. The shift in thinking will be from 'timely' management to 'early' management. This will be most critical shift of thinking for eradication of RVOT dysfunction disease.

There has been a modest degree of success in reducing reintervention rates following TPVI. The hammock effect resulting in acute RVOT obstruction has been effectively eliminated. Stent fractures will be preventable with application of pre-stenting and use of newer more durable stents with enhanced radial strength. Even as the true profile of long term outcomes is being delineated, we expect that with earlier TPVI, there will be preservation of RV function and RV functional longevity will normalize with improved quality of life and survival.

References

1. Bonhoeffer P, Boudjemline Y, Saliba Z, et al. Percutaneous replacement of pulmonary valve in a right-ventricle to pulmonary-artery prosthetic conduit with valve dysfunction. Lancet. 2000;356:1403–5.
2. Khambadkone S, Coats L, Taylor A, et al. Percutaneous pulmonary valve implantation in humans: results in 59 consecutive patients. Circulation. 2005;112:1189–97.
3. Lurz P, Coats L, Khambadkone S, Nordmeyer J, Boudjemline Y, Schievano S, Muthurangu V, Lee TY, Parenzan G, Derrick G, Cullen S, et al. Percutaneous pulmonary valve implantation: impact of evolving technology and learning curve on clinical outcome. Circulation. 2008;117:1964–72.
4. Zahn EM, Hellenbrand WE, Lock JE, McElhinney DB. Implantation of the melody transcatheter pulmonary valve in patients with a dysfunctional right ventricular outflow tract conduit early results from the U.S. Clinical trial. J Am Coll Cardiol. 2009;54:1722–9.
5. McElhinney DB, Hellenbrand WE, Zahn EM, et al. Short- and medium-term outcomes after transcatheter pulmonary valve placement in the expanded multicenter US melody valve trial. Circulation. 2010;122:507–16.
6. Eicken A, Ewert P, Hager A, et al. Percutaneous pulmonary valve implantation: two-centre experience with more than 100 patients. Eur Heart J. 2011;32:1260–5.
7. Fraisse A, Aldebert P, Malekzadeh-Milani S, Thambo JB, Piéchaud JF, Aucoururier P, Chatelier G, Bonnet D, Iserin L, Bonello B, Assaidi A, Kammache I, Boudjemline Y. Melody transcatheter pulmonary valve implantation: results from a french registry. Arch Cardiovasc Dis. 2014;107:607–14.
8. Butera G, Milanesi O, Spadoni I, et al. Melody transcatheter pulmonary valve implantation. Results from the registry of the Italian Society of Pediatric Cardiology. Catheter Cardiovasc Interv. 2013;81:310–6.
9. Kenny D, Hijazi ZM, Kar S. Percutaneous implantation of the Edwards SAPIEN transcatheter heart valve for conduit failure in the pulmonary position: early phase 1 results from an international multicenter clinical trial. J Am Coll Cardiol. 2011;58:2248–56.
10. Haas NA, Moysich A, Neudorf U, et al. Percutaneous implantation of the Edwards SAPIEN(™) pulmonic valve: initial results in the first 22 patients. Clin Res Cardiol. 2013;102:119–28.
11. Rubio-Alvarez V, Limon R, Soni J. [Intracardiac valvulotomy by means of a catheter]. Arch Inst Cardiol Mex. 1953;23:183–92.
12. Kan JS, White Jr RI, Mitchell SE, Gardner TJ. Percutaneous balloon valvuloplasty: a new method for treating congenital pulmonary-valve stenosis. N Engl J Med. 1982;307:540–2.
13. Zeevi B, Keane JF, Perry SB, et al. Balloon dilation of postoperative right ventricular outflow obstructions. J Am Coll Cardiol. 1989;14:401–8.
14. Almagor Y, Prevosti LG, Bartorelli AL, et al. Balloon expandable stent implantation in stenotic right heart valved conduits. J Am Coll Cardiol. 1990;16:1310–4.

15. Ovaert C, Caldarone CA, McCrindle BW, et al. Endovascular stent implantation for the management of postoperative right ventricular outflow tract obstruction: clinical efficacy. J Thorac Cardiovasc Surg. 1999;118:886–93.
16. Sugiyama H, Williams W, Benson LN. Implantation of endovascular stents for the obstructive right ventricular outflow tract. Heart. 2005;91:1058–63.
17. McElhinney DB, Hennesen JT. The Melody® valve and Ensemble® delivery system for transcatheter pulmonary valve replacement. Ann N Y Acad Sci. 2013;1291:77–85.
18. Garay F, Webb J, Hijazi ZM. Percutaneous replacement of pulmonary valve using the Edwards-Cribier percutaneous heart valve: first report in a human patient. Catheter Cardiovasc Interv. 2006;67:659–62.
19. Cheatham SL, Holzer RJ, Chisolm JL, Cheatham JP. The Medtronic Melody® transcatheter pulmonary valve implanted at 24-mm diameter – it works. Catheter Cardiovasc Interv. 2013;82:816–23.
20. Boone RH, Webb JG, Horlick E, et al. Transcatheter pulmonary valve implantation using the Edwards SAPIENTM transcatheter heart valve. Catheter Cardiovasc Interv. 2010;75:286–94.
21. Feltes TF, Bacha E, Beekman RH, et al. Indications for cardiac catheterization & and intervention in pediatric cardiac disease. Circulation. 2011;123:2607–52.
22. Gillespie MJ, Rome JJ, Levi DS. Melody valve implant within failed bioprosthetic valves in the pulmonary position: a multicenter experience. Circ Cardiovasc Interv. 2012;5:862–70.
23. Meadows JJ, Moore PM, Berman DP. Use and performance of the melody transcatheter pulmonary valve in native and postsurgical, nonconduit right ventricular outflow tracts. Circ Cardiovasc Interv. 2014;7:374–80.
24. Malekzadeh-Milani S, Ladouceur M, Cohen S, Iserin L, Boudjemline Y. Results of transcatheter pulmonary valvulation in native or patched right ventricular outflow tracts. Arch Cardiovasc Dis. 2014;107:592–8.
25. Berman DP, McElhinney DB, Vincent JA, Hillenbrand WE, Zahn EM. Feasibility and short-term outcomes of percutaneous transcatheter pulmonary valve replacement in small (<30 kg) children with dysfunctional right ventricular outflow tract conduits. Circ Cardiovasc Interv. 2014;7:142–8.
26. Schievano S, Coats L, Migliavacca F, et al. Variations in right ventricular outflow tract morphology following repair of congenital heart disease: implications for percutaneous pulmonary valve implantation. J Cardiovasc Magn Reson. 2007;9:687–95.
27. Boudjemline Y, Agnoletti G, Bonnet D, et al. Percutaneous pulmonary valve replacement in a large right ventricular outflow tract: an experimental study. J Am Coll Cordial. 2004;43: 1082–7.
28. Boudjemline Y, Brugada G, Van-Aerschot I. Outcomes and safety of transcatheter pulmonary valve replacement in patients with large patched right ventricular outflow tracts. Arch Cardiovasc Dis. 2012;105:404–13.
29. Fraisse A, Assaidi A, Mauri L, et al. Coronary artery compression during intention to treat right ventricle outflow with percutaneous pulmonary valve implantation: Incidence, diagnosis and outcome. Catheter Cardiovasc Interv. 2014;83:E260–8.
30. Morray BH, McElhinney DB, Cheatham JP, et al. Risk of coronary artery compression among patients referred for transcatheter pulmonary valve implantation: a multicenter experience. Circ Cardiovasc Interv. 2013;6:535–42.
31. Daskalopoulos DA, Edwards WD, Driscoll DJ, Danielson GK, Puga FJ. Coronary artery compression with fatal myocardial ischemia. J Thorac Cardiovasc Surg. 1983;85:546–51.
32. Lurz P, Puranik R, Nordmeyer J, et al. Improvement in left ventricular filling properties after relief of right ventricle to pulmonary artery conduit obstruction: contribution of septal motion and interventricular mechanical delay. Eur Heart J. 2009;30:2266–74.
33. Schievano S, Taylor AM, Capelli C, et al. First-in-man implantation of a novel percutaneous valve: a new approach to medical device development. EuroIntervention. 2010;5:745–50.
34. Cao QL, Kenny D, Zhou D, Pan W, Ge J, Hijazi ZM. Early experience with a novel self-expanding percutaneous stent-valve in the native right ventricular outflow tract. Catheter Cardiovasc Interv. 2014;84:1131–7.

35. Demkow M, Rużyłło W, Biernacka EK, et al. Percutaneous Edwards SAPIEN(™) valve implantation for significant pulmonary regurgitation after previous surgical repair with a right ventricular outflow patch. Catheter Cardiovasc Interv. 2014;83:474–81.
36. Nordmeyer J, Khambadkone S, Coats L, et al. Risk stratification, systematic classification, and anticipatory management strategies for stent fracture after percutaneous pulmonary valve implantation. Circulation. 2007;115:1392–7.
37. McElhinney DB, Cheatham JP, Jones TK, et al. Stent fracture, valve failure, and right ventricular outflow tract reintervention after transcatheter pulmonary valve implantation: patient-related and procedural risk factors in the US melody valve trial. Circ Cardiovasc Interv. 2011;4:602–14.
38. Nordmeyer J, Lurz P, Khambadkone S, et al. Prestenting with a bare metal stent before percutaneous pulmonary valve implantation: acute and 1-year outcomes. Heart. 2011;97:118–23.
39. Balzer DT. Percutaneous pulmonary valve implantation: fixing the problems and pushing the envelope. Curr Opin Pediatr. 2012;24:565–8.
40. Nordmeyer J, Coats L, Lurz P, et al. Percutaneous pulmonary valve-in-valve implantation: a successful treatment concept for early device failure. Eur Heart J. 2008;29:810–5.
41. Atamanyuk I, Raja SG, Kostolny M. Bartonella Henselae endocarditis of percutaneously implanted pulmonary valve: a case report. J Heart Valve Dis. 2011;20:94–7.
42. Patel M, Iserin L, Bonnet D, Boudjemline Y. Atypical malignant late infective endocarditis of Melody valve. J Thorac Cardiovasc Surg. 2012;143:e32–5.
43. Alsoufi B, Al-joufan M, Al-Omrani A, Bulbul Z. Obstruction of a percutaneous pulmonary valve by an aspergillus mycotic thrombus mimicking massive pulmonary embolus. Ann Thorac Surg. 2012;94:e5–6.
44. Bhat D, Forbes TJ, Aggarwal S. A case of life-threatening Staphylococcus aureus endocarditis involving percutaneous transcatheter prosthetic pulmonary valve. Congenit Heart Dis. 2013;8:E161–4.
45. Buber J, Bergersen L, Lock JE. Bloodstream infections occurring in patients with percutaneously implanted bio-prosthetic pulmonary valve: a single-center experience. Circ Cardiovasc Interv. 2013;6:301–10.
46. McElhinney D, Benson L, Eicken A, Kreutzer J, Padera RF, Zahn EM. Infective endocarditis after transcatheter pulmonary valve replacement using the melody valve: combined results of 3 prospective North American and European Studies. Circ Cardiovasc Interv. 2013;6: 292–300.
47. Villafañe J, Baker GH, Austin EH, Miller S, Peng L, Beekman R. Melody® pulmonary valve bacterial endocarditis: experience in four pediatric patients and a review of the literature. Catheter Cardiovasc Interv. 2014;84:212–8.
48. Tiete AR, Sachweh S, Roemer U, Kozlik-Fredmann R, Reuchart B, Daebritz SH. Right ventricular outflow tract reconstruction with the Contegra bovine jugular vein conduit: a word of caution. Ann Thorac Surg. 2004;77:2151–6.
49. Shebani SO, McGuirk S, Baghai M, et al. Right ventricular outflow tract reconstruction using Contegra valved conduit: natural history and conduit performance under pressure. Eur J Cardiothorac Surg. 2006;29:397–405.
50. Baslaim G. Bovine valved xenograft (Contegra) conduit in the extracardiac Fontan procedure: the preliminary experience. J Card Surg. 2008;23:146–9.
51. Bajraktari G, Olloni R, Daullxhiu I, Ademaj F, Vela Z, Pajaziti M. MRSA endocarditis of bovine Contegra valved conduit: a case report. Cases J. 2009;2:57.
52. Stefanidis C, Benahmed-Mostafa A, Sanoussi A, Quiriny M, Demanet H, Theunissen C, et al. Edocarditis of bovine jugular vein conduit due to Q fever. Ann Thorac Surg. 2011;91: 1990–2.
53. Prior N, Alphonso N, Arnold P, et al. Bovine jugular vein valved conduit: up to 10 years follow-up. J Thorac Cardiovasc Surg. 2011;141:983–7.
54. Breymann T, Blanz U, Wojtalik M, et al. European Contegra Multicenter Study: 7-year results after valved bovine jugular vein graft implantations. Thorac Cardiovasc Surg. 2009;57: 257–69.

55. Albanesi F, Sekarski N, Lambrou D, Von Segesser LK, Berdajs DA. Incidence and risk factors for Contegra graft infection following right ventricular outflow tract reconstruction: long-term results. Eur J Cardiothorac Surg. 2014;45:1070–4.
56. Cheung G, Vejlstrup N, Ihlemann N, et al. Infective endocarditis following percutaneous pulmonary valve replacement: diagnostic challenges and application of intra-cardiac echocardiography. Int J Cardiol. 2013;169:425–9.
57. Lee C, Park CS, Lee CH. Durability of bioprosthetic valves in the pulmonary position: long-term follow-up of 181 implants in patients with congenital heart disease. Cardiovasc Surg. 2011;142:351–8.
58. Murphy JG, Gersh BJ, Mair DD, et al. Long-term outcome in patients undergoing surgical repair of tetralogy of Fallot. N Engl J Med. 1993;329:593–9.
59. Gatzoulis MA, Till JA, Somerville J, Redington AN. Mechanoelectrical interaction in tetralogy of Fallot. QRS prolongation relates to right ventricular size and predicts malignant ventricular arrhythmias and sudden death. Circulation. 1995;92:231–7.
60. Plymen CM, Bolger AP, Lurz P, et al. Electrical remodeling following percutaneous pulmonary valve implantation. Am J Cardiol. 2011;107:309–14.
61. Therrien J, Siu S, Harris L, et al. Impact of pulmonary valve replacement on arrhythmia propensity late after repair of tetralogy of Fallot. Circulation. 2001;103:2489–94.
62. Lurz P, Giardini A, TayloR AM, et al. Effect of altering pathologic right ventricular loading conditions by percutaneous pulmonary valve implantation on exercise capacity. Am J Cardiol. 2010;105:721–6.
63. Diller GP, Kempny A, Liodakis E, et al. Left ventricular longitudinal function predicts life-threatening ventricular arrhythmia and death in adults with repaired tetralogy of Fallot. Circulation. 2012;125:2440–6.
64. Ortega M, Triedman JK, Geva T, et al. Relation of left ventricular dyssynchrony measured by cardiac magnetic resonance tissue tracking in repaired tetralogy of fallot to ventricular tachycardia and death. Am J Cardiol. 2011;107:1535–40.
65. Harrild DM, Marcus E, Hasan B, et al. Impact of transcatheter pulmonary valve replacement on biventricular strain and synchrony assessed by cardiac magnetic resonance feature tracking. Circ Cardiovasc Interv. 2013;6:680–7.
66. Eyskens B, Reybrouck T, Bogaert J, et al. Homograft insertion for pulmonary regurgitation after repair of tetralogy of Fallot improves cardiorespiratory exercise performance. Am J Cardiol. 2000;85:221–5.
67. Müller J, Engelhardt A, Fratz S, Eicken A, Ewert P, Hager A. Improved exercise performance and quality of life after percutaneous pulmonary valve implantation. Int J Cardiol. 2014;173: 388–92.
68. Batra AS, McElhinney DB, Wang W, et al. Cardiopulmonary exercise function among patients undergoing transcatheter pulmonary valve implantation in the US Melody valve investigational trial. Am Heart J. 2012;163:280–7.
69. Lutter G, Metzner A, Jahnke T, Bombien R, Boldt J, Iino K, Cremer J, Stock UA. Percutaneous tissue-engineered pulmonary valved stent implantation. Ann Thorac Surg. 2010;89:259–63.
70. Boldt J, Lutter G, Pohanke J, Fischer G, Schoettler J, Cremer J, Metzner A. Percutaneous tissue-engineered pulmonary valved stent implantation: comparison of bone marrow-derived CD133+-cells and cells obtained from carotid artery. Tissue Eng Part C Methods. 2013;19: 363–74.

Chapter 14
Arterial Switch in TGA-IVS: Coronary Transfer

Francois Lacour-Gayet

Abstract The arterial switch operation has become the standard operation for transposition of the great arteries. This chapter focuses on coronary transfer and proposes a uniform and simplified technique of coronary transfer applicable to both simple and complex coronary patterns. The Marie Lannelongue coronary classification based on the course of coronary arteries, is convenient because the coronary transfer depends upon the various courses. A single ostium group is identified in this chapter. The uniform surgical technique of coronary transfer is to control the kinking of the posterior looping vessel and the stretching of the anterior looping vessel. In complex forms, the coronary trunks need to be well dissected. Intramural coronary, single ostium as well as malaligned commissure remain challenging, and demand a second learning curve. Late complications requires long term follow up to detect: pulmonary branches stenosis, coronary anomalies, and occurrence of aortic regurgitation or aortic root dilation. The arterial switch operation stands as a remarkable success of pediatric cardiac surgery of the last decades.

Keywords Transposition of the great arteries • Arterial switch operation • Coronary anomaly • Cono-truncal anomaly • Congenital heart surgery • Cyanotic heart disease

---

F. Lacour-Gayet, MD
Department of Pediatric Cardiac Surgery, National Heart and Lung Institute,
Royal Brompton Hospital, Imperial College University, Sydney Street, London SW3 6NP, UK
e-mail: flacourgayet@mac.com

F. Lacour-Gayet et al. (eds.), *Surgery of Conotruncal Anomalies*,
DOI 10.1007/978-3-319-23057-3_14

Introduction

The arterial switch operation (ASO) [1] is today the operation of choice for patients with Transposition of the Great Arteries (TGA); either in TGA with intact ventricular septum (TGA-IVS), in TGA-VSD or in TGA-VSD with aortic arch obstruction (see Chap. 15). The arterial switch operation has become, with time, a simplified and safe operation, with very low operative mortality in many centers [2]. Most technical problems raised by complex coronary artery patterns and by associated cardiac lesions have found adapted solutions. This first chapter on TGA addresses: –the coronary arteries classification in TGA, – the ASO surgical technique in TGA-IVS in focusing on the transfer of the coronary arteries. The technique presented thereafter is a uniform and reproducible method [3]. At a time, when a learning curve is hardly accepted, it is believed that this uniform technique described with many practical details will be useful, especially for complex coronary transfer.

Classification of Coronary Arteries

Magdi Yacoub and Radley-Smith published the first classification of the coronary arteries anatomy in TGA [4]. The Leiden classification [5] based on the origin of the coronary arteries, recognizes: – a sinus 1 located on the right hand-side of an observer sitting in the aortic non-coronary sinus and a sinus 2 on the left hand-side.

We are following the Marie Lannelongue classification [3, 6] that is based on the course of the coronary arteries vessels more than on their origin. The main interest of this classification is that the coronary relocation techniques are contingent upon these different courses. The vessels are frequently antero-posterior or oblique but can be side by side. If the aorta is usually located on the right of the PA in situs solitus, it can be exceptionally slightly located on the left [7]. The classification recognizes, in anatomic position and in situs solitus: – a left and anterior facing sinus (Leiden sinus 1) and a right and posterior facing sinus (Leiden sinus 2). When the vessels are side-by-side the right sinus becomes anterior and the left sinus become posterior. We consider that 20 % of the coronary artery patterns deserve to be called complex. Four groups, are identified according to the coronary courses and the number of ostium:

- Normal course. Two ostia
- Looping courses. Two ostia
- Intramural course. Two ostia
- Single ostium, Miscellaneous course.

Normal Course, Two Ostia (60 %) (Fig. 14.1)

The Normal Course of the coronary arteries is the most frequent and represents 60 % of cases. The left ostium (Sinus 1) gives the left anterior descending (LAD) and the circumflex artery (Cx), and the right ostium (Sinus 2) gives the right coronary artery

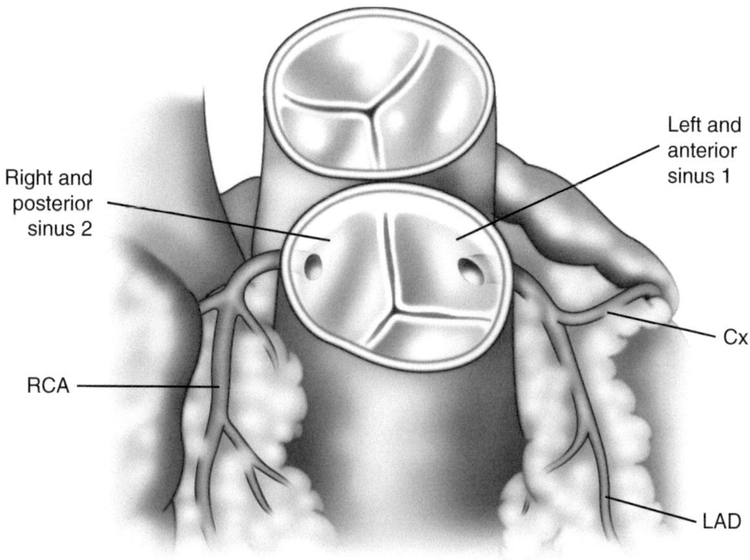

Fig. 14.1 Normal course, two ostia (60 %)

(RCA). No vessel is crossing either in front of or behind the great vessels. It corresponds to: –Yacoub type A – Leiden 1 LAD, Cx; 2 RCA.

Looping Courses, Two Ostia (29.5 %) (Fig. 14.2)

The Looping Courses with two ostia, are those in which a coronary runs in front of and/or behind the great vessels, and represent 29.5 % of the cases. Three subgroups are identified: the posterior looping course, the double looping course, and the anterior looping course.

Posterior Looping Course (20 %) (Fig. 14.2, Top)

The posterior looping course is one in which the circumflex artery arise from the RCA and loops behind the pulmonary artery to reach the lateral wall of the left ventricle. It is the second most frequent coronary pattern with a prevalence around 20 %. We don't consider this isolated posterior course with the Cx from the RCA as a complex coronary anatomy. It corresponds to Yacoub type D and Leiden 1 LAD; 2 RCA, Cx.

Double Looping Course (9 %) (Complex Fig. 14.2, Medium)

In double looping courses with two ostia, the anterior loop is always the RCA, which arose from the left sinus (Sinus 1) and cross the aortic root to reach the right AV groove. The posterior loop is made by two different coronary arteries: – either

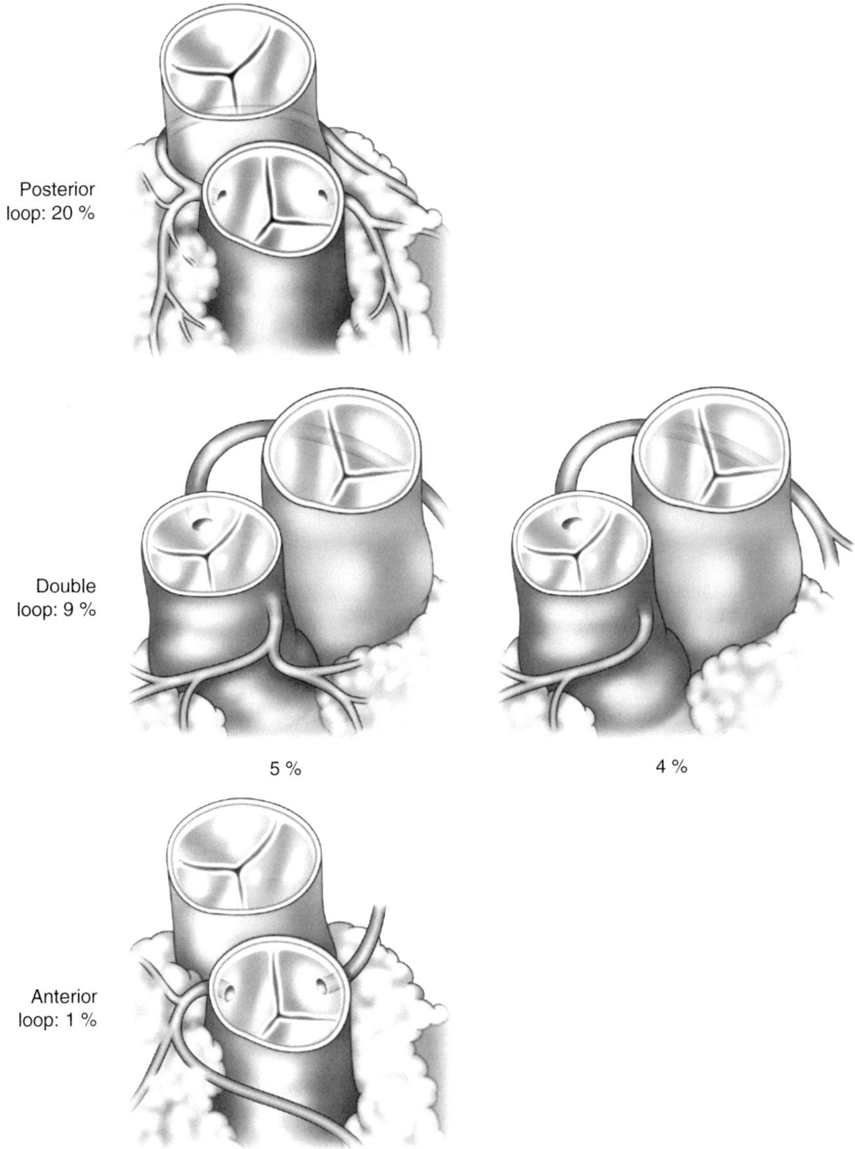

Fig. 14.2 Looping courses, two ostia (29.5 %). *Top*: Posterior loop. *Medium*: Double loop, complex. *Bottom*: Anterior loop, complex

by the left main trunk (6 %), recognized as "inverted coronary arteries anatomy" by Aldo Castaneda (S1: RCA; S2: LAD, Cx) – or by the circumflex alone (4 %) (S1: RCA, LAD; S2: Cx). The great vessels are constantly side-by-side located in double loops; the aorta being on the right. Double loops are frequent in the Taussig-Bing anomaly. *This group is complex.*

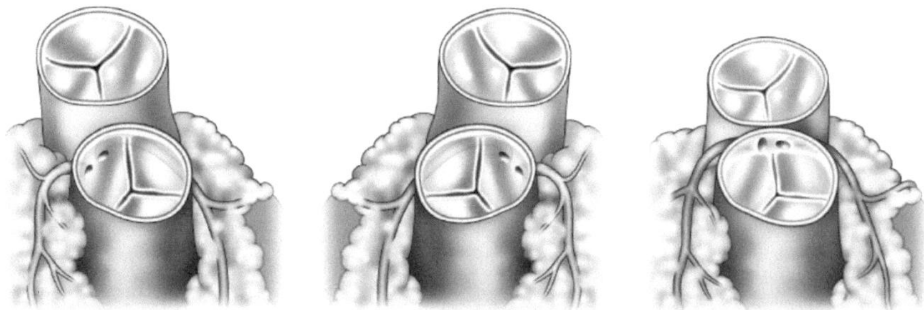

Fig. 14.3 Intramural course, two ostia (5 %). complex

Anterior Looping Course (0.5 %) (Complex Fig. 14.2, Bottom)

The anterior looping course with two ostia is one pattern in which the LAD arise from the RCA and crosses anteriorly the aorta to reach the anterior inter-ventricular groove. An isolated anterior looping is very rare, around 0.5 %. It corresponds in the Leiden classification to: S1 Cx; S2 RCA, LAD. *It is complex.*

Intramural Course, Two Ostia (5 %) (Complex Fig. 14.3)

The intramural course with two ostia, is one in which, one or both coronary arteries has an abnormal intramural course in the posterior aortic wall. Three forms are seen.

Intramural left coronary is the most frequent, with *the left coronary ostium arising from the right sinus* and being frequently stenotic.
The RCA could be intramural arising from the left sinus.
The two ostia can arise above the posterior commissure, with an intra mural course of the two coronary arteries. Very frequently the left coronary ostium is stenotic. In addition, the intra-mural course can be associated with looping courses, increasing even more the technical difficulty. It corresponds to Yacoub type C. No intra-mural course is identified in the Leiden classification. The intramural course group is *complex.*

Single Ostium. Miscellaneous Course. (5.5 %) (Complex Fig. 14.4)

We modified the Marie Lannelongue classification [6] in this publication and identified a specific group of single ostium with miscellaneous course. There are three groups:

Single right coronary ostium is the most frequent (4 %), with three forms. One with a posterior loop made by the entire left main trunk. One with double loop, with the posterior loop made by the Cx and the anterior loop made by the LAD and one, very rare, with the anterior loop made by the entire left main trunk. All three forms correspond Leiden : S1:0; S2: LAD, Cx, RCA, but have different courses.
Single left coronary ostium is less frequent (1 %). It is an anterior looping of the RCA that crosses in front of the aorta, with side by side great vessels. It corresponds to Leiden S1: LAD, Cx, RCA, S2: 0
Para-commissural single ostium. This exceptional coronary pattern (0.5 %), identified as type B by Yacoub, is the most challenging to repair. One para-commissural ostium gives rise to two intramural coronary arteries.

Diagnosis. Imaging

As most of the Conotruncal Anomalies (CTA), TGA can be diagnosed by fetal echocardiography with a high degree of accuracy. TGA is usually not associated with chromosomic abnormalities except for those with aortic arch obstruction (see Chap. 15)

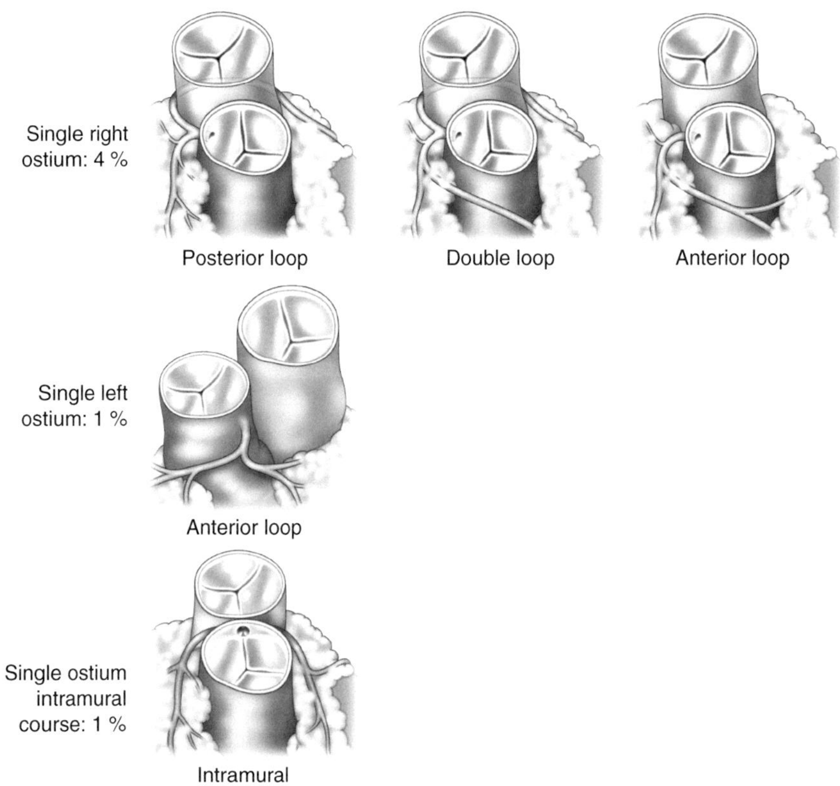

Fig. 14.4 Single ostium. Miscellaneous course. (5.5 %). Complex

where a Di George syndrome is frequent. The development of fetal diagnosis has been a significant improvement, allowing a delivery next to a pediatric heart center.

The diagnosis relies essentially on the post-natal echocardiography, which rules out in TGA-IVS the coronary anatomy, the absence of one or several VSDs, the aortic arch anatomy and the absence of LVOT obstruction.

The complexity of the ASO [2, 8] should be evaluated before surgery. Simple coronary patterns (80 %) include: normal course (60 %) and posterior loop with two ostia (circumflex coming from the right) (20 %). All other coronary patterns (20 %) are complex as well as severe maligned commissures (5 %). All together, around 75 % of the ASO in TGA-IVS are named simple.

No angiography is usually needed. Echocardiography is superior, particularly for the diagnosis of intramural coronary and malaligned commissure. A neonatal Rashkind atrial septostomy and/or a Prostaglandin E1 infusion is the most frequent pre-operative practice.

Pre-Operative Check List for an Arterial Switch in TGA-IVS
Coronary anatomy defining: simple and complex coronary patterns.
Absence of significant VSD (>3 mm)
Absence of aortic arch obstruction
Absence of LVOT obstruction
Absence of intra-cranial bleeding
Absence of ongoing feto-maternal infection

Indication

The arterial switch operation (ASO) in TGA-IVS is electively undertaken at the end of the first week of life. Rarely, the presence of a perinatal damage (intra-cranial bleeding, infection, etc.) requires delaying the operation for several weeks. Birth weight <2 kg remains in several centers an indication to delay the surgery. The ASO is then performed later with or without a left ventricular remodeling (see Chap. 16).

Surgical Technique

Cardio-Pulmonary Bypass and Myocardial Protection

The ASO for TGA-IVS is undertaken under full cardio-pulmonary bypass at a flow of 100–150 cc/kg/min, with bi-caval canulation and moderate hypothermia (28–32 °C). The priming volume is currently around 150 cc, using short tubing and miniaturized membrane oxygenators. It includes fresh frozen plasma and red blood cells, to obtain a hematocrit around 30 %. Our preference for myocardial protection uses Custodiol HTK© crystalloid cardioplegia first injected at a dose of 30 mL/kg, and repeated every 40–60 min at a dose of 10 mL/kg by direct injection in the coronary ostia, using a DLP olive-tip cannula. Others are using blood cardioplegia, either cold or warm. Modified ultra filtration and steroids are rarely used.

Uniform Coronary Transfer Technique Described in Normal Coronary Anatomy

The technique of coronary transfer described here, in TGA-IVS, with normal coronary pattern is applicable to all coronary anatomy. This technique was described in other publications [3, 9].

Surgical Technique I: Normal Coronary Arteries Course (Fig. 14.5)

After median sternotomy, the thymus gland is partially resected, keeping a residual superior segment. A large rectangular patch of *pericardium is harvested* and kept in iced-cold saline solution. The pericardium is used *fresh*. The patient pericardium is suspended, avoiding undue traction. The first step is a carefully *inspection* of the anatomy, evaluating the origin and the courses of the coronary arteries, recognizing abnormal looping and single ostium. Full recognition of intra mural course requires intra-aortic inspection. In TGA-IVS the great vessels are usually located in antero-posterior relationship, with the aorta slightly located on the right. Side by side vessels are more common in TGA VSD and Taussing-Bing. *The control of the aorta and the right and left PA branches* is carefully achieved with vessel lops. The ductus arteriosus wall is extremely fragile under PGE1; its dissection is started on the right side of the ascending aorta. Traction on the left PA vessel loop helps to dissect the left border. *The PDA is carefully controlled* by two silk sutures, which will be tied when going on bypass. The *cannulation of the aorta* (1) is high and close to the brachiocephalic artery, using a straight cannula. The *superior vena cava venous cannula* (2) is introduced into the atrial appendage and placed in the right atrium. CPB is instituted with one venous cannula. The *inferior vena cava venous cannula* (3) is introduced close to the inferior vena cava and snared. A *left atrial venting cannula* (4) (Medtronic©) is placed through the Sondergaard sulcus. The superior venous cannula is then introduced into the superior vena cava and snared. Others vent the LA through the ASD. The *division of the PDA* requires an accurate technique. The ductus is doubly ligated and then divided, with suturing of both ends. A vascular clip is often used to occlude the aortic end. Any tear or needle puncture of the ductal wall proximal to the ligation should be avoided, as a tear of the origin of the ductus arteriosus is difficult to control. Additional direct stitching usually worsens the bleeding, or may create an isthmus stenosis. Serious bleeding at this stage is better controlled under circulatory arrest.

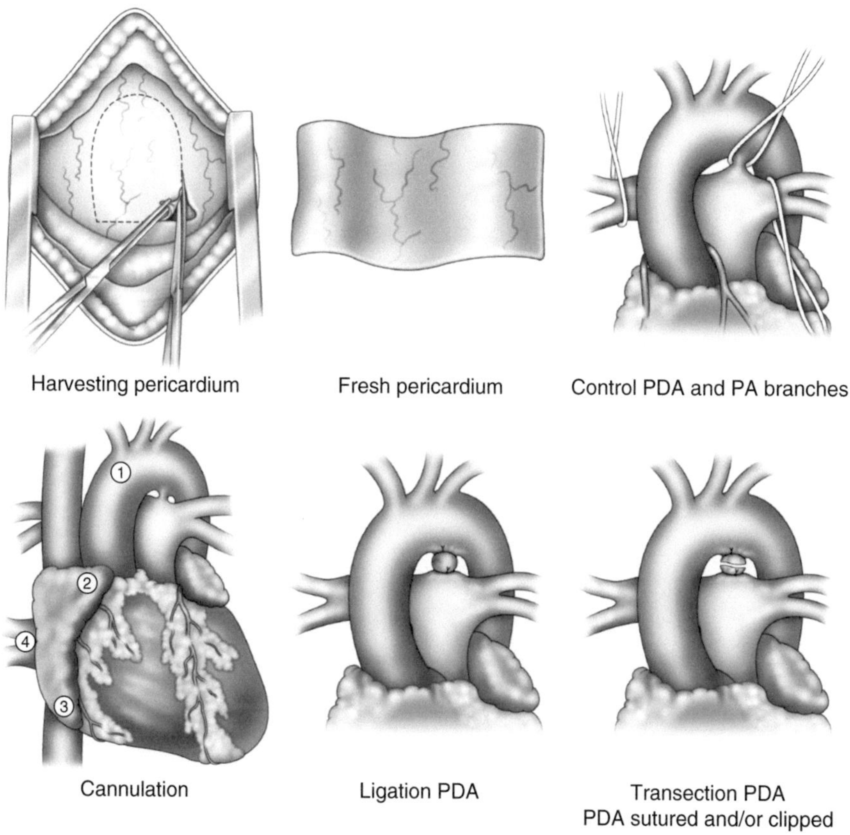

Fig. 14.5 Surgical technique I. Normal coronary arteries course

Surgical Technique II. Normal Coronary Arteries Course (Fig. 14.6)

The space between the aortic and pulmonary roots is carefully dissected. This dissection runs close to the origin of the coronary trunks that are dissected carefully, using very low coagulation intensity. When the coronary trunks are not well seen, this dissection should not be done. The *aortic cross-clamp* is placed close to the aortic cannula. The *cardioplegia is injected* through a needle placed at the level of the aortotomy. A short, longitudinal, right atriotomy allows suctioning of the cardioplegia return and give access to the *atrial septal defect, which is closed using running suture.* In case of a large atrial septal defect, patch closure is preferred to prevent arrhythmias.

The transection of the great vessels is a crucial step of the ASO. The objective is to *reduce the length of the aorta* that will stand behind the PA following the Lecompte maneuver. *The aorta is divided in high position* at a middle point between the clamp

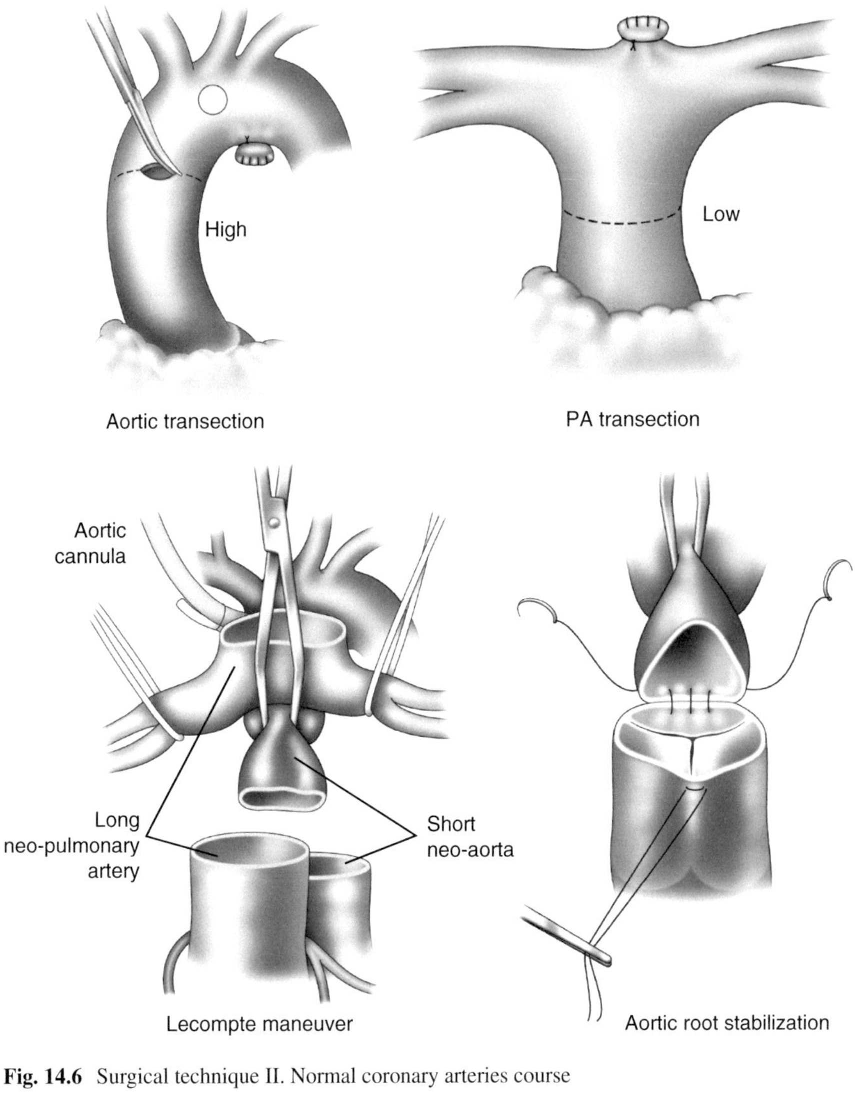

Fig. 14.6 Surgical technique II. Normal coronary arteries course

and the aortic annulus. The anatomy is explored and the alignment of the commissures is checked. T*he PA trunk is transected in a low position*, 2 mm above the pulmonary commissures.

The Lecompte maneuver is then performed. The PA branches are fully dissected until the lobar branches are clearly seen. The pulmonary bifurcation is then pulled up in front of the distal ascending aorta. Using a second cross-clamp, the aortic cross-clamp is mobilized and placed below the pulmonary bifurcation, closely in contact with the aortic cannula, to expose the maximum length of distal ascending aorta. Following a high division of the aorta and a low division of the

PA, the posterior neo-aorta length is reduced, and the anterior neo-pulmonary artery is long. The pulmonary bifurcation should be free floating on the aorta. If the aorta seems to compress from behind the PA branches, additional dissection of the distal PA should be done until the PA bifurcation is free.

To prevent undue movements, *the aorta is stabilized*. The aortic clamp is blocked on the surgical field at "12 o'clock" to stabilize the distal aorta. The neo-aortic root is placed so that the anterior commissure is standing exactly at "6 o'clock" Then the anastomosis between the distal aorta and the neo-pulmonary artery is partially performed posteriorly to stabilize the neo-aortic root in good place.

Surgical Technique III. Normal Coronary Arteries Course (Fig. 14.7)

The *harvesting of coronary buttons* is an important step. To allow safe buttons anastomoses, it is crucial to *take the largest possible button*, removing nearly the entire sinus of Valsalva. *The arterial switch operation is aortic surgery, not coronary surgery*. Two traction sutures, one anterior and one posterior, help exposure. The location of the ostia is carefully evaluated, particularly their relationship with the commissures and with the aortic annulus. Using microsurgery scissors the first incisions are vertical, one anterior and one posterior, pushing away the aortic leaflets. The last incision is horizontal and follows the aortic annulus. Then the button is detached from the myocardium using electrocoagulation. The coronary trunks are mobilized on a few millimeters, and generously in case of looping courses.

Following evidence that the neo-aortic root is enlarging with time [10]; the re-implantation of the coronary buttons should *avoid increasing the neo-aortic root diameter*, which is already large in TGA. In this regard, *we avoid using the trap-door incision* that increases the root diameter. Instead, we resect a fragment of the neo-aortic wall and place the button in the space created. Others are using the technique of closed aorta, with first reconstructing the aorta, and then checking the location of the buttons. This closed aorta technique also avoids enlarging the aortic root.

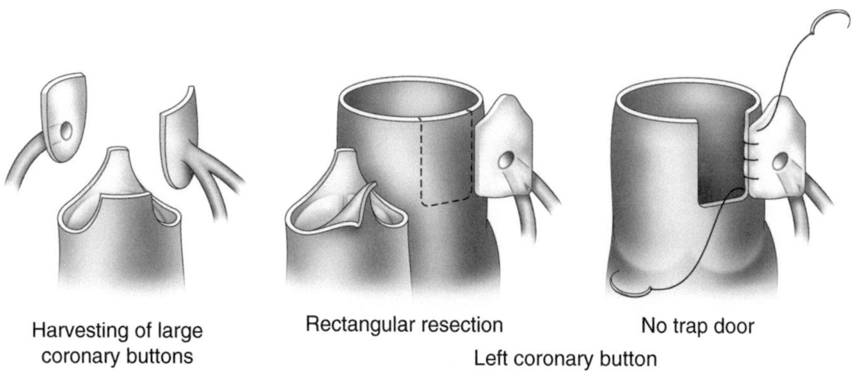

Fig. 14.7 Surgical technique III. Normal coronary arteries course

The *left coronary button is placed in low position*. The location of the left button is quite constant, in the neo-aorta left-anterior sinus, as lateral as possible. A *quadrangular resection* of the neo-aortic wall is performed. The anastomosis is then performed and the button is incorporated.

Surgical Technique IV. Normal Coronary Arteries Course (Fig. 14.8)

The *right coronary button is placed in a higher position*. The bottom of right button is placed in the right aortic root sinus, as lateral as possible. The rectangular or semi lunar resection of the aortic wall is more superficial than in the left side.

In order to correct the diameter mismatch between the neo-aortic root and the distal aorta, the superior part of the button is included into the ascending aorta. *The distal end-to-end aortic anastomosis* is performed, starting on the left. The aortic anastomosis should be permanently controlled and adjusted so that the anterior commissure remains exactly at "6 o'clock". When reaching the right side, the *distal ascending aorta is incised vertically* toward the clamp and the superior end of *the right button is used to enlarge the distal aorta*, and to gently pull up the right coronary trunk. It is anticipated that limiting the diameter mismatch between the neo-aortic root and the distal aorta prevents further dilation of the aortic root. The right button will be placed higher in cases with posterior and double looping courses.

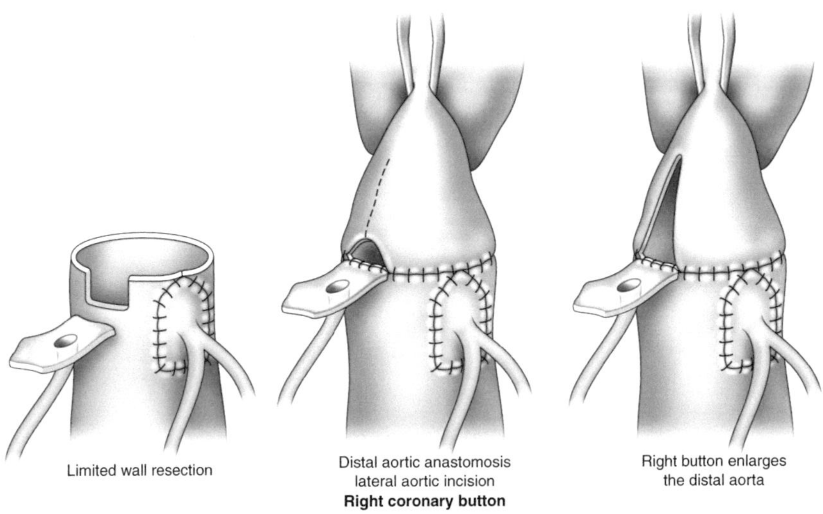

Fig. 14.8 Surgical technique IV. Normal coronary arteries course

Surgical Technique V. Special Features (Fig. 14.9)

Three special features can be seen in all coronary patterns.

Ostium next to a commissure. Sometimes, one ostium is located next to the posterior commissure, rarely to the lateral one. In order to take a safe and large button, the commissure is taken down and will be re-implanted later on the pericardial patch.

Early infundibular branch. Frequently, an early infundibular branch coming from the left main trunk can block the transfer of the left button and stenose the left main trunk. When large, this branch is dissected to release the tension. When small, this infundibular branch is divided. This generates a limited ischemia of the infundibulum that will fully recover within hours. To notice that the kinking of the left coronary is not obvious by inspection and could be only suspected on ECG changes or hemodynamic instability. Division of the infundibular branch will immediately resolve the issue. Rarely a branch can block the right coronary artery.

Commissures malalignment. Fig. 14.10. When significant, this is a major abnormality that is *complex* TGA [2]. It can be seen in all coronary patterns. The malalignment impacts on the coronary relocation. Not really on the right button that could be placed above the commissure, but very much on the left button that cannot be re-implanted in usual position. We have used a technique of *commissures re-alignment*.

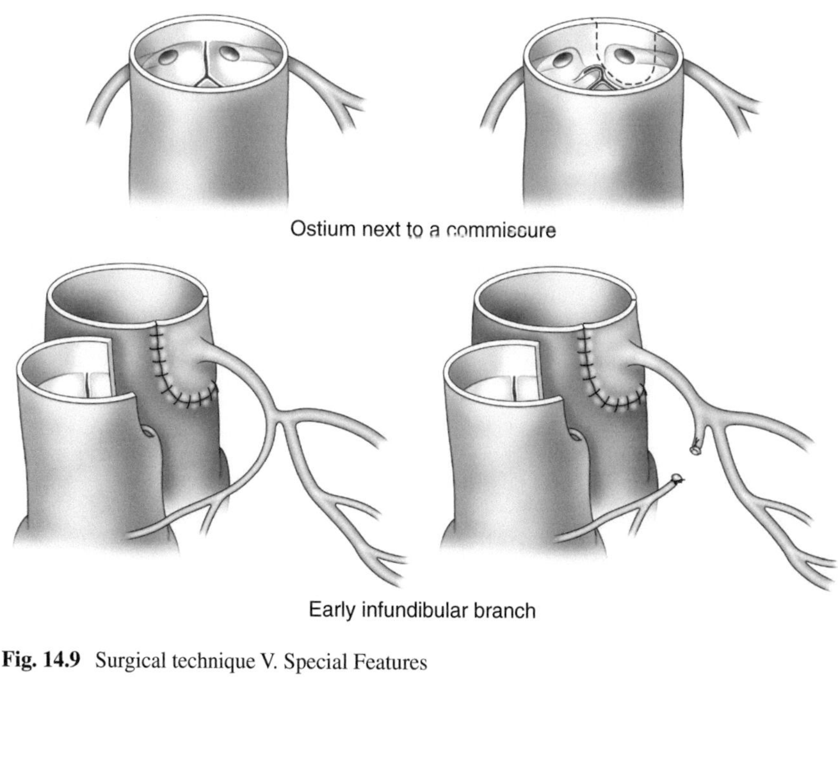

Fig. 14.9 Surgical technique V. Special Features

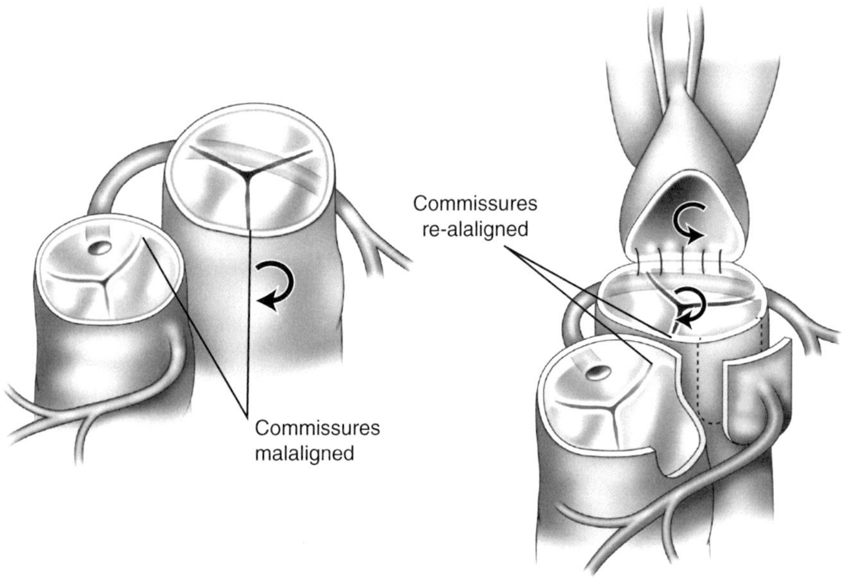

Fig. 14.10 Surgical technique V. Commissures malalignment

Prior to transferring the coronary, the distal ascending aorta and the pulmonary artery trunk are *rotated in opposite direction in order to realign the anterior and posterior commissures*. As the rotations are distributed evenly on the two vessels, the torsion is well tolerated. Then the aortic clamp is repositioned at 12H to stabilize the new setting.

Surgical Technique VI. Pulmonary Trunk Reconstruction (Fig. 14.11)

It is safer to perform the *reconstruction of the PA trunk* with the aorta cross-clamped. A rectangular fresh autologous pericardial patch will fill in the spaces created by the harvesting of the coronary buttons. The suture line follows the remnant of the PA wall or of the aortic annulus. The patch is running behind the posterior commissure, which is then *attached on the pericardial patch.*

Surgical Technique VII. Normal Coronary Arteries. Final Result (Fig. 14.12)

The *final coronary transfer result* is shown on Fig. 14.9. This uniform technique [3] is used *for nearly all coronary patterns*. The aortic cross-clamp is removed and the quality of the reperfusion is carefully evaluated, based on the coloration of the myocardium and on the normal filling of the coronary arteries. The distal pulmonary anastomosis is done under beating heart.

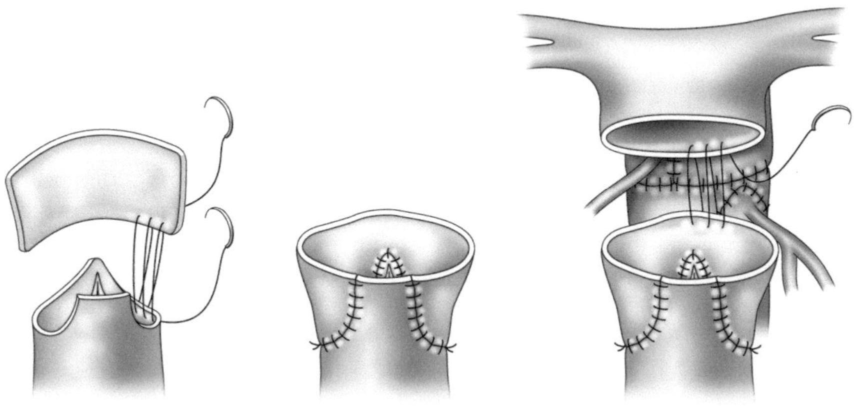

Fig. 14.11 Surgical technique VI. Pulmonary trunk reconstruction

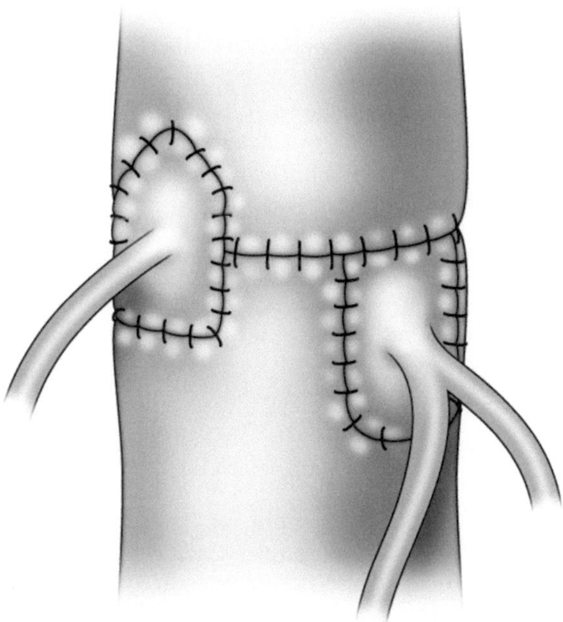

Fig. 14.12 Surgical technique VII. Normal coronary arteries. Final result

Surgical Technique VIII. Complex Coronary Transfer (Fig. 14.13)

It is important to understand the risk inherent to coronary transfer in complex coronary patterns. *The posterior loop is associated with a risk of kinking and the anterior loop with a risk of stretching. Generous dissection of the coronary trunks is necessary* to avoid kinking or stretching of the coronary trunks. As a rule, when there is a posterior looping vessel, the right button needs to be re-implanted in high position to prevent the kinking of the posterior vessel. (circumflex or left main trunk). When there is an anterior looping vessel (RCA), it should be dissected extensively to prevent stretching. Others are using trap-door.

Surgical Technique VIII Posterior Loop. Two Ostia (Fig. 14.14)

The circumflex is dissected posteriorly from the PA trunk and the right button is placed in high position and included in the aortic anastomosis. Circumflex coming off the RCA is not considered as a complex coronary pattern.

Surgical Technique VIII. Anterior Loop. Two Ostia (Fig. 14.15, Bottom)

This is an exceptional pattern. Trap door may be useful.

Surgical Technique VIII. Double Loop. Two Ostia (Fig. 14.15, Top)

The anterior looping vessel, always the RCA, is *extensively dissected* free from the aorta. As well the posterior looping vessel, either the circumflex or the left main trunk, is dissected free for the PA trunk. *The right button is placed in high position*, above the aortic anastomosis. The left button is placed in low position. Others are using a trapdoor on the left button.

Side-by-side vessels are almost constant in double loop. Fig. 14.15 Top. This pattern seen in Taussig-Bing hearts (see Chap. 15) and rare in TGA-IVS. After the Lecompte maneuver, the reconstruction of the pulmonary bifurcation can compress

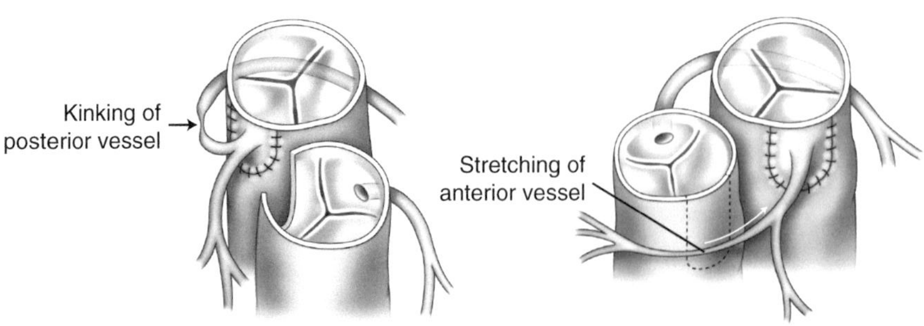

Fig. 14.13 Surgical technique VIII. Complex coronary transfer

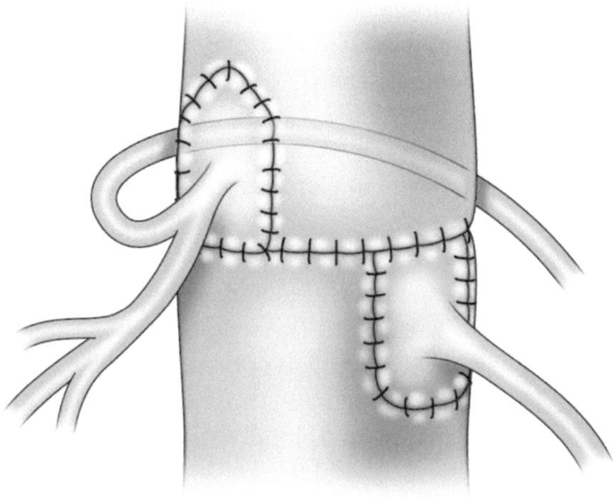

Fig. 14.14 Surgical technique VIII posterior loop. Two ostia

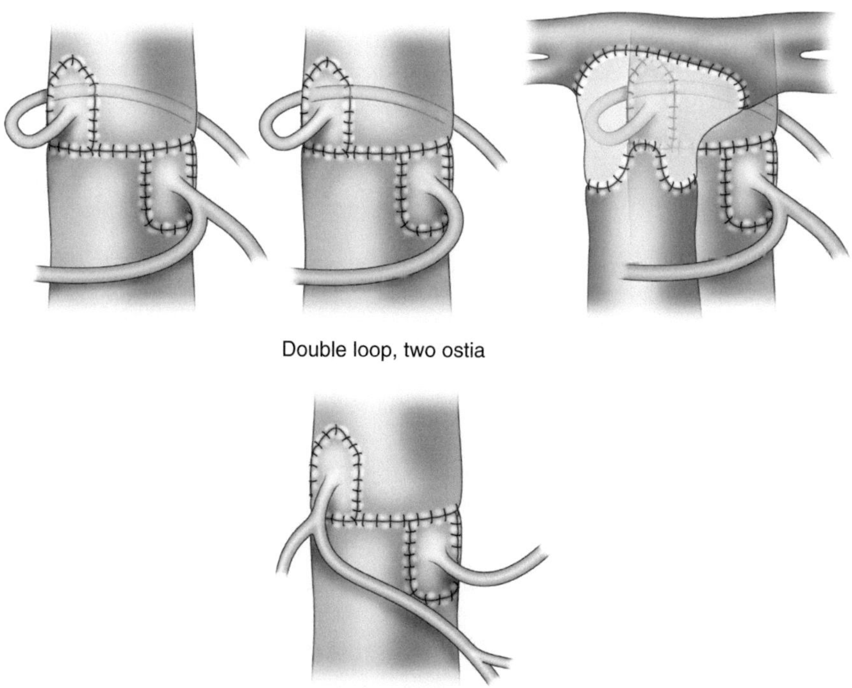

Fig. 14.15 Surgical technique VIII. Complex coronary transfer. *Bottom*: Anterior loop. Two ostia. *Top*: Double loop. Two ostia

the right coronary that is looping anteriorly. Mobilization of the pulmonary bifurcation to the right is necessary to prevent a compression of the RCA. The right PA is incised for 20 mm, and the PA trunk is directly anastomosed to the right PA to *translate the PA trunk to the right*. The left part of the PA trunk is then patched. The other option is not to perform a Lecompte maneuver.

Surgical Technique IX. Intra Mural Coronary Arteries. Two Ostia (Fig. 14.16)

Coronary transfer with intramural course is challenging. The technique is to *create two buttons* as described by R. Mee and T. Asou [11]. The technique is shown for Type II A, with intra-mural course of the left coronary artery. It is similar in Type II B and C (Fig. 14.1). The ostia are found very close to each other, either in the right sinus or above the posterior commissure. First, the posterior commissure is totally detached. The intramural course is evaluated using a coronary probe. It can be extremely long, measuring more than 20 mm. The *two ostia are harvested* "*en bloc*". The harvesting of the left button should be very cautious, considering the very long intramural course. It is the entirety of the sinus that is harvested. The left ostium, which is frequently stenotic, is incised and "unroofed" on a distance of 5 mm. After this opening, the two ostia are sufficiently distant to create two buttons. Then, the common button is incised in its middle to create two buttons. The incision should stay distant from the ostia to allow a safe suturing. Using 8/0 Prolene, the two buttons are relocated on each sinus according to the basic technique. The posterior commissure will be reattached on the pericardial pulmonary patch.

Surgical Technique X. Single Ostium. Miscellaneous Course (Fig. 14.17)

Single coronary ostium patterns have mixed courses: either looping or intramural course, knowing that both courses could be associated.

The *three single right coronary* (Fig. 14.17, top) are relocated following the same principles. Their relocation follows the same principles. Extensive dissection of the looping coronary trunks is essential. The right button is transferred in a high position. Trapdoor may be useful.
Single left coronary (Fig. 14.17, medium) is re-implanted in low position.
The case of *single ostium with intramural* course, Yacoub type B, raises a maximum of problems (Fig. 14.17, bottom)

- *Creating two buttons* is the most appealing technique. From the single ostium, the intramural course of the right and left coronary are unroofed of a few millimeters. This allows creating two buttons that are re-implanted following the uniform technique [12].
- The *other technique* described by Moat et al. [13] It is to create a fistula between the posterior wall of the aortic root and the anterior wall of the pulmonary root,

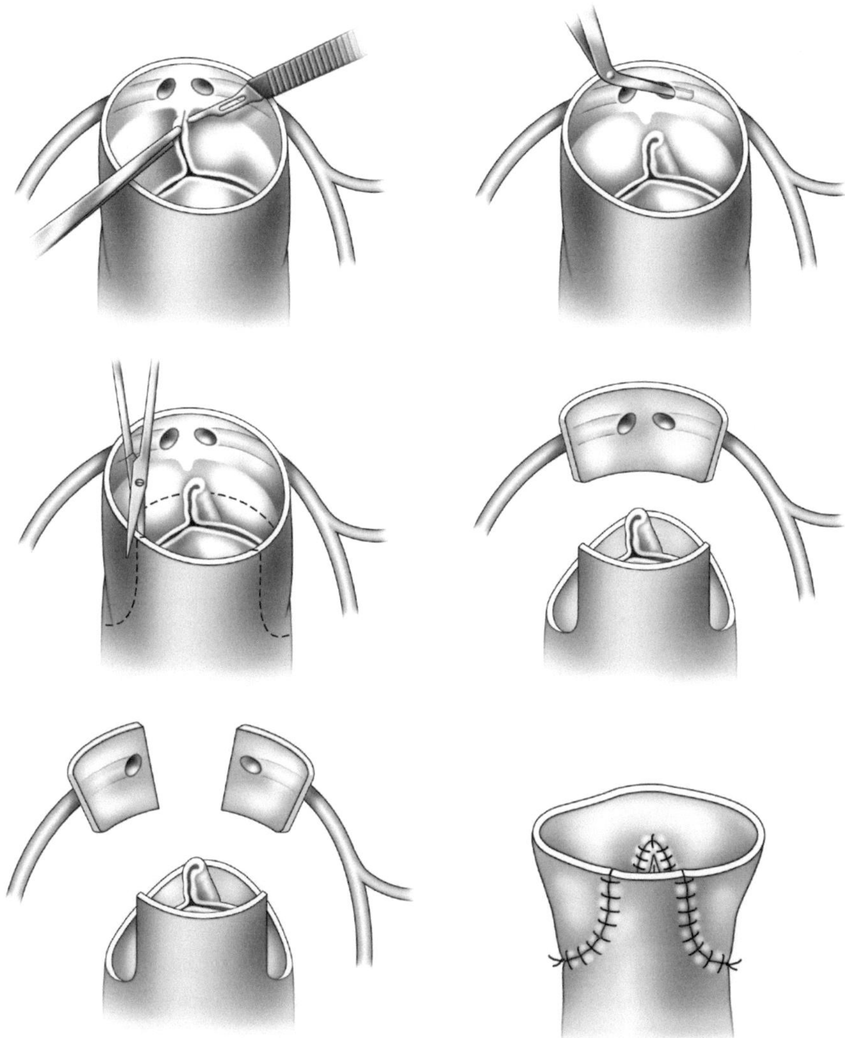

Two buttons are created. The left ostium is opened

Fig. 14.16 Surgical technique IX. Intra mural coronary arteries. Two ostia

in order to reroute the coronary flow without doing a coronary relocation. The risk is to leave the coronary arteries between the aorta and PA with ultimate risk of compression.

- Another technique described by Yacoub and Radley-Smith [4] is to rotate the button on 180° and relocate it behind. The risk is again that the coronary arteries remain between the aorta and PA
- Finally, this anatomy could be the only indication for an atrial switch.

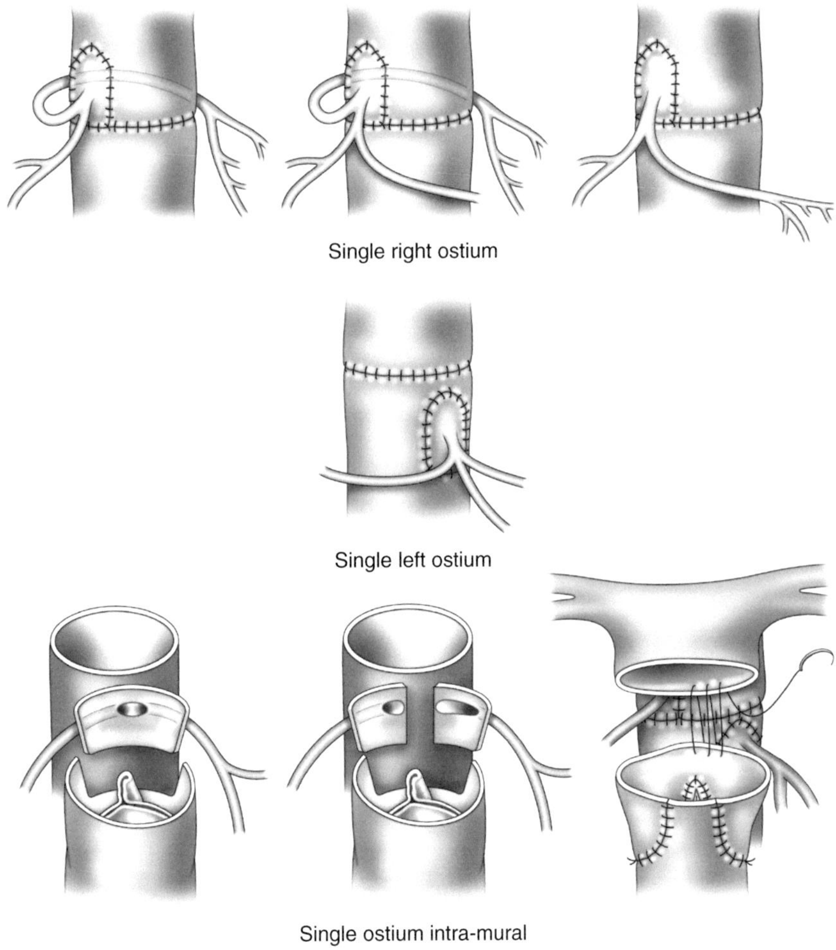

Fig. 14.17 Surgical technique X. Single ostium. Miscellaneous course. *Top*: Single right coronary arteries

Outcome

The early mortality of ASO for TGA-IVS is today very low [2] and is as low as 2.2 % in the Society of Thoracic Surgeons congenital database (See Chap. 4). Depending on publications, the risk factors for early death remain: intra-mural coronaries, single ostium, malaligned commissure and very low birth weight. Other risks are association with coarctation of the aorta (see Chap. 15) and TGA-IVS seen late (see Chap. 16).

The early morbidity of ASO for TGA-IVS is limited and includes in a recent publication [2]: 15 % of sternum left open, 12 % occurrence of complication and an average length of hospital stay around 10 days.

The long-term outcome of the arterial switch operation is available today, with many patients having reached the adult age. Generally, the results are very satisfactory with most patients leaving a normal life, including sports. Impaired neurodevelopment is exceedingly rare in ASO with TGA-IVS as the operation is undertaken on full flow CPB. The late mortality is exceptional after 1 year and is in relation with re-operation.

Right ventricular outflow tract obstruction is the most frequent complication [14, 15], 5–15 %. The compression of PA branches by the aorta following the Lecompte maneuver can be prevented, as shown above. When severe, the RVOT requires reintervention. Balloon dilation and stenting are not ideal and a surgical reoperation can better correct the RVOT obstruction with patch enlargement of the PA branches and trunk.

Late coronary complication rate is 2–5 % [14–16] and is associated with intramural course and single ostium [14]. Stenosis or occlusion of coronary arteries can be asymptomatic, which justifies [16] coronary evaluation by coronary angiogram or CT scan-angiography in patients with complex coronary anatomy. Coronary bypass graft or ostium enlargement are performed [15].

Late aortic root dilation and aortic valve regurgitation [10, 14–16] is observed in ASO performed on TGA-VSD. In TGA-IVS, aortic root dilation is rare as the native neo-aortic root is moderately dilated in TGA-IVS.

References

1. Jatene AD, Fontes VF, Paulista PP, et al. Anatomic correction of transposition of the great vessels. J Thorac Cardiovasc Surg. 1976;72:364–70.
2. Stoica S, Campbell D, Lacour-Gayet F, et al. Morbidity of the arterial switch operation. Ann Thorac Surg. 2012;93:1977–83.
3. Lacour-Gayet F, Anderson RH. A uniform surgical technique for transfer of both simple and complex patterns of the coronary arteries during the arterial switch procedure. Cardiol Young. 2005;15(S1):93–101.
4. Yacoub M, Radley-Smith R. Anatomy of the coronary arteries in transposition of the great arteries and methods for their transfer in anatomical correction. Thorax. 1978;33:418–24.
5. Gittenberger-de Groot AC, Sauer U, Oppenheimer-Dekker A, et al. Coronary artery anatomy in transposition of the great arteries: a morphologic study. Pediatr Cardiol. 1983;4(Suppl):I15–24.
6. Planche C, Lacour-Gayet F, Serraf A. Arterial switch. Pediatr Cardiol. 1998;19:297–307.
7. Houyel L, Van Praagh R, Lacour-Gayet F, Serraf A, Petit J, Bruniaux J, Planché C. Transposition of the great arteries [S, D, L]. Pathologic anatomy, diagnosis, and surgical management of a newly recognized complex. J Thorac Cardiovasc Surg. 1995;110:613–24.
8. Lacour-Gayet F. Complexity stratification of the arterial switch operation: a second learning curve. Cardiol Young. 2012;22:739–44.
9. A Lacour-Gayet F, natomical repair of transposition of the great arteries. In: Gardner T, Spray T, editors. Operative cardiac surgery. 5th ed. London: Arnold; 2004. p. 769–91.
10. Schwartz ML, Gauvreau K, del Nido P, Mayer JE, Colan SD. Long-term predictors of aortic root dilation and aortic regurgitation after arterial switch operation. Circulation. 2004;110(11 Suppl 1):II128–32.
11. Asou T, Karl TR, Pawade A, Mee RB. Arterial switch: translocation of the intramural coronary artery. Ann Thorac Surg. 1994;57:461–5.

12. Cuttone F, Lacour-Gayet F, et al. Arterial Switch Operation in Single Coronary Ostium With Intramural Course: Subclavian Artery Patch Angioplasty. Ann Thorac Surg. 2015;100: 1084–6.
13. Moat N, Pawade A, Lamb R. Complex coronary arterial anatomy in transposition of the great arteries. Arterial switch procedure without coronary relocation. J Thorac Cardiovasc Surg. 1992;103:872–6.
14. Pasquali SK, Hasselblad V, Li JS, Kong DF, Sanders SP. Coronary artery pattern and outcome of arterial switch operation for transposition of the great arteries: a meta-analysis. Circulation. 2002;106:2575–80.
15. Angeli E, Raisky O, Bonnet D, Sidi D, Vouhé PR. Late reoperations after neonatal arterial switch operation for transposition of the great arteries. Eur J Cardiothorac Surg. 2008;34:32–6.
16. Losay J, Touchot A, Serraf A, Litvinova A, Lambert V, Piot JD, Lacour-Gayet F, Capderou A, Planche C. Late outcome after arterial switch operation for transposition of the great arteries. Circulation. 2001;104(12 Suppl 1):121–6.

Chapter 15
Arterial Switch for TGA or DORV and VSD, with and Without Aortic Arch Obstruction

Francois Lacour-Gayet, Emre Belli, and Olivier Ghez

Abstract Arterial switch operations undertaken in transposition of the great arteries (TGA) and Taussig Bing with ventricular septal defect (VSD) are complex. The association with an aortic arch obstruction (AAO), seen predominantly in Taussig-Bing increased significantly the complexity of the operation. One-stage neonatal repair has become the technique of reference. However, palliation remains indicated in newborns presenting with Swiss cheese VSDs, small birth weight and extra cardiac damages.

The increasing difficulties of the arterial switch operation in TGA/DORV-VSD are: the important diameter mismatch between the aorta and the pulmonary root, – the closure of the VSD, – the management of more complex coronary artery patterns, the association with AAO and the presence of a subaortic obstruction.

The ASO mortality, reported by the STS database congenital database is respectively 5 % for TGA/DORV-VSD without AAO and 12.6 % when an AAO is associated.

Late reoperations occur in 30 %, either: re-coarctation, right ventricular obstruction, aortic valve regurgitation, aortic root dilation and coronary stenosis. Long-term actuarial survival is 85 % at 15 years; nevertheless, close lifelong surveillance of these patients is necessary.

Complex arterial switch remain challenging and require a second learning curve.

Keywords Congenital heart disease • Congenital cardiac surgery • Transposition of the great arteries • Arterial switch operation • Double outlet right ventricle • Taussig-Bing • Ventricular septal defect • Aortic arch obstruction • One stage repair

F. Lacour-Gayet, MD (✉)
Department of Pediatric Cardiac Surgery, National Heart and Lung Institute,
Royal Brompton Hospital, Imperial College University, Sydney Street, London SW3 6NP, UK
e-mail: flacourgayet@mac.com

E. Belli, MD
Department of Pediatric Cardiac Surgery, Hôpital Jacques Cartier, Massy 92000, France

O. Ghez, MD
Department of Pediatric Cardiac Surgery, Royal Brompton Hospital, Sydney Street, London SW3 6NP, UK

F. Lacour-Gayet et al. (eds.), *Surgery of Conotruncal Anomalies*,
DOI 10.1007/978-3-319-23057-3_15

Background

This chapter will address the anatomical repair of complex switch, which include arterial switch undertaken in TGA-VSD and in Taussig-Bing with and without AAO.

The arterial switch operation (ASO), was first published by Adib Jatene [1, 2] in 1975 in two patients with transposition of the great vessels with ventricular septal defect (TGA-VSD). VSD is the most frequent associated lesion in complete transposition of the great arteries, with an incidence around 30 %. Taussig-Bing, defined as a double outlet right ventricle (DORV) subpulmonary VSD (see Chap. 23) is a more complex condition than TGA-VSD.

The association with an aortic arch obstruction (AAO) is seen in 20 % of TGA with VSD, and in 60 % of Taussig-Bing. AAO is also observed in 3 % of TGA with intact ventricular septum (TGA-IVS).

The association with AAO is a severe condition with a significant higher risk at repair. These complex lesions are today optimally treated by one stage neonatal ASO, requiring a well-experienced team. However palliation remains indicated in particular conditions.

Anatomic Classification

TGA- VSD

In TGA-VSD, the VSD can be located in any part of the inter-ventricular septum as in normally related great arteries; but is more frequently peri-membranous (Fig. 15.1a, b). Multiple and Swiss Cheese VSD represent 10 % and raise specific surgical issues. The aorta is usually anterior and to the right of the PA. Rarely the

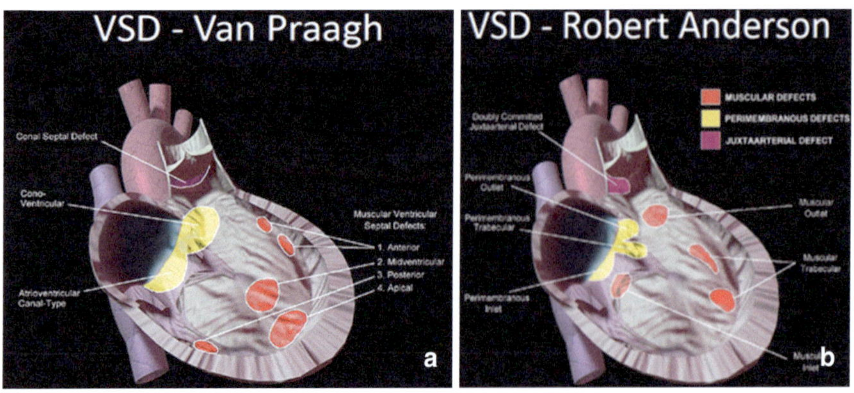

Fig. 15.1 Definition of VSD according to R. Van Praagh (**a**) and RH Anderson (**b**)

aorta can be partially located to the left of the PA [3]. There is always a significant aorto-pulmonary mismatch diameter, with the PA trunk being significantly larger than the diameter of the aorta. The PA is entirely located on the left ventricle and there is a mitro-pulmonary continuity. The coronary anatomy is similar to TGA-IVS (see Chap. 14).

Taussig-Bing *(Figs. 15.2, 15.3, and 15.4)*

Taussig Bing (TB) is a form of DORV (see Chap. 23). The VSD is subpulmonary, close to the pulmonary annulus, and is located above the anterior limb of the trabecula septo marginalis (TSM) (Fig. 15.2). The aorta always arises totally from the RV and the pulmonary artery arises either partially [4, 5] or entirely [6] from the RV. There is constantly a double conus (Figs. 15.2 and 15.4). Mitro-pulmonary discontinuity is required for the diagnosis of TB [4, 6]. TB is different from DORV-non-committed VSD because in TB, the VSD is located close to the PA annulus and separated only by a distance less than an aortic annulus diameter [7]. The aorta is always located side by side to the PA with an important aorto-pulmonary diameter mismatch (Fig. 15.3). The coronary arteries patterns are more complex with

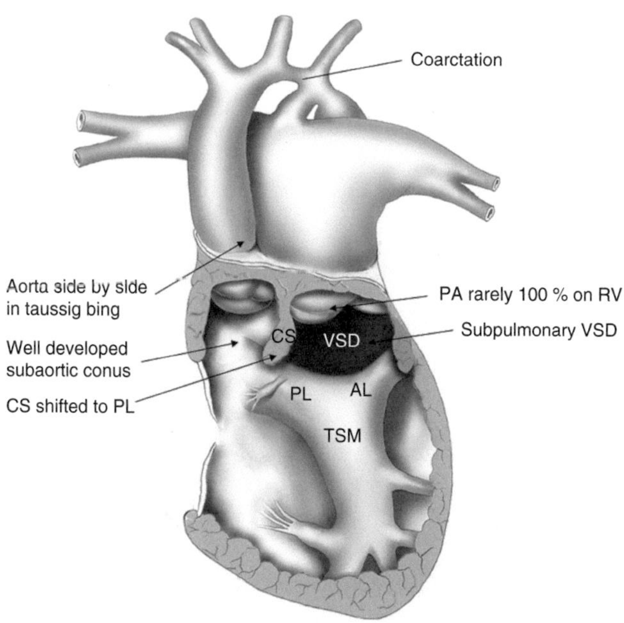

Fig. 15.2 DORV-TGA (Taussig Bing). Subpulmonary VSD. Cono-ventricular VSD above the anterior limb of the TSM. The great vessels are side by side. Large aorto-pulmonary diameter mismatch. Aortic arch obstruction. Shifting of the conal septum toward the subaortic conus. Double conus. The PA is partially "levoposed" on the left ventricle

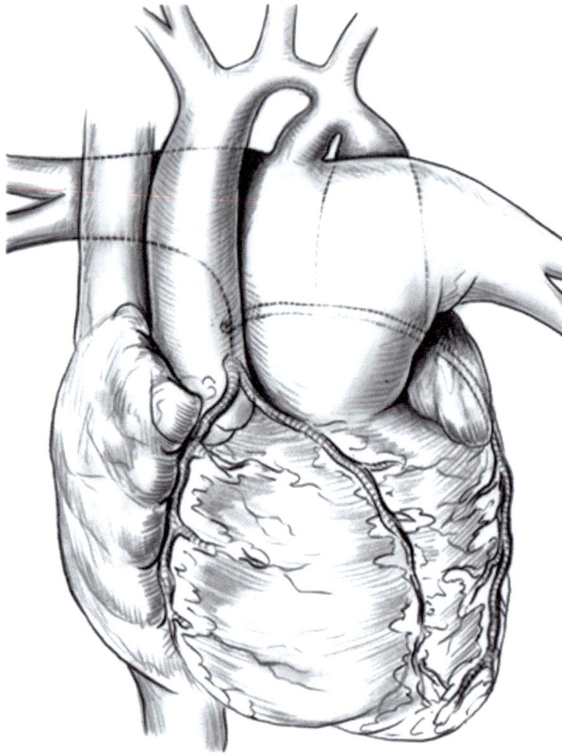

Fig. 15.3 Taussig Bing. Important Aorto-Pulmonary diameter mismatch. Coarctation. Abnormal coronary pattern. Side by side vessels

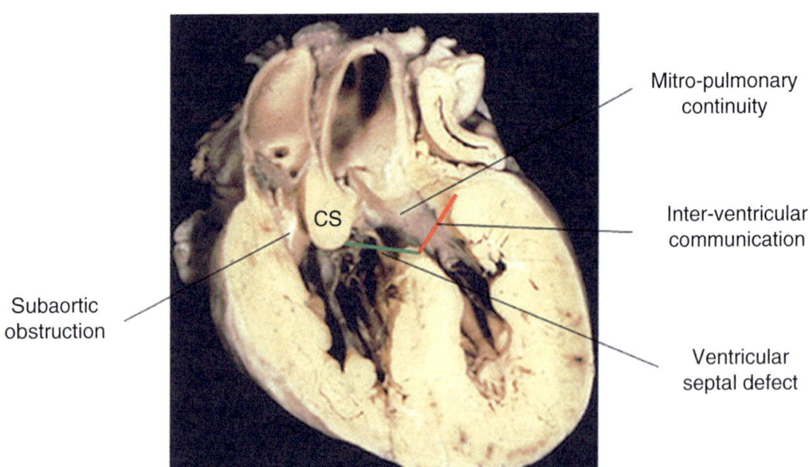

Fig. 15.4 Taussig Bing. Notice that the two great vessels are nearly 200 % on the right ventricle and that there is a mitro-pulmonary continuity. Anterior shifting of the conal septum. In green the ventricular septal defect with malaligned conal septum: the "hole" to close. In red the interventricular communication (RH Anderson): the "hole" not to close (Courtesy of Pr Yen Ho, Royal Brompton Hospital, London)

frequent double looping courses (see Chap. 14). Either (Fig. 15.5a) with the RCA coming from the left-anterior sinus (sinus 1) and crossing in front of the aorta with the common left coronary trunk coming from the right-posterior sinus (sinus 2) and running behind the PA; sometimes named "inverted coronary arteries". Or (Figs. 15.3 and 15.5b); with the LAD and RCA arising from the anterior sinus (sinus 1) and the circumflex arising alone from the posterior sinus (sinus 2) running behind the PA.

The right ventricle is sometimes "smallish" (Fig. 15.3), but exceptionally hypoplastic in neonates in absence of associated organic tricuspid stenosis [12].

Multiple VSD are seen in 10 % of TB. Swiss cheese VSDs, defined as more than two VSD, should be detected prior to surgery because this association may contraindicate one stage repair.

The two most specific cardiac associations in Taussig Bing are the presence of – an aortic arch obstruction and – a subaortic obstruction.

Aortic Arch Obstruction (AAO)

AAO is present in around 60 % of TB [8, 9] (Figs. 15.2 and 15.3). Less frequently, AAO is associated with TGA-VSD and TGA-IVS. The AAO is usually a coarctation with hypoplasia of the transverse arch or more rarely an interrupted aortic arch (10 %). The mismatch (Figs. 15.2 and 15.3) between the ascending aorta and the pulmonary artery is massive, with the pulmonary artery being twice or more than the diameter of the aorta.

Depending on publications, *a subaortic obstruction* is observed in 10 % [10] to 60 % [11], of the Taussig-Bing presenting with an AAO. It is in relation with: – a RVOT obstruction due the anterior shifting of the conal septum (Figs. 15.2 and

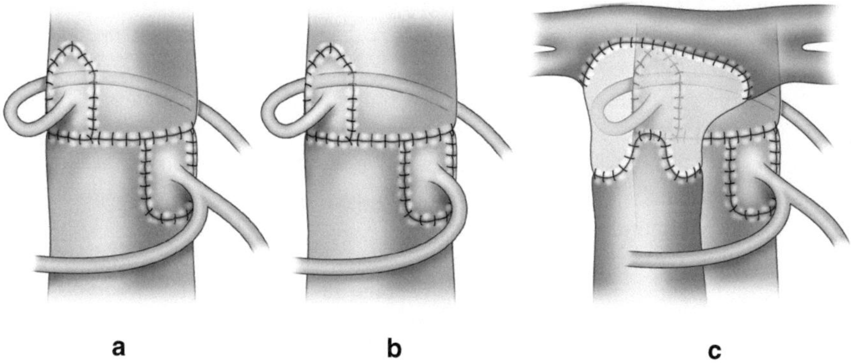

Fig. 15.5 Double loop coronary artery patterns. Side by side vessels. (**a**) Inverted coronary arteries. RCA sinus 1: anterior loop. Common left trunk sinus 2: posterior loop. (**b**) RCA, LAD sinus 1: anterior loop. CX sinus 2: posterior loop. (**c**) The pulmonary trunk is transferred to the right PA to avoid a right coronary artery compression

15.4) – and a potential hypoplasia of the aortic annulus. This subaortic obstruction will be "switched" into a subpulmonary obstruction after anatomical repair, which could require late reoperation [8].

Other Associated Lesions

Straddling AV valve is associated in 5 % of Taussig-Bing, involving either the tricuspid valve or the mitral valve. Only type C straddling [13] is an absolute contra-indication to anatomical repair.

Accessory mitral tissue, creating a subpulmonary obstruction is possible.

Di George syndrome with 22q11 deletion is observed in 10–20 %, and is more frequent in cases with aortic arch obstruction.

Imaging and Diagnosis

Echocardiography alone almost always provides a good anatomical evaluation of TGA-VSD [14] and Taussig Bing. The segmental and sequential analysis confirms the diagnosis of TGA. The location, size and numbers of VSD are defined. The diameter of the VSD is important information. When the VSD is less than 4 mm, the hemodynamics is similar to a TGA with intact septum, requiring an arterial switch within the first 2 weeks of life. The anatomy of the pulmonary valve is analyzed and the absence of LVOT obstruction confirmed. The magnitude of the trans-atrial shunting is assessed. An experienced echocardiography operator is able to describe with a good degree of accuracy the coronary anatomy and particularly detect the intramural courses.

In Taussig Bing [15], the echocardiography confirms: – the subpulmonary VSD, – the origin of both great vessels from the right ventricle and the partial levoposition of the PA when present, – the mitro-pulmonary discontinuity – and the presence of a double infundibulum.

The diagnosis of subaortic obstruction is only made by echography or CT scan, showing an anterior shifting of the conal septum toward the subaortic conus. The smallest size of the subaortic area is accurately measured to evaluate the severity of the subaortic stenosis. The catheterization will not show any obvious gradient, due to the large VSD shunt.

The diagnosis of aortic arch obstruction is also obtained by echocardiography. In newborn under Prostaglandin, the isthmus could be maintained open without evidence of isthmic coarctation. The presence of a hypoplasia of the transverse aortic arch is a clear landmark for an aortic arch obstruction.

Multiple or Swiss cheese VSD is a *difficult diagnosis*. It can be missed by the echocardiogram because the shunting from the large subpulmonary VSD masks any shunting in the muscular septum. Doppler could be misleading. The diagnostic of multiple muscular VSD relies on the presence of structural defects in analyzing all the muscular septum from the posterior to the anterior area, close to the anterior wall. Once suspected, the final diagnosis may require catheterization. CT scan could be also contributing.

Catheterization is useful to confirm multiple and Swiss cheese VSDs. It is requested in patients seen late, with suspicion of pulmonary vascular obstructive disease (see Chap. 16)

The indication of a *Balloon Atrial Septostomy* (BAS) depends on the quality of the atrial shunting and on the size of the VSD. In TGA-VSD without aortic arch obstruction (AAO), many centers perform a BAS and stop the Prostaglandin infusion in order to delay the surgery in insuring a good atrial mixing.

Prenatal diagnosis of TGA-VSD is achieved in more than half of the pregnancies. In utero transport, followed by delivery in a center close to a pediatric heart center, has decreased the mortality and the morbidity of the neonatal surgical repair [16]. Di George is frequent in presence of aortic arch obstruction.

Check List

- Ventriculo arterial alignment (TGA or Taussig Bing)
- Location of aorta (anterior and to the right, side by side)
- Aorto-pulmonary diameter mismatch
- Morphology of pulmonary valve
- VSD location, diameter, VSDs number
- Patency of ductus arteriosus
- Coronary anatomy
- Type of conus, mitro-pulmonary connection
- Aortic arch obstruction, coarctation, hypoplastic arch, IAA
- Subaortic obstruction: aortic valve and LVOT diameter
- Straddling, overriding AV valves
- Weight, prematurity, extra cardiac pathology
- Di George
- Irradiated blood

Surgical Techniques

Today the operation of reference for TGA-VSD and Taussig Bing, with or without AAO is a one-stage neonatal arterial switch operation (ASO) with VSD closure, with or without aortic arch repair. However, two stage operation remain indicated, depending on the center's strategy, in presence of Swiss cheese VSD, very small weight and extracardiac damages.

Palliative Procedures

PA trunk banding by left thoracotomy [16] or sternotomy, has progressively been abandoned due to the risk of late aortic valve regurgitation after ASO [14, 15, 19]. It remains indicated in very small birth weight, or in patients presenting with associated extra cardiac lesions like intra cranial bleeding, necrotizing entero-colitis, major infections. It is contra-indicated in presence of subaortic obstruction.

The increased experience with *PA branches banding*, developed with the Hybrid type I palliation of HLHS, has been applied to TGA-VSD in order to preserve the future aortic valve. It has been used in presence of Swiss cheese VSD [20].

Aortic arch repair by left thoracotomy ± PA Banding was used at the beginning of the ASO experience in patients with TGA/DORV-VSD with aortic arch obstruction. The repair of the nearly constant hypoplasia of the aortic arch by thoracotomy is challenging and is frequently complicated by recurrent arch obstruction. The second stage ASO is often made more challenging. Due to the frequently associated subaortic obstruction, a PA banding is usually poorly tolerated.

Arterial switch with aortic arch repair associated with PA banding by sternotomy is the technique that we favor in case of Swiss Cheese VSD. See below.

One Stage Anatomical Repair of TGA-VSD and Taussig Bing

Cardio-Pulmonary Bypass (CPB) and Myocardial Protection

The CPB is run on full flow, with bicaval canulation and with antegrade cerebral perfusion when an arch repair is needed. The priming of the circuit today is less than 200 ml and includes packed red cells, plasma and/or albumin. Our preference is to use NTK-Custodiol crystalloid cardioplegia [12, 17]. Others favors warm blood cardioplegia and strict normothermia. Modified Ultra Filtration (MUF) is rarely used, while Conventional Ultra Filtration (CUF) is routinely applied.

ASO in TGA – VSD

The one stage repair is undertaken in the first 2 weeks of life.

The operation starts with the VSD patch closure. It is similar than in any VSD surgery. Perimembranous, outlet and mid trabecular VSD are closed through the tricuspid valve (Fig. 15.1). Different patch materials are used (Goretex, bovine pericardium, Dacron, etc…). Due to the fragility of the neonatal myocardium, a small needle is favored (7/0 Prolene, 6.5 needle, or 6/0 Prolene, 9 needle). Several pledgeted separate stitches, using 6/0 Premio ©, are useful. The rest of the patch is secured with a running suture. The ASO follows and needs to deal with an important mismatch in diameter between the aorta and the PA (See Chap. 14). TGA-VSD and Taussig Bing share the risk of late neo-aortic root dilation due to the large native pulmonary annulus. In this regard, we believe that the "trap-door" technique, which enlarges even more the neo-aortic root, should not be used.

ASO in Taussig Bing

The management of the VSD is clearly the most challenging part of the arterial switch operation. Due to the malalignement of the conal septum, the VSD is more difficult to treat. As shown in Fig. 15.4, the baffle patch needs to connect the left ventricle to the pulmonary artery, in closing the ventricular septal defect represented in green on Fig. 15.4; and not the interventricular communication, represented in red. Sometimes, the VSD could be closed through the tricuspid valve only. The trans-tricuspid approach, in incising the anterior tricuspid leaflet, offers a good access to the superior border of the VSD. In many instances, a double or triple approach is needed. We favor a technique with dual approach through the tricuspid and aortic valve after harvesting of the coronary buttons. Starting from the top, the superior part of the large patch is secured to the conal septum; then the operation is completed through the TV and the patch is secured to the inferior rim of the VSD with a running suture. We have abandoned the approach through the native pulmonary valve, which was associated with impairment of the neo-aortic valve [18].

The coronary transfer in Taussig-Bing is more complex due to the frequent presence of a double looping course (Fig. 15.5a, b). Due to the side by side vessels relationship, the right coronary (RCA) that is running in front of the reconstructed PA trunk, could be compressed. It is useful to transfer the pulmonary trunk to the right PA to prevent a compression of the RCA (Fig. 15.5c).

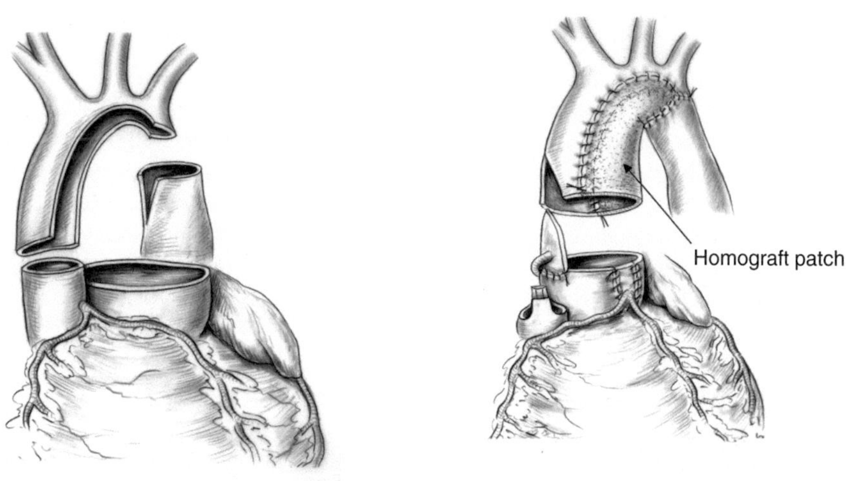

Fig. 15.6 Aortic arch repair. The coarctation is resected with all ductal tissue. The descending aorta is partially anastomosed directly to the transverse arch. A large patch of either pulmonary homograft or bovine pericardium is used to enlarge the arch and the ascending aorta so as to control the mismatch between the ascending aorta and the neo-pulmonary root

ASO in Taussig Bing with Aortic Arch Obstruction (Figs. 15.5 and 15.6)

The one stage repair of ASO + AAA repair and VSD closure is undertalken in the first week of life, through sternotomy.

We routinely used antegrade cerebral perfusion and have abandoned circulatory arrest. The CPB is run around 20–25° Celsius at a flow of 50 ml/kg/min. The arch is repaired first. As shown in Fig. 15.6, a large patch of either homograft or bovine pericardium is used to enlarge together the transverse aortic arch and the ascending aorta; so as to normalize the diameter of the distal ascending aorta to fit the enlargement of the pulmonary artery.

The subaortic obstruction (Figs. 15.2 and 15.4) could be absent or reduced [8, 12] to small muscular bands in the subaortic infundibulum that are resected through the native aortic valve [10, 15, 17]. Elsewhere it can be important, requiring a right ventriculotomy with resection of the parietal band and patch enlargement of the infundibulum [12]. The challenge is major in some interrupted arch with hypoplasia of the aortic annulus. The presence of an anterior loop with the RCA crossing the infundibulum, close to the aortic annulus forbids a transection of the annulus and force is to place a small RV to PA conduit, usually a Goretex 5 [12]. In any case, the small aortic annulus will become a small PA annulus with ultimate risk of RVOT obstruction [12, 21].

Management of TGA/DORV with Multiple VSD

Apical muscular VSD and Swiss cheese VSD, defined as more than two VSDs, are very challenging to repair in neonates. Our strategy has been to perform a *palliative first stage arterial switch*. The ASO is performed, the arch is repaired accordingly and a PA banding on the reconstructed PA trunk is applied. The VSDs are left intact. There is a *triple advantage of doing an arterial switch*: – first the PA banding is placed on the final PA and preserve the neo-aortic valve, – second, the shifting of the conal septum is no more a contra-indication to PA banding and –third, a normal physiology and mixing are restored. The second stage, undertaken several months later, is to close the multiple VSD. The ultimate Swiss cheese VSD closure is frequently a hybrid procedure, with surgical closure of the cono-ventricular VSD and device closure of the muscular VSDs. Due to the PA banding, late re-operation on the RVOT could not be excluded.

The Case of TGA-IVS Associated with AAO

This association is rare and a source of complication. The presence of a coarctation could be "missed" because the isthmus is maintained opened under Prostaglandin. The only landmark of an associated coarctation could be some hypoplasia of the transverse arch and a smallish isthmus. The coarctation may then become obvious in the hours or days following the post-operative course, with elevated arterial pressure , absent of femoral pulses and low cardiac output syndrome. Urgent coarctation repair is requested by left thoracotomy without CPB.

This association is to be detected prior to the ASO. Our strategy to interrupt the Prostaglandin in TGA-IVS when the atrial mixing is satisfactory gives time for the isthmus to narrow and secure the diagnosis. When the SaO2 is to low, due to poor atrial mixing, a balloon atrial septostomy is routinely performed.

Kawashima Operation

This technique proposed for Taussig-Bing, which tunnelized the VSD to the aorta, requires the resection of the conal septum and is therefore very challenging in neonates. It was abandoned by most centers in favor of one-stage ASO [14, 15].

Outcomes

The hospital mortality of the arterial switch at the EACTS-ECHSA Congenital Database [22] (see Chap. 4), for the period 2010–2013, is: *2.6 % for TGA-IVS, 5 % for TGA-VSD* and 11.3 % for TGA/DORV-VSD with AAO.

The striking five times increased mortality of TGA/DORV-VSD with AAO compared to TGA-IVS reflects the challenge of the ASO in presence of aortic arch obstruction. The two times elevated hospital mortality of ASO in TGA-VSD compared to ASO in TGA-IVS is believed to be related to the VSD closure particularly in Taussig-Bing [23].

In recent series, the hospital mortality of the ASO in TGA – VSD and Taussig Bing with and without AAO is below 5 % [17, 19]. Swiss cheese VSDs and small birth weight remain risk factors [23] for early mortality. The complexity of the coronary artery patterns is not anymore a risk factor in most centers [24].

The long term results of ASO for Taussig-Bing are today available [11, 19]. Survival is over 85 % at 15 years. Most patients are in NYHA class 1, they are in sinus rhythm and the biventricular function is preserved in 95 %. Nevertheless, the risk of reoperation either surgery or interventional cardiology, is significant and is around 30 %. Mainly due to RVOT obstruction [21], re-coarctation, coronary stenosis, aortic valve regurgitation. Aortic root dilation is favored by the aorto-pulmonary diameter mismatch [11, 25], it may require re-operation in the long term, No aortic rupture are so far described (see Chap. 34).

Performing a control coronarography or CT angiogram in patients with complex coronary anatomy (double loop and intramural course) is our current practice. Therefore, close lifelong surveillance of these patients is necessary.

References

1. Jatene AD, Fontes VF, Paulista PP, de Souza LC, Neger F, Galantier M, Souza JE. Successful anatomic correction of transposition of the great vessels. A preliminary report. Arq Bras Cardiol. 1975;28:461–4.
2. Jatene AD, Fontes VF, Paulista PP, Souza LC, Neger F, Galantier M, Sousa JE. Anatomic correction of transposition of the great vessels. J Thorac Cardiovasc Surg. 1976;72:364–70.
3. Houyel L, Van Praagh R, Lacour-Gayet F, Serraf A, Petit J, Bruniaux J, Planché C. Transposition of the great arteries [S, D, L]. Pathologic anatomy, diagnosis, and surgical management of a newly recognized complex. J Thorac Cardiovasc Surg. 1995;110:613–24.
4. Taussig HB, Bing RJ. Complete transposition of aorta and levoposition of pulmonary artery. Am Heart J. 1949;37:551–7.
5. Stellin G, Zuberbuhler JR, Anderson RH, Siewers RD. The surgical anatomy of the Taussig-Bing malformation. J Thorac Cardiovasc Surg. 1987;93:560–9.
6. Van Praagh R. What is the Taussig Bing malformation? Circulation. 1968;38:445–9.
7. Belli E, Lacour-Gayet F, Serraf A, et al. Double-outlet right ventricle with non-committed ventricular septal defect. Eur J Cardiothorac Surg. 1999;15:747–52.
8. Lacour-Gayet F, Serraf A, Galletti L, et al. Biventricular repair of conotruncal anomalies associated with aortic arch obstruction: 103 patients. Circulation. 1997;96(Suppl II):328–34.
9. Alsoufi B, Cai S, Williams WG, Coles JG, Caldarone CA, Redington AM, Van Arsdell GS. Improved results with single-stage total correction of Taussig-Bing anomaly. Eur J Cardiothorac Surg. 2008;33:244–50.
10. Comas JV, Mignosa C, Cochrane AD, Wilkinson JL, Karl TR. Taussig-Bing anomaly and arterial switch: aortic arch obstruction does not influence outcome. Eur J Cardiothorac Surg. 1996;10:1114–9.
11. Schwarz F, Blaschczok HC, Sinzobahamvya N, Sata S, Korn F, Weber A, Asfour B, Hraska V. The Taussig-Bing anomaly: long-term results. Eur J Cardiothorac Surg. 2013;44:821–7.
12. Lacour-Gayet F. Arterial switch operation with VSD and aortic arch reconstruction. Semin Thorac Cardiovasc Surg. 2007;19:245–8.
13. Piot JD, Rey C, Serraf A, Touchot A, Sousa Uva M, Lacour-Gayet F, Planché C. Transposition of great vessels with anomaly of the atrioventricular valves or chordae: echocardiographic aspects and surgical correlations. Arch Mal Coeur Vaiss. 1995;88:699–704.
14. Serraf A, Comas JV, Lacour-Gayet F, Bruniaux J, Bouchart F, Planché C. Neonatal anatomic repair of transposition of the great arteries and ventricular septal defect. Eur J Cardiothorac Surg. 1992;6:630–4.
15. Serraf A, Lacour-Gayet F, Bruniaux J, Losay J, Petit J, Touchot-Kone A, Bouchart F, Planche C. Anatomic repair of Taussig-Bing hearts. Circulation. 1991;84(5 Suppl):III200–5.
16. Bonnet D, Coltri A, Butera G, Fermont L, Le Bidois J, Kachaner J, Sidi D. Detection of transposition of the great arteries in fetuses reduces neonatal morbidity and mortality. Circulation. 1999;99:916–8.
17. Stoica S, Campbell D, Lacour-Gayet F, et al. Morbidity of the arterial switch operation. Ann Thorac Surg. 2012;93:1977–83.
18. Mohammadi S, Belli E, Aupecle B, Lacour-Gayet F, et al. Left-sided lesions after anatomic repair of transposition of the great arteries, ventricular septal defect, and coarctation: surgical factors. J Thorac Cardiovasc Surg. 2004;128(1):44–52.
19. Hayes D, Jones S, Bacha E, Richmond ME, Andrews HF, Glickstein JS, Chen JM, Liberman L. Primary arterial switch operation as a strategy for total correction of Taussig – Bing anomaly: a 21-year experience. Circulation. 2013;128:S194–8.
20. Weinstein S, Liveris A, Shenoy RU, Lacour-Gayet F. Bilateral pulmonary arterial banding for complex transposition of the great arteries. J Thorac Cardiovasc Surg. 2013;145(3):876–8.
21. Sinzobahamvya N, Blaschczok HC, Asfour B, Arenz C, Jussli MJ, Schindler E, Photiadis J, Urban AE. Right ventricular outflow tract obstruction after arterial switch operation for the Taussig-Bing heart. Eur J Cardiothorac Surg. 2007;31(5):873–8.

22. EACTS-ECHSA congenital database. Free access on line http://www.eactscongenitaldb.org/index.php?LANG=en&level=2&struct=14_1.
23. Lacour-Gayet F. Complexity stratification of the arterial switch operation: a second learning curve. Cardiol Young. 2012;22(6):739–44.
24. Lacour-Gayet F, Anderson RH. A uniform surgical technique for transfer of both simple and complex patterns of the coronary arteries during the arterial switch procedure. Cardiol Young. 2005;15(S1):93–101.
25. Koolbergen DR, Manshanden JS, Yazdanbakhsh AP, Bouma BJ, Blom NA, de Mol BA, Mulder BJ, Hazekamp MG. Reoperation for neoaortic root pathology after the arterial switch operation. Eur J Cardiothorac Surg. 2014;46(3):474–9.

Chapter 16
TGA-IVS and TGA-VSD Seen Late

Shoujun Li and Kai Ma

Abstract Late referral of patients with complete transposition of the great arteries (TGA) is common in developing countries. However, outcomes of these patients who undergo surgical correction late remain unclear. To obtain favorable outcomes in these "late" patients, understanding of the surgical indications, management and specific surgical techniques is essential. Although the anatomical and hemodynamic features of 'TGA- intact ventricular septum (IVS)' and 'TGA-ventricular septal defect (VSD)' seen late are different, arterial switch operation (ASO) generally remains the prevailing surgical procedure for both of them. According to the pathophysiological changes, we define 'TGA-IVS seen late' as refer to therapy beyond the age at 1 month and 'TGA-VSD seen late' as refer to therapy beyond the age at 6 months.

In TGA-IVS seen late, favorable left ventricular (LV) geometry is the prerequisite. Age, LV shape, pressure ratio between the two ventricles and LV mass index are the determinants for primary or two-stage ASO. In general, overall outcomes of ASO undertaken for TGA-IVS seen late are favorable. Two-stage ASO is associated with higher late mortality and more neo-aortic regurgitation. Later age at retraining is associated with higher late mortality. Age beyond 3 months at retraining is associated with impaired LV function.

In TGA-VSD, pulmonary vascular obstructive disease is the main challenging feature associated with late presentation, particularly with respect to late operability and postoperative safety. Moreover, accompanying diameter mismatch between the pulmonary trunk and aorta needs surgical attention, i.e. neo-aortic sinotubular reconstruction, to minimize postoperative neo-aortic regurgitation. Outcomes are satisfactory when ASO performed before 3 years of age. In the contrary, sub-optimal outcomes, including high prevalence of pulmonary hypertension crisis and valve insufficiency, will present if the ASO performed beyond 3 years of age. Palliative ASO with a fenestration on the VSD patch has proven to provide a more safety postoperative course.

S. Li, MD (✉) • K. Ma, MD, PhD
Pediatric Cardiac Surgery Center, National Center for Cardiovascular Disease and Fuwai Hospital, Chinese Academy of Medical Sciences, Peking Union Medical College, Beijing 100037, PR China
e-mail: drlishoujun@yahoo.com

F. Lacour-Gayet et al. (eds.), *Surgery of Conotruncal Anomalies*,
DOI 10.1007/978-3-319-23057-3_16

Keywords Complete transposition of the great arteries • Surgical management • Arterial switch operation • Late referral • Left ventricular retraining • Pulmonary vascular obstructive disease

The management of TGA-IVS and TGA-VSD seen late are different and the chapter will study the two conditions in two separate parts.

Part 1: Surgery of Transposition of the Great Arteries with Intact Ventricular Septum Seen Late

Introduction and Definition

Nearly 75 % of complete TGA patients present with an intact ventricular septum (IVS) or a very small (<3 mm) ventricular septal defect (VSD), a patent foramen ovale (PFO) or an atrial septal defect (ASD), and many times a patent ductus arteriosus (PDA). As discussed in previous chapters (Chaps. 15, 16 and 17), the arterial switch operation (ASO) has become the prevailing surgical procedure for the various forms of complete TGA. The current operative mortality is low and the late results are satisfactory [1].

In many developing countries, late diagnosis of congenital heart disease is a significant issue, and up to 95 % of infants go untreated. Likewise, some circumstances may arise that will cause delaying the safe period for an arterial switch in both northern America and Europe. A neonate with TGA-IVS – may be seriously ill, with necrotizing enterocolitis, renal failure and intra cranial bleeding, – or may be premature or have low birth weight. Moreover, the geographical distance between the patients and a center offering ASO may be too long to opportune surgical therapy.

The LV ability to sustain a systemic function is slowly decreasing after 1 month of age in TGA-IVS. It is obvious that LV regression will raise the risk for uneventful arterial switch. Therefore, in this chapter, we will address surgical management, indications and outcome of TGA-IVS patients presenting beyond 1 month of age.

Morphological and Pathophysiological Features of the Regressing LV

When the ventricular septum is intact and no significant pulmonary stenosis is present, the LV morphology and function are normal at birth. However, LV will regress within a few weeks after birth following the gradually decrease of pulmonary vascular resistance. The LV wall thickness, LV end diastolic volume, LV cavity will be less than normal as a response to after-load reduction. In infants with TGA-IVS, the LV cavity is the usual ellipsoid at birth but soon becomes banana shaped [2]. Accompanying LV regression, both the function of deconditioned LV and its ability to sustain systemic circulation are slowly decreasing [3]. As a result, patients with TGA-IVS presenting for surgery beyond the first month of life have been considered at high risk for ASO. There is increasing likelihood that the regressed LV will be unable to accommodate the acute increased workload of systemic pressure [4].

In TGA/IVS, a dynamic type of LVOT obstruction is frequent, usually mild and not readily apparent. Leftward bulging of the ventricular septum toward the lower-pressure LV, which narrows the LV outflow tract during systole but opens widely during diastole, is clearly seen at echocardiography.

Favorable LV geometry is an essential prerequisite for optimal ASO outcomes. Two groups of TGA patients seen late (>1 month) can be recognized depending on LV morphology.

"Late" TGA-IVS Patients with Favorable LV Morphology

LV ability to sustain a systemic function is slowly decreasing after 2 weeks of age in TGA-IVS and depends upon the patency of the ductus arteriosus, the level of the pulmonary resistances, the size of intra-atrial communication and the presence of a dynamic left ventricular outflow tract obstruction. There is a wide variation in the level of preoperative LV deconditioning. Other factors, possibly genetically predetermined, might also play a role in dictating the regression of pulmonary vascular resistance and LV performance. In presence of favorable LV geometry at echocardiography (see below), primary ASO should be attempted as soon as possible without LV reconditioning.

"Late" TGA-IVS Patients with Regressed LV Morphology

In presence of regressed LV morphology at echocardiography, we believed empirically that at approximately 1 month of age a significant number of children with TGA-IVS is at too great a risk for one stage ASO.

Diagnosis and Imaging

Echocardiography has become the diagnostic method of choice to evaluate the capability of the LV to sustain the systemic circulation. The anatomic structure of TGA-IVS is best evaluated from the subcostal four-chamber view, which allows all the great vessels and their connections to be displayed. The LV morphology evaluation requires accurate measurements of: – the LV end diastolic diameter, – the shape of the interventricular septum, – and the size of ASD and PDA. It is also necessary to measure the degree of dynamic left ventricular outflow tract obstruction, as well as the presence of atrioventricular valve (AV) anomalies.

The LV myocardial mass and mass index are quantitative parameters for LV myocardial evaluation. Both of them are calculated at echocardiography. The formulas issued by the American Society of Echography [5] are used. According to the experience of Marie Lannelongue Hospital, Paris [6] and our institution [7], a LV mass <35 g/m^2 index is a strong indication for LV failure after ASO.

In addition, the echocardiogram defines with reasonable accuracy the coronary arteries pattern and the presence of aortic arch obstruction.

Magnetic Resonance Imaging (MRI) is considered a more reliable method [8, 9] to evaluate the LV performance. But it is a complex and expensive technology, requiring intubation of the patient.

Surgical Indications

It has been our strategy to offer ASO to nearly all patients with TGA-IVS seen late. However, associated severe pulmonary valve anomalies remain a contraindication for ASO.

Primary ASO

Even beyond 1 month of age, patients with favorable LV performance are considered good candidates for primary ASO [10]. It has been reported that 70–80 % of patients who referred beyond the age at 2 months required no LV preparation. However, the need for mechanical support (e.g. extra corporeal membrane oxygenation.) in some of the older patients may limit the widespread adoption of extending the boundaries of primary ASO.

LV Retraining

As shown in Fig. 16.1, LV retraining is indicated according to a combination of different factors [6, 7]:

- Age >1 month
- LV mass index <35 g/m^2
- Right to left bulging of the interventricular septum with a "banana" LV shape, designating a low LV pressure
- LV/RV wall thickness ratio
- LV/RV systolic pressure ratio <0.5 (age <3 months) or 0.6 (age >3 months).

4–3 Atrial switch option.

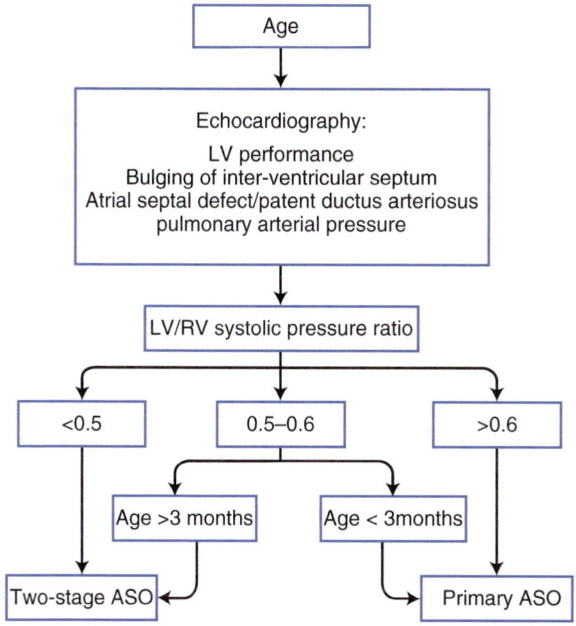

Fig. 16.1 Indication for primary and staged ASO

To avoid long-term impaired LV systolic function, some surgeons prefer the atrial switch (Senning/Mustard operation) in very late presenting patients whose LV myocardium is considered not anymore qualified for successful retraining. Our preference has been to avoid atrial switch.

Timing of Second Stage ASO

The second-stage ASO was performed once the LV mass index had reached 50 g/m^2, and when the interventricular septum resumed a straight shape, indicating an increased LV pressure [6, 7]. In majority of cases, LV in TGA-IVS has the ability to hypertrophy rapidly, achieving a plateau within 7–14 days and meeting the criteria for the second stage ASO after PA banding. However, 2–3 months duration of retraining is usually necessary for patients beyond 6 months of age, in presence of severely unprepared LV.

Check List Prior to Surgery for Late TGA-IVS Patients

- Age
- Diameter of the ASD and PDA
- LV mass, LV end diastolic volume, LV geometry, interventricular septum

- LV/RV systolic pressure ratio
- LV/RV wall thickness ratio
- Potential left ventricular outflow tract obstruction can modify the LV preload and afterload
- Annulus and morphology of the pulmonary valve
- Diameter of pulmonary artery branches
- Complex coronary anatomy
- Aortic arch obstruction
- Anatomy of atrioventricular valves

ASO Surgical Technique

One Stage ASO

The technique is similar to neonatal ASO (Chap. 15). Mechanical support with extracorporeal membrane oxygenation (ECMO) was not required in our group of TGA-IVS with good LV morphology.

Postoperative ECMO represents a postoperative LV preparation and is currently used by several centers [10–13]. Nevertheless, ECMO remains logistically a difficult procedure associated with an elevated cost in relation with the technical staff required, the expensive long-lasting oxygenator membrane and the important quantity of blood products. So far, ECMO support is used more as a rescue method than an elective indication of LV retraining.

Two Stage ASO

This procedure includes a first stage of LV retraining followed by a second stage ASO.

LV Retraining Procedure (Pulmonary Artery Banding and Modified B-T Shunt)

The procedure is carried out through median sternotomy. The left ventricle and right ventricle pressures are measured by direct manometry confirming the low LV pressure and the reduced LV/RV pressure ratio. The modified Blalock-Taussig shunt is first performed and implanted between the innominate artery and the right pulmonary artery branch. When present, the patent ductus arteriosus is ligated. The size of the Gore-Tex conduit was 3.5, 4, and 5 mm, depending on the body weight. Then a banding of the pulmonary trunk is performed with continuous measurement of LV and arterial systolic pressure. The band is placed medially in a way to preserve together the pulmonary valve and the pulmonary artery bifurcation (Fig. 16.2). The aim of the banding is to obtain an intraoperative LV/RV between 0.65 and 0.75.

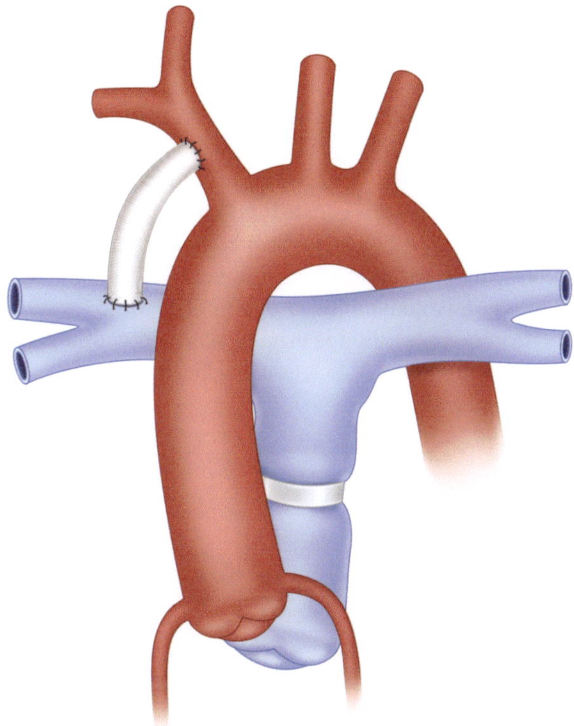

Fig. 16.2 Retraining technique (pulmonary artery banding & modified B-T shunt)

There are several principles of retraining technique to be respected. Before banding the surgeon must ensure that there is a good size interatrial communication. If not, it can be produced by balloon atrial septostomy or atrioseptectomy under cardiopulmonary bypass. Banding in the absence of an inadequate interatrial communication may increase cyanosis to an unacceptable level. For this reason, when banding cyanotic patients, the authors monitor arterial pO_2 and arterial saturation and try to avoid any reduction in PaO_2 below 35 mmHg. A decrease in systemic oxygen saturation is anticipated during the procedure. Achieving stable hemodynamic balance is currently the greatest technical difficulty. In our experience, a relatively small diameter of the modified B-T shunt is always pursued even though the banding may be forcibly loose. Inotropic support was always required, including variously: milrinone, dopamine, or epinephrine.

Second Stage ASO

Although the surgical technique is almost same for one-stage and two-stage ASO, the second-stage ASO is technically more challenging owing to the presence of adhesions. The Blalock-Taussig shunt is ligated and transected at the beginning of the cardiopulmonary bypass, and the pulmonary artery trunk is divided at the site of the previous pulmonary artery band. The fibrotic tissue of the distal pulmonary artery at the site of the banding is excised, but the thickened tissue on the proximal pulmonary trunk (neo-aortic root) is carefully preserved in the contrary. The reading of the coronary arteries course and the mobilization of the pulmonary branches required particular attention. Bovine pericardium is utilized to reconstruct the neo-pulmonary root.

In patients with TGA-IVS seen late, it is common for mean arterial pressure to hover at 40–45 mmHg for 2 or 3 days, in the presence of peripheral warmth. In such patients, scrupulous care is taken to avoid volume overloading and, if possible, the mean left atrial pressure is maintained at 6–8 mmHg while awaiting the development of LV hypertrophy. Extubation is usually achieved within 3–6 days after surgery based on the quality of the LV function at echocardiogram.

Outcomes

Outcomes of One Stage ASO

In general, the younger the patient with TGA-IVS at arterial switch repair, the safer the operation. In the author's institution, 78 patients beyond the age of 1 month with favorable LV geometry underwent one-stage ASO between 2000 and 2011 [7]. The median age at one-stage ASO was 1.9 months (range, 31 days to 6.8 months). The in-hospital mortality was 2.6 % and the late mortality was 2.7 %, with two deaths associated with impaired LV function. *No ECMO was required.* At follow-up, there were seven significant late neo-aortic regurgitations (9.8 %). The mean left ventricular ejection fraction was 67±9 %. These encouraging results were actually similar to neonatal ASO outcomes.

Outcomes of Two-Stage ASO

The regressed LV can be well prepared by pulmonary artery banding and modified Blalock-Taussig shunt. The LV mass index, LV/RV wall thickness ratio, LV to RV pressure ratio, LV mass and volume, and mass to volume ratio will increase significantly within a week after retraining [14, 15]. Although the LV is responsive, numerous complications are still challenging. The band will cause scarring that complicate pulmonary artery reconstruction. Scarring also can distort the neo-aortic valve and substantially increase the incidence of neo-aortic valve regurgitation [16]. Adhesions, caused by the band, obscure coronary artery anatomy and make the coronary transfer more difficult.

In consecutive 31 patients who underwent two-stage ASO at our institution, the median age at training was 5.2 months. The median duration of LV retraining was 18 days. Prior to retraining, the median LV mass index and median LV/RV systolic pressure ratio was 26 g/m^2 and 0.36, respectively. There was no death at LV retraining. Two patients required revision of a too-tight PA banding with low oxygen saturation. . All the 31 patients with LV retraining underwent anatomical repair at our institution [7]. At the time of the second stage ASO, the LV mass index increased to median 57 g/m^2 and the LV/RV systolic pressure ratio rose to 0.62.

Median age at second stage ASO was 6.0 months (range, 37 days to 10.4 years). Cross-clamp times were longer owing to adhesions. Two in-hospital deaths were caused by septicemia, and the other was caused by low cardiac output syndrome. Overall survival for the total two-stage ASO population was 89.3 % at 6 months, and 75.0 % at 1 year and 5 years. Age at LV retraining, as a continuous value, was the only risk factor for late mortality [7].

Long-Term Outcome of Second-Stage ASO

Long-term follow-up results have shown less well-preserved ventricular function in patients who underwent two-stage switch. Diastolic function impairment [17] was observed, due to sub-endocardial ischemia probably induced by too a rapid LV hypertrophy after banding with reduced coronary flow reserves.

Obviously, subendocardial ischemia and edema are correlated with the degree of pulmonary artery banding. However, less-aggressive banding techniques have also been correlated with inadequate LV preparation. The adjustable banding technique [18–21] is an appealing proposition requiring further evaluation.

Impact of Age >3 months at Retraining

In our experience [7], all the in-hospital mortality, late mortality, and at least moderate neo-aortic regurgitation were observed in patients who had their LV retrained beyond 3 months of age. So we further compared the outcome between patients less than 3 months of age and patients greater than 3 months. There were seven patients in the less than 3 months group and 24 patients in the more than 3 months group. The long-term LVEF was significantly lower in patients who retrain the LV beyond 3 months of age. Estimated overall survival for the more than 3 months population was 85.7 % at 6 months, 66.7 % at 1 year, and 66.7 % at 5 years.

Part 2: TGA-VSD Seen Late

Introduction and Definition

Around 25 % of patients with complete TGA (without LVOT obstruction) have associated ventricular septal defect (VSD) [22]. The VSD is the most common associated anomaly in patients with TGA. The VSD may be small, large, multiple, and occur anywhere within the interventricular septum, and will substantially influence the pathophysiological features, natural history and surgical management.

Favorable outcomes have been achieved through proper surgical repair during neonatal period or early infancy, avoiding pulmonary vascular obstructive disease (PVOD) [23]. However, some adverse issues are deteriorating the surgical outcomes of ASO performed beyond 6 months of age.

According to the satisfactory blood mixing, late referral of patients with TGA-VSD is common in many developing countries. The main challenging features [24] associated with late presentation are: the development of PVOD and severe great vessels diameter discrepancy.

In this chapter, we will address the surgical management of patients with TGA, unrestrictive VSD and absent LVOT obstruction, presenting beyond 6 months of age.

Morphological and Pathophysiological Features Of TGA-VSD beyond 6 Months of Age

Great Vessels

The pulmonary artery tends to be significantly larger than the aorta in presence of a VSD, and the discrepancy between the great vessels is even greater with anterior malalignment of the conal septum [25]. More important, the diameter mismatch of the two great arteries is correlated with the pulmonary blood flow increase and pulmonary vascular pathology. In TGA-VSD, especially with maligned VSD, the great vessels may be side by side, with the aorta to the right (Fig. 16.3). In the cohort of TGA-VSD patients who underwent surgical repair in the author's institution, the incidence of side by side great arteries was nearly 20 %. The mean diameter ratio between the aorta and pulmonary artery was 1:1.8.

Pulmonary Vascular Obstructive Disease (PVOD)

When pulmonary vascular disease develops in TGA, pathologic, cellular and molecular changes in the pulmonary arteries are variable. Pulmonary microthrombi are present in about 25 % of lungs [26]. A variety of intimal lesions, including eccentric cushion lesions and occlusion with recanalization of nonlaminar intimal fibrosis, have been clearly identified. In one of our study [27], we directly acquire lung specimens from both TGA-VSD and simple VSD patients during cardiac surgery. Expression of eNOS and MMP-2 was significantly lower in the TGA+VSD group than in the VSD alone group. Interestingly, both eNOS and MMP-2 are involved in the interaction with hypoxia-induced factor, which suggests that high oxygenation in the pulmonary circulation may affect the progress and reversibility of pulmonary hypertension [28, 29].

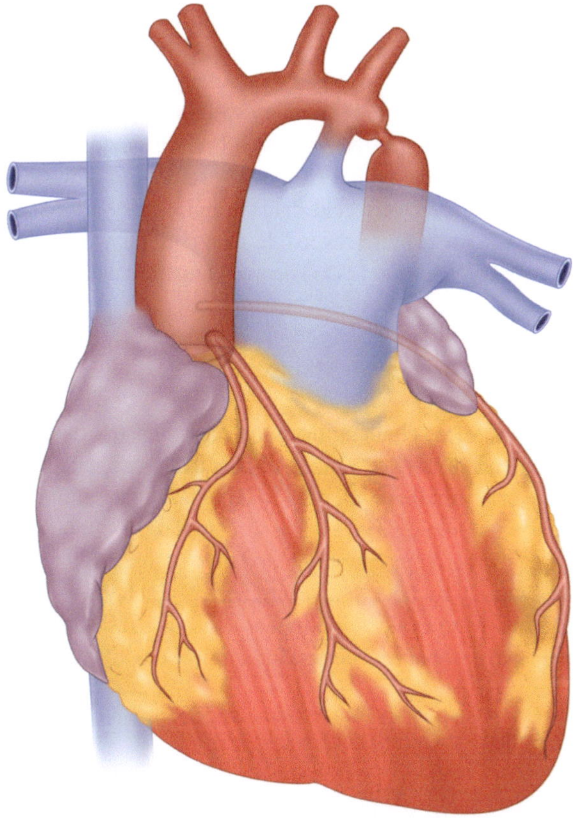

Fig. 16.3 Side-by-side great vessels & aorta/pulmonary trunk discrepancy

Main Clinical Manifestation

Because of the satisfactory inter-circulatory blood mixing, the newborns with TGA and a large VSD may have no clinical symptoms initially. Cyanosis is commonly mild, most evident with stress and crying.

At the age of 2–3 weeks, the symptoms of heart failure, such as tachycardia, tachypnea, and liver enlargement began to develop and become prominent. Cardiac murmurs mainly arise from significant VSD or PDA. Moreover, additional gallop rhythm and narrow splitting of the second heart sound with accentual pulmonary component will eventually emerge. When pulmonary vascular resistance rises probably around 6 months of age, the main manifestation will transfer to cyanosis again with mild heart failure.

The early development and widespread presence of PVOD in patients with TGA-VSD have been widely documented by hemodynamic measures and biopsy studies [30]. Patients with TGA and large VSD have moderate pulmonary vascular changes occurring in 20 % before 2 months of age, 25 % from 3 to 12 months, and 78 % after

12 months of age. The data from the author's institution suggests that PVOD will be irreversible or partial reversible after 3 years of age. In general, associated coarctation accelerates the progress of pulmonary vascular obstruction.

Comparing to isolated VSD, the pulmonary vascular disease of TGA-VSD is more severe. The potential mechanisms may include (1) erythrocytosis, (2) high O_2 saturation of the pulmonary circulation and (3) low O_2 saturation of systemic circulation. However, with great surprise we found that the pulmonary arterial hypertension in patients with TGA-VSD was more reversible than patients with simple VSD in one study conducted by our institution [27]. The mechanism remains largely unclear.

Physiopathology Based on Age >6 Months at Surgery

In our experience, the most challenging issue regarding the overall operative outcomes of ASO undertaken in "late" TGA-VSD is the occurrence of PVOD which is correlated with age at repair. It is important to recognize that pulmonary hypertension is not synonymous with pulmonary vascular disease. High pulmonary artery pressure is either made up of increased pulmonary blood flow or increased pulmonary vascular resistance, but very rarely by both. However, there is much yet to be analysed before we fully understand how to evaluate pulmonary vascular resistances. As a result, the age is considered as a reasonable criterion for surgical classification.

ASO Within 6 Months of Age

Progressive PVOD is infrequent when performing arterial switch in TGA-VSD within 6 months of age. ASO is considered safe with low risk of irreversible pulmonary vascular resistance.

ASO Beyond 6 Months of Age

Although the quantitative assessment of pulmonary vascular resistance is surrounded with uncertainty, it has been repeatedly reported [31–33] that patients with TGA and large VSD have pulmonary vascular changes grade 3 or greater occurring in more than 40 % after 6 months of age. Elevated pulmonary vascular resistance and irreversible pulmonary artery obstructive disease dominate the early and late outcome of ASO performed beyond 6 months of age.

Diagnosis and Imaging

The diagnosis of TGA-VSD may be delayed because of obscure clinical manifestations. Chest radiography, electrocardiography, echocardiography, cardiac catheterization and angiography may be more or less beneficial in the diagnosis and surgical decision-making.

Imaging and Pulmonary Vascular Resistance Evaluation

Chest radiography shows cardiomegaly, pulmonary plethora, and a wide superior mediastinum in TGA-VSD who present late. Evidence of elevated pulmonary vascular resistance will progressively appear, such as fewer plethoras, particular in the peripheral lung fields. Regarding the pulmonary vascular hyperplasia, regular radiography is essential when evaluate the long-term surgical benefits.

Echocardiography is particularly valuable in evaluating the surgical anatomy of TGA with unrestrictive VSD; defining the diameter and location of the VSD, the great vessels mismatch as well as association with multiple VSD, abnormal pulmonary valve, aortic arch obstruction, AV valve anomalies and others. Another significant information is the estimation of the pulmonary artery pressure to guide the surgical decision.

Cardiac catheterization is strongly indicated if there is evidence of pulmonary vascular disease shown in clinical manifestations, radiography or echocardiography, to measure pulmonary vascular resistance.

Because of intracardiac communications in patients with TGA, the Fick method is usually the only practical way of measuring pulmonary and systemic blood flow. However, when pulmonary blood flow is elevated and therefore pulmonary arterial oxygen saturation high, the Fick calculation tends to be inaccurate for its inherent errors [34]. Fortunately, calculations are more accurate when the pulmonary blood flow is low and pulmonary vascular resistance correspondingly high. Potential for error also exists when the pulmonary blood flow is nearly fully saturated.

Surgical Indication

In our clinical experience, performing ASO beyond the age at 6 months requires an optimal postoperative management to control PVOD.

Indication for Pulmonary Artery Banding

For TGA-VSD patients presenting late, surgical constriction of the pulmonary artery can provide effective palliation for both heart failure and pulmonary vascular disease. Pulmonary artery banding may be indicated when complex multiple VSDs are present or in presence of medical conditions delaying open-heart surgery. However, elective arterial switch and VSD partial or total closure is currently the procedure of choice. Since TGA physiology requires a somewhat higher pulmonary blood flow for optimum inter-circulatory mixing, the pulmonary artery banding in TGA-VSD should be less tight than in infants with normally related great arteries.

Indication for Palliative Arterial Switch

In TGA-VSD with elevated pulmonary vascular resistance, the total closure of the VSD markedly increases the risk of mortality. Palliative arterial switch has been accomplished with low surgical risk and substantial hemodynamic and clinical benefit. It is presumed that the VSD fenestration during ASO could decompress the right ventricle if the pulmonary arteriolar resistance suddenly increases. However, PVOD usually continually progresses and late mortality related to pulmonary hypertension crisis is high.

Advanced PVOD characterized by calculated pulmonary vascular resistances greater than eight Wood Units/m^2 is considered a contraindication to closure of the VSD and an indication for palliative ASO with VSD fenestration. Those with a resistance of 6–8 units/m^2 are evaluated individually. However, more recent experience suggests that full repair can be achieved with good long-term outcome, including regression of pulmonary hypertension, even when initial pulmonary resistances calculations show levels of 10–20 U/m^2. Consequently, with general improvements in preoperative and postoperative care and the availability of pulmonary vasoactive agents, palliative procedures are less indicated.

When ASO is performed beyond 3 years of age, the pulmonary vascular disease is rarely completely reversible, resulting in a high mortality. Thus in our clinical practice, an appropriate VSD fenestration is strongly indicated in patients older than 3 years.

Indication for Neo-aortic Sinotubular Junction Reconstruction

Pulmonary trunk dilation is certainly considered as an important cause for postoperative neo-aortic regurgitation. Neo-aortic sinotubular junction reconstruction is regularly performed in our institution when the diameter ratio between aortic and pulmonary trunk less than 1:1.6–2.0. For patients who undergo ASO beyond 6 months of age, simple neo-aortic wall folding at the sinotubular junction level (Figs. 16.4 and 16.5) is usually indicated. Moreover, preoperative pulmonary valve regurgitation may be seen in patients older than 3 years, thus additional valve annulus plasty is considered.

Check List Prior to Surgery for Late TGA-VSD >6 Months

- Age at repair
- VSD diameter and location
- Great vessels diameter mismatch
- Pulmonary artery hypertension and pulmonary vascular resistance
- Annulus and morphology of the pulmonary valve
- Complex coronary anatomy
- Aortic arch obstruction
- Anatomy of atrioventricular valves

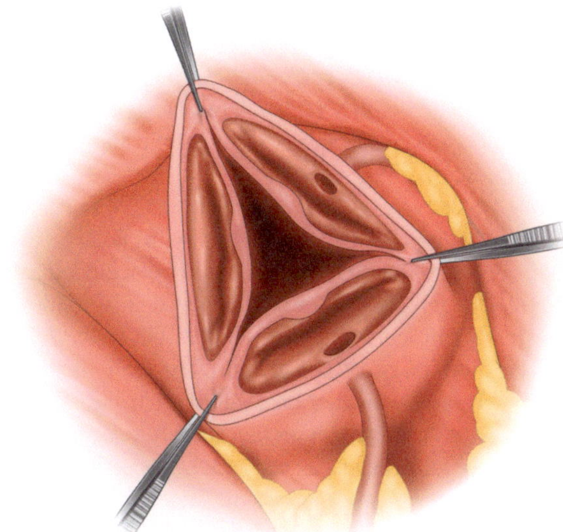

Fig. 16.4 Neo-aortic sinotubular junction plasty. Before plasty

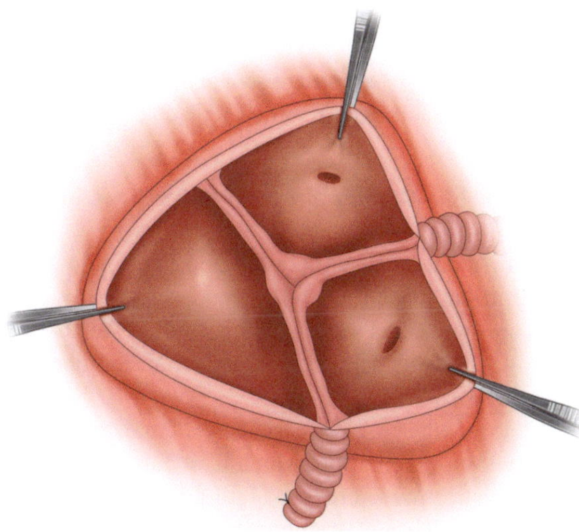

Fig. 16.5 Neo-aortic sinotubular junction plasty. After fold the aortic wall at the level of sinotubular junction

Surgical Technique

The differentiations between "early" and "late" ASO for TGA-VSD mainly regard the pathophysiology of pulmonary vascular disease and great vessels discrepancy. So we will only discuss these specific issues. ASO techniques have been described in previous chapters.

VSD Patch Fenestration

When severe PVOD is suspected, the patients will benefit from a palliative arterial switch operation with VSD patch fenestration [35]. Decision to size the fenestration is based on one half of the expected aortic annulus diameter that is large enough to decompress the right ventricle.

In patients without valved VSD patch, when a sizable and stable left-to-right shunt is defined by echocardiography, indicating a regression of the pulmonary artery pressure, the fenestration could be occluded safely using interventional procedure. The indications for percutaneous closure [36] are (1) stable hemodynamics and good ventricular function and (2) persistent left-to-right shunt and estimated systolic pulmonary arterial pressure less than 50 mmHg.

In patients with unidirectional valved patch, the valve closes itself off [37, 38] allowing unidirectional flow only, preventing any left-to-right shunt. Hence, the burden of an additional procedure can be avoided [39]. Using this kind of technique, the VSD was approached through the right atrium. After inspecting the VSD, the unidirectional valved patch is prepared. A Dacron patch to match the width of the defect and approximately 1.5 times longer than the desired length is chosen, and a suitable fenestration is made using standard aortic punch. The patch is then folded on itself in such a way that after it is folded, the dimensions are adequate for closure of the septal defect. The flap created by the folding of the patch should cover the fenestration. The patch is then sutured to the edges of the septal defect using interrupted or continuous sutures in such a way that the flap lies toward the left ventricular apex to avoid left ventricular outflow tract obstruction.

Neo-aortic Sinotubular Junction Reconstruction

When the diameter ratio between aorta and pulmonary trunk is less than 1.6–2.0, neo-aortic sinotubular junction remodeling may be added to decrease the regurgitation. The goal of this technique, i.e. folding the aortic wall at the level of sinotubular, is to ensure that the ratio of diameter at sinotubular junction to the aortic annulus is 0.8 (Figs. 16.4 and 16.5).

Moreover, the technique is more demanding in presence of pulmonary (neo-aortic) valve regurgitation, which is mainly secondary to the annulus dilatation. In our experience, we prefer to suture a prosthetic (Gore-Tex) ring onto the valvular annulus in addition to simply folding the sinotubular junction. Sixteen to 18 mm prosthetic ring implantation is recommended for patients who are older than 3 years. However, we suggest that partial anuloplasty using a segmental prosthetic ring is advisable for infants and young children.

Medications to Reduce Pulmonary Pressure

There is obviously a role for drugs like Bosentan or Sildenafil in reducing the pulmonary pressures and pulmonary vascular resistance both preoperatively and postoperatively. However, for many reasons, there is no specific protocol at this time for using these drugs properly. Although the optimal duration of this therapy is uncertain, Bosentan, Sildenafil or in combination was utilized postoperatively in further reducing pulmonary arterial pressure and avoiding pulmonary hypertension crisis. Retrospective cohort studies, randomized control trials and other clinical studies are desirable to provide sufficient evidence in guidelines making.

Outcomes

Outcomes of ASO

In the author's institution, the early mortality rate was 5 % among a total cohort of 173 TGA-VSD patients who underwent arterial switch from 2003 to 2012. Among the 121 patients who underwent ASO beyond the age of 6 months, 52 patients who underwent ASO between the age at 6 months and 1 year achieved favorable outcomes. However, the outcomes of 35 patients who underwent ASO beyond the age at 3 years were obviously suboptimal, with a high mortality (35.5 %). In the multivariate analysis of this cohort, higher pre-operative pulmonary artery pressure was identified as a potent predictor for late mortality (unpublished data). In a subgroup analysis, it was concluded that patients with mean pulmonary artery pressure less than 50 mmHg could achieve satisfying results after an ASO. However, even though the operation can decrease pulmonary artery pressure, patients with preoperative mean pulmonary artery pressure greater than 50 mmHg still suffered from high midterm mortality.

Most long-term death is correlated with pulmonary arterial hypertension crisis [40]. Unsurprisingly, majority of death occur within the first year after anatomical repair. Compliance of oral drugs therapy targeting PVOD is essential to maintain an uneventful postoperative course [41].

Neo-aortic Regurgitation

For patients with unrestrictive VSD, especially who referred late, the pulmonary (neo-aortic) valve is continuously exposed in a high pulmonary pressure, resulting in numerous histopathological changes. Moreover, pulmonary (neo-aortic) root dilation usually associated, substantially enlarge the valve annulus. For these mechanisms, neo-aortic regurgitation after arterial switch is more commonly seen in TGA-VSD than simple TGA [16, 42, 43].

In our experience, at 5 years follow up the incidence of at least moderate neo-aortic regurgitation is between 10 and 20 %. Unsurprisingly, higher age at repair, as a continuous variable, was identified as an independent predictor for neo-aortic regurgitation in multivariate analysis (unpublished data). At 3 years follow-up, moderate or severe neo-aortic regurgitation was noted in 5.8 % patients who underwent ASO between the age at 6 months and 1 year, as well as in 8.0 % patients who underwent ASO between the age at 6 months and 3 years. However, among the 31 survivors who underwent anatomical repair beyond the age at 3 years, eight (26 %) of them developed a significant neo-aortic regurgitation.

In the author's institution, a prospective randomized control trial was conducted to investigate the outcomes of neo-aortic sinotubular junction plasty. Both the hospital mortality and the incidence of neo-aortic regurgitation were lower in the patients who underwent additional sinotubular junction plasty.

Outcomes of Palliative ASO

Hospital mortality rates after palliative arterial switch have been favorable (0–14.3 %). The improvement in arterial oxygen saturation and quality of life in selected patients with TGA-VSD and severe PVOD is significant. Lei et al. [12] evaluated a group of 21 consecutive patients who had undergone palliative arterial switch operation. Mean postoperative systemic arterial oxygen saturation increased significantly. One late death occurred 3 months after surgery. Early death occurs in three patients. In their series, except the two patients early in their learning curve whose VSD were left open, all the other patients had their VSD closed using both surgical and interventional approach.

References

1. Tobler D, Williams WG, Jegatheeswaran A, Van Arsdell GS, McCrindle BW, Greutmann M, et al. Cardiac outcomes in young adult survivors of the arterial switch operation for transposition of the great arteries. J Am Coll Cardiol. 2010;56(1):58–64.
2. Huhta JC, Edwards WD, Feldt RH, Puga FJ. Left ventricular wall thickness in complete transposition of the great arteries. J Thorac Cardiovasc Surg. 1982;84:97–101.
3. Maroto E, Fouron JC, Douste-Blazy MY, Carceller AM, van Doesburg N, Kratz C, et al. Influence of age on wall thickness, cavity dimensions and myocardial contractility of the left ventricle in simple transposition of the great arteries. Circulation. 1983;67:1311–7.
4. Yacoub MH, Radley-Smith R, Maclaurin R. Two-stage operation for anatomical correction of transposition of the great arteries with intact interventricular septum. Lancet. 1977;1(8025):1275–8.
5. Devereux RB, Alonso DR, Lutas EM, Gottlieb GJ, Campo E, Sachs I, et al. Echocardiography assessment of LV hypertrophy: comparison to necropsy findings. Am J Cardiol. 1986;57:450–8.
6. Lacour-Gayet F, Piot D, Zoghbi J, Serraf A, Gruber P, Mace L, et al. Surgical management and indication of left ventricular retraining in arterial switch for transposition of the great arteries with intact ventricular septum. Eur J Cardiothorac Surg. 2001;20(4):824–9.
7. Ma K, Hua Z, Yang K, Hu S, Lacour-Gayet F, Yan J, et al. Arterial switch for transposed great vessels with intact ventricular septum beyond one month of age. Ann Thorac Surg. 2013. doi:10.1016/j.athoracsur.2013.09.011.
8. Nikitin NP, Huan Loh P, de Silva R, Witte KK, Lukaschuk EI, Parker A, et al. Left ventricular morphology, global and longitudinal function in normal older individuals: a cardiac magnetic resonance study. Int J Cardiol. 2006;108:76–83.
9. Wood PW, Choy JB, Nanda NC, Becher H. Left ventricular ejection fraction and volumes: it depends on the imaging method. Echocardiography. 2014;31(1):87–100.

10. Kang N, de Leval MR, Elliott M, Tsang V, Kocyildirim E, Sehic I, et al. Extending the boundaries of the primary arterial switch operation in patients with transposition of the great arteries and intact ventricular septum. Circulation. 2004;110(11 Suppl 1):I123–7.
11. Foran JP, Sullivan ID, Elliott MJ, de Leval MR. Primary arterial switch operation for transposition of the great arteries with intact ventricular septum in infants older than 21 days. J Am Coll Cardiol. 1998;31:883–9.
12. Davis AM, Wilkinson JL, Karl TR, Mee RB. Transposition of the great arteries with intact interventricular septum. Arterial switch repair in patients 21 days of age or older. J Thorac Cardiovasc Surg. 1993;106:111–5.
13. Sarris GE, Chatzis AC, Giannopoulos NM, et al. The arterial switch operation in Europe for transposition of the great arteries: a multi-institutional study from the European Congenital Heart Surgeons Association. J Thorac Cardiovasc Surg. 2006;132:633–9.
14. Jonas RA, Giglia TM, Sanders SP, Wernovsky G, Nadal-Ginard B, Mayer Jr JE, et al. Rapid, two-stage arterial switch for transposition of the great arteries and intact ventricular septum beyond the neonatal period. Circulation. 1989;80:I203–8.
15. Boutin C, Jonas RA, Sanders SP, Wernovsky G, Mone SM, Colan SD. Rapid two-stage arterial switch operation. Acquisition of left ventricular mass after pulmonary artery banding in infants with transposition of the great arteries. Circulation. 1994;90:1304–9.
16. Schwartz ML, Gauvreau K, Del NP, Mayer JE, Colan SD. Long-term predictors of aortic root dilation and aortic regurgitation after arterial switch operation. Circulation. 2004;110(11 Suppl 1):I128–32.
17. Poirier NC, Mee RB. Left ventricular reconditioning and anatomical correction for systemic right ventricular dysfunction. Semin Thorac Cardiovasc Surg. 2000;3:198–215.
18. Bonnet D, Corno AF, Sidi D, Sekarski N, Beghetti M, Schulze-Neick I, et al. Early clinical results of the telemetric adjustable pulmonary artery banding FloWatch-PAB. Circulation. 2004;110 Suppl 1:II158–63.
19. Corno AF, Prosi M, Fridez P, Zunino P, Quarteroni A, von Segesser LK. The non-circular shape of FloWatch-PAB prevents the need for pulmonary artery reconstruction after banding. Computational fluid dynamics and clinical correlations. Eur J Cardiothorac Surg. 2006;29:93–9.
20. Dibardino DJ, Kleeman K, Bove EL. A method of transcutaneously adjustable pulmonary artery banding for staged left ventricular retraining. J Thorac Cardiovasc Surg. 2012;144:553–6.
21. Sekarski N, Hurni M, von Segesser LK, Meijboom EJ, Di Bernardo S. Adaptable pulmonary artery band for late arterial switch procedure in transposition of the great arteries. Ann Thorac Surg. 2012;94:1311–6.
22. Norwood WI, Dobell AR, Freed MD, Kirklin JW, Blackstone EH. Intermediate results of the arterial switch repair. J Thorac Cardiovasc Surg. 1988;96:854–62.
23. Khairy P, Clair M, Fernandes SM, Blume ED, Powell AJ, Newburger JW, et al. Cardiovascular outcomes after the arterial switch operation for D-transposition of the great arteries. Circulation. 2013;127(3):331–9.
24. Lalezari S, Bruggemans EF, Blom NA, Hazekamp MG. Thirty-year experience with the arterial switch operation. Ann Thorac Surg. 2011;92(3):973–9.
25. Kirklin JW, Blackstone EH, Tchervenkov CI, Castaneda AR. Clinical outcomes after the arterial switch operation for transposition. Patient, support, procedural, and institutional risk factors. Circulation. 1992;86:1501–15.
26. Newfeld EA, Paul MH, Muster AJ, Idriss FS. Pulmonary vascular disease in transposition of the great vessels and intact ventricular septum. Circulation. 1979;59(3):525–30.
27. Pan X, Zheng Z, Hu S, Li S, Wei Y, Zhang Y, et al. Mechanisms of pulmonary hypertension related to ventricular septal defect in congenital heart disease. Ann Thorac Surg. 2011;92(6):2215–20.
28. Hänze J, Weissmann N, Grimminger F, Seeger W, Rose F. Cellular and molecular mechanisms of hypoxia-inducible factor driven vascular remodeling. Thromb Haemost. 2007;97:774–87.
29. Lehoux S, Lemarié CA, Esposito B, Lijnen HR, Tedgui A. Pressure-induced matrix metalloproteinase-9 contributes to early hypertensive remodeling. Circulation. 2004;109:1041–7.

30. Nakajima Y, Momma K, Seguchi M, Nakazawa M, Imai Y. Pulmonary hypertension in patients with complete transposition of the great arteries: midterm results after surgery. Pediatr Cardiol. 1996;17(2):104–7.
31. Ferencz C. Transposition of the great vessels. Pathophysiologic considerations based upon a study of the lungs. Circulation. 1966;33:232.
32. Newfeld EA, Paul MM, Muster AJ, Idriss FS. Pulmonary vascular disease in complete transposition of the great arteries: a study of 200 patients. Am J Cardiol. 1974;34:75–82.
33. Wagenvoort CA, Nauta J, van der Schaar PJ, Weeda HW, Wagenvoort N. The pulmonary vasculature in complete transposition of the great vessels, judged from lung biopsies. Circulation. 1968;38:746–54.
34. Bush A, Busst CM, Knight WB, Carvalho JS, Rigby ML, Shinebourne EA. Preoperative measurement of pulmonary vascular resistance in complete transposition of the great arteries. Br Heart J. 1990;63(5):300–3.
35. Burkhart HM, Dearani JA, Williams WG, Puga FJ, Mair DD, Ashburn DA, et al. Late results of palliative atrial switch for transposition, ventricular septal defect and pulmonary vascular obstructive disease. Ann Thorac Surg. 2004;77(2):464–9.
36. Lei BF, Chen JM, Cen JZ, Lui RC, Ding YQ, Xu G, et al. Palliative arterial switch for transposition of the great arteries, ventricular septal defect, and pulmonary vascular obstructive disease: midterm outcomes. J Thorac Cardiovasc Surg. 2010;140(4):845–9.
37. Novick WM, Sandoval N, Lazorhysynets VV, Castillo V, Baskevitch A, Mo X, et al. Flap valve double patch closure of ventricular septal defects in children with increased pulmonary vascular resistance. Ann Thorac Surg. 2005;79(1):21–8.
38. Talwar S, Choudhary SK, Nair VV, Chauhan S, Kothari SS, Juneja R, et al. Arterial switch operation with unidirectional valved patch closure of ventricular septal defect in patients with transposition of great arteries and severe pulmonary hypertension. World J Pediatr Congenit Heart Surg. 2012;3(1):21–5.
39. Choudhary SK, Talwar S, Airan B. A simple technique of unidirectional valved patch for closure of septal defects. J Thorac Cardiovasc Surg. 2007;134(5):1357–8.
40. Fan H, Hu S, Zheng Z, Li S, Zhang Y, Pan X, et al. Do patients with complete transposition of the great arteries and severe pulmonary hypertension benefit from an arterial switch operation? Ann Thorac Surg. 2011;91(1):181–6.
41. Nemoto S, Sasaki T, Ozawa H, Katsumata T, Kishi K, Okumura K, et al. Oral sildenafil for persistent pulmonary hypertension early after congenital cardiac surgery in children. Eur J Cardiothorac Surg. 2010;38(1):71–7.
42. Pan X, Hu S, Li S, Zheng Z, Wang Y, Zhang Y, et al. Predictors for late insufficiency of the neo-aortic valve after the switch procedure. J Heart Valve Dis. 2010;19(6):731–5.
43. Losay J, Touchot A, Capderou A, Piot JD, Belli E, Planche C, Serraf A. Aortic valve regurgitation after arterial switch operation for transposition of the great arteries: incidence, risk factors, and outcome. J Am Coll Cardiol. 2006;47(10):2057–62.

Chapter 17
TGA-VSD and LVOTO: Rastelli Procedure

Christian Kreutzer

Abstract The Rastelli procedure has been, for the last 45 years, the most common technique used for the surgical treatment of transposition of the great arteries (TGA), ventricular septal defect (VSD, and left ventricular outflow tract obstruction (LVOTO). The fundamental parts of the procedure are the baffling of the VSD to the aorta and the reconstruction of the right ventricle outflow tract (RVOT). In spite of low early morbidity and mortality (M/M), substantial late M/M has been reported due to left and right sided obstruction with a late survival of only 48 % at 20 years follow up. Indications of alternative procedures such as Arterial Switch operation with LVOTO resection, the REV procedure and aortic translocation procedure have been described with the aim of improving late survival. In the same way, modifications of the original Rastelli technique have been postulated to diminish such fate. These include improving patient selection by meticulous anatomic diagnosis, early repair and avoidance of long standing palliative systemic to pulmonary shunts, routine enlargement of the VSD by resection of the conal septum, and use of fresh pericardial valved conduits in the pulmonary position. In conclusion, the Rastelli procedure still provides excellent early and late results in selected patients with TGA-VSD and LVOT obstruction.

Keywords TGA • Rastelli operation • Arterial switch • Congenital heart surgery • Cardiac surgery

Introduction

Giancarlo Rastelli [1] was a bright young Italian cardiac surgeon who devised extraordinary contributions to the field of congenital heart disease from common AV canal to conotruncal malformations. After graduating from the University of Parma, Dr Rastelli was granted a North Atlantic Treaty Organization (NATO) scholarship in 1961, which allowed him a fellowship in cardiac surgery at the Mayo Clinic, under the mentorship of pioneer John W. Kirklin. During his 9 years there, Rastelli participated in the

C. Kreutzer, MD
Department of Pediatric Cardiac Surgery, Hospital Universitario Austral, Pilar, Province of Buenos Aires, Argentina
e-mail: ckreutze@cas.austral.edu.ar

F. Lacour-Gayet et al. (eds.), *Surgery of Conotruncal Anomalies*,
DOI 10.1007/978-3-319-23057-3_17

cardiac catheterization laboratories as well as the surgical ward and was eventually appointed as the Head of the cardiovascular research laboratory.

In 1968, Rastelli described the most commonly performed procedure for TGA, VSD and LVOTO, the Rastelli procedure. In the original description, the procedure involved baffling of the VSD to the aorta and connection of the right ventricle to the pulmonary arteries with a homograft conduit. The first operation was performed by Dr. Robert B. Wallace in July, 1968 and soon after published as a milestone paper [2]. This operation was the first ever described with the theoretic advantage of incorporating the left ventricle into the systemic circulation for correction of TGA, and it was widely applied to treat this subset of patients. Its use was also expanded to other anatomic variants of TGA, such as TGA and VSD without pulmonary stenosis as well as double-outlet right ventricle (DORV) until the arterial switch operation (ASO) emerged in 1975. Dr Rastelli died prematurely from Hodgkin's Disease at the age of 36 years, but his legacy of outstanding contributions remains celebrated worldwide in the congenital heart surgery community.

Anatomy

Left ventricular ouflow tract obstruction (LVOTO) is present in 20 % of cases of TGA with VSD [3]. The ventricular septal defect is single and subaortic or conoventricular in the vast majority of patients, with malalignement of the conal septum producing posterior deviation, resulting in a tunnel-like narrowing of the left ventricular outlow (LVOT) that increases with time. The VSD is usually non restrictive, however enlargement at the time of the Rastelli procedure is generally performed, since the defect may become restrictive after biventricular repair because of a decrease in left ventricular volume load [4]. Other types of VSDs such as the atrioventricular canal type may be present. Inlet extension of the subaortic VSD is present in 4 % of cases. Multiple VSDs rare and located in the muscular and apical portions of the septum [5].

Typically, the ventricles are well balanced. However, a hypoplastic LV or RV might be present particularly in patients with AV valve abnormalities such as straddling or overriding.

The pulmonary valve is often bicuspid and the annulus hypoplastic. However, in almost one third of the cases the pulmonary valve and annulus are normal. In one report [5], 18 % of patients with TGA-VSD, and LVOTO had no anatomic LVOTO when they were newborn infants. Furthermore, 29 % had a normal pulmonary valve.

Anomalies of the tricuspid valve are common, especially in cases with remote VSD, and include abnormal attachments and straddling valves in 5 % of the cases. These anatomic variants are important because these attachments may interfere in baffling the VSD from the LV to the aorta. These abnormalities have been described as a risk factor for early and late mortality after the Rastelli procedure [5].

The diagnostic landmarks that differentiate d-TGA from DORV are the presence, in DORV, of a subaortic and subpulmonary conus with absence of continuity between the mitral and pulmonary valves as well as alignment of the pulmonary root relative to the ventricular septum [6].

Diagnosis and Imaging

Preoperative evaluation requires a thorough understanding of the intracardiac, great vessels and coronary anatomy. Echocardiographic examination is adequate in most cases, although in special circumstances a cardiac catheterization might be required. These circumstances include presence of a previous systemic to pulmonary artery shunt to rule out pulmonary artery distortion and stenoses, aorto-pulmonary collaterals, unclear coronary anatomy and increased pulmonary vascular resistance. A complete Doppler echocardiogram is performed to examine the volume of the ventricles, VSD size and location relative to the position of the great vessels, and the anatomy of the pulmonary root, including leaflet characteristics and annulus size. Echocardiography is also useful to describe coronary artery anatomy and abnormal AV valve attachments. Preparing a check list is important in determining clear indications for the Rastelli procedure.

Check List

- Appropriate LV and RV volume.
- VSD location and size (subaortic, inlet extension, AV canal type). Multiple VSD
- AV valve morphology.
  - AV valve straddling and overriding
  - Abnormal tricuspid chordae insertion onto conal septum
  - Accessory AV valve tissue protruding in LVOT
- Pulmonary valve morphology.
  - Leaflet anatomy (bicuspid, tricuspid).
  - Pulmonary annulus diameter
  - Pulmonary branches. (stenosis post BT shunt, hypoplasia)
- LVOT obstruction mechanisms

Indications and Surgical Technique in the Current Area

Indications

Current early and late results with the arterial switch in TGA and VSD are excellent with a late survival of more than 90 % at 20 years; therefore, the arterial switch operation is the procedure of choice for those forms of TGA with LVOT obstruction amenable to subaortic resection. An early ASO eliminates dynamic LVOT gradients commonly seen in TGA and VSD by connecting the LV to the systemic circulation. It is important at the time of the repair to examine the pulmonary valve, since the presence of a mildly stenotic bicuspid valve *is not* a contraindication for an arterial switch repair. The presence of anatomic features that may produce LVOTO by a different mechanism, such as small left ventricular–pulmonary junction and abnormal mitral valve attachments, will not be influenced by an early arterial switch operation. A cleft mitral valve, abnormal papillary muscle or valve attachment to the conal septum, and accessory mitral valve tissue are anatomic features that will not be affected by a dynamic element. In a series of 43 patients with TGA/VSD and LVOTO, Belli and colleagues [6] have concluded that a "lower preoperative pulmonary valve z-score and complex multilevel atrioventricular valve-related LVOTO are independent predictors of recurrent LVOTO and LVOT reoperation. TGA/ LVOTO patients with pulmonary valve z-score exceeding −1.8 and resectable valvular or subvalvular LVOTO, or both, should be candidates for ASO, regardless of the severity of the LVOT peak gradient" [7].

When the LVOTO is fixed the arterial switch is contraindicated and therefore a Rastelli procedure or other form of VSD baffling to aorta, such as a REV [8] or an aortic root translocation [9] may be performed.

In this matter it is imperative to note that the size of the left ventricular–pulmonary junction is of much importance in the selection of the procedure. Performance of a Rastelli procedure in patients with a moderately stenotic pulmonary annulus results in malalignement of the neo-LVOT, since it is standing anteriorly to the RVOT resulting in a long, tortuous baffle that may contribute to the late development of LVOTO. Complete resection of the conal septum was described as a fundamental step in the REV operation with the aim of eliminating this potential complication [10]. Moreover, moderate pulmonary annular stenosis is the optimal scenario for the aortic root translocation procedure, because the root moves posteriorly with better alignment in the LVOT without the need for a large prosthetic patch. This may improve long-term left ventricular function and decreases the substrate for ventricular arrhythmias.

In addition, aortic root translocation may be indicated in cases with TGA and LVOTO with a remote VSD.

Correspondingly, a severely hypoplastic annulus and/or pulmonary atresia are the optimal anatomic settings for constructing the LVOT by using the Rastelli procedure.

Finally, when a reparative biventricular procedure for TGA is likely to be complicated due to morphologic risk factors, (hypoplastic RV or LV, non-committed or multiple VSD's, abnormal AV valve septal attachments) alternative procedures such as one and a half ventricle repair, or a Fontan-Kreutzer procedure should be considered. As reported by de Leval, [11] a high-risk biventricular repair is not always preferable to a single ventricle repair in terms late morbidity and mortality.

The optimal age for the performance of a Rastelli repair remains controversial. Palliation with a systemic to pulmonary artery shunt allows for the performance of Rastelli repair at an older age with larger conduits, therefore reducing the need for reoperations.

In summary, the optimal setting for a Rastelli procedure is: balanced ventricles, severe pulmonary annular stenosis or atresia, subaortic conoventricular VSD, and normal AV valve anatomy.

Surgical Technique

Through a median sternotomy the thymus is excised. If the use of a pericardial valved conduit is planned [12], the pericardium is dissected free from left to right phrenic nerves. With the aid of a ruler, measurements are performed to prepare a conduit according to the body surface area of the patient (Table 17.1), a portion of the pericardium is harvested and the conduit is constructed by another surgeon (Fig. 17.1).

If a homograft or a heterograft is preferred the pericardium is opened in the usual fashion and a small rectangular piece is resected for hood augmentation of the proximal anastomosis of the conduit. After standard bicaval cannulation, CPB is conducted under mild hypothermia, with myocardial protection insured by crystalloid cardioplegia.

A transverse incision is made in the pulmonary artery at the level of the bifurcation (Fig. 17.2) to examine the pulmonary valve. If the pulmonary valve is considered adequate for an arterial switch, the Rastelli procedure is abandoned, and preparation for an ASO with VSD closure and LVOTO resection is commenced.

If the pulmonary valve is not suitable to function as the systemic semilunar valve, the Rastelli technique is performed. The site of the right ventriculotomy is carefully selected to avoid sternal compression of the conduit. It is important to emphasize that the ventriculotomy should be performed *as leftward as possible very close to the anterior descending coronary artery*. The VSD is explored and a VSD enlargement by complete resection of the conal septum [8] is carried out almost always to prevent late LVOT obstruction since the LV to aorta baffle may become restrictive after volume unloading [4, 5, 13, 14] (Fig. 17.3). A pledgeted traction suture at the crest of the conal septum and introduction of a Hegar dilator in the left ventricular cavity through the pulmonary valve may facilitate the resection.

The main pulmonary artery is transected and over sewn, incorporating the pulmonary valve, with a double running suture (Fig. 17.4a). In adolescents and adults it is advisable to reinforce this suture with pericardium. To construct the intracardiac baffle an oval piece of glutaraldehyde-treated autologous pericardium (preferred in newborns and infants) or a 0.6-mm thick Gore-Tex patch (W.L. Gore and Associates, Flagstaff, Arizona) (for older children) is prepared. For adolescents and

Table 17.1 Size of the pericardium required according to the selected conduit diameter

Rectangle trapezoid				
D(mm)	Width (mm) (A–A′)	H of valves (h) a–a′	Lesser base (mm)	Wider base (mm)
10.0	31.4	10.0	31.4	35.0
12.0	38.0	11.0	38.0	42.0
14.0	44.0	12.5	44.0	48.5
16.0	51.0	13.5	51.0	56.0
18.0	56.5	15.0	56.5	62.0
20.0	63.0	16.0	63.0	69.0

adults, a section of a large Gore-tex conduit can be used as well. Continuous 6/0 polypropylene suture with a half circle 8 mm needle is favored in neonates and infants to suture the patch from the edges of the VSD to the aortic annulus. The suture line may go into the tricuspid septal leaflet annulus in cases in which a muscle band is not present. Special care is taken to avoid intramural residual VSD's, by

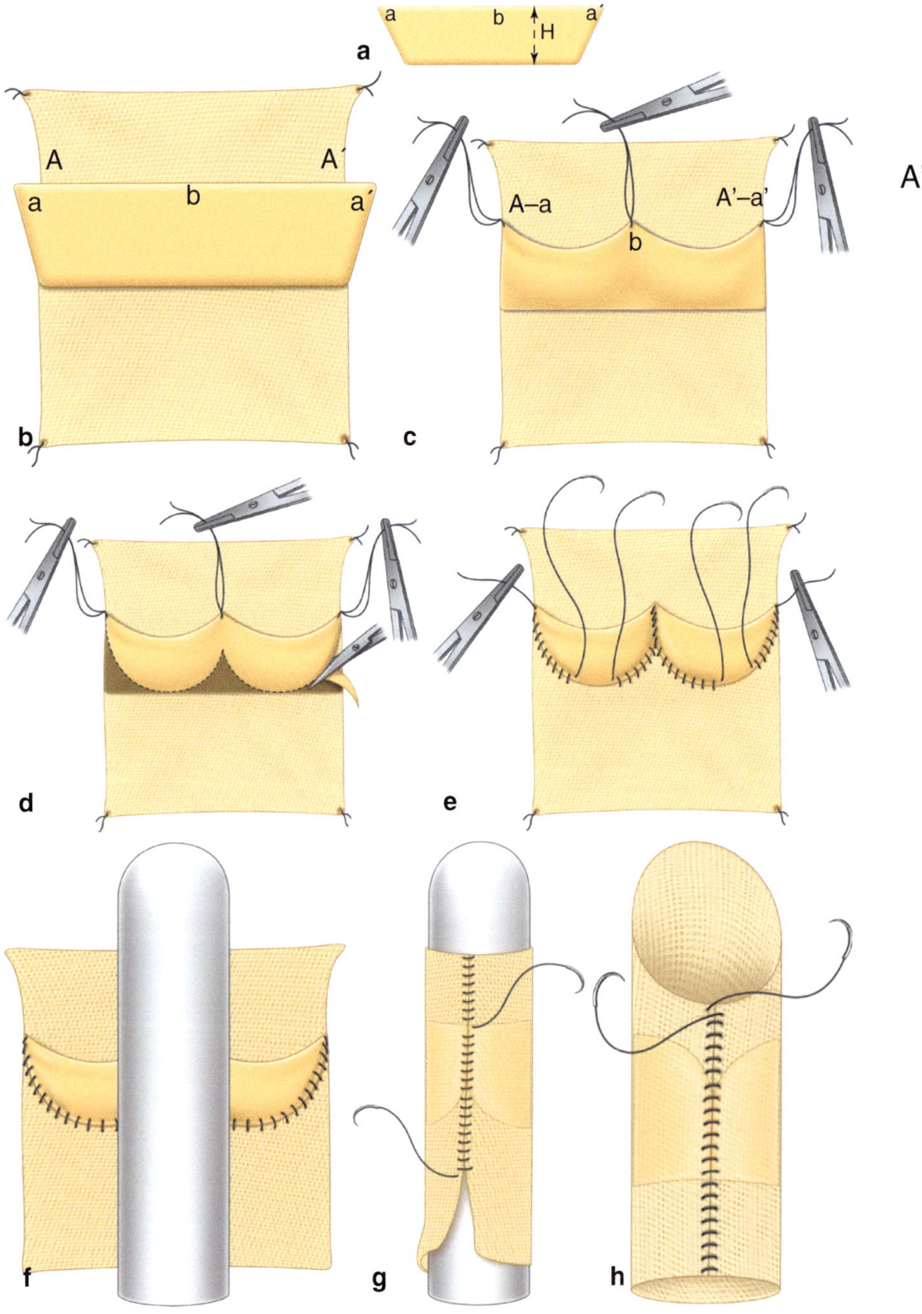

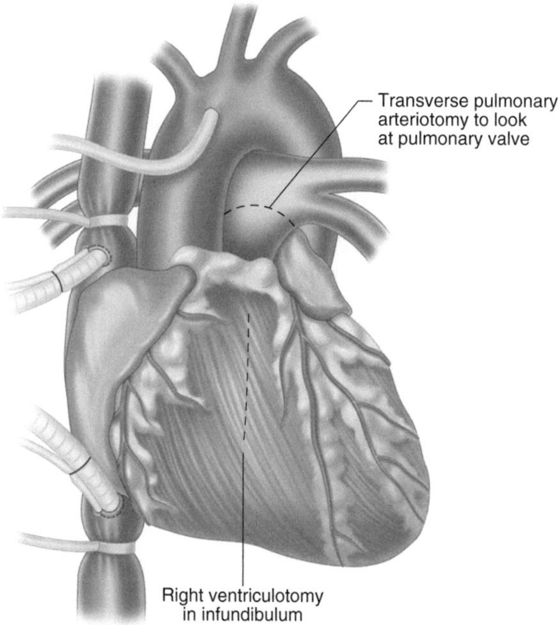

Fig. 17.2 The incisions in the pulmonary artery and right ventricle are highlighted in black dashes. The incision in the pulmonary artery allows inspection of the pulmonary valve to determine its suitability for use as a systemic semilunar valve and the performance of an arterial switch

suturing the patch close to the aortic "annulus." In older patients, standard 5/0 or 4/0 interrupted sutures are preferred. The patch should be wide enough to allow appropriate and not excessive bowing in RVOT (Fig. 17.4b).

RV to PA continuity is then established with the aid of a conduit that should be lying on the left away from the sternal wall (Fig. 17.5). We favor the use of a pericardial conduit in children above 3 months of life. Its use in neonates is not recommended because neonates suffer from increased pulmonary vascular resistance and,

Fig. 17.1 Surgical technique for autologous pericardial valved conduit construction: (**a**) pericardial trapezoid: *a–a′* is the wider base; *b* is the midpoint, and *H* is the height of the future valve (Table I). (**b**) pericardial rectangle (note the wider distal end): *A–A′* is the base of the rectangle; the trapezoid has been superimposed (note that the wider base of trapezoid [*a–a′*] is 10 % wider than the base of the rectangle *[A–A′]*). (**c**) Three double-armed sutures have been placed to secure the trapezoid to the rectangle at *A–a, A′–a′*, and *b* to the midpoint of the rectangle. (**d**) The form of the cusps is given by trimming the three triangles at the base of the trapezoid. (**e**) The running suture is performed from *A* and *A′*, suturing the trapezoid to the edge of the rectangle in the first 3 mm and then from *b* to secure the cusps to the rectangle (note that the first 3 mm of the suture stated at *b* is double). (**f**) The pericardial rectangle with the cusps is wrapped around the corresponding Hegar dilator. (**g**) The conduit is closed with a 6–0 double running suture. The suture is started at the distal end, and the proximal end remains untied. (**h**) The completed valved conduit

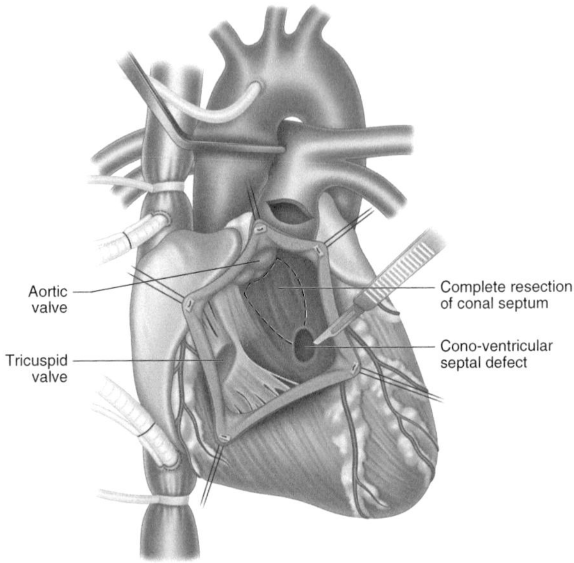

Fig. 17.3 The ventriculotomy appears larger than real for demonstration purposes. The *dotted lines* mark the resection of the conal septum, which is performed in almost all patients

therefore, a reliable competent pulmonary valve is necessary. After completion of the proximal and distal anastomoses the heart is deaired and the aortic cross clamp is removed. The patient is then weaned from cardiopulmonary by-pass in the usual fashion.

Outcomes

Several large series of Rastelli procedures have been reported, [5, 15, 16]. In all of these series the early mortality has been low, but all have shown substantial late morbidity and mortality (Fig. 17.6).

The group at Boston Children's [5] reported the results on 101 consecutive patients with TGA/VSD ± LVOTO and demonstrated disappointing late results of this procedure. Early mortality was 7 %, with no deaths in the last 7 years of the study. Complete AV block, ($p=0.004$), straddling tricuspid valve ($p=0.04$), use of a Carpentier Edwards conduit ($p=0.02$), and longer aortic cross clamping times ($p=0.04$) were identified as risk factors for early mortality. Late survival was only 52 % at 20 years, with 17 late deaths (five sudden) and one heart transplant. Most common causes of death included LV failure and arrhythmias. There was no difference in terms of late morbidity and mortality for decade of the study and age at repair. Freedom from RVOTO reintervention was 57 %, 53 %, 24 % and 21 % at 5, 10, 15 and 20 years, respectively. Risk factors for re-intervention included the per-

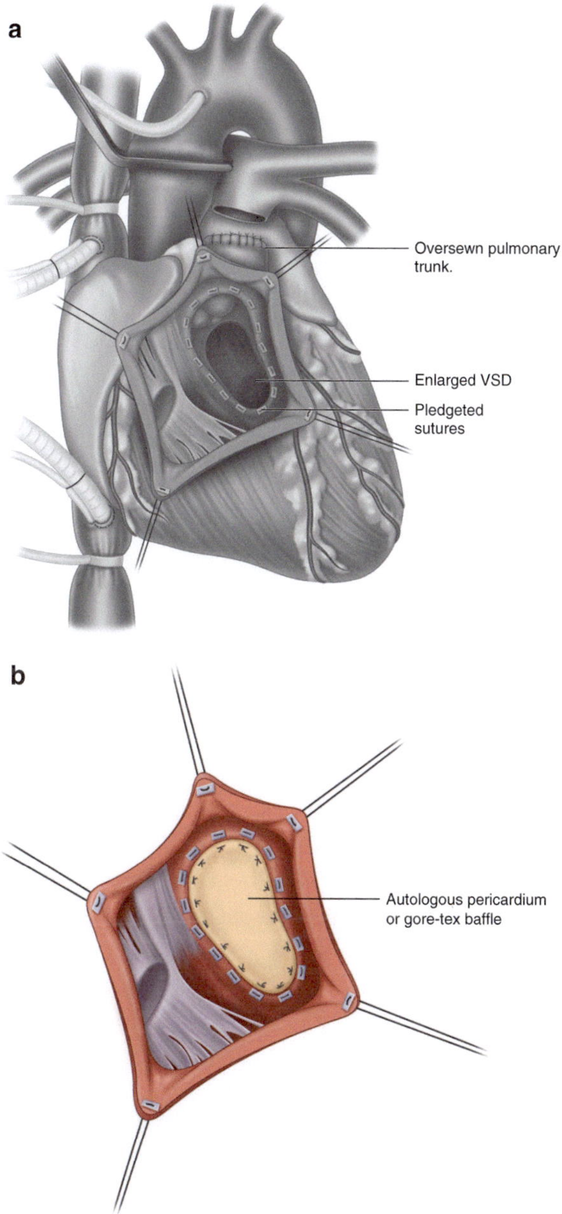

Fig. 17.4 (**a**) After oversewing the pulmonary trunk, the baffle from the LV to the aorta is constructed. A running suture (for infants) or pledgeted interrupted sutures (for older infants) are used to secure the pericardium or Gore-tex baffle. (**b**) The complete baffle should bow into the RV infundibulum

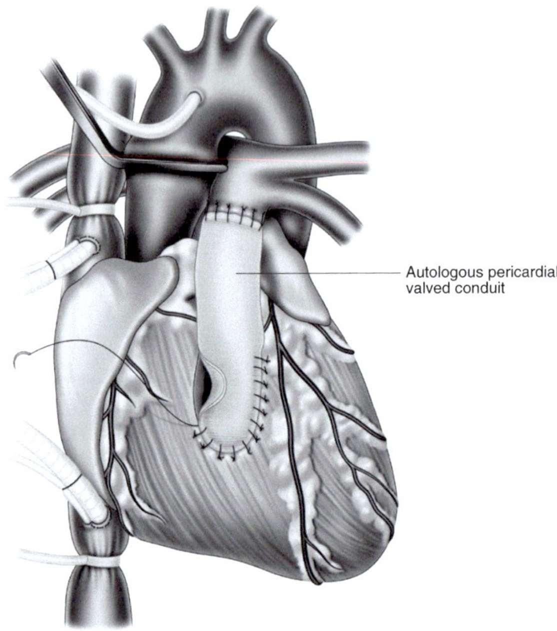

Fig. 17.5 Right ventricle to pulmonary artery continuity is established with the use of a conduit

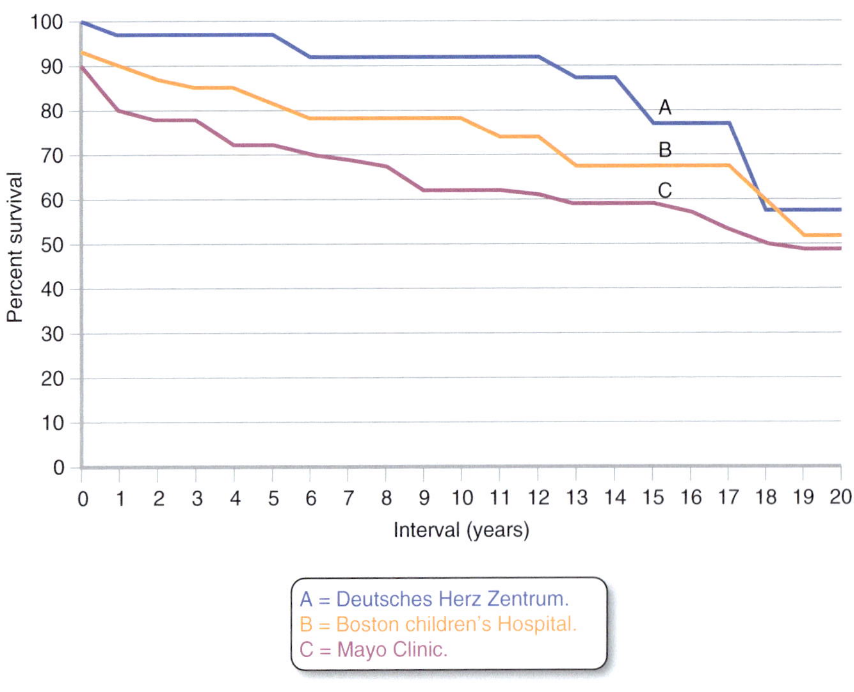

Fig. 17.6 Overall survival for Rastelli. *A* Deutsches Herz Zentrum. *B* Boston Children's Hospital. *C* Mayo Clinic

formance of the Rastelli procedure in infancy ($p=0.0001$), weight less than 9 kg at repair ($p=0.001$) and placement of the conduit to the right side of the aorta ($p=0.02$) (Fig. 17.7).

Freedom from LVOTO reintervention, was 88 %, 82 %, 82 % and 82 % 5, 10, 15 and 20 years, respectively. Risk factor for reintervention included absence of VSD enlargement at Rastelli ($p=0.02$), longer CPB time ($p=0.02$) and longer length of stay ($p=0.02$).

The Mayo Clinic study [15] is the largest published series encompassing more than 30 years of experience and 231 patients (Fig. 17.6). Early mortality was 10 %, but late survival only 48 % at 20 years. Again, the most common causes of death were arrhythmias and LV failure. Freedom from reintervention was only 18 % at 20 years.

Hörer published a 27-year experience with the Rastelli repair with 39 consecutive patients [16]. There was no early mortality. At a median follow-up of 8.9 years (range, 0–25 years), two patients died of sudden death, and two received heart transplantation. Freedom from death or transplantation was 93.8 ± 4.3 % and 57.5 ± 15.1 % at 10 and 20 years, respectively (Fig. 17.6). Freedom from conduit replacement was 48.8 ± 10.3 % and 32.5 ± 10.3 % at 10 and 20 years, respectively. Subvalvular and valvular left ventricular outflow tract obstruction ($p=.012$), peripheral pulmonary artery stenosis ($p<.001$), enlargement of the ventricular septal defect ($p=.030$), and longer ischemic time ($p=.015$) were predictive for death or transplantation. Patients younger than 4 years at repair demonstrated a trend toward a lower freedom from death or transplantation ($p=.068$), but needed significantly more conduit replacements ($p=.038$) compared with patients 4 years or older. In contrast to the Boston and Mayo Clinic studies, peripheral pulmonary stenosis appeared as a risk factor for

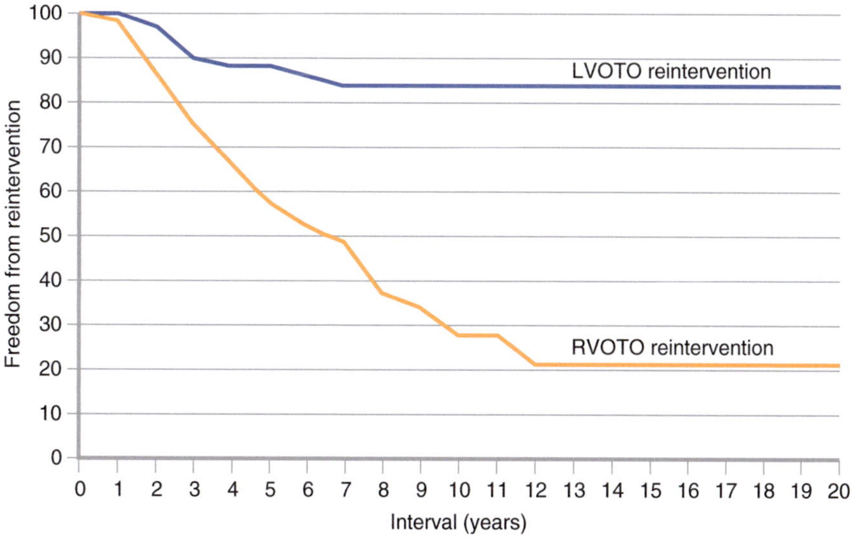

Fig. 17.7 Freedom from LVOTO and RVOTO reinterventions, Boston Children's Hospital Study

late death or transplant. Of note, peripheral pulmonary stenosis is rarely seen in TGA VSD and LVOTO at birth, and only develops as a complication of palliative systemic to pulmonary artery shunts.

Schlichter and Kreutzer [12, 17]. reported their experience with the Rastelli procedure utilizing fresh autologous pericardial valved conduits in 45 patients with an early mortality 16 % and a freedom from reoperation from conduit stenosis of 75 % at 10, 15 years and 20 years. These conduits have shown growth capacity and may exhibit viability as living tissue. In those conduits that were replaced, the pericardial tissue was normal at histological examination with two layers: a endothelized neointima and a fibrous layer with collagen and fibroblasts. The main disadvantage of this conduit is severe pulmonary regurgitation that appeared by 3 months after implantation.

Comments

The late outcome in terms of LVOT obstruction and LV dysfunction and its association with the absence of VSD enlargement at the time of the Rastelli, has motivated the modification of the surgical technique for VSD baffling. The routine resection of the conal septum as described by Lecompte [8] for the REV procedure has been widely adopted and its use produces a more “straight” and short LVOT. However it is important to differentiate REV and Rastelli. The RVOT reconstruction is established with a valved conduit in Rastelli and without conduit in REV, where the PA trunk is directly reimplanted following a Lecompte maneuver.

Most patients with TGA, VSD and LVOTO present cyanosis and/or heart failure soon after birth, therefore requiring surgical treatment. Palliation with a BT shunt allows delaying the repair and implanting a larger conduit at the time of the Rastelli procedure. However, palliation also leads to hemodynamic deterioration, pulmonary artery distortion, volume overload, and ongoing cyanosis. In the other hand early correction in the first month of life requires the use of small homografts, requiring early replacement typically in the second year of life [5]. Although correction early in life is our preferred method; palliation or correction for the symptomatic infant should be decided based on institutional policies, conduit availability, and experience of the unit with complex infant heart surgery.

The late results of the arterial switch for TGA and VSD are outstanding with late survival and freedom from reoperation above 90 % at 20 years. Therefore it is mandatory nowadays to perform an arterial switch whenever possible, including cases with mild pulmonary stenosis and/or bicuspid pulmonary valves. Although these valves may eventually fail in the systemic circulation, it seems preferable to have an aortic valve replacement in adulthood than multiple RV-PA conduit replacements, and multiple catheter interventions the first two decades of life and development of RV failure.

The aortic root translocation [18] is part of the surgical armamentarium in TGA-VSD and LVOTO. However one should be cautious in widespread indications of this procedure since there are only short series published without long term outcome. The main advantage of the aortic root translocation is a perfectly aligned LVOT. However, late aortic regurgitation has been reported and a longer follow up is requested [19].

In summary, the Rastelli operation is a low-risk procedure. Nevertheless, substantial late morbidity and mortality have been reported due to anatomical variations and surgical techniques. However, it is often possible to neutralize those variables in a subset of patients in whom the Rastelli procedure can be applied with excellent early and late results.

References

1. Squarcia U, Squarcia A. Giancarlo Rastelli: the scientist, the man. Clin Cardiol. 2007;30:485–7.
2. Rastelli GC, Wallace RB, Ongley PA. Complete repair of transposition of the great arteries with pulmonary stenosis: a review and report of a case corrected by using a new surgical technique. Circulation. 1969;39:83–95.
3. Castaneda AR, Jonas RA, Mayer JE, Hanley FL. D-transposition of the great arteries. In: Cardiac surgery of the neonate and infant. Philadelphia: WB Saunders; 1994.
4. Rychik J, Jacobs ML, Norwood WI. Early changes in ventricular geometry and ventricular septal defect size following Rastelli operation or intra-ventricular baffle repair for conotruncal anomaly: a cause for development of sub-aortic stenosis. Circulation. 1994;90(5 Pt 2):II13–9.
5. Kreutzer C, De Vivie J, Oppido G, Kreutzer J, Gauvreau K, Freed M, Mayer Jr JE, Jonas R, del Nido PJ. Twenty-five-year experience with Rastelli repair for transposition of the great arteries. J Thorac Cardiovasc Surg. 2000;120:211–23.
6. Pasquini L, Sanders SP, Parness IA, Colan SD, Van Praagh S, Mayer JE, et al. Conal anatomy in 119 patients with D-loop transposition of the great arteries and ventricular septal defect: an echocardiographic and pathologic study. J Am Coll Cardiol. 1993;21:1712–21.
7. Kalfa DM, Lambert V, Baruteau AE, Stos B, Houyel L, Garcia E, Ly M, Belli E. Arterial switch for transposition with left outflow tract obstruction: outcomes and risk analysis. Ann Thorac Surg. 2013;95(6):2097–103.
8. Lecompte Y, Neveux JY, Leca F, Zannini L, Tu TV, Buboys Y, et al. Reconstruction of the pulmonary outflow tract without a prosthetic conduit. J Thorac Cardiovasc Surg. 1982;84:727–33.
9. Nikaidoh H. Aortic translocation and biventricular outflow tract reconstruction: a new surgical repair for transposition of the great arteries associated with ventricular septal defect and pulmonary stenosis. J Thorac Cardiovasc Surg. 1984;88:365–72.
10. Lecompte Y. Rastelli repair for transposition of the great arteries: still the best choice? J Thorac Cardiovasc Surg. 2002;123(1):192–3.
11. Delius RE, Rademecker MA, de Leval MR, Elliott MJ, Stark J. Is a high-risk biventricular repair always preferable to conversion to a single ventricle repair? J Thorac Cardiovasc Surg. 1996;112(6):1561–8.
12. Kreutzer C, Kreutzer GO, De C, Mayorquim R, Roman MI, Vazquez H, Simon JL, Kreutzer EA, Schlichter AJ. Early and late results of fresh autologous pericardial valved conduit. Semin Thorac Cardiovasc Surg Pediatr Card Surg Annu. 1999;2:65–76.
13. Alsoufi B, Awan A, Al-Omrani A, Al-Ahmadi M, Canver CC, Bulbul Z, Kalloghlian A, Al-Halees Z. The Rastelli procedure for transposition of the great arteries: resection of the infundibular septum diminishes recurrent left ventricular outflow tract obstruction risk. Ann Thorac Surg. 2009;88(1):137–42.
14. Navabi MA, Shabanian R, Kiani A, Rahimzadeh M. The effect of ventricular septal defect enlargement on the outcome of Rastelli or Rastelli-type repair. J Thorac Cardiovasc Surg. 2009;138(2):390–6.

15. Dearani JA, Danielson GK, Puga FJ, Mair DD, Schleck CD. Late results of the Rastelli operation for transposition of the great arteries. Semin Thorac Cardiovasc Surg Pediatr Card Surg Annu. 2001;4:3–15.
16. Hörer J, Schreiber C, Dworak E, Cleuziou J, Prodan Z, Vogt M, Holper K, Lange R. Long term results after the Rastelli repair for transposition of the great arteries. Ann Thorac Surg. 2007;83(6):2169–75.
17. Kreutzer C, Blunda C, Kreutzer G, Schlichter AJ. The autologous pericardial valved conduit for right ventricular outflow tract reconstruction. Oper Tech Thorac Cardiovasc Surg. 2003;8(3):146–14.
18. Morell VO, Jacobs JP, Quintessenza JA. Aortic translocation in the management of transposition of the great arteries with ventricular septal defect and pulmonary stenosis: results and follow-up. Ann Thorac Surg. 2005;79:2089–92.
19. Prêtre R. Editorial comment: arterial switch, reparation a l'etage ventriculaire, Rastelli or Nikaidoh? Eur J Cardiothorac Surg. 2013;44:1094–5.

Chapter 18
TGA-VSD-LVOT Obstruction : REV (Réparation à l'Etage Ventriculaire) Procedure

Pascal R. Vouhé and Olivier Raisky

Abstract *Background:* Anomalies of the ventriculo-arterial connection with ventricular septal defect (VSD) and left ventricle outflow tract obstruction (LVOTO) are often repaired by using the Rastelli procedure. To obviate the main drawbacks of the Rastelli operation, Lecompte described in 1988 a new procedure called REV (Réparation à l'Etage Ventriculaire), which includes two major modifications: routine excision of the conal septum and reconstruction of the right ventricular outflow tract without conduit.

Technique: In all patients with a conal septum interposed between the VSD and the aortic orifice, the conal septum is excised extensively, even if the VSD is not restrictive; this allows the construction of a large and straight left ventricle-to-aorta tunnel. The pulmonary artery is reimplanted directly onto the right ventricle, typically after anterior translocation (French maneuver).

Indications: The REV operation is indicated in hearts characterized by malposition of the great arteries with a short (or absent) subpulmonary conus and a severe pulmonary outflow tract obstruction involving the pulmonary valve. In contrast, the presence of a remote VSD, abnormal insertion of the mitral valve and major abnormal insertions of the tricuspid valve on the conal septum are contraindications to a REV operation. Most of these latter malformations can be repaired using a Bex-Nikaidoh procedure. (See Chaps. 22 and 23)

Results: The current operative risk is low (<5 %). At 25 years, the probability of survival is 85 % whereas survival without reoperation is 45 %. In addition, the probability of reoperation for right ventricular outflow tract obstruction is 33 %, and for left ventricular outflow tract obstruction, 5 %.

Conclusions: The REV operation provides better results than the classical Rastelli procedure in terms of survival and need for reoperation for right or left ventricular outflow tract obstruction.

P.R. Vouhé, MD, PhD (✉) • O. Raisky, MD, PhD
Necker Hospital, Paris, France

Department of Pediatric Cardiac Surgery, APHP – Hôpital Universitaire Necker – Enfants Malades, University Paris Descartes, Sorbonne Paris Cité,
149 rue de Sèvres, Paris 75015, France
e-mail: pascal.vouhe@nck.aphp.fr

F. Lacour-Gayet et al. (eds.), *Surgery of Conotruncal Anomalies*,
DOI 10.1007/978-3-319-23057-3_18

Keywords Transposition of the great arteries • Malposition of the great arteries • REV procedure • Rastelli procedure

Introduction

Most anomalies of ventriculoarterial connection with ventricular septal defect (VSD) and pulmonary stenosis are repaired by use of the Rastelli operation. In the classic Rastelli procedure, the left ventricle is connected to the aorta through the VSD, which is enlarged anteriorly if needed, and an extracardiac valved conduit is used to connect the right ventricle to the pulmonary artery. Although this procedure represented a major breakthrough in the history of congenital heart surgery, the late results are not optimal (see Chap. 19). To reduce some of the adverse late consequences of the Rastelli operation (namely, need for reoperation on the right ventricular outflow tract (RVOT) and risk of subaortic stenosis), Lecompte published a new procedure in1988 [1] which includes two major modifications: routine excision of the conal septum and reconstruction of the RVOT without conduit insertion.

Lecompte called this procedure REV (for Réparation à l'Etage Ventriculaire), which means repair at the ventricular level. This was also a play on words, because the meaning of the French word "rêve" is "dream". However, this name introduced some confusion with the intraventricular repair procedure (IVR), a completely different operation.

Classification

The classification of anomalies of ventriculo-arterial connection remains a matter of debate. Between normal connection (characterized by mitral-aortic fibrous continuity, such as in tetralogy of Fallot) and classical transposition (with mitral-pulmonary continuity), there is a spectrum of malformations with two subarterial (subaortic and subpulmonary) conus and a VSD. The development of each conus is extremely variable from short or even absent to very long. Because of this variability, the VSD may be described as subaortic (short subaortic conus and long subpulmonary conus), subpulmonary (long subaortic conus and short subpulmonary conus), doubly-committed (two short conuses), and non-committed (two long conuses). This spectrum of malformations includes anomalies classically called double outlet right ventricle, double outlet left ventricle or complex transposition with VSD .

From a surgical point of view, it is more important to determine the optimal reparative procedure than to give a precise name to the malformation. With this concept in mind, it has been shown [2, 3] that two anatomic factors are paramount in the decision: the length of the subpulmonary conus and the anatomy of the pulmonary outflow tract (POT) [4]. A well-developed subpulmonary conus allows intraventricular repair, whatever the anatomy of the POT. On the contrary, a short subpulmonary conus, as seen in transposition where the subpulmonary conus is absent, prohibits IVR and indicates a surgical repair which is dependent on the anatomy of the POT. Our current decision tree is depicted in Table 18.1.

Imaging

The information which is necessary to plan the surgical procedure can almost always be provided by complete transthoracic echocardiographic evaluation alone. The echocardiographer should have extensive experience with the diagnosis and repair of conotruncal anomalies. Most importantly, the examination should be performed in the presence of the attending surgeon. The anatomy of the malformation should be fully delineated and the surgical repair carefully planned. Occasionally, other preoperative studies (transesophageal echocardiography, CT scan, MRI, cardiac catheterization) are necessary to define some features, such as anomalies of the atrioventricular valves, pulmonary artery anatomy, pulmonary vascular resistances or extracardiac anomalies. Preoperative work-up must be complete in order to avoid, as far as possible, unexpected intraoperative findings and the need for unplanned decisions.

Check-List

Feasibility of Biventricular Repair

size of both ventricles
major anomalies of atrioventricular valves (straddling)
multiple VSD's ("swiss-cheese")

Table 18.1 Surgical management of patients with anomalous ventriculoarterial connection and VSD

	"Long" subpulmonary conus (> aortic valve diameter)	"Short" subpulmonary conus (< aortic valve diameter)
Normal pulmonary outflow tract	IVR	Arterial switch
Subnormal pulmonary valve	IVR (+ infundibular patch)	Rotation of truncus arteriosus
Severe pulmonary outflow tract stenosis	IVR (+ transannular patch)	**REV** Bex – Nikaidoh Rastelli

Feasibility of REV Procedure

1. Connect the left ventricle to the aorta through the VSD:

   conoventricular VSD (not trabecular or inlet)
   other VSDs
   in presence of a conal septum:

   – no mitral insertions
   – no major tricuspid insertions (if any, importance)

   in absence of a conal septum: size of the VSD (anterior enlargement)
   size of the residual right ventricular cavity after construction of the intracardiac tunnel

2. Achieve valveless direct reconstruction of the right ventricular outflow tract:

   low pulmonary vascular resistances
   anatomy and size of the proximal pulmonary arteries (hypoplasia, localized stenosis needing repair)
   presence and size of a pulmonary trunk
   relationship between the great arteries (side by side or more-or-less anteroposterior).

Preference Card

bovine pericardium (intracardiac tunnel and pulmonary patch)
glutaraldehyde tanned autologous pericardium (pulmonary patch in small babies)
pledgetted sutures (intracardiac tunnel)
transesophageal echocardioghraphy

Indications

Selection of Patients

The REV operation, undertaken in TGA-VSD- LVOT obstruction, is indicated in patients with a short (or absent) subpulmonary conus and severe POT stenosis. Careful Doppler echocardiographic examination provides the information. The length of the subpulmonary conus is evaluated by the tricuspid-to-pulmonary distance; it is less than the diameter of the aortic valve. The POT obstruction is usually valvar and subvalvar; Doppler echocardiographic evaluation demonstrates that the subvalvar obstruction cannot be relieved adequately and that the pulmonary valve cannot be preserved (even after surgical repair).

There is a small group of patients in whom the subpulmonary conus is asymmetric; the mitral-to-pulmonary distance is shorter than the tricuspid-to-pulmonary distance. The tricuspid-to pulmonary distance may be long enough to allow IVR, but, because of the shorter mitral-to-pulmonary distance, the RVOT (with the pulmonary orifice in its native position) is long, angulated and potentially stenotic. A REV procedure is then indicated.

Contra-indications

In some potential candidates for a REV operation, this option should be abandoned for anatomic reasons.

- Remote position of the VSD (inlet or trabecular) without conoventricular extension. Resection of the conal septum (an essential step of the REV operation) cannot be performed without inducing surgical heart block. Separate closure of the VSD and a Bex-Nikaidoh procedure is indicated [5, 6].
- Abnormal insertions of the mitral valve apparatus on the conal septum. Resection of the conal septum is impossible or dangerous. Often, the abnormal conal insertions are associated with other severe malformations of the mitral valve such as straddling or parachute valve. A univentricular approach should be preferred if possible or, alternatively, biventricular repair may be performed with a prosthetic replacement of the mitral valve. In some patients, there are only abnormal chordae attached onto the conal septum, and some of them are not essential for mitral valve function. The Bex-Nikaidoh operation [5, 6], with preservation of the essential chordae, may offer a potential solution.
- Abnormal insertions of the tricuspid valve apparatus on the conal septum. When there are only a few chordae involved, this can be dealt with, as described below. However, when a major part of the tricuspid subvalvar apparatus is included, it is better to abandon the REV operation and to utilize the Bex-Nikaidoh option [5, 6].

Inadequate Pulmonary Vascular Bed

Because of diffuse hypoplasia of the pulmonary arteries or increased pulmonary vascular resistances, the presence of a competent pulmonary valve may be necessary. A modified Rastelli procedure is indicated; the intracardiac step is identical to that of the REV operation and a prosthetic valved conduit is used to reconstruct the right ventricular outflow tract [7].

Optimal Age

The intracardiac part of the REV operation may be difficult to perform in small babies. A minimum of 6 months – 6 kg is usually considered necessary to achieve a safe repair. A primary palliative approach may be indicated (systemic-pulmonary shunt with or without atrial septectomy). Bilateral systemic-to-pulmonary shunts should, however, be avoided because extensive mobilization of the pulmonary arteries may be more difficult.

Surgical Technique

Initiation of Cardiopulmonary Bypass

The procedure is performed through a median sternotomy, using conventional cardiopulmonary bypass with bicaval cannulation and a vent in the left atrium. Normothermic bypass and intermittent warm blood cardioplegia [8] are used; the cardioplegia is delivered every 10–12 min into the aortic root.

Palliative aorto-pulmonary shunts or a patent ductus arteriosus are dissected and ligated immediately after initiation of bypass. Before aortic cross-clamping, the ascending aorta, the pulmonary trunk and its branches are mobilized and care is taken to divide the pericardial attachments of all the vessels to facilitate their mobilization.

Cardiac Incisions

The right atrium is opened. An atrial septal defect, if present, is closed either directly or with a prosthetic patch; in most cases, a small calibrated ASD is left in order to allow temporary left or right ventricular unloading during the postoperative period. Through the tricuspid orifice, the intraventricular anatomy is inspected and the feasibility of a REV operation is confirmed. The right atrial approach may subsequently be used to secure to the inferior margin of the VSD the prosthetic patch used to construct the intracardiac tunnel.

The ascending aorta is divided close to the aortic clamp, leaving most of the proximal ascending aorta into which cardioplegia can be administered at regular intervals. The intracardiac anatomy is inspected through the aortic orifice. The pulmonary trunk is divided as close as possible to the valvar commissures.

The right ventricle is then opened. In most, the aorta is anterior to the pulmonary artery and the pulmonary bifurcation needs to be translocated anteriorly (French maneuver); the right ventricle is then opened longitudinally below the aortic valve (incision 1). Care is taken to preserve as many coronary arteries as possible; a large conal coronary artery is often present and should be preserved. The identification of the coronary arteries may be difficult in the presence of epicardial adhesions due to previous operations. The incision is started at its caudal end and extended upwards, taking great care to preserve the aortic leaflets. When the great arteries are strictly side by side, the pulmonary bifurcation should be left in its native position on the left side (and more rarely on the right side) of the aorta; the ventricular incision must be modified accordingly (incisions 2 and 3). In all cases, the incision must be planned and performed to provide excellent exposure of the aortic orifice and perfect assessment of the intracardiac anatomy (Fig. 18.1).

Resection of the Conal Septum (Fig. 18.2)

In all patients with a conal septum interposed between the VSD and the aortic orifice, the conal septum must be resected extensively; adequate alignment of the aortic orifice with the newly created left ventricular outflow tract depends upon the extensiveness of the septal resection. This step is greatly facilitated by the introduction of a Hegar dilator through the pulmonary orifice into the left ventricular cavity. This maneuver improves the exposure of the conal septum and protects the mitral valve apparatus.

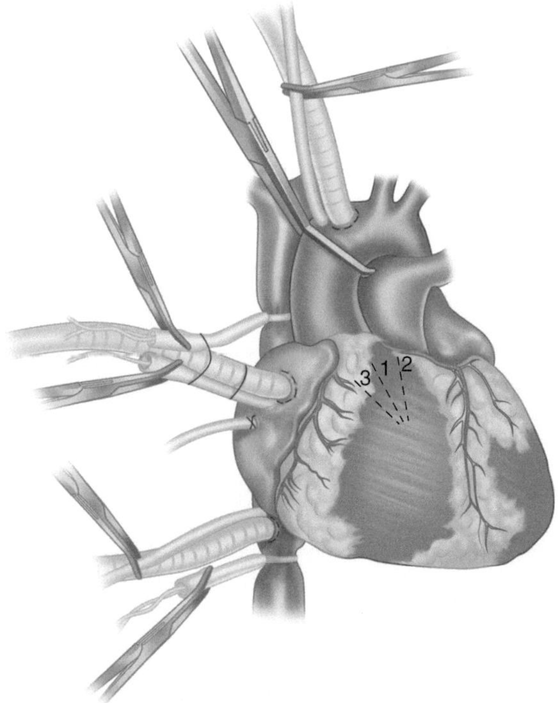

Fig. 18.1 Right ventricular incision. In most cases, the pulmonary bifurcation will be translocated in front of the aorta; the right ventricle is opened below the aortic valve (incision 1). When the great arteries are side by side, the pulmonary artery will be left in its native position on one side of the aorta. The incision is made accordingly (incisions 2 or 3). In all cases, the coronary arteries are preserved carefully (Reprinted with permission from Ref. [9])

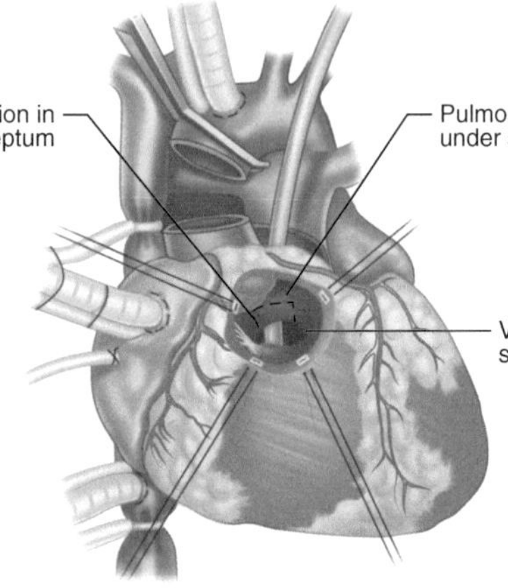

Fig. 18.2 Resection of the conal septum. The exposure of the conal septum is improved by the introduction of a Hegar dilator into the pulmonary orifice. The conal septum, interposed between the VSD and the aortic orifice, is resected extensively "en bloc" (Reprinted with permission from Ref. [9])

Three incisions are then made: one anterior and one posterior from the upper margin of the VSD up to the aortic annulus, and one parallel to the aortic annulus. The conal septum is resected "en bloc". It is crucial to carry out the upper incision in an oblique plane (and not in a horizontal plane) to avoid injury to the ventricular wall between both arterial orifices or to proximal coronary arteries (Fig. 18.3). When the conal resection is correct, it always permits the construction of a large tunnel from the left ventricle to the aorta, even if the VSD is initially restrictive; it is pointless to extend the resection anteriorly.

However, there are rare patients in whom the VSD is restrictive and the conal septum absent or small. It is then necessary to incise or resect the anterior margin of the VSD to avoid postoperative subaortic obstruction. This type of septal resection is hazardous, as this portion of the interventricular septum may include large septal coronary arteries supplying the conduction tissue.

When there is a papillary muscle of the tricuspid valve abnormally inserted onto the conal septum, the papillary muscle (and its chordae) are detached and subsequently reattached on the prosthetic patch, after the construction of the intracardiac tunnel. At the end of the operation, the function of the tricuspid valve must be evaluated and significant regurgitation should be corrected.

Construction of the Intracardiac Tunnel

In most cases, the construction of the intracardiac tunnel can be achieved through the ventriculotomy alone. However, when the exposure is not adequate, a part of the construction should be carried out through either the right atrium or the aortic orifice.

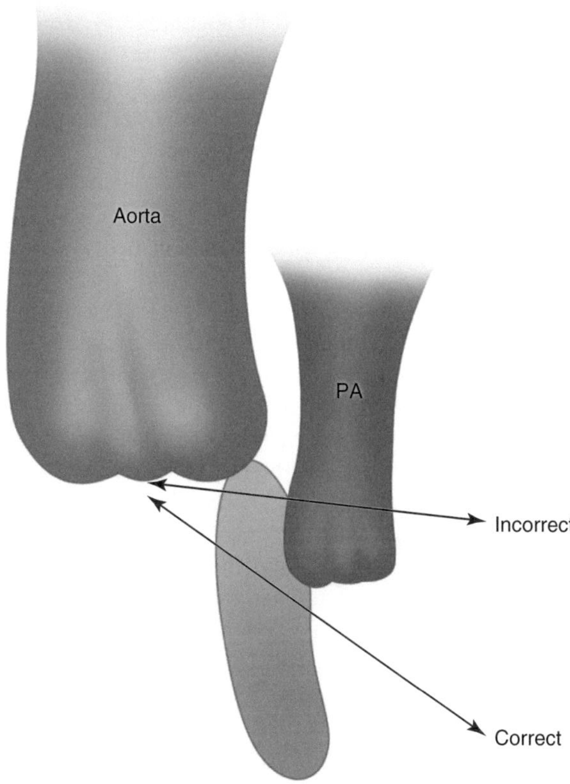

Fig. 18.3 Resection of the conal septum (cont'd). As the pulmonary orifice is usually lower than the aortic orifice, the subaortic line of resection must be carried out in an oblique plane, to avoid injury of the cardiac wall between the great arteries (Reprinted with permission from Ref. [9])

The intracardiac tunnel is constructed using a prosthetic patch made of heterologous bovine pericardium. The important technical point is a perfect tailoring of the patch. It is often recommended to oversize the patch, in order to prevent the development of subaortic stenosis. Actually, oversizing is ineffective, and potentially harmful. In most cases, there is an angulation between the lower part of the tunnel close to the tricuspid valve and the upper part close to the aortic valve. If the patch is oversized, the summit of the angulation may protrude to the left side and cause subaortic obstruction. Extensive resection of the conal septum and perfect tailoring of the prosthetic patch are the best ways to avoid subaortic obstruction, not oversizing of the patch.

The distance between the inferior margin of the VSD and the anterior margin of the aortic annulus is precisely measured. A circle having this distance as its circumference is tailored in the prosthetic patch. The future right-sided margin of the patch (between the tricuspid valve and the aortic valve) is trimmed straight, whereas the left-sided margin is temporarily left intact and round.

The patch is then secured to the inferior margin of the VSD using interrupted pledgetted mattress sutures. The approach may differ according to the anatomy. When the margin is formed by the tricuspid annulus itself, the sutures are passed through the base of the septal leaflet of the tricuspid valve and we prefer to do it through the right atrium; great care is taken to avoid injury to the conduction tissue. Alternatively, if there is a muscular rim between the VSD and the tricuspid annulus, the sutures are placed in that rim through the right ventricular approach.

The suture line then goes up on the right side to reach to right portion of the aortic annulus. Along this portion, a continuous running suture is used, reinforced with a few interrupted pledgetted stitches (Fig. 18.4).

At this point, the patch must be tailored definitively. This is done by trimming the left-sided margin of the patch such that it reaches the anterior limit of the tunnel without tension, but also without bulging (Fig. 18.5). A running continuous suture is used to join the left portion of the aortic annulus.

The final step of the construction of the intracardiac tunnel is to secure the patch around the anterior margin of the aortic annulus. This is done using a series of interrupted pledgetted mattress sutures. To prevent the occurrence of "intramural" residual VSDs, the sutures must be placed very close to the aortic annulus, and not on trabeculations within the right ventricle. When the aortic annulus is not exposed adequately through the right ventricle, the sutures along the superior aspect of the VSD should be inserted through the aortic orifice. Mattress sutures are placed in the base of the aortic leaflets; pledgets are then avoided to prevent any distortion of the valve.

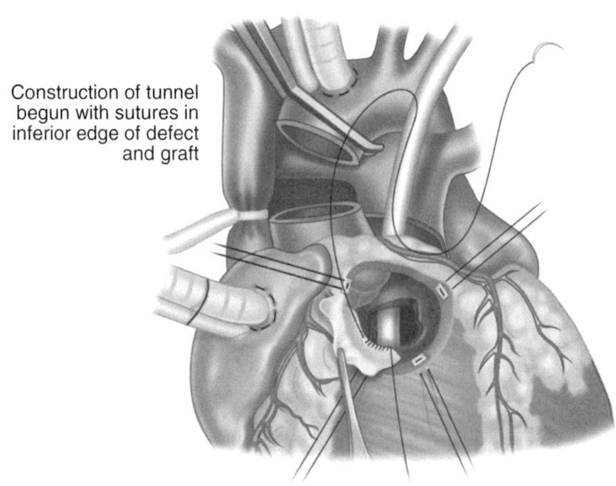

Fig. 18.4 Construction of the intracardiac tunnel. The pericardial patch is secured first to the inferior border of the VSD, using continuous or interrupted mattress sutures. Injury to the conduction tissue must be avoided. Often it is better to do it through the right atrial approach. Using a running suture, the patch is secured in straight line from the tricuspid annulus up to the right angle of the aortic orifice (Reprinted with permission from Ref. [9])

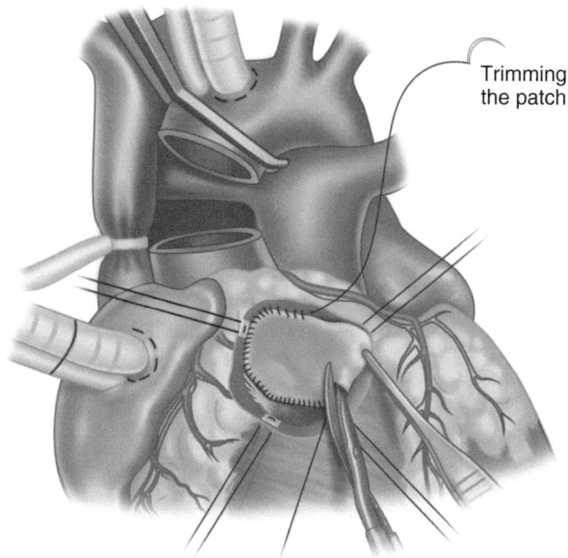

Fig. 18.5 Construction of the intracardiac tunnel (cont'd). After adequate trimming of the left-sided margin of the patch, the construction of the intracardiac tunnel is completed. Around the aortic orifice, it is often useful to place interrupted sutures through the aortic orifice (Reprinted with permission from Ref. [9])

Reconstruction of the Right Ventricular Outflow Tract

The cardiac end of the pulmonary orifice is closed primarily using a series of interrupted sutures. Care is taken not to distort the proximal coronary arteries which may course very close to the pulmonary annulus and be difficult to identify in case of previous operations. The patency of the proximal coronary arteries must be ascertained.

As previously stated, in most patients, the spatial relationship between the great arteries is more or less anteroposterior. In this situation (approximately 75 % of cases), the pulmonary bifurcation must be translocated anterior to the ascending aorta. The pulmonary branches are mobilized extensively, well beyond the pericardial reflection, down to the second order branches. The pulmonary bifurcation is translocated in front of the ascending aorta (French maneuver). The ascending aorta is reconstructed by end-to-end anastomosis. It is essential to remove a generous piece of ascending aorta in order to shorten and relocate the aorta more posteriorly, thus leaving more space anteriorly for the reimplanted pulmonary artery. The piece of ascending aorta may subsequently be interposed between the pulmonary artery and the right ventriculotomy to facilitate the direct reimplantation of the pulmonary artery (particularly when there is an abnormal coronary artery coursing in front of the aortic orifice) (Fig. 18.6) (see Chap. 19).

When the great arteries are strictly side-by-side the French maneuver is potentially harmful. After adequate mobilization of the pulmonary branches, the main pulmonary artery is left in its anatomical position (on the left or on the right of the reconstructed ascending aorta) and reimplanted directly onto the right ventricle.

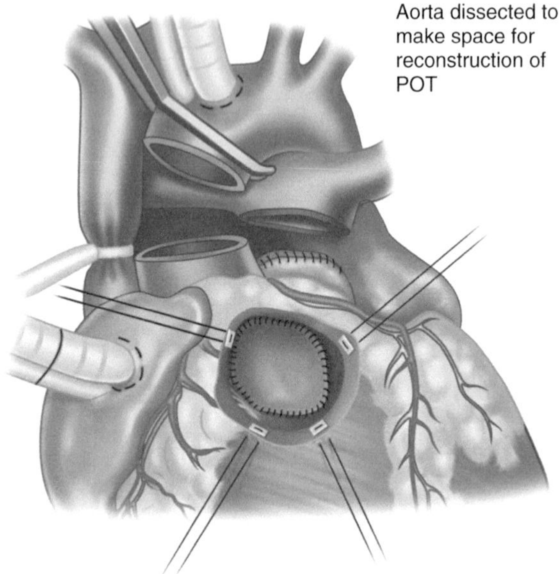

Fig. 18.6 Reconstruction of the ascending aorta. The cardiac end of the pulmonary orifice is closed. Care is taken to avoid injury to the coronary arteries. The pulmonary bifurcation is translocated in front of the aorta when the aorta is anterior to the pulmonary artery. A generous piece of ascending aorta is resected and the aorta is reconstructed (Reprinted with permission from Ref. [9])

The posterior half the circumference of the distal pulmonary trunk is directly anastomosed to the upper part of the right ventricular incision. The anterior wall of the pulmonary trunk is incised vertically up to the bifurcation. A prosthetic patch (heterologous or autologous pericardium), calibrated according to the patient's body surface area, is inserted to reconstruct the right ventricular outflow tract (Fig. 18.7).

It has been our practice to routinely implant a monocusp pulmonary valve, made of heterologous pericardium, autologous pericardium or PTFE membrane. Most of these valves function for only a limited period of time and eventually calcify and become stenotic, thus representing a major cause of reoperation. For those patients with low pulmonary artery pressure and resistances we recommend a valveless reconstruction.

Unlike the intracardiac patch, the patch that reconstructs the right ventricular outflow tract must be generous, particularly in its longitudinal axis. An obligatory angulation exists between the intracardiac portion of the right ventricular outflow tract and the extracardiac portion. If the anterior patch is too flat, this may create an obstruction at the level of the summit of this angulation.

Outcomes

Early Outcome

Patients undergoing REV operation must be evaluated using intraoperative trans-esophageal echocardiography following separation from cardiopulmonary bypass. Potential residual defects are multiple: obstruction of the intraventricular

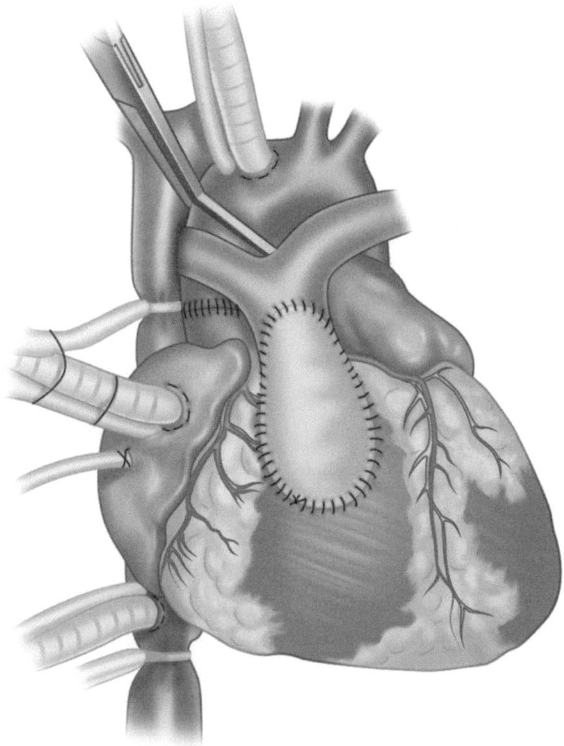

Fig. 18.7 Reconstruction of the pulmonary trunk. The posterior half of the circumference of the pulmonary trunk is reimplanted on the right ventriculotomy directly. The right ventricular outflow tract is completed using an anterior generous pericardial patch (Reprinted with permission from Ref. [9])

tunnel (inadequate enlargement of a restrictive VSD or distortion of the prosthetic patch), residual VSD, obstruction of the right ventricular outflow tract. Such residual anomalies must be recognized and corrected prior to leaving the operative theater.

The REV procedure usually requires a prolonged period of aortic cross-clamping, and temporary myocardial dysfunction may occur. Allowing residual shunting at the atrial level may be useful to maintain adequate systemic cardiac output, at the expense of some arterial desaturation. If the hemodynamic status is marginal, delayed sternal closure and ECMO assistance may be necessary.

The current mortality rate is low. Between 2007 and 2013, 28 patients underwent REV procedure in our institution without early mortality. During the same period, 132 patients were reported to the EACTS database with an early mortality rate of 5.3 % (7 patients) [10].

Late Outcome

The late outcome of 181 patients who underwent a REV procedure, with a mean follow-up of 12.3 ± 7.1 years, was recently reported [11]. The probability of survival at 25 years was 85 % (Fig. 18.8). Reoperation was required for right ventricular outflow tract obstruction in 36 patients (20 %) and for left ventricular outflow tract obstruction in 3 patients (1.7 %). By using cumulative method analysis the probability of being alive without reoperation at 25 years was 45 %, that of reoperation for right ventricular outflow tract obstruction was 33 % and that of reoperation for left ventricular outflow tract obstruction was 5 % (Fig. 18.9). Most patients (87 %) were asymptomatic and leading a normal life; 72 % were free of rhythm disturbances.

These results compare favorably with those of the classical Rastelli operation [12–15]. However, the long-term fate of the reconstructed right ventricular outflow tract remains a matter of concern. Many reoperations were necessary because of stenosis resulting from the insertion of a prosthetic monocusp. Valveless reconstruction, as it is now performed, may decrease this problem. Interestingly, the need for pulmonary valve implantation has been, to date, very rare (6 patients – 3.3 %). However, this will undoubtedly increase with longer follow up.

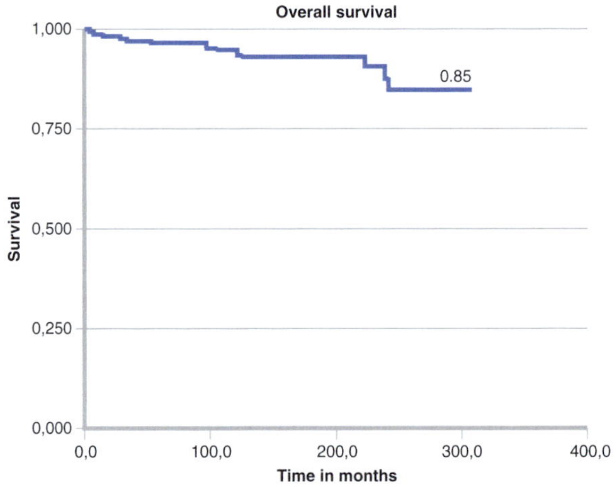

Fig. 18.8 Overall survival at 25 years, using the Kaplan-Meier method (Reprinted with permission from Ref. [11])

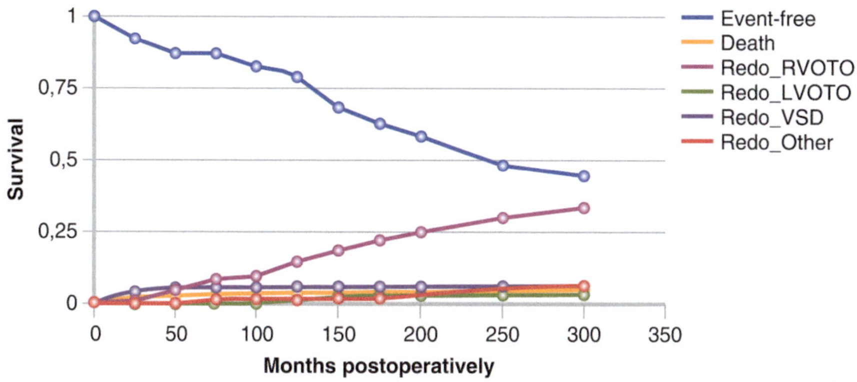

Fig. 18.9 Probability of different outcomes at 25 years, using cumulative method analysis (Reprinted with permission from Ref. [11])

References

1. Rubay J, Lecompte Y, Batisse A, Durandy Y, Dibie A, Lemoine G, Vouhé P. Anatomic repair of anomalies of ventriculo-arterial connection (REV). Results of a new technique in cases associated with pulmonary outflow tract obstruction. Eur J Cardiothorac Surg. 1988;2(5):305–11.
2. Borromée L, Lecompte Y, Batisse A, Lemoine G, Vouhé P, Sakata R, Leca F, Zannini L, Neveux JY. Anatomic repair of anomalies of ventriculoarterial connection associated with ventricular septal defect. II. Clinical results in 50 patients with pulmonary outflow tract obstructionJ. Thorac Cardiovasc Surg. 1988;95(1):96–102.
3. Lecompte Y. Réparation à l'Etage Ventriculaire – the REV procedure: technique and clinical results. Cardiol Young. 1991;1:63–70.
4. Lecompte Y, Batisse A, Di Carlo D. Double-outlet right ventricle: a surgical synthesis. Adv Card Surg. 1993;4:109–36.
5. Bex JP, Lecompte Y, Baillot F, Hazan E. Anatomical correction of transposition of the great arteries. Ann Thorac Surg. 1980;29:86–8.
6. Nikaidoh H. Aortic translocation and biventricular outflow tract reconstruction. A new surgical repair for transposition of the great arteries associated with ventricular septal defect and pulmonary stenosis. J Thorac Cardiovasc Surg. 1984;88:365–72.
7. Morell VO, Jacobs JP, Quintessenza JA. Surgical management of transposition with ventricular septal defect and obstruction to the left ventricular outflow tract. Cardiol Young. 2005;15 Suppl 1:102–5.
8. Durandy YD, Younes M, Mahut B. Pediatric warm open heart surgery and prolonged cross-clamp time. Ann Thorac Surg. 2008;86:1941–7.
9. Lecompte Y, Vouhé P. Réparation à l'Etage Ventriculaire (REV procedure): not a Rastelli procedure without conduit. Oper Tech Thorac Cardiovasc Surg. 2003;8:150–9.
10. EACTS Congenital Database http://www.eactscongenitaldb.org/index.php?LANG=en&level=2&struct=14_1
11. Di Carlo D, Tomasco B, Cohen L, Vouhé P, Lecompte Y. Long-term results of the REV (réparation à l'étage ventriculaire) operation. J Thorac Cardiovasc Surg. 2011;142:336–43.
12. Kreutzer C, De Vive J, Oppido G, Kreitzer J, Gauvreau K, Freed M, Layer JE, Jonas R, del Nido PJ. Twenty-five-year experience with Rastelli repair for transposition of the great arteries. J Thorac Cardiovasc Surg. 2000;120:211–23.

13. Dearani JA, Danielson GK, Puga FJ, Mair DD, Schleck CD. Late results of the Rastelli operation for transposition of the great arteries. Semin Thorac Cardiovasc Surg Pediatr Card Surg Annu. 2001;4:3–15.
14. Hörer J, Schreiber C, Dworak E, Cleuziou J, Prodan Z, Vogt M, Holper K, Lange R. Long-term results after the Rastelli repair for transposition of the great arteries. Ann Thorac Surg. 2007;83:2169–75.
15. Vouhé PR, Tamisier D, Leca F, Ouaknine R, Vernant F, Neveux JY. Transposition of the great arteries, ventricular septal defect, and pulmonary outflow tract obstruction. Rastelli or Lecompte procedure? J Thorac Cardiovasc Surg. 1992;103:428–36.

Chapter 19
Transposition of the Great Arteries with VSD and LVOTO. The Autograft Procedure for RVOT (the "DREAM")

Dominique Metras

Abstract In transposition of the great arteries, ventricular septal defect and LVOTO (pulmonary stenosis or atresia), the classical procedures described (Rastelli and REV) can lead to late complications like LV outflow tract obstruction and even more RV outflow tract obstruction leading to reoperations (almost 100 % in Rastelli, 33 % in REV).

This chapter deals with a surgical procedure we have developped combining features of both procedures and using the concept of autograft to decrease the rate of reoperations in the RV outflow.

We perform an intracardiac procedure as in REV, with resection of conal septum, to avoid LV outflow obstruction and the main feature is to use a cylinder of autologous aorta to extend the main PA, located like a Rastelli conduit, avoiding all Lecompte manoeuvers with anterior transfer of pulmonary bifurcation.

Thus the RV outflow and the autograft conduit sutures are free from tension and possible compression, and being an autologous living tissue, the conduit is susceptible to grow. Due to the growth of this autograft, early primary correction is allowed even under 1 year of age.

In our series reported here, half of the patients had a primary procedure without preliminary shunt, and there was an actuarial freedom from RV outflow reoperation of 95 % at 16 years and more.

Keywords Transposition-VSD-LVOTO surgery • Aortic autograft conduit

---

DREAM is an acronym for: Direct REpair with an Autograft from Marseille

D. Metras, MD
Department of Cardio-Thoracic Surgery, Children's Hospital La Timone, University Marseille-Aix, Marseille, France
e-mail: metrasd@yahoo.fr

F. Lacour-Gayet et al. (eds.), *Surgery of Conotruncal Anomalies*,
DOI 10.1007/978-3-319-23057-3_19

Background

In TGA with VSD and LVOTO (stenosis or atresia) the Rastelli procedure described in 1969 [1] has provided the possibility of a correction including rerouting the blood from the LV to the aorta with a patch and creating a RV-PA connection with a valve conduit.

However this pioneer strategy had some inconvenients: the need of a conduit led to replacements and repeated operations, practically in all patients [2, 3] preliminary palliative surgery was most often necessary to allow growth of the patient and implantation of a sizeable conduit, and among reoperations some were necessary due to LV-Aorta pathway progressive stenosis.

Lecompte [4] reported a new procedure, the REV (Reconstruction Endo Ventriculaire) aiming at avoidance of these inconvenients. The LV-Ao pathway is rendered more direct and straight by resection of the conal septum (free from conducting tissue), the main pulmonary artery is directly anastomosed to the right ventriculotomy, after a Lecompte manoeuver, so that the pulmonary bifurcation is brought anterior to the aorta. Finally, this procedure, creating an autologous tissue RV-PA connection, allows early surgery, without systematic need for preliminary palliative surgery. With time, however, reoperations have proven to be necessary : some rare LV outflow obstruction, but mostly RV-PA obstruction 33 % in the Lecompte-Vouhé series [5].

Another concept described long ago by Bex in TGA without VSD and LVOTO [6], with posterior translocation of the transposed aorta with coronaries on the LV outflow was adapted by Nikaidoh [7], with the RV outflow repaired with a conduit or a patch, and recently this procedure regained interest [8, 9]. However, although the LV outflow is probably best repaired with the Bex-Nikaidoh procedure, there are still 30 % reoperations reported on the RV outflow for secondary stenosis. In addition the transfer of aortic valve and coronaries has been also the reason for occasional morbidity and reoperations.

By present time, with the improvement in post-operative care, the morbimortality has been considerably improved in all kinds of procedures, so that the more complex procedures have now a very low mortality rate.

In 1993, we have started to use a new operation [10], fundamentally to improve and decrease the late RV outflow problems. Basically it uses the autograft concept with a procedure combining:

1. The intra-cardiac REV procedure for better LV-Ao connection
2. The Rastelli procedure using a cylinder of aorta of the patient, extending the pulmonary trunk with a living tissue with growth potential. The reconstruction can be done leaving the pulmonary artery bifurcation orthotopically posterior to the aorta avoiding tension on the anastomosis or possible anterior compression.

Anatomic Classification Used

The anatomic classification we use is basically as taught by R. Van Praagh, derived from the Farre description in 1814 [11],meaning that the great arteries arise from the wrong ventricle, being displaced across the septum. The concept was clarified by R. Van Praagh in 1966, in a basic paper [12] where all the concepts of D or L-transposition, of ventricular D and L–loop, and also the idea of malposition was proposed where both great arteries fail to be actually displaced across the ventricular septum.

As very well described in the textbook of Kirklin and Barratt-Boyes (edition 2013) [13], the VSD is usually cono-ventricular, and occasionally in the inlet septum. This rare location never occurred in our series of patients. Not rarely, the VSD is partially obstructed by fibrous tissue developed from the tricuspid valve leaflets. In one of our case, it was almost closed with, as a result, a supra-systemic LV pressure.

The LVOTO can be valvar, often bicuspid, annular, or sub-valvular, with often combination of the three.

The combination of VSD and LVOTO in TGA requires a particular procedure, our modification described in this chapter being one of them.

However, it must be mentioned that according to an anatomical study on specimens [14], some cases could have benefited from Arterial Switch Operation (ASO), VSD closure and pulmonary valvotomy. Despite the interest of the concept, we doubt that a surgeon would accept to do an ASO associated with an aortic valve procedure.

Diagnosis Imaging

As most congenital heart diseases, the diagnostic and the evaluation of TGA with VSD and LVOTO are presently done with 2-D echography, NMR and CT scan. A diagnostic catheterisation is no more performed, except if a doubt on some morphology or more importantly on the pulmonary vascular resistances (PVR) exist. As in the DREAM procedure there is no permanent valvulation of the pulmonary artery, and only occasional monocusp use, a somehow elevated PVR might then change the choice of procedure to a Rastelli procedure using a valve conduit.

Surgical Technique

The basic steps of the operation are the followings:

(a) after usual monitoring and lines insertion (arterial and central venous catheter, urinary catheter, percutaneous O_2 saturation, NIRS when available…), a median sternotomy is performed. After vertical incision and suspension of the pericardium, a large piece of pericardium is harvested and treated with glutaraldehyde.

The external anatomy of the heart is analysed, in particular the respective position of the ascending aorta and the main pulmonary, and the coronary branches disposition. This is important in view of the decision of the right or left-sided connection of the MPA to the RV, relative to the aorta. Also the location and direction of the right ventriculotomy is decided according to the same criteria.

One other aspect to analyse is the length of the ascending aorta, since the procedure includes a harvesting of a cylinder of ascending aorta for the MPA extension.

(b) Before starting canulations and cardio-pulmonary by-pass (CPB), several preliminary surgical manoeuvers are accomplished without CPB, provided they are tolerated. As soon as they are not tolerated, they are done after institution of CPB.

These manoeuvers are :

Ascending aorta is dissected free from the main pulmonary artery (MPA), and if it is felt that the length might be insufficient for harvesting of the cylinder and end-to-end anastomosis with the intra-pericardial portion, the dissection is extended reaching the origin of the innominate artery, in view of a distal canulation or canulation in the aortic arch.

Both pulmonary branches and the bifurcation are dissected free as for an arterial switch operation.

The PDA or ligamentum arteriosum is divided after ligation or suture.

If a modified Blalock-Taussig shunt (MBTS) with a PTFE has been performed it is dissected and controlled, the division and suture being done under CPB.

(c) After the usual purse-strings, heparin administration, aortic and bicaval canulation are performed, and CPB is started.

Our current policy is a normothermic CPB and warm blood intermittent cardioplegia in the ascending aorta and directly in the coronary ostia when the aorta is opened.

The first step is then division and suture of the MBTS.

The RA is then opened vertically to analyse the intra-cardiac anatomy, with special attention to the location and size of the VSD, to the possible narrowing of the VSD by fibrous tissue. The AV valve anatomy is analized, ruling out any straddling of papillary muscle rendering hazardous the insertion of the patch conduit restoring LV-Aorta continuity.

The presence and thickness of the infundibular septum under the vessels is also evaluated.

The interatrial septum is also analysed. A LA vent is inserted through the septum or through an ASD, if present.

(d) Then, if the decision of performance of the procedure is taken, (in one of our case, a straddling of the mitral valve being discovered, the decision was to rather perform a birectional superior cavo-pulmonary anastomosis) the subsequent steps are followed, all the initial steps being described in the REV operation [4].

1. Right ventriculotomy.

   In general oblique, avoiding the coronary branches, directed upwards to the right or left-side according to the side of the future

   RV-PA connection respective to the aorta (Fig. 19.1).

Through the ventriculotomy, the VSD position is identified, the possible fibrous tissue obliteration, the infundibular septum …and all other features of interest are also visualised.

2. Transversal MPA division.

   It is done as low as possible. Through the opening and the pulmonary valve, a Hegar bougie is located in the LV as described in the REV operation. In case of pulmonary atresia this cannot be done.

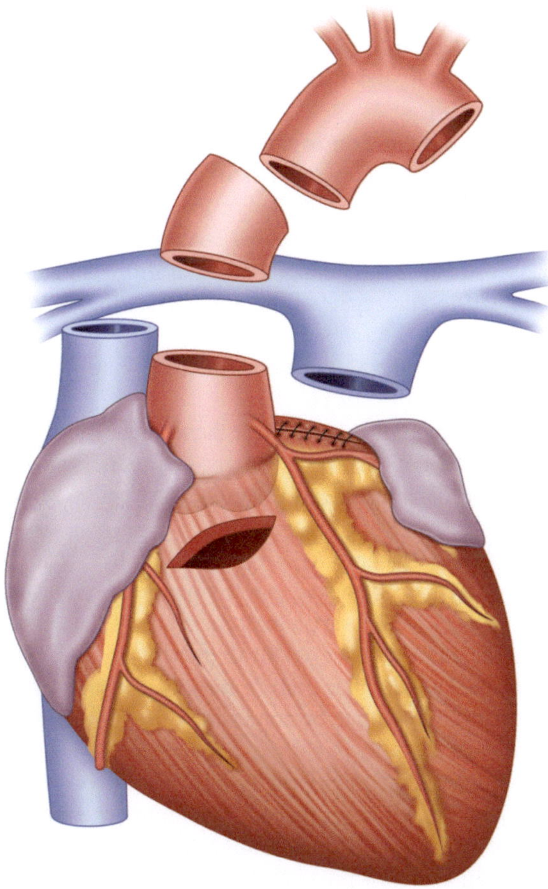

Fig. 19.1 Free dissection of the pulmonary arteries. A cylindric segment of ascending aorta is detached. The proximal aspect of the main pulmonary artery is closed after having contructed the LV-Aorta patch, and intra-cardiac REV procedure. In this case the oblique ventriculotomy has been made to connect the extended MPA on the left side of the Aorta

3. Through the ventriculotomy, with the control of the bougie, a large resection of the conal (or infundibular) septum is performed

   The mitral valve being hidden and protected by the bougie.

   The pathway between LV and aorta having been made more direct after this conal resection, a LV-Aorta channel is constructed. A large patch (using dacron or pericardium, either autologous treated with glutaldehyde or equine) is inserted. It is attached on the RV edge of the VSD in general with interrupted mattress sutures, then in the RV, directed towards the aortic orifice. The space between the two lines must be wide enough to obtain an unobstructed LV-Aorta channel. The anterior and superior final part is sutured using part of the free wall of the RV, to avoid the aortic annulus, often very close to the incision. Subsequently, after transversal division of the aorta during aortic autograft harvesting, the diameter of this channel can be evaluated through the aortic valve.
4. The proximal end of the transected pulmonary artery is closed with a double running suture. The pulmonary valve, usually stenotic and thickened is sutured also with the pulmonary wall.

   This is done to avoid creation of a cul-de-sac communicating with the LV, with potential thrombus formation and risk of embolism.
5. The aortic autograft cylinder is then harvested. A transverse incision is performed, close to the top of the aortic valve commissures, after having checked that the coronary ostia are not in danger, and that sufficient aortic wall tissue is provided for the end-to-end repair of the aorta. Then the upper division of the cylinder is performed.

   Due to the curvature of the ascending aorta, this cylinder has an anterior wall higher than the posterior (Fig. 19.1).

   After inspecting through the aortic valve the adequacy of the LV-Aorta channel (some more resection of the conal septum can be done, with caution, through the aortic valve, if necessary), an end-to-end reconstruction of the aorta is done with a running suture.
6. Extension of the Main Pulmonary Artery (MPA) with the aortic autograft.

The aortic autograft is then anastomosed in a termino-terminal fashion to the MPA using a running suture. If necessary, small incisions of the MPA walls are performed to accomodate the largest possible diameter.

The longer aspect of the cylinder, the anterior wall, is inserted posteriorly, to allow the suture to the ventriculotomy to be done without tension, and without a risk of coronary compression.

The RV-PA connection is then constructed by suturing the posterior aspect of the extended MPA to the upper part of the ventriculotomy, the reconstruction being located to the right or the left of the ascending aorta (Figs. 19.2 and 19.3).

The final reconstruction is done with a hood of pericardium, using or not a monocusp patch. The use of this monocusp is decided according to the supposed pulmonary vascular resistance, the post-operative RV function and the availability of a competent monocusp device. It was rarely used in our experience.

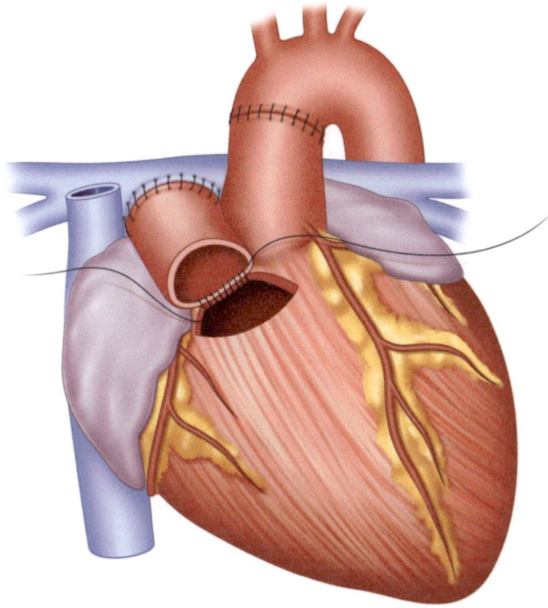

Fig. 19.2 The MPA is extended with the aortic autograft cylinder is sutured to the right ventriculotomy, located on the right side of the aorta

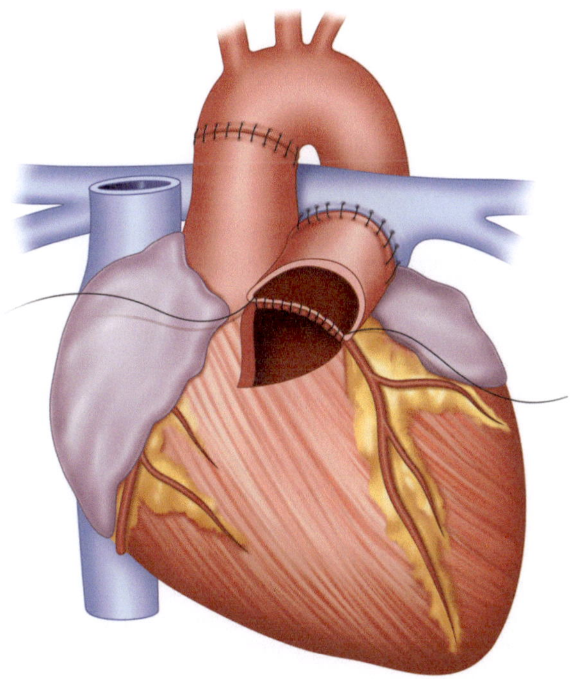

Fig. 19.3 The reconstruction is made on the left side of the aorta

Outcomes

Between 1993 and 2005 we have performed 25 procedures in the University Children's Hospital La Timone, Marseille. The results have been reported in the EJCTS [15] and we shall concentrate on RV outflow result, since this is basically the aim of our procedure.. There were 19 patients with pulmonary stenosis, and 6 with pulmonary atresia. Patient's age ranged from 2.5 months to 11 years (mean 2.2 years), 13 patients had undergone previous palliative operation, and 12 had a primary correction.

The connection between the RV and the extended main pulmonary pulmonary was brought to the right of the aorta in 13 cases and to the left in 12 cases. Accordingly, the right ventriculotomy had been done obliquely directed on the right or the left.

In 5 cases a monocusp pulmonary or aortic homograft was added in the proximal pericardial hood reconstruction.

Aortic cross-clamping duration ranged from 90 to 140 mn (mean 113 mn). One patient, 1 year old, died on post-operative day 3, due to severe RV failure, before we had started our program of post-operative ECMO. Mean hospital stay was 16 days.

All patients were followed by regular echocardiogram, occasional catheterisation, and more recently by NMR when possible.

All patients were under class I category, in sinus rhythm.

One female patient died 15 years after surgery. She had multiple other non-cardiac problems and at the last echographic evaluation she had a satisfactory result with a RV pressure of 50 mmHg and a RV-PA gradient of 12 mmHg, with moderate pulmonary insufficiency

Overall, the late survival after a mean follow-up of 12.8 years (maximum 17 years) was 92 % as reported in 2011. At echocardiogram, if one exclude the patient reoperated for stenosis, the RV pressures ranged from 30 to 55 mmHg (mean: 41).

The RV-PA gradient evaluated by echocardiogram ranged from 8 to 44 mmHg (mean 17 mmHg).

As seen in some patients having a late catheterisation (Fig. 19.4), and more recently by NMR (Fig. 19.5) the RV outflow stayed wide open, without aspect of compression.

Pulmonary regurgitation was evaluated appropriately in 14 patients : 3 important, three moderate, 8 mild.

Three patients underwent a reoperation for sub-aortic stenosis. In one of them no resection of the infundibular septum had been made, in one other there were abnormal chordae creating turbulences in the LV outflow, in the third one there was a LSVC, factor found to be associated with the occurrence of late development of subaortic stenosis [16]. Successful reoperation were performed 4, 5, and 6 years after initial surgery. The patients are now more than 10 years after this reoperation.

Only one patient has undergone a reoperation for RV outflow stenosis. The patients had undergone surgery at the age of 2.5 months, weight 4 kg, after neonatal MBTS. Due to restrictive VSD and supra systemic LV pressures the corrective

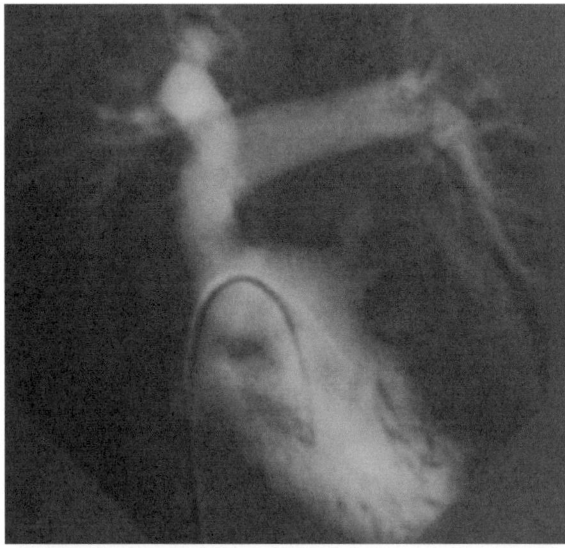

Fig. 19.4 Right ventricular angiogram late after surgery

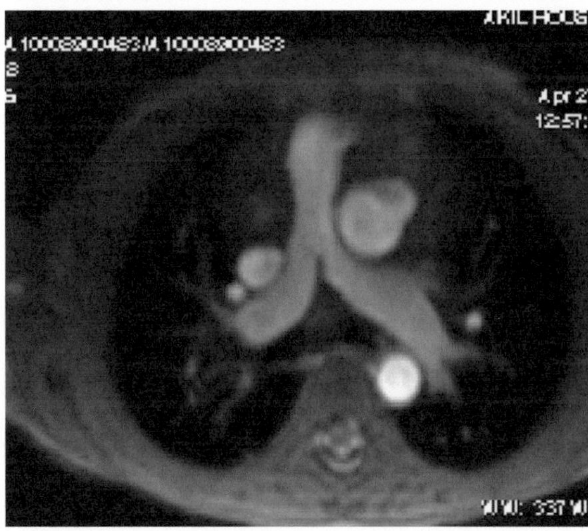

Fig. 19.5 NMR aspect of the RV outflow reconstruction

procedure was planned. The procedure included VSD enlargement by resection of fibrous tissue.

At the age of 13 years, he underwent patch enlargement of the RV outflow, found with a calcification and retraction of the pericardial hood associated with severe stenosis and high RV pressures. The autograft tissue was pliable, and found to be normal tissue at microscopic pathology and the postoperative course was uneventful, with adequate relief of the stenosis. Subsequently, at the age of 18 years he underwent a valvulation by insertion of a homograft, in view of the presence of a massive pulmonary regurgitation.

Therefore, in the entire series, presently with a follow-up of 19 years (mean 13 years) there is a freedom of reoperation for RV-PA stenosis of 90 % (Fig. 19.6).

Without entering in too much details, it is by far a procedure giving the best late results in RV outflow freedom of reoperation [17] compared to the Rastelli procedure, the REV and more recently the Bex-Nikaidoh procedures, with 30 % (minimum) to almost 100 % of RV outflow reoperations [2, 3, 5, 7–9].

Conclusion

Our "DREAM" procedure, representing a combination of REV (in view of the LV outflow) and a modified Rastelli procedure using a living tissue (ascending aorta), combines the advantages of both procedures and avoid their drawbacks:

1. the correction can be done early, without previous shunt procedure (as REV)
2. the LV outflow has the features of the REV, but does not avoid totally reoperations. The Bex-Nikaidoh is probably best concerning this issue.
3. The RV –PA connection is done without tension and possible anterior compression. The tissue is a living tissue, susceptible to grow.

   The rate of RV outflow reoperation is the lowest among other procedures as studied in a multicentric experience [17].
4. Due to the longterm valveless system, as many other operations, it might however lead to the need of valvulation, possibly in the future done without surgery.

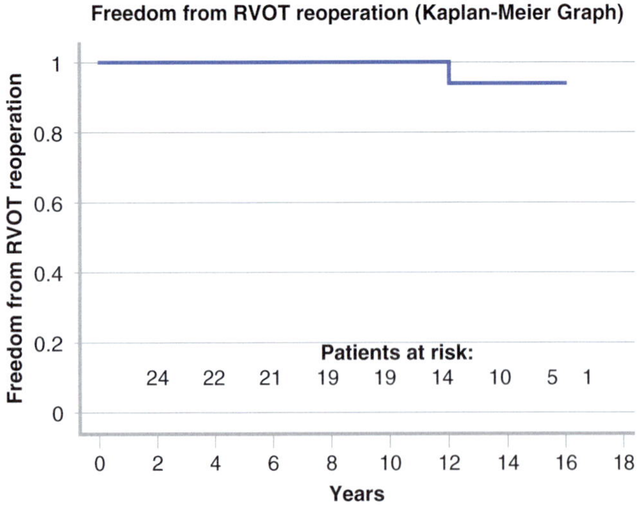

Fig. 19.6 Actuarial Kaplan-Meier

References

1. Rastelli GC, McGoon DC, Wallace RB. Anatomic correction of transposition of the great arteries with ventricular septal defect and subpulmonary stenosis. J Thorac Cardiovasc Surg. 1969;48:545–52.
2. Dearani JA, Davidson GK, Pupa FJ, Mast DD, Schleck CD. Results of Rastelli operation. Semin Thorac Cardiovasc Surg. 2001;4:3–15.
3. Kreutzer C, De Vive J, Oppido G, Kreutzer J, Gauvreau K, Freed M, Mayer Jr JE, Jonas R, Del Nido PJ. Twenty-five-year experience with Rastelli repair for transposition of the great arteries. J Thorac Cardiovasc Surg. 2000;120:211–23.
4. Lecompte Y. Réparation à l'étage ventriculaire. The REV procédure: technique and clinical results. Cardiol Young. 1991;1:63–70.
5. Vouhé P. Malposition of the great arteries. Paris: Course on Congenital heart Surgery; 2009.
6. Bex JP, Lecompte Y, Baillot F, Hazan E. Anatomical correction of transposition of the great arteries. Ann Thorac Surg. 1980;29:86–8.
7. Yeh Jr T, Ramaciotti C, Leonard SR, Roy L, Nikaidoh H. The aortic translocation (Nikaidoh) procedure: midterm results superior to the Rastelli procedure. J ThoracCardiovasc Surg. 2007;133:461–9.
8. Morell VO, Jacobs JP, Quintessenza JA. Aortic translocation in the management of transposition of the great arteries with ventricular septal defect and pulmonary stenosis: results and follow-up. Ann Thorac Surg. 2005;79:2089–92.
9. Bautista-Hernandez V, Marx GR, Bacha EA, Del Nido PJ. Aortic root translocation plus arterial switch for transposition of the great arteries with left ventricular outflow tract obstruction: intermediate-term results. J Am Coll Cardiol. 2007;49:485–90.
10. Metras D, Kreitmann B, Riberi A, Wernert F, Pannetier-Mille A. Extending the concept of the autograft for complete repair of transposition of the great arteries with ventricular septal defect and left ventricular outflow tract obstruction: a report of ten cases of a modified procedure. J Thorac Cardiovasc Surg. 1997;114:746–54.
11. Farre JR. Pathological researches. Essay 1: on malformation of the human heart. London: Longman, Hurst, Rees, Orme, Brown; 1814. p. 28.
12. Van Praagh R, Van Praagh S. Isolated ventricular inversion. Am J Cardiol. 1966;17:395.
13. Kirklin, Barratt-Boyes. Complete transposition of the great arteries. Cardiac Surgery. Elsevier Saunders; 2013. p. 1863.
14. Lalezari S, Mahtab EA, Bartelings MM, Wisse LJ, Hazekamp MG, Gittenberger-de Groot AC. The outflow tract in transposition of the great arteries: an anatomic and morphologic study. Ann Thorac Surg. 2009;88(4):1300.
15. Metras D, Fouilloux V, Mace L, Alain F. Bernard Kreitmann Right ventricular outflow repair: the aortic autograft technique procures the best late results in the transposition complex. Eur J Cardiothorac Surg. 2011;40(3):614–8.
16. Kalfa D, Ghez O, Kreitmann B, Metras D. Secondary subaortic stenosis in heart defects without any initial subaortic obstruction: a multifactorial postoperative event. Eur J Cardiothorac Surg. 2007;32:582–7.
17. Hazekamp MG, Gomez AA, Koolbergen DR, Hraska V, Metras DR, Mattila IP, Daenen W, Berggren HE, Rubay JE, Stellin G. Surgery for transposition of the great arteries, ventricular septal defect and left ventricular outflow tract obstruction: European Congenital Heart Surgeons Association Multicentre Study. Eur J Cardiothorac Surg. 2010;38:699–706.

Chapter 20
The Aortic Translocation (Nikaidoh) Procedure

Victor O. Morell

Abstract The Nikaidoh procedure was introduced for the management of patients with transposition of the great arteries (TGA) with a ventricular septal defect (VSD) and pulmonary stenosis (PS). The technique has proven especially useful in the subset of patients with anatomic variables that complicate the performance of a Rastelli repair, which include: an inlet, distant or restrictive VSD, a hypoplastic right ventricle, and a straddling atrioventricular valve.

Keywords Transposition of the great arteries • Ventricular septal defect • Pulmonary stenosis • Aortic translocation • Nikaidoh

Introduction

In 1980, Bex et al. [1] reported a new surgical technique for the management of transposition of the great arteries. They described moving the aortic root together with the coronary arteries to the pulmonary position as a way to provide a true 'anatomic correction' for TGA. The procedure was perfected in anatomical specimens before performing it successfully in a 3-year-old girl with TGA and pulmonary stenosis. In 1984, Nikaidoh [2] described and popularized the concept of aortic translocation for the management of TGA with a ventricular septal defect and pulmonary stenosis.

V.O. Morell, MD
Department of Cardiothoracic Surgery, University of Pittsburgh Medical School, Children's Hospital of Pittsburgh of UPMC, One Children's Hospital Drive, 4401 Penn Ave., Pittsburgh, PA 15224, USA
e-mail: victor.morell@chp.edu

F. Lacour-Gayet et al. (eds.), *Surgery of Conotruncal Anomalies*,
DOI 10.1007/978-3-319-23057-3_20

Diagnosis and Imaging

Cyanosis is the most common presenting clinical symptom with this cardiac lesion. Echocardiography is the preferred diagnostic tool. It is important to identify the anatomy of the left ventricular outflow tract obstruction, great vessels relationship, coronary anatomy, location of the ventricular septal defect, and the presence of straddling atrioventricular valve tissue. Cardiac catheterization is not routinely utilized for diagnostic purposes.

Anatomy, Indications and Check List Prior to Surgery

When to proceed with a Nikaidoh procedure? Well, there is a body of evidence, based on anatomical studies and clinical experience, that has identified specific morphological characteristics that when present appear to be better managed with the aortic translocation technique [1–16]. These important anatomic features need to consider preoperatively and/or intraoperatively. They include the following:

I. *The location of the VSD:* Restrictive, inlet type or more apically located defects are better managed with aortic translocation. The subvalvar apparatus of the atrioventricular valves commonly interfere with the creation of an unobstructed intraventricular tunnel. For some patients, it may be the only surgical approach that allows a biventricular repair.

II. *The size of the Right Ventricle:* The Nikaidoh procedure does not negatively affect the RV volume because it avoids the creation of an intraventricular tunnel. Therefore, the presence of RV hypoplasia is an indication for the aortic translocation technique.

III. *Abnormal AVV attachments or straddling:* The surgical approached used for the Nikaidoh procedure allows much better visualization and management of abnormal chordal attachments, specially to the outlet septum. Tricuspid valve straddling has been identified as a risk factor for death in patients undergoing a Rastelli [17].

IV. *Size of the pulmonary valve annulus*: In aortic translocation, the distance travelled by the translocated aorta is directly related to the size of the PV annulus (Fig. 20.1). If the PV annulus is too small then there is not much to be gained by moving the aortic root closer to the left ventricle. Therefore, patients with pulmonary atresia are not considered to be candidates for this procedure. At our institution patients with a PVa diameter > or = 5 mm are considered to be candidates for aortic translocation.

V. *Coronary artery anatomy*: In our experience, the most common reason to "abort" a Nikaidoh procedure has been epicardial course of a major coronary artery preventing the safe harvesting of the aortic root from the RV. Also, the presence of a posterior looping coronary is of concern because of the possibility of injury when suturing the aortic root to the pulmonary annulus. When present, we have opted to leave a small segment of the pulmonary artery wall in continuity with the pulmonary valve annulus to which the posterior aspect of the aortic root is sutured,

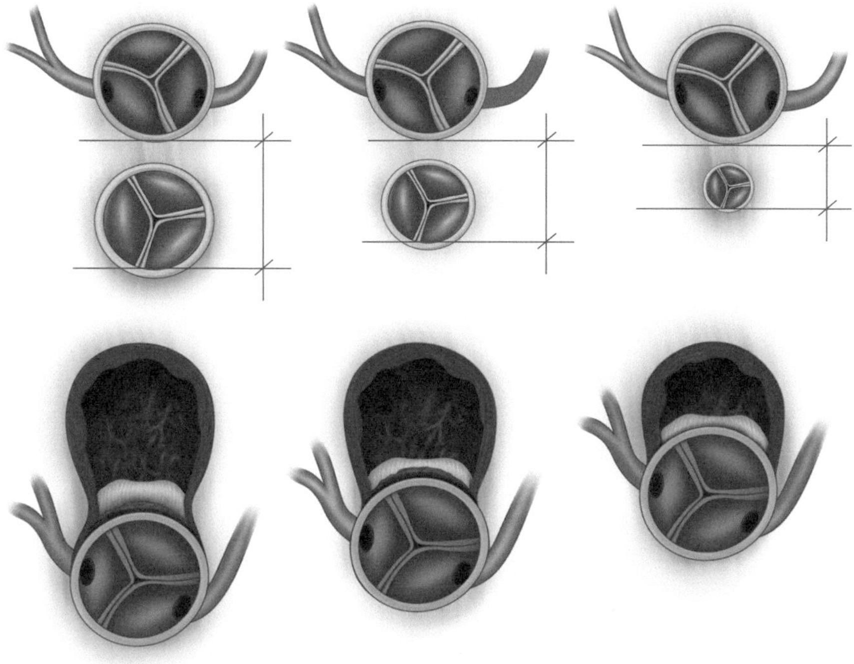

Fig. 20.1 The size of the pulmonary valve annulus clearly impacts the distanced traveled by the aortic root during the posterior translocation of the root when performing a Nikaidoh procedure in patients with D-TGA

thus avoiding a suture line in close proximity to the course of the coronary artery. The presence of "very complex" coronary anatomy (i.e. a single posterior intramural coronary artery) should be considered a relative contraindication.

VI. *The "great vessels" relationship*: In the presence of true "anterior-posterior" great vessels relationship the aortic root and coronary arteries could be harvested and moved "en block". When the relationship is more "side-by-side" it becomes more challenging and frequently require coronary artery harvesting and reimplantation in order to prevent coronary artery kinking or torsion leading to myocardial ischemia.

Surgical Technique

Technique in TGA-VSD-LVOTO

At Children's Hospital of Pittsburgh, cyanotic neonates are initially palliated with a systemic to pulmonary artery shunt via a median sternotomy incision. Elective repair is then performed at 6–12 months of age. Unpalliated patients are considered candidates for complete repair at 2–6 months of age.

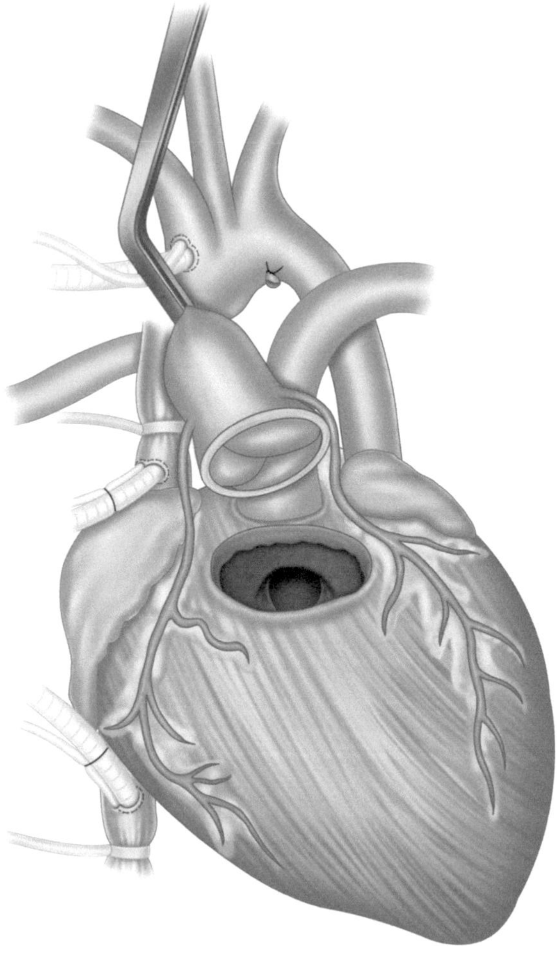

Fig. 20.2 Aortic root harvesting. The aortic root is circumferentially harvested from the right ventricle after mobilizing the proximal aspects of the coronary arteries

The operative management usually involves bi-caval cannulation with mild to moderate hypothermia (30 to 32° Centigrade). An LV-vent is always used as well as antigrade blood cardioplegia. A segment of autologous pericardium is commonly harvested for the reconstruct the right ventricular outflow tract (RVOT).

The surgical technique involves (Figs. 20.2, 20.3, 20.4, 20.5 and 20.6):

I. ***Mobilization of proximal coronary arteries:*** It is vital to identify and extensively dissect the proximal segments of the coronary arteries in order to allow for "en block" translocation or for eventual coronary reimplantation.

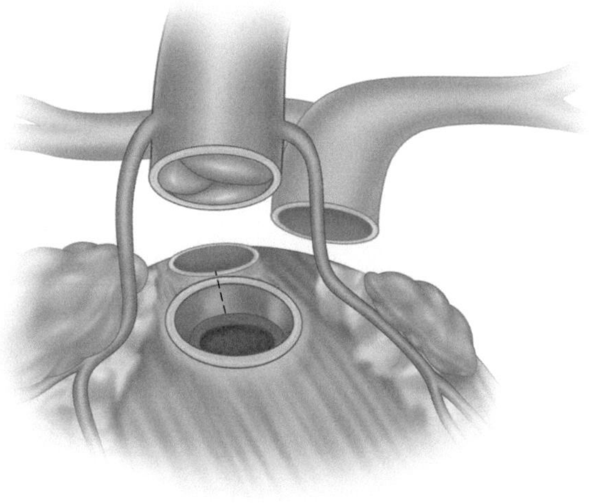

Fig. 20.3 Division of outlet septum. After transection of the proximal MPA the outlet septum is divided along the doted lines

II. ***Harvesting of the aortic root from the right ventricle***. It is important to avoid injuring the aortic valve during harvesting. We initially make a curvilinear incision in the anterior wall if the RV, parallel to the aortic annulus, in order to visualize the valve. The aortic root is then circumferentially dissected from the RV. The harvesting of one or both coronary buttons can facilitate this segment of the operation.

III. ***Transection of the proximal main pulmonary artery***. The main pulmonary artery is transected proximally, preserving the length of the vessel.

IV. ***Division of the outlet septum***. This maneuver results in the division of the hypoplastic pulmonary valve annulus and the usually posteriorly deviated outlet septum resulting in the creation of a widely patent left ventricular outflow tract (LVOT). The edges of the divided outlet septum are frequently resected in order to prevent protrusion into the reconstructed LVOT.

V. ***Translocation of the aortic root***. The posterior aspect of the aortic root is the suture to the residual pulmonary annulus using a running suture. If harvested, the coronary artery buttons can be reimplanted at this time.

VI. ***VSD closure***. The VSD patch is sutured inferiorly and laterally to the edges of the VSD defect and superiorly to the aortic root. Occasionally, in the presence of a "shallow" VSD there is no need for a patch.

VII. ***RVOT reconstruction***. There are several techniques utilized, including: (1) keeping the native pulmonary arteries posterior to the aorta and using a conduit to reestablish continuity, (2) performing a LeCompte maneuver with or without a conduit. Our preference is to perform a Lecompte maneuver with a direct RV to PA connection with an anterior pericardial patch.

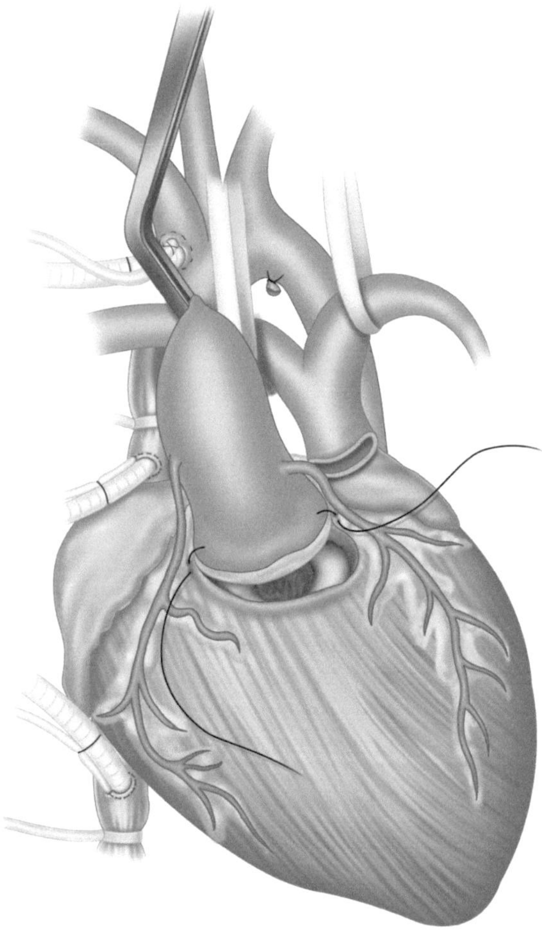

Fig. 20.4 Posterior translocation of the aorta. The aortic root is sutured to the pulmonary annulus posteriorly and laterally

Technique in Corrected TGA-VSD-LVOTO

In patients with congenitally corrected transposition, the atrioventricular conduction axis runs anterior and cephalad to the pulmonary valve, and then descends along the anterior margin of the ventricular septal defect before diverging into the bundle branches [18]. *Division of the muscular outlet septum, therefore, does not result in complete heart block*, but care should be taken when suturing the patch around the ventricular septal defect so as not to injure the conduction tissue (Fig. 20.7). In these patients the great vessels tend to be side-by side, therefore, coronary reimplantation is a necessity. In my experience I have found that the RCA can often be left attached to the aorta only requiring reimplantation of the left main

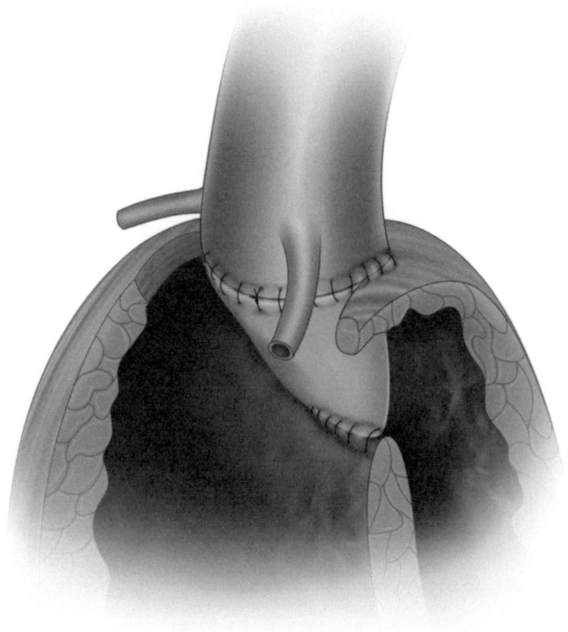

Fig. 20.5 VSD closure. Note that the superior aspect of the patch is sutured to the anterior aspect of the aortic root

coronary artery. An atrial switch procedure is also required; my preference is the Senning procedure.

Outcomes

The Nikaidoh procedure is slowly gaining popularity among congenital cardiac surgeons for the management of patients with complex transposition. The most recent Society of Thoracic Surgery Congenital Database report reveals that approximately 10–15 % of all patients with TGA/VSD/LVOTO are being managed with an aortic translocation procedure, while the great majority is still undergoing a Rastelli procedure [19]. Interestingly, both surgical options had similar in-hospital mortality rates, approximately 5 %.

Aortic translocation avoids the creation of a tortuous intraventricular tunnel, which should result in a much lower incidence of postoperative left ventricular outflow tract obstruction. To date, as far as I know, there has been no reported case of such obstruction after aortic translocation, be it performed for physiologically uncorrected or congenitally corrected transposition.

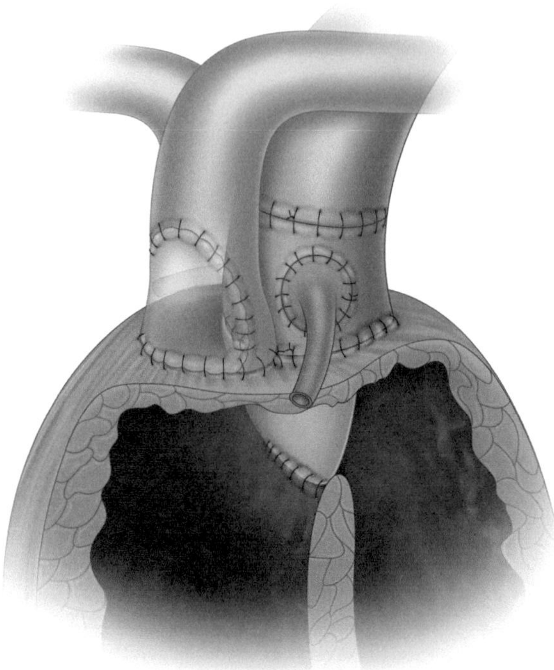

Fig. 20.6 RVOT reconstruction. A LeCompte maneuver with direct RV to PA connection is our preferred approach

This repair also allows for the RV to PA connection to sit in a more posterior position in the mediastinum (Fig. 20.8). We anticipate that this might reduce the incidence of right ventricular outflow tract obstruction secondary to sternal compression, this being a well-documented problem of the Rastelli repair. Also, using a direct RV to PA connection should reduce the number of reoperations as suggested by the REV operation or "réparation à l'étage ventriculaire" published data [20, 21].

Aortic translocation results in more normally aligned right and left ventricular outflow tracts, which theoretically should result in better intracardiac flow dynamics, and should, in turn, result in improved outcomes over the longer term (Fig. 20.4). Yeh and Nikaidoh reported no mortality in 18 patients with a median follow-up of 11.4 years [8]. Bautista reported no late deaths in 11 patients with a median follow-up of 59 months [10]. Clearly, longer follow-up is required to better assess the perceived benefits of this surgical technique.

Significant aortic root dilatation and/or aortic valve insufficiency has been observed in some patients after the Nikaidoh procedure [3, 10]. In our initial publi-

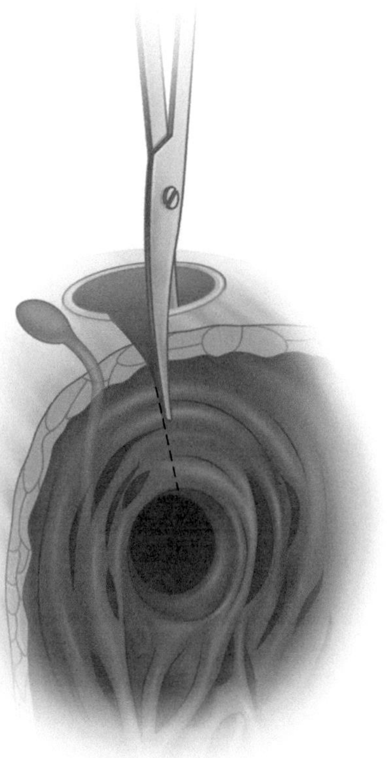

Fig. 20.7 Division of outlet septum in congenitally corrected transposition of the great arteries. Note that the conduction system runs anterior and cephalad to the pulmonary valve, and then descends along the anterior margin of the ventricular septal defect

cation [3], we reported the presence of at least moderate aortic insufficiency in 3 out of 11 survivors. The etiology of this finding is still unclear, but it must be assumed that technical factors play a role, like the disruption of the sinotubular junction during coronary reimplantation. In our experience aortic valve insufficiency has only developed in patients in which both coronary arteries required reimplantation. Emani and associates described a 25 % incidence of aortic root dilatation, with a Z score >3, in their aortic translocation series [22]. Nikaidoh has not reported significant AI in any of his patients despite the fact that root dilatation was noted in the majority of the patients (63 %) [8].

In conclusion, the Nikaidoh procedure for complex TGA and with anomalies of the LVOTO can be achieved with low morbidity and mortality and good relief of the left ventricular outflow tract and right ventricular outflow tract obstruction in intermediate-term follow-up.

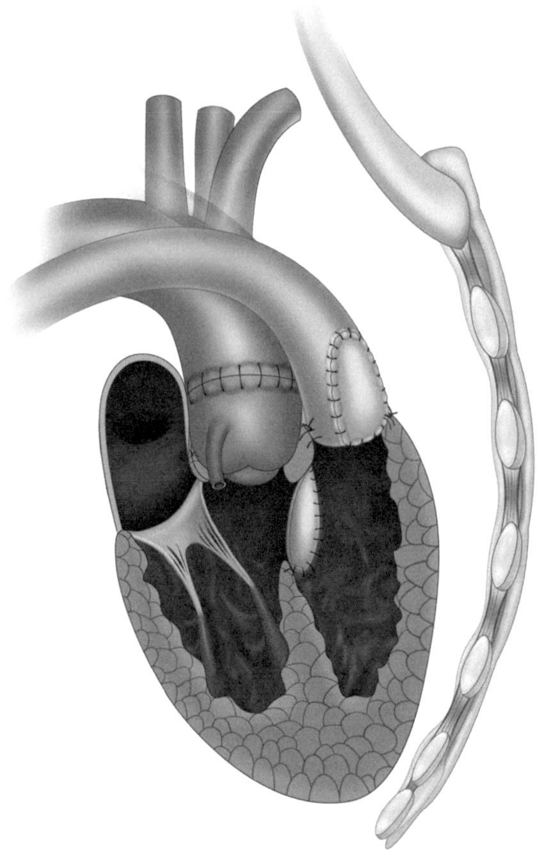

Fig. 20.8 The Nikaidoh procedure allows for a "normal" anatomical repair when compared to a Rastelli. The RV to PA connection is not prone to sternal compression and both ventricular outflow tracks are straighter

References

1. Bex JP, Lecompte Y, Baillot F, Hazan E. Anatomic correction of transposition of the great arteries. Ann Thorac Surg. 1980;29:86–8.
2. Nikaidoh H. Aortic translocation and biventricular outflow tract reconstruction: a new surgical repair for transposition of the great arteries associated with a ventricular septal defect and pulmonary stenosis. J Thorac Cardiovasc Surg. 1984;88:365–72.
3. Morell VO, Jacobs JP, Quintessenza JA. The role of aortic translocation in the management of complex transposition of the great arteries. Semin Thorac Cardiovasc Surg Pediatr Card Surg Annu. 2004;7:80–4.
4. Morell VO, Jacobs JP, Quintessenza JA. Surgical management of transposition with ventricular septal defect and obstruction to the left ventricular outflow tract. Cardiol Young. 2005;15 Suppl 1:102–5.

5. Morell VO. Aortic translocation for TGA with VSD and PS. Cardiothoracic Surgery Network, Expert Techniques, Congenital Cardiac; 2005.
6. Morell VO, Wearden PD. Aortic translocation for the management of transposition of the great arteries with a ventricular septal defect, pulmonary stenosis and hypoplasia of the right ventricle. Eur J Cardiothorac Surg. 2007;31:552–4.
7. Morell VO, Jacobs JP, Quintessenza JA. Aortic translocation and biventricular outflow tract reconstruction in the management of complex transposition of the great arteries with ventricular septal defect and pulmonary stenosis: results and follow-up. Ann Thorac Surg. 2005;79:2089–93.
8. Yeh T, Ramaciotti C, Leonard SR, Roy L, Nikaidoh H. The aortic translocation (Nikaidoh) procedure: midterm results superior to the Rastelli procedure. J Thorac Cardiovasc Surg. 2007;133:461–9.
9. Sayin OA, Ugurlucan M, Saltik L, Sungur Z, Tireli E. Modified Nikaidoh procedure for transposition of great arteries, ventricular septal defect and left ventricular outflow tract obstruction. Thorac Cardiovasc Surg. 2006;54:558–60.
10. Bautista-Hernandez V, Marx GR, Bacha EA, del Nido PJ. Aortic root translocation plus arterial switch for transposition of the great arteries with left ventricular outflow tract obstruction. J Am Coll Cardiol. 2007;49:485–90.
11. Hu S, Li S, Wang X, et al. Pulmonary and aortic translocation in the management of transposition of the great arteries with ventricular septal defect and left ventricular outflow tract obstruction. J Thorac Cardiovasc Surg. 2007;133:1090–2.
12. Hazekamp M, Portela F, Bartelings M. The optimal procedure for the great arteries and left ventricular outflow tract obstruction. An anatomical study. Eur J Cardiothorac Surg. 2007;31:879–87.
13. Yamagishi M, Shuntoh K, Matsushita T, et al. Half-turned truncal switch operation for complete transposition of the great arteries with ventricular septal defect and pulmonary stenosis. J Thorac Cardiovasc Surg. 2003;125:966–8.
14. Kandeel M, Kumar N, Prabhakar G, et al. Aortic Translocation for D-TGA Associated with LVOTO and VSD. Ann Thorac Surg. 1995;59:515–8.
15. Hass GS. Advances in pediatric cardiovascular surgery: anatomic reconstruction of the left ventricular outflow tract in transposition of the great arteries with pulmonic valve abnormalities. Curr Opin Pediatr. 2000;12:501–4.
16. Jacobs ML, Pelletier G, Wearden PD, Morell VO. The role of Fontan's procedure and aortic translocation in the surgical management of patients with discordant atrioventricular connections, interventricular communication, and pulmonary stenosis or atresia. Cardiol Young. 2006;16 Suppl 3:97–102.
17. Kreutzer C, De Vine J, Oppido G, et al. Twenty-five-year experience with Rastelli repair for transposition of the great arteries. J Thorac Cardiovasc Surg. 2000;120:211–23.
18. Anderson RH, Arnold R, Wilkinson JL. The conduction tissue in congenitally corrected transposition. Lancet. 1973;1:1286–7.
19. Data Analyses of The Society of Thoracic Surgeons (STS) Congenital Heart Surgery Database; 2013.
20. Lee JR, Lim HG, Kim YJ, Rho RR, Bae EJ, Noh CI, Yun YS, Ahn C. Repair of transposition of the great arteries, ventricular septal defect and left ventricular outflow tract obstruction. Eur J Cardiothorac Surg. 2004;25:735–41.
21. Van Son JAM, Sim EKW. Lecompte operation with preservation of the pulmonary valve for anomalies of ventriculoarterial connection. Eur J Cardiothorac Surg. 1996;10(7):585–9.
22. Emani SM, Beroukhim R, Zurakowski D, Pigula FA, Mayer JE, del Nido PJ, Geva T, Bacha EA. Outcomes after anatomic repair for D-transposition of the great arteries with left ventricular outflow tract obstruction. Circulation. 2009;120:S53–8.

Chapter 21
Double Root Translocation Operation for Complete Transposition of Great Arteries with Ventricular Septal Defect and Pulmonary Stenosis & Double-Outlet Right Ventricle with Non-committed Ventricular Septal Defect and Pulmonary Stenosis

Shengshou Hu

Abstract The abnormal connection of the ventricle and great arteries is a commonly seen congenital heart disease. It becomes even more clinically complicated when combined with pulmonary stenosis (PS) and ventricular septal defect (VSD). DORV with non-committed ventricular septal defect (DORVncVSD) represents the extreme end of DORV anatomical spectrum. There are problems for classic Rastelli (or REV) or Nikaidoh operations, such as long-term obstruction of left and right ventricle outflow tract and problems due to narrowing of the left ventricle to aorta tunnel. In 2004, double root translocation (DRT) was initially performed in Fuwai Hospital. It aims at retrieving the normal geometry of the left and right ventricle outflow tract, while at the same time maximally preserving function and growth potential of the aortic and pulmonary valves. Until May, 2013, 100 patients have undergone DRT operation in Fuwai Hospital and the early and late results were satisfactory.

Keywords TGA-VSD-LVOTO • DORV • DORV-non-committed VSD • Nikaidoh procedure • Aortic translocation • Double root translocation • Congenital heart surgery • Complex CHD • Conotruncal anomaly

---

S. Hu, MD
Department of Cardiovascular Surgery, National Center for Cardiovascular Diseases and Fuwai Hospital, 167 Beilishi Road, Beijing 100037, China
e-mail: shengshouhu@yahoo.com

F. Lacour-Gayet et al. (eds.), *Surgery of Conotruncal Anomalies*,
DOI 10.1007/978-3-319-23057-3_21

Background

The abnormal connection of ventricle and great arteries is commonly seen in congenital heart disease, which becomes even more clinically complicated when combined with pulmonary stenosis (PS). Ventricular septal defect (VSD) is usually the associated abnormality, for which surgical treatment is complicated. TGA with intact ventricular septum are rarely seen and satisfactory treatment effect could be obtained by performing arterial switch operation (ASO) after previous pulmonary artery angioplasty or relief of outflow tract [1]. Complete transposition of great arteries combined (TGA) with ventricular spetal defect and pulmonary stenosis is defined as the aorta taking its origin completely from the right ventricle while the pulmonary artery from the left ventricle, combined with isolated or multiple VSD. Pulmonary stenosis refers to stenosis occuring valvularly or subvalvularly, which is usually associated with bicuspid pulmonary valve deformity and obstruction of left ventricle outflow tract (LVOTO) due to fibrosis or muscular pulmonary subvalvular hypertrophy.

The birth ratio of TGA is about 1:2100 to 1:4500. The ratio is low for those with intact ventricular septum who have stenosis of left ventricle outflow tract, the ratio of which at birth is only 0.7 %. As for TGA patients with VSD, up to 20 % of them are born with LVOTO. This ratio could add to 30–35 % as a certain number of patients develop secondary LVOTO with their growing up [2].

In 1969, Rastelli and colleagues [2] initially developed surgical approach by means of applying intracardiac and extracardiac tunnel for treatment of this deformity, with satisfactory results obtained (see Chap. 19). Ever since then, the Rastelli operation and the modified réparation à l'étage ventriculaire (REV) procedure [2, 3] have been the standard surgical approach for this disease [2, 3]. However there are disadvantages for both of these operations. The intracardiac tunnel used by Rastelli procedure would cause long-term obstruction of left and right ventricle outflow tract and problems due to involution of the artificial tunnel, leading to a high rate of a reoperation of more than 40 % [4, 5]. As for REV operation, because of absence of valvulation in the reconstructed outflow tract of right ventricle, severe regurgitation would occur and influences function of the right ventricle [6]. Therefore, the long term prognosis is questionable for Rastelli and REV operation.

In 1984, Nikaidoh [7] operation was initially used in clinical practice, which reimplants the dislocated aortic root into the outflow tract of the left ventricle as a treatment for patients with TGA combined with LVOTO. However, integrity the outflow tract of the left ventricle, in spite of the anatomical correction by Nikaidoh operation, was ruined by the incision during the procedure. Moreover, when reconstructing the outflow tract of the right ventricle, the native pulmonary valve was not preserved, which may cause severe post-operative regurgitation and influence the function of the right ventricle. Although artificial or bioprosthetic outflow tunnels have been used for reconstruction of the outflow tract of the right ventricle in some sick children, there is still an issue with reoperations because of failure of growth of the reconstructed tissue [8].

Double-outlet right ventricle (DORV) is defined as a type of ventriculo-arterial connection in which both great vessels arise either entirely or predominantly from the right ventricle. As a primitive mode of ventriculo-arterial connection corresponding to an early stage of the embryologic development, DORV represents a spectrum of various morphologic subgroups, and therefore a wide spectrum of different surgical techniques has been adopted for repair. DORV with non-committed ventricular septal defect (DORVncVSD) represents the extreme end of the anatomical spectrum. More importantly, the VSD lies at a distance from both the aortic and pulmonary annulus that is greater than the aortic annulus diameter [9]. This anatomical characteristic led to the difficulty of intracardiac tunnel repair associated with an important and inevitable risk of late subaortic obstruction. Furthermore, the biventricular repair of DORVncVSD or DORV with subpulmonary VSD, associated with pulmonary stenosis (PS), needs to meet the challenge of complete reconstruction of the two ventricular outflow tracts and remains a procedure of high risk. Moreover, the Rastelli procedure has proved to be an unsatisfactory solution owing to its disappointing long-term results; and the presence of a remote VSD is an anatomical contraindication to the REV procedure, which is an alternative to the Rastelli Procedure. Nikaidoh procedure, with the evolution of aortic translocation techniques, has exceptionally been performed in cases of DORV with subpulmonary VSD and PS; however, its clinical application to DORVncVSD with severe right ventricular outflow tract (RVOT) obstruction has never been reported [10].

Just as Prof. Reddy said on the 88th American Association for Thoracic Surgery (AATS) annual meeting, "If there is something left to be most challenging to pediatric cardiac surgeons in the new century, it is ventricular-aortic discordance with ventricular septal defect and pulmonary stenosis." In view of all the issues above, in 2004, double root translocation (DRT) was initially performed in Fuwai Hospital, which aims at retrieving the normal geometry of the left and right ventricle outflow tract, while at the same time maximally preserving the long-term function and growth potential of the aortic and pulmonary valves, for which there has been better clinical results [10–12].

Anatomical Classification

Type of VSD

In TGA, the VSD morphology is similar to isolated VSD. The type of VSD most frequently seen occurs at the infundibular part, which is not adjacent to the pulmonary valve and lies a certain distance from the tricuspid valve, which is different from the Tetralogy of Fallot. The infundibular VSD is associated with a leftwards displacement of the conal septum, causing LVOTO. When it moves rightwards, double outlet right ventricle (DORV) is formed, or in other words, Taussig-Bing anomaly, which is usually associated with subaortic obstruction or aortic arch obstruction. When the VSD lies underneath the aorta, the infundibulum could become restrictive or even atretic. VSD located in the inflow tract (perimembranous VSD) is commonly seen, with the conductive bundle running at its posterior and inferior border. Muscular and multiple VSD could also be present. The non-committed VSD refers to those lying at a distance from both the aortic and pulmonary annulus that is greater than the aortic annulus diameter, which brings difficulty to intracardiac tunnel repair, for it is associated with an important and inevitable risk of late subaortic obstruction [10].

Classification of LVOTO (Pulmonary and Subpulmonary Stenosis)

The mechanism of LVOTO is often multifactorial including pulmonary valvular stenosis (bicuspid pulmonary valve), pulmonary annulus hypoplasia and subpulmonary stenosis. LVOTO could be either functional or anatomic. Functional LVOTO is usually seen in TGA without VSD, caused by the leftward move of muscular septum due to increase of pressure within the right ventricle, which is similar with hypertrophic obstructive myocardiopathy but without asymmetrical septal hypertrophy. Anatomical LVOTO is usually seen in TGA patients associated with VSD. Stenosis occurs either valvular or subvalvular. The subvalvular stenosis could be muscular or fibrous. Abnormal fibrous or tendinous tissue adhesion could sometimes be detected between the anterior leaflet of mitral valve and the muscular septum of outflow tract. Other causes of LVOTO include deformity of mitral valve apparatus and formation of membranous septum aneurysm which protrudes into the outflow tract of the left ventricle [2]. The DRT operation requires that the pressure gradient of pulmonary valve is larger than 35 mmHg and that diameter of pulmonary annulus larger than at least one third of the aortic valve. Excessive hypoplasia of pulmonary valve resulting in insufficient pulmonary valvular diameter is unsuitable for DRT operation, which is an indication for "palliative" Rastelli.

Existence of Bilateral Conal Structure

Subaortic conus exists in most TGA or TGA-type DORV patients, and subpulmonary conus exists in most DORV conditions, forming a bilateral conal structure. Up to May 2013, 106 patients underwent DRT operation in Fuwai Hospital, among whom 67 patients were found to have bilateral conal structure. The fibrous structure between the pulmonary and the mitral valve is generally larger than 10 mm in patients weighing more than 10 kg, which is a significant anatomical basis for DRT operation, since both aortic and pulmonary artery roots could be cut off from the outflow tract of left ventricle, which allows subsequent biventricular reconstruction of the outflow tracts.

Anomaly of Coronary Artery Patterns

Coronary ostial abnormalities result embryologically from a failure of the normal fusion of the main coronary trunks with the sinus of Valsalva bud emerging from the aorta. Most TGA patients, whether simple TGA or with coexisting VSD, have the left anterior descending and circumflex coronary arteries arising from a common trunk in sinus 1 (left anterior facing sinus) and the right coronary artery arising from sinus 2 (right posterior facing sinus) [13]. Among the 100 patients who underwent DRT operation in Fuwai hospital, 11 patients were diagnosed of single coronary ostium (11 %). The coronary artery pattern is the major risk factor specifically related to the malformation of TGA. The origin of the left main coronary artery or only the left anterior descending or circumflex coronary artery from sinus 2 was a risk factor for death [13].

Diagnosis and Imaging

Echocardiography

A preliminary anatomical diagnosis could be achieved by echocardiography. 2D echocardiogram could clearly demonstrate the positional relationship of the great arteries, as well as defining the cause and extent of pulmonary or subpulmonary stenosis. Developmental condition of pulmonary valve could be well-judged by measurement of the diameter of valvular ring and identification of the number and shape of valve leaflets. Moreover, the connection and distance between pulmonary and mitral valvular rings was also able to be identified. Meanwhile, echocardiogram could reveal the developmental condition of the two ventricles, including the structure and function of atrio-ventricular valves, chordae straddling and malformation of coronary arteries.

Cardiac Catheter Imaging (*Figs. 21.1 and 21.2*)

Cardiac catheter imaging is an important supplement for echocardiography, which provides more direct and numerical anatomical information. Both right and left ventricles volume are assessed as well as alignment with the great arteries. Muscular and multiple VSD are better obviated by angiogram than by echocardiography. Moreover, angiography provides clear information on pulmonary artery branches size, pulmonary annulus diameter, subvalvular muscular obstruction, associated PDA, and presence of aorta-pulmonary collateral arteries which may require intraoperative occluding in a hybrid operating room. The course of the coronary arteries could be well identified. In general, cardiac imaging is an important preoperative examination of these complex patients guiding the operating strategy in providing critical anatomic information.

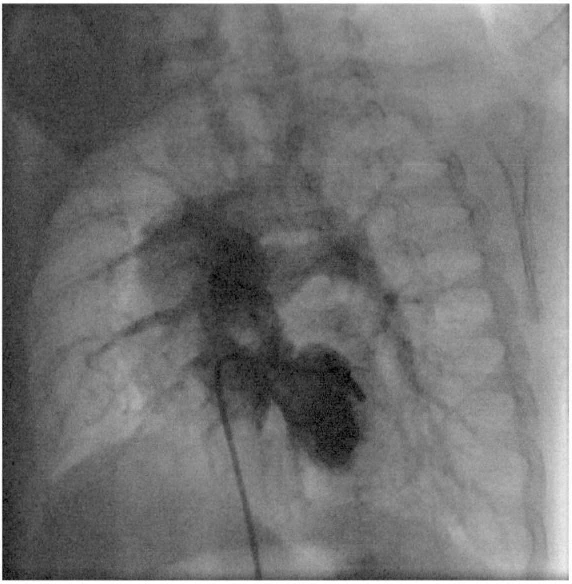

Fig. 21.1 Catheter Imaging of left ventricle: The contrast medium was injected into the left ventricle, which developed an image first. With systole of the heart, the contrast medium passed into the right ventricle through VSD, developing image of the RV. Both great arteries arise from RV, with the aorta lying anteriorly and the PA posteriorly. VSD is remote from both great arteries

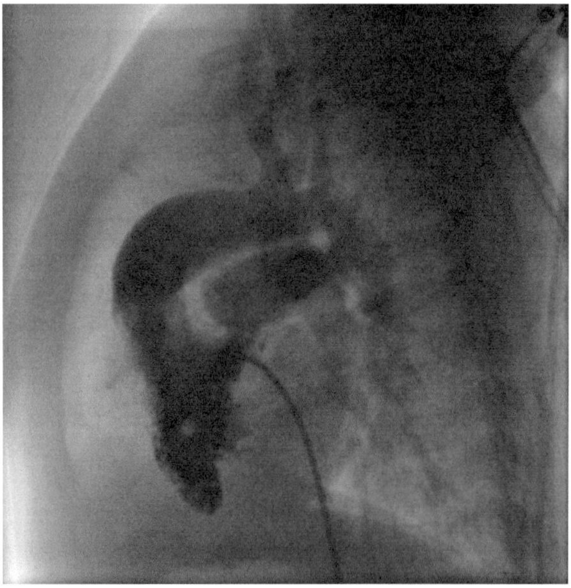

Fig. 21.2 Catheter Imaging of right ventricle: The contrast medium was injected into the right ventricle, which developed an image first. With systole of the heart, both great arteries developed image simultaneously. A minority of medium passed into LV. Subaortic as well as subpulmonary stenosis could be detected in the image. Bilateral conal structure of the great arteries could be identified

Cardiovascular Computer Tomography (CT) and Magnetic Resonance Imaging (MRI)

These two imaging techniques are more accurate than echocardiography in spatial resolution but not routinely used as pre-operative assessment, only serving as supplements. MRI requires usually general anesthesia which complicates the pre-operative management

Check List Prior to DRT

1. Age > 6 months and weight > 8 kg
2. Diagnosis of TGA- VSD-LVOTO or DORVncVSD-PS confirmed
3. Two good size ventricles.
4. RV to PA systolic gradient > 35 mmHg.
5. Morphology of PA valve, pulmonary annulus and PA branches. Presence of MAPCAs
6. Coronary anatomy
7. Absence of severe associations (CAVSD, AV valve straddling, and swiss cheese VSD)

Indications

For patients under 6 month of age and with asymmetrical growth of two ventricles, or with severe cyanosis and hypoplastic pulmonary arteries, we recommend an systemico-pulmonary shunt operation with aim of alleviating patient's hypoxia and promoting development of pulmonary arteries and ventricles. Radical operation is advisable when patient grows up to 6 month or older, when his pulmonary arteries have been well developed.

For patients with TGA, VSD and PS, DRT could be generally applied. However, the REV procedure is an alternative consideration: in patients with subaortic VSD or a side by side great arteries relationship, and in patients with a small conal septum, making it easy to reroute the aorta through an intra-ventricular tunnel. In the case of subpulmonary VSD or VSD distant from the aorta, along with an antero-posterior relationship of the two great arteries, DRT can be the optimal choice.

Considering patients with DORVncVSD and PS, the indication mainly depends on the location of VSD and its relationship with the outlets of the great arteries. The procedure of DORV with a subaortic VSD is routinely performed with Fallot repair technique. For patients with subpulmonary VSD, closing VSD and reconstructing outlet of left ventricle are subsequent to translocation of aortic and pulmonary roots. In other case with intact bilateral muscular conus, VSD is remote from both great arteries (or slightly closer to the pulmonary artery), and the conal septum would be widely resected during mobilization of the aortic and pulmonary root, and the part of conal septal tissue of the upper edge of the VSD is reserved as the neo-left ventricular outflow tract, which is for reconnection to the aortic root (Fig. 21.3).

In summary, the best indication for DRT operation is patients aged older than 6 months, who are diagnosed with TGA-VSD-PS, or DORVncVSD-PS, with subpulmonary VSD or VSD remote from both great arteries. Both ventricles shall be well-developed and without severe associating deformities (CAVSD, AV valve straddling, and Swiss cheese VSD, etc).

Atrio-ventricular discordance is not a contra-indication for DRT. Under this circumstance, however, the pulmonary root shall not be completely harvested, and certain portion of the pulmonary annular need to be preserved to avoid injury to the conduction tissue traveling underneath. Moreover, the timing of surgery should be delayed due to atrial switch procedures such as Senning or Mustard.

Among all the 106 patients who underwent DRT in Fuwai Hospital, 9 cases received concomitant atrial switch procedures because of anomalous atrio-ventricular connection, with operation time as well as recovery stay much longer than those receiving simple DRT. Surgical risk is especially high for those with severe cyanosis due to severe pulmonary stenosis, who have been long enduring chronic hypoxia preoperatively. Existence of aorto-pulmonary collateral vessels is not contraindi-

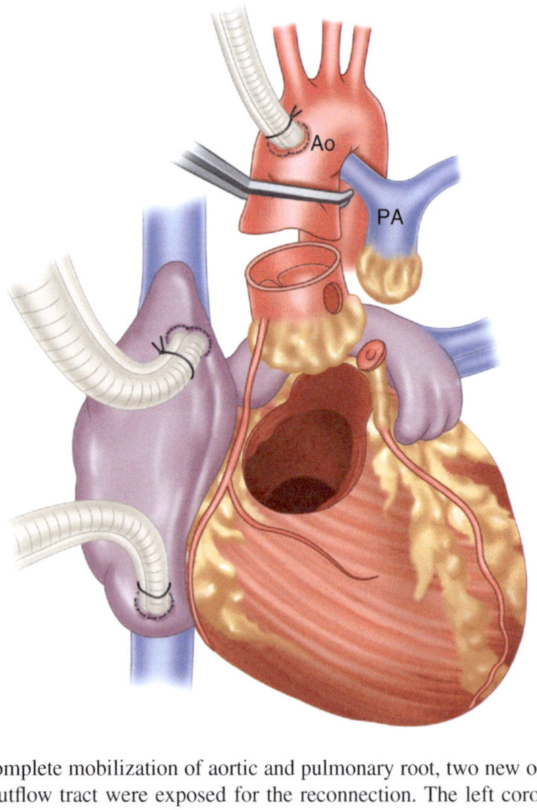

Fig. 21.3 After complete mobilization of aortic and pulmonary root, two new orifices of left and right ventricular outflow tract were exposed for the reconnection. The left coronary ostium was harvested and prepared for reimplantation at a favorable site in the aortic sinus. The VSD was repaired with a Dacron patch to make an intracardiac tunnel from LV to the neoaorta. The aorta was transected for a subsequent Lecompte maneuver (*Ao* aorta, *MV* mitral valve, *PA* pulmonary artery)

cated for DRT either, for which a hybrid procedure is advisable, with interventional embolization of collateral vessels being done prior to performing DRT.

Surgical Techniques

DRT for TGA-VSD-LVOTO

1. The operation is performed under general anesthesia and hypothermic cardiopulmonary bypass with aortic and bicaval cannulation. Before setting up bypass, the aortopulmonary septum and both left and right pulmonary arteries should be fully mobilized, and the ductus arteriosus shall be ligated and divided. Modified balanced ultrafiltration was applied and Cold HTK cardioplegia was infused through the aortic root every 2 h and ice was placed around the epicardium for myocardial protection.
2. After dividing the aorta 1 cm above the level of aortic sinotubular junction (Fig. 21.4), aortic valve and orifice of the coronary arteries were explored. Both the left and right

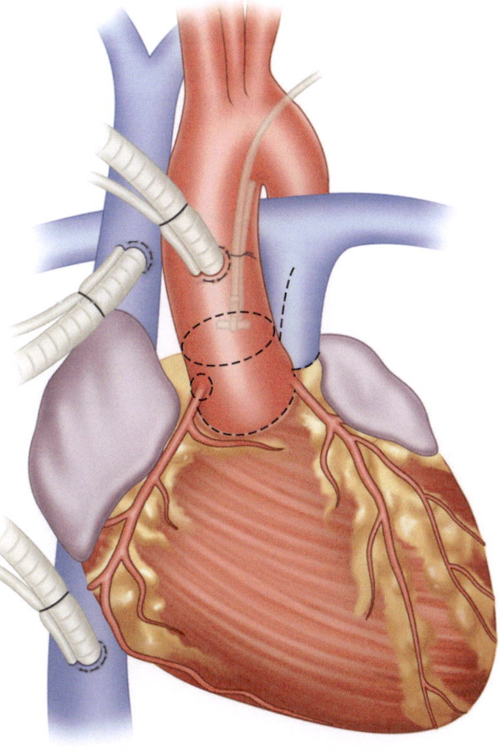

Fig. 21.4 Both aortic and pulmonary root were excised and harvested, *5 to 8* mm below the aortic annulus and 4 to 6 mm below the pulmonary annulus respectively. The narrowed LVOT was opened and VSD was repaired

coronary artery trunks were mobilized from the aortic root. Then the aortic root was resected from the outflow tract of the right ventricle 0.5 cm below the aortic valve, and one side of the coronary artery orifice was excised (Fig. 21.5) (normally the right side).

3. The VSD was repaired by a patch. Interrupted suture with 5-0 prolene lines was made at the inferior border of the VSD next to the annulus of the tricuspid valve from incision of right ventricle outflow tract, with the rest border repaired by continuous suture to close the VSD.
4. The main pulmonary artery (MPA) was dissected to explore the pulmonary valve. Then the root of MPA was amputated from the left ventricle outflow tract after dissecting along the commissure of two anterior leaflets. Attention shall be paid to avoid damaging the mitral valve annulus. Subpulmonary residual fibrous stenosis was excised and along with some muscle on the side of the ventricular septum if necessary, in order to relief obstruction of the outflow tract of the left ventricle.
5. The defect left on the aortic sinus wall after excising of coronary artery orifice was then repaired by autologous glutaraldehyde-tanned pericardial patch. The aortic root was then rotated backwards with the unmoved orifice of the coronary artery (usually the left one) as a foothold to the opening of the left ventricular outflow tract (be cautious not to twist the coronary artery) (Fig. 21.5). 5-0 prolene stitches with patches were applied to complete anastomosis of the aortic root and the left ventricular outflow tract with a U-shape interrupted sutures (Fig. 21.6). The excised coronary artery orifice was then transplanted to corresponding position of aortic root with continuous suture using a 6-0 prolene stitch, termed as button technique. After Lecompte maneuver (Figs. 21.7 and 21.8) was per-

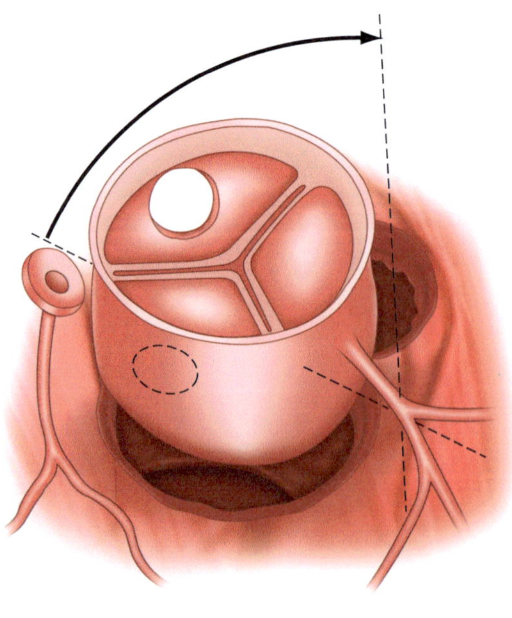

Fig. 21.5 Both the left and right coronary artery trunks were mobilized from the aortic root. Then the aortic root was amputated from the outflow tract of the right ventricle 0.5 cm below the aortic valve, and one side of the coronary artery orifice was excised (normally the right side)

formed, anastomosis of the proximal and distal end of the aorta was then completed.

6. The pulmonary artery root was reconstructed with allogeneic pulmonary or bovine jugular monovalvular patch (Fig. 21.7), and the hypertrophic parietal band of right ventricular outflow tract was excised. The opening of the outflow tract of right ventricle was then constricted to the size of the neopulmonary root diameter. Then 6-0 prolene stitch was used to complete the anastomosis of MPA root and right ventricular outflow tract, with a continuous suture (Fig. 21.8).

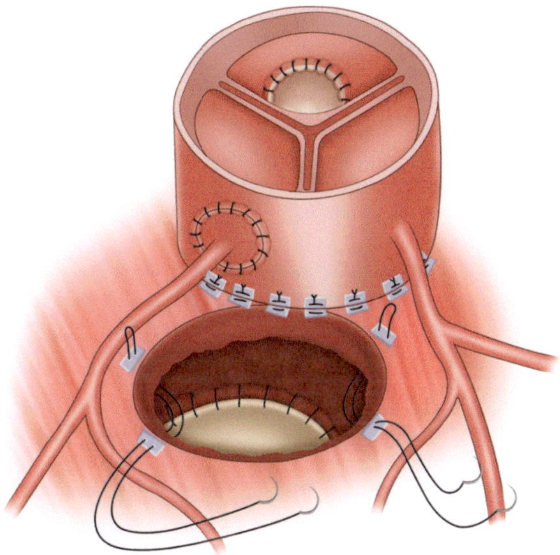

Fig. 21.6 The excised CA was selectively transferred to a favorable site (Button technique). The VSD was repaired by a patch from incision of right ventricle outflow tract. The opening of the outflow tract of right ventricle was constricted to the size of the neopulmonary root diameter

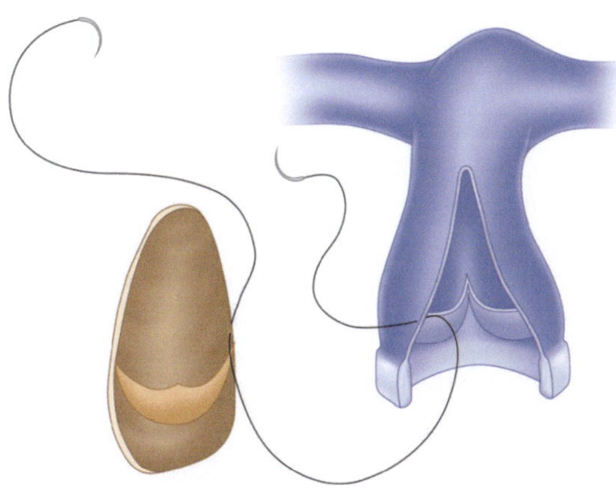

Fig. 21.7 A free pulmonary root with monovalve patch was reconstructed, making 3 valves in the same plane for a competent valvular apparatus

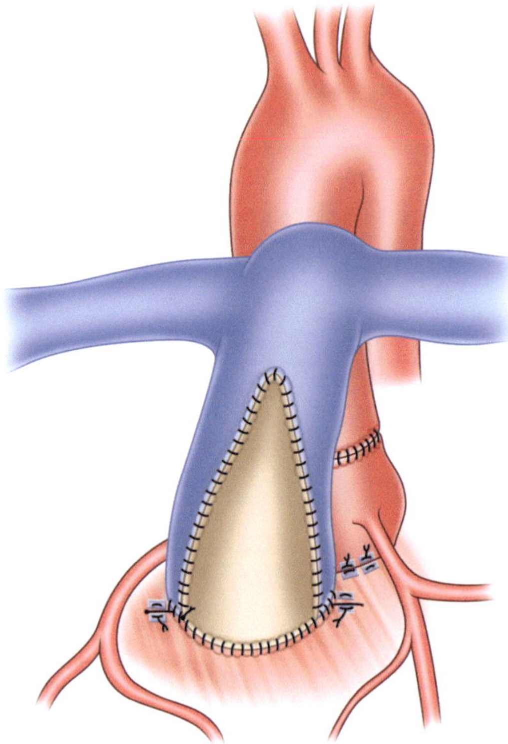

Fig. 21.8 After Lecompte maneuver was performed, anastomosis of the proximal and distal end of the aorta was then completed. The pulmonary artery root was reconstructed with allogeneic pulmonary or bovine jugular monovalvular patch, after which anastomosis of MPA root and right ventricular outflow tract was then completed

DRT Procedure for DORV

There is no essential difference between surgical procedures for patients with DORVncVSD-PS and TGA-VSD-PS. Presence of well-shaped bilateral conus in DORV patients facilitate the harvesting of the aortic and pulmonary roots en bloc, without injury to peripheral tissue. Competence of the neo-aortic and pulmonary valves could be better preserved with sufficient muscular support from great vessel roots during their reimplantation (Fig. 21.9). The LVOT was reconstructed by suturing the upper half of the VSD patch to the remaining conal septum, which is widely resected during mobilization of the pulmonary root, while the lower half sutured to the bottom edge of the septal defect (Fig. 21.10).

Technical Highlights

There has been a number of modifications of the initial Nikaidoh operation. For instance, Morrell et al suggested that much attention shall be paid to the coronary artery transfer so as to avoid twisting or stretching. He also emphasized the importance of the Lecompte maneuver for preserving the competence of RVOT [14]. However, since the conal septal tissue of VSD was dissected anyway, the LVOT would become forwards and enlarged, which may cause post-operative aortic insufficiency. Meanwhile the RVOT was completely replaced by foreign tissue, losing its long-term valve function and growth potential. DRT operation is different from the classic Nikaidoh or the modified surgeries in following aspects.

(a) The autologous pulmonary valve was well preserved. In DRT operation, pulmonary artery root was completely harvested from the LV and transplanted onto the reconstructed RVOT, constituting its posterior and lateral wall, while a monovalve allogeneic pulmonary artery conduit served as the anterior wall of RVOT. In this way, the hemodynamics of the neo-constructed RVOT was most close to normal and at the same time theoretically preserved the growth potential and avoided calcification or obstruction of RVOT.
(b) After harvesting the pulmonary artery root from the LV, LVOTO was further alleviated, which spared the majority of patients from having their conal septum dissected in order to enlarge the LVOT, thus preserved the LV function as much as possible and maintained the almost normal hemodynamics of LVOT. Therefore, the possibility of post-operative aortic insufficiency due to enlargement of LVOT was greatly reduced.
(c) Coronary artery transplantation was not included in the classic Nikaidoh operation [7]. In modified operations it was suggested that transplantation of coronary arteries could prevent coronary artery related incidents [8, 14]. In DRT operation, normally one of the coronary arteries was fully mobilized. Then with the other coronary artery as a foothold, the aortic root was rotated to the posterior, rather than moving in parallel, which ensured the preserved coronary artery to be avoided from twisting or stretching. For those with single coronary artery, rotating could be performed with the only coronary artery as foothold after being fully mobilized. If necessary, bilateral coronary artery transfer should be performed.

Outcomes

From March, 2004 to May, 2013, up to 100 dTGA or TGA type DORV combined with VSD and PS patients underwent DRT operation in Fuwai Hospital (63 cases of dTGA, 28 cases of DORV and 9 cases of cTGA). Concomitant procedures included: Senning procedure in 9 cases, transcatheter aortic-pulmonary collateral artery occlusion in 9 cases, angioplasty of left and right pulmonary arteries in 16 cases,

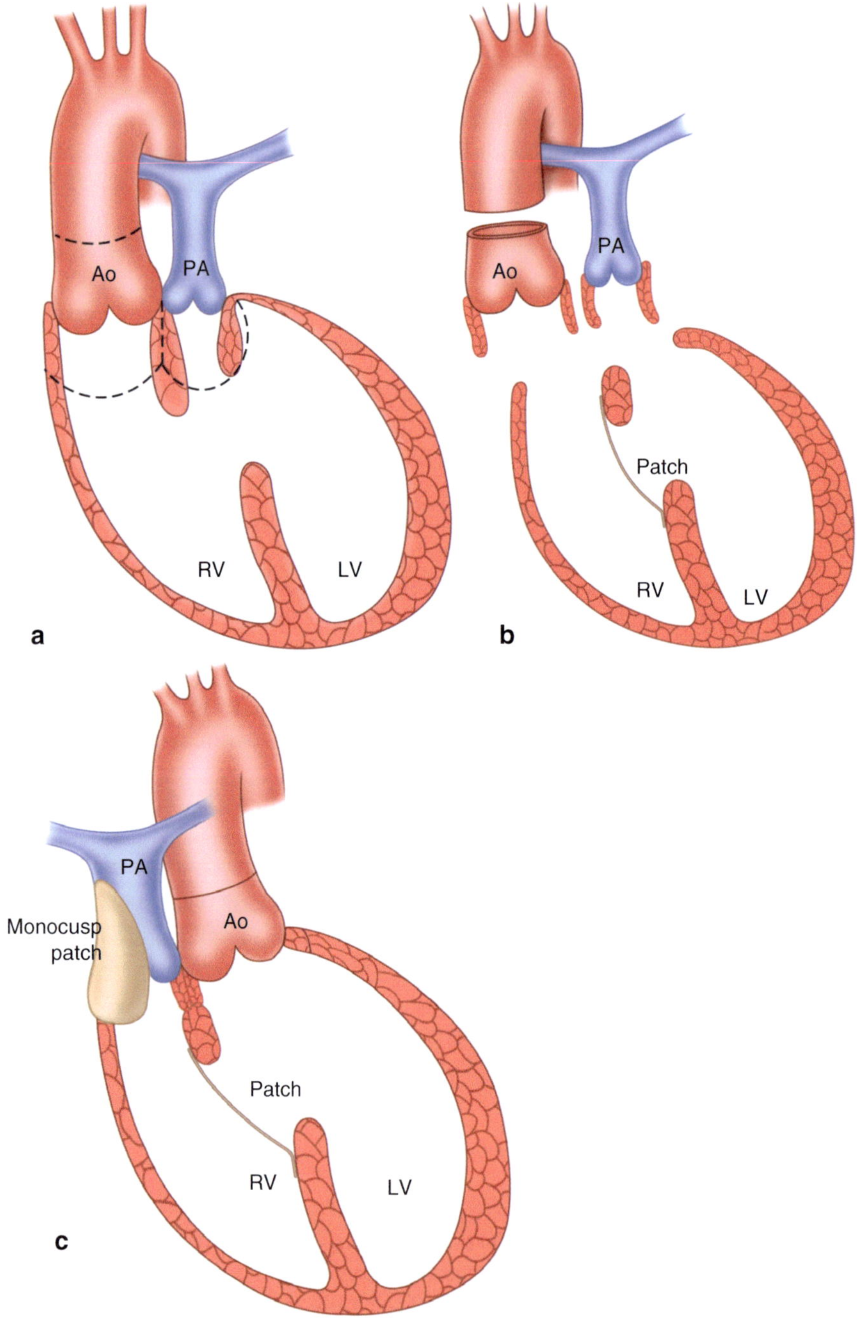
Ao
PA
RV
LV
a
Ao
PA
Patch
RV
LV
b
PA
Ao
Monocusp
patch
Patch
RV
LV
c

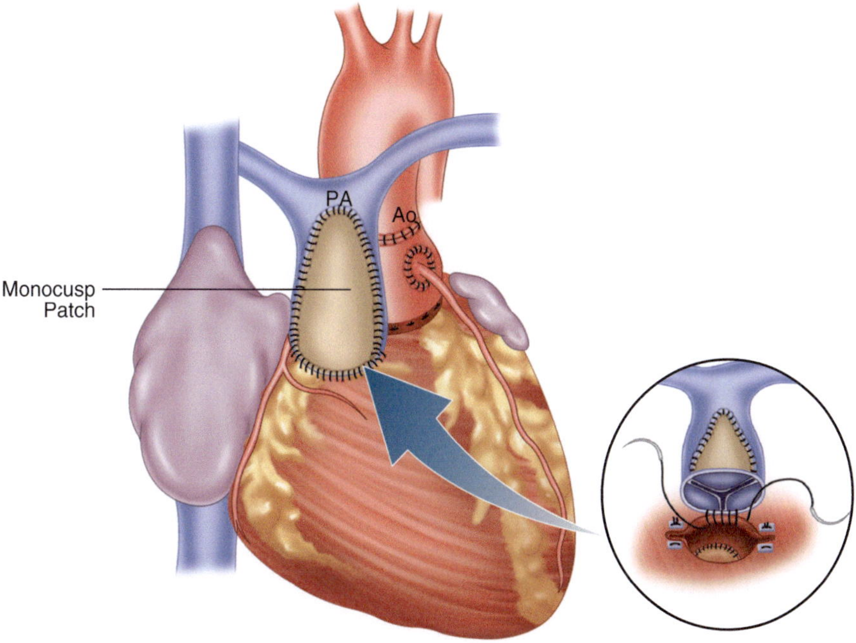

Fig. 21.10 Reconstruction of the left ventriculoaorta and right ventriculopulmonary trunk continuity. The aortic roots were connected to the neo-orifice of the left ventricular outflow tract, followed with left coronary artery reimplantation. After the Lecompte maneuver, a monocusp bovine jugular vein patch or a homograft pulmonary patch was tailored to reconstruct a neopulmonary root and connected to the reshaped orifice of the right ventricular outflow tract (*Ao* aorta, *LV* left ventricle, *PA* pulmonary artery, *RV* right ventricle)

and delayed sternal closure in 12 cases. The mean CPB time was 305.5 ± 64.2 min, and the mean aortic time was 208.6 ± 40.8 min. Average mechanical ventilating time was 6.5 ± 9.4 days. Mortality rate during hospital stay was 5% (5 cases), of which 4 patients died of low cardiac output syndrome (all within the first 40 cases), 1 case died on the 16th day postoperatively. 12 cases had to receive Extracorporeal

Fig. 21.9 The anatomy of double-outlet right ventricle with noncommitted ventricular septal defect (VSD) associated with pulmonary stenosis features with (1) a VSD distant from both aortic and pulmonary annulus by a length superior to an aortic diameter; (2) both great vessels arising 200 % from the right ventricle; (3) a double conus; and (4) pulmonary stenosis with hypoplasia trunk. The dashed line illustrates the area of mobilization of aortic and pulmonary root. The ventricular septal tissue of the upper edge of the VSD was reserved as the ventricular septum of the neo–left ventricular outflow tract for after reconnection to aortic root (*Ao* aorta, *LV* left ventricle, *MV* mitral valve, *PA* pulmonary artery, *RV* right ventricle

Membrane Oxygenation (ECMO) support perioperatively due to low cardiac output syndrome (8 occurring within the first 40 cases), of whom 9 patients successfully weaned off after 6.2 ± 4.0 days in average. 8 cases had to undergo hemofiltration therapy due to renal failure, and 23 patients received peritoneal dialysis. Tracheostomy was performed in 8 patients because of long-time mechanical ventilation. Permanent pacemaker was installed in 2 cases due to complete atrioventricular block (both cases underwent concomitant Senning procedure). The DRT operation is complicated in steps and brings large trauma to patients. The operation itself involves a number of intracardiac key structures and thus requires a thorough understanding of the anatomy of complicated congenital heart disease as well as excellent surgical skills of the operator. As a new type of operation, a learning curve is necessary. There are obvious differences for results between the early and late cases. Of all the 5 death cases of our 100 patients who received DRT, 4 occurred within the first 40 cases, and for those 12 cases requiring ECMO assistance, 8 were found among the first 40 cases.

Post-operative following-up was taken with a successful rate of 96.9. During the 2 ~ 85 month (median 44 months) follow-ups, there were 5 late death, 3 of which died suddenly and 2 died of heart failure. The LVOT pressure gradient was 4.03 ± 1.84 mmHg in average, with trivial AI occurring in 8 cases (8 %). The mean RVOT pressure gradient was 14.32 ± 17.04 mmHg, and only 6 patients showed moderate or severe PI. 1 patient underwent reoperation due to PS. Middle and long-term follow up demonstrated good function of both LVOT and RVOT.

In 2005, Morell and colleagues reviewed 12 TGA patients who had received Nikaidoh operation. There was 1 hospital death (8.3 %) and during a median follow-up of 33 months, 3 patients (25 %) developed moderate aortic insufficiency, and late RVOTO occurred in 2 cases (17 %). 4 (33 %) late reoperation were performed in three patients for reasons such as conduit replacement and valve repair [14]. In 2006, Yeh et al reviewed 19 patients who underwent Nikaidoh operations. There was 1 hospital death (5 %) and during a follow-up of 11.4 years in median, 3 patients (16 %) developed moderate aortic insufficiency, 9 patients (47 %) developed moderate pulmonary insufficiency, and late RVOTO occurred in 3 cases (16 %). Up to 5 cases (26 %) required late reoperations for RVOT reasons, among whom 4 received homograft replacement and 1 patient underwent pulmonary valve replacement [8]. In the study carried out by Hernandez and colleagues in 2007, up to 11 patients diagnosed of dTGA with LVOTO or TGA type DORV underwent Nikaidoh plus arterial switch operation. During the follow-up of 59 months, 1 patients (10 %) developed moderate aortic insufficiency, 5 patients (45 %) developed moderate pulmonary insufficiency, and late RVOTO occurred in 5 cases (45 %). 5 cases (45 %) required reoperation for reason of RV-to-PA conduit obstruction [15]; In 2013, Honjo et al reviewed 28 TGA with LVOTO or DORV patients who received surgical repair in there center, among whom 8 patients underwent Nikaidoh operation. Others received ASO plus LVOTO resection (n = 12), Rastelli (n = 6), or single ventricle palliation (n = 2). The median follow-up period was 65 months, during which 3 patients (38 %) developed mild aortic insufficiency. There was no hospital death or late LVOTO [16].

Table 21.1 Outcomes comparison between DRT and cther surgical procedures performed at different centers

Author	Case number	Follow-up time	In-hospital death	LVOT	AI	RVOT	PI	Redo-operation
Morell and Quintessenza [14]	12	33 M	1(8.3%)	Stenosis 1(8%)	Moderate 3(25 %)	Stenosis 2(17 %)	N/A	4(33 %)
Yeh (2006) [8]	19	11.4 Y	1(5%)	N/A	Moderate 3(16 %)	Stenosis 3(16 %)	Moderate 9(47 %)	5(26 %)
Bautista-Hernandez et al. (2007) [15]	11	59 M	0	N/A	Moderate 1(10 %)	Stenosis 5(45 %)	Moderate 5(45 %)	5(45 %)
Honjo et al. (2013) [16]	8	65 M	0	N/A	Moderate 3(38 %)	N/A	N/A	N/A
Our Group (2013)	106	44 M	3	PG 4–16 mm Hg (median: 5)	Mild 11(11 %)	PG 4–24 mm Hg (median : 10)	moderate 11(11 %) moderate 6(6 %)	1(1 %)

Compared with the surgical outcomes for treatment of d-type TGA with VSD and PS along with DORVncVSD in other centers, our patients have generally low percentage for postoperative aortic insufficiency, RVOTO, pulmonary insufficiency, and reoperation (Table 21.1).

References

1. Hazekamp M, Portela F, Bartelings M. The optimal procedure for the great arteries and left ventricular outflow tract obstruction. An anatomical study. Eur J Cardiothorac Surg. 2007;31(5):879–87.
2. Rastelli GC, Wallace RB, Ongley PA. Complete repair of transposition of the great arteries with pulmonary stenosis. A review and report of a case corrected by using a new surgical technique. Circulation. 1969;39(1):83–95.
3. Rastelli GC, McGoon DC, Wallace RB. Anatomic correction of transposition of the great arteries with ventricular septal defect and subpulmonary stenosis. J Thorac Cardiovasc Surg. 1969;58(4):545–52.
4. Kreutzer C, De Vive J, Oppido G, et al. Twenty-five-year experience with rastelli repair for transposition of the great arteries. J Thorac Cardiovasc Surg. 2000;120(2):211–23.
5. Lee JR, Lim HG, Kim YJ, et al. Repair of transposition of the great arteries, ventricular septal defect and left ventricular outflow tract obstruction. Eur J Cardiothorac Surg. 2004;25(5):735–41.
6. Pretre R, Gendron G, Tamisier D, et al. Results of the Lecompte procedure in malposition of the great arteries and pulmonary obstruction. Eur J Cardiothorac Surg. 2001;19(3):283–9.
7. Nikaidoh H. Aortic translocation and biventricular outflow tract reconstruction. A new surgical repair for transposition of the great arteries associated with ventricular septal defect and pulmonary stenosis. J Thorac Cardiovasc Surg. 1984;88(3):365–72.
8. Yeh Jr T, Ramaciotti C, Leonard SR, et al. The aortic translocation (Nikaidoh) procedure: midterm results superior to the Rastelli procedure. J Thorac Cardiovasc Surg. 2007;133(2):461–9.
9. Belli E, Serraf A, Lacour-Gayet F, et al. Double-outlet right ventricle with non-committed ventricular septal defect. Eur J Cardiothorac Surg. 1999;15:747–52.
10. Hu S, Xie Y, Li S, et al. Double-root translocation for double-outlet right ventricle with noncommitted ventricular septal defect or double-outlet right ventricle with subpulmonary ventricular septal defect associated with pulmonary stenosis: an optimized solution. Ann Thorac Surg. 2010;89(5):1360–5.
11. Hu SS, Li SJ, Wang X, et al. Pulmonary and aortic root translocation in the management of transposition of the great arteries with ventricular septal defect and left ventricular outflow tract obstruction. J Thorac Cardiovasc Surg. 2007;133(4):1090–2.
12. Hu SS, Liu ZG, Li SJ, et al. Strategy for biventricular outflow tract reconstruction: rastelli, REV, or Nikaidoh procedure? J Thorac Cardiovasc Surg. 2008;135(2):331–8.
13. Walters HL, Mavroudis C, Tchervenkov CI, Jacobs JP, Lacour Gayet F, Jacobs ML. Congenital heart surgery nomenclature and data base project: double outlet right ventricle. Ann Thorac Surg. 2000;69(Suppl):249–63.
14. Morell VO, Jacobs JP, Quintessenza JA. Aortic translocation in the management of transposition of the great arteries with ventricular septal defect and pulmonary stenosis: results and follow-up. Ann Thorac Surg. 2005;79(6):2089–92; discussion 2092–3.
15. Bautista-Hernandez V, Marx G, Bacha EA, del Nido PJ. Aortic root translocation plus arterial switch for transposition of the great arteries with left ventricular outflow tract obstruction: intermediate-term results. J Am Coll Cardiol. 2007;49(4):485–90.
16. Honjo O, Yasuhiro K, Bharucha T, Mertens L, Caldarone CA, Redington AN, Van Arsdell G. Anatomical factors determining surgical decision-making in patients with transposition of the great arteries with left ventricular outflow tract obstruction. Eur J Cardiothorac Surg. 2013;44(6):1085–94; discussion 1094.

Chapter 22
Transposition of the Great Arteries with Ventricular Septal Defect and Left Ventricle Outflow Tract Obstruction: Pulmonary Valve Translocation

Jose Pedro da Silva

Abstract The surgical technique choice for the treatment of transposition of the great arteries (TGA) with ventricular septal defect (VSD) and left ventricle outflow tract obstruction (LVOTO) has varied at different heart centers. Since April 1994, we have used the pulmonary root translocation (PRT) to approach this malformation as part of its anatomical repair. Afterwards, we extended its application to other types of congenital heart disease involving malposition of the great arteries, VSD and pulmonary ventricle outflow tract obstruction. We describe the detailed steps of this operation which consists of: removal of the pulmonary artery (PA) with the pulmonary valve from the left ventricle, resection of some conal septum, closure of the pulmonary root hole with autologous pericardial patch, construction of an intraventricular tunnel that diverted blood flow from the left ventricle to the aorta and connection of the pulmonary artery root to the right ventricle. Up to December 2013, 62 patients were subjected to PRT, being the TGA, VSD and PS the most frequent diagnosis (42 patients). Overall, there were 3 (4.8 %) early deaths and 2 (4.4 %) late death. Echocardiographic and follow-up studies on the initial series of 44 consecutive patients showed nonlinear growth of the pulmonary root and good performance of the valve at 10 years. Only 4 patients required reinterventions owing to right ventricular outflow tract problems.

In conclusion: PRT is a good surgical alternative for treatment of patients with TGA complexes, VSD, and LVOTO, with acceptable operative risk, high long-term patient survival, and few reinterventions. Most patients had adequate pulmonary root growth and performance.

Keywords Transposition of the great arteries • Ventricular septal defect • Pulmonary stenosis • TGA-VSD-LVOTO • Ventricular outflow tract obstruction • Congenital heart disease • Cardiac surgery

---

J.P. da Silva, MD
Heart Surgery Service, Department of Cardiovascular Surgery, Hospital Beneficencia Portuguesa of São Paulo, Rua Maestro Cardim, 769, Sala 221, Sao Paulo 01323-900, Brazil
e-mail: dasilvajp@uol.com.br

F. Lacour-Gayet et al. (eds.), *Surgery of Conotruncal Anomalies*,
DOI 10.1007/978-3-319-23057-3_22

Introduction

Pulmonary valve (or root) translocation is a technique that we have used since April 1994 as an alternative treatment for transposition of the great arteries (TGA) with ventricular septal defect (VSD) and pulmonary stenosis (PS) and for selected cases of double-outlet right ventricle with a subpulmonary VSD [1]. More recently, we have extended its use as part of the anatomic repair procedure in patients with congenitally corrected transposition, pulmonary stenosis, and large VSD [2]. The surgical technique consisted of: removal of the pulmonary artery (PA) with the pulmonary valve from the left ventricle, resection of some conal septum, closure of the pulmonary root hole with autologous pericardial patch, construction of an intraventricular tunnel that diverted blood flow from the left ventricle to the aorta and anterior pulmonary artery translocation to construct a new right ventricle outflow tract. In patients presenting with important pulmonary valve stenosis (After repair Intraoperative right ventricle – pulmonary artery systolic gradient superior to 35 mmHg) the pulmonary artery was enlarged with a monocusp valve pericardial patch.

This technique was aimed at maintaining pulmonary valve function, as much as possible, including the capacity for growth, as an attempt to avoid the problems inherent in a right ventricle to pulmonary artery conduit. Furthermore, by not incising or mobilizing the aorta, we have attempted to preserve aortic valve anatomy and function as an important measure to improve the patient's clinical outcome.

Anatomical Classification and Definitions

The anatomical classification that we use is based in Congenital Heart Surgery Nomenclature and Database Project: Transposition of the Great Arteries, published in year 2000 by members of the STS-Congenital Heart Surgery Database Committee and representatives from the European Association for Cardiothoracic Surgery [3]. Also, we used the sequential segmental approach recommended by Anderson et al. [4]. Therefore, we have utilized the following terminology: atrio-ventricular connection types: concordant, discordant, ambiguous, double inlet, absent right connection, or absent left connection; ventriculo-arterial connection [concordant], discordant [transposition], double outlet.

Malposition of great arteries is used as a general expression to describe all defects with abnormal position of the great arteries, regardless of ventricular origin, while transposition of the great arteries refers only to left ventricular origin of the pulmonary artery and right ventricular origin of the aorta. In cases of double outlet right ventricle, malposition is a more accurate term than transposition to describe the anatomical situation of the great arteries, as proposed by Van Praagh [5], since both arteries rise from the RV.

In this chapter, we will describe pulmonary valve translocation in TGA with VSD and PS, the more common form of great arteries malposition with VSD and pulmonary stenosis, which can be also described as: atrioventricular concordance, ventriculoarterial discordance, subaortic VSD and left ventricle outflow tract obstruction (LVOTO). The procedure was indicated to patients with significant pulmonary valve stenosis. Two patients who presented with predominant subvalvar obstruction were subjected to the Jatene's switch operation after resection of the subvalvar stenosis.

Anatomic and Hemodynamic Diagnosis

The anatomic and hemodynamic information needed prior to surgery were obtained by echocardiogram, CT scan angiography and, occasionally by heart catherization. In some patients who presented with radiological signs of pulmonary over circulation and little cyanosis in combination with severe LVOTO, the presence of excessive systemic to pulmonary arterial collateral circulation is suspected and heart catheterization is indicated to determine its importance and anatomical position. Also, in cases of severe cyanosis associated to less severe LVOTO, heat catheterization is indicated in order to rule out pulmonary hypertension.

The main anatomical details to be evaluated are listed below.

Check List Prior to Surgery

(a) The pulmonary valve diameter and the correspondent Z value, as well as, the presence of subpulmonary obstruction. Also, the relationship of the pulmonary root with the anterior leaflet of the mitral valve and the aortic root and, if possible, the coronary arteries situation.
(b) Diameter of pulmonary branches and presence of stenosis
(c) Presence of a PDA or Blalock-Taussig shunt
(d) Abnormal coronary anatomy
(e) The size and position of the VSD
(f) Presence of multiple VSD
(g) Elevated lung resistances

The Surgical Technique

The operation is performed via median sternotomy. Cardiopulmonary bypass is instituted with aortic and bicaval cannulation. Systemic hypothermia (23–25 °C) and cold antegrade blood cardioplegia (30 mL/kg), followed by subsequent doses (10–15 mL/kg) at 20- to 30-min intervals during the cross-clamp period, is used for myocardial protection.

The main operative steps are:

- The pulmonary artery mobilization begins before cardiopulmonary bypass. This includes the dissection of any previously placed systemic-pulmonary shunt, to be divided on the initiation of cardiopulmonary bypass. The pulmonary trunk is separated from the aorta, and a plane of dissection developed close to the pulmonary artery wall, staying away from the coronary arteries. This dissection advances toward the left ventricle and stops when it is 2–3 mm inside the myocardium (Fig. 22.1). Also, the pulmonary artery branches are extensively mobilized from their distal attachments. The completion of the pulmonary root harvesting is resumed once the heart is arrested and the right ventriculotomy is done. So this surgical step can be controlled from both outside and inside the heart.

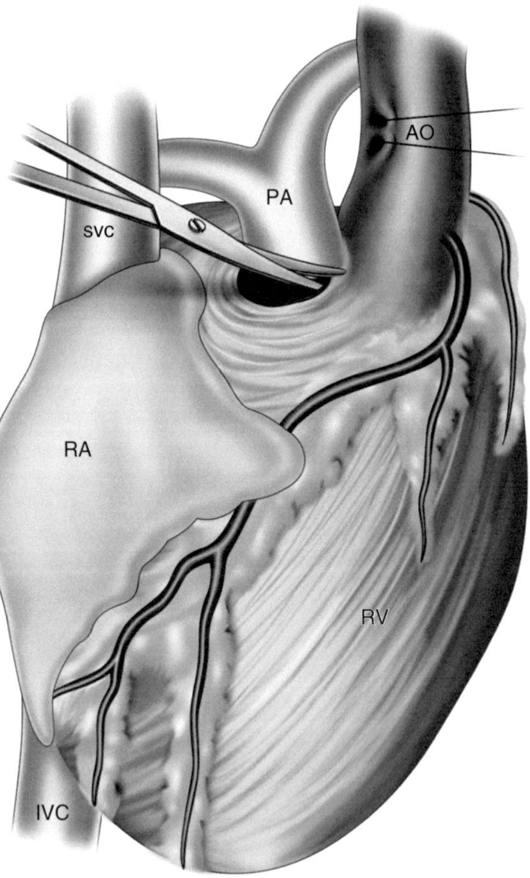

Fig. 22.1 The initial dissection of the pulmonary artery root after the mobilization of the pulmonary artery branches. *RV* right ventricle, *Ao* aorta, *PA* pulmonary artery, *RA* right atrium, *IVC* inferior vena cava, and *SVC* superior vena cava

– A vertical right ventriculotomy is performed (Fig. 22.2a), with care taken to avoid injury to large conal right ventricular branches and the left anterior descending coronary artery, especially if intrapericardial adhesions obscure visu-

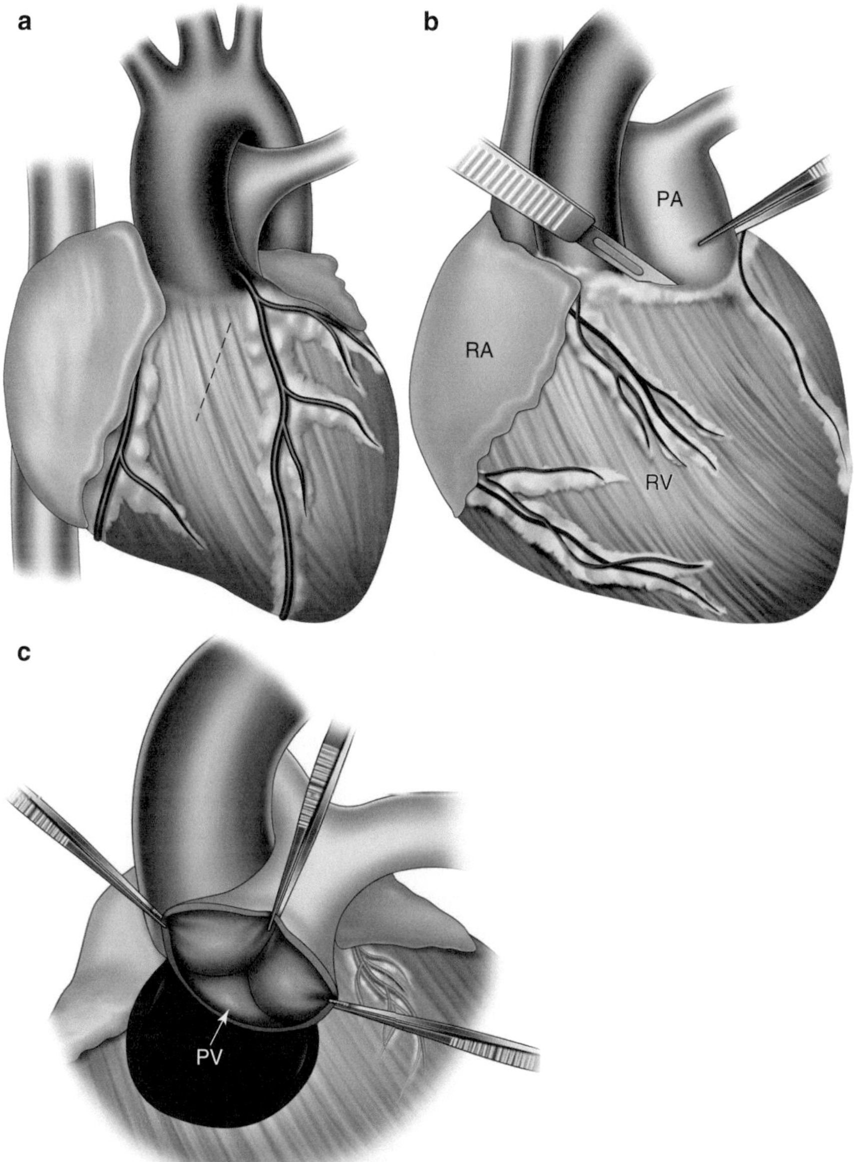

Fig. 22.2 Preoperative heart anatomy in transposition of the great arteries with ventricular septal defect and pulmonary stenosis: the right ventriculotomy place (*dashed line*) (**a**), or double outflow tract right ventricle with sub aortic ventricular septal defect and pulmonary stenosis (**b**), pulmonary valve (**c**). *Ao* aorta, *PA* pulmonary artery, *RA* right atrium, *RV* right ventricle, *LV* left ventricle

alization of their courses. The tissue underlying the pulmonary valve is inspected and an incision around it is made (Fig. 22.2b). This dissection from inside the ventricles will meet the outside dissection completing the pulmonary artery removal with the intact pulmonary valve and the subvalvar myocardium and fibrotic tissue (Fig. 22.2c). These careful steps are important to harvest the pulmonary artery root with an intact valve and to prevent damage to the adjacent aortic sinus of Valsalva and the mitral valve annulus. It is also important to avoid entering the interventricular septum, which can occur if the dissection is performed solely from outside of the heart. The pulmonary valve is inspected; any remaining subvalvar fibrous tissue and excessive myocardial muscle are removed.

- After the removal of the pulmonary valve from the left ventricle, the conal septum (CS) interposed between the superior margin of the VSD and the aortic valve is excised. This accomplished by making a vertical incision on the conal septum, from the VSD to near aortic valve, followed by another horizontal incision, paralleling the aortic valve (dashed line). Some myocardial tissue is maintained near the aortic valve and little excision of the remaining conal septum is performed (Fig. 22.3a). In case of restrictive VSD, the conal septum is removed more extensively and some more anterosuperior septum is removed in order to enlarge the VSD (Fig. 22.3b).
- The resultant opening in the left ventricle from the pulmonary root harvesting is checked for mitral valve disruption and closed using a glutaraldehyde treated autologous pericardial patch with 6-0 polypropylene running suture technique (Fig. 22.4).
- The size and location of the VSD are inspected, paying particular attention to its relation to the aortic valve. Obstructing right ventricular muscle bundles are resected. (B) An intracardiac tunnel, connecting the left ventricle to the aorta, is created using a Dacron patch (Fig. 22.5). The suture line is carried away from the edge of VSD along its postero-inferior margin to avoid damage to the conduction system and is reinforced with interrupted sutures in any area of possible weakness. Generally, the patch is sutured to the base of the septal leaflet of the tricuspid valve, to avoid the posteroinferior margin of the VSD, in order to prevent heart block. In some instances, a papillary muscle of the tricuspid valve can be standing on the conal septum. This type of anatomy requires the detachment of that papillary muscle from the septum in order to clear space for the construction of an effective left ventricle to aorta tunnel. Next, the anteroseptal commissure of TV is sutured and the Dacron patch anterior side is placed in a way that it crosses the distal end of this commissural suture. This maneuver facilitates the tunnel construction and gives support for the anteroseptal commissure, preventing prolapse and insufficiency of the TV. The setback of this approach for the tricuspid valve is that it cause some tricuspid valve orifice reduction. Therefore, it can be used only in patients who presents dilated TV. Alternatively, the papillary muscle can be re-implanted on the Dacron patch, dispensing the TV anteroseptal commissure suture.
- The intact pulmonary artery with valve is translocated anteriorly, to the left side of the aorta, to be connected to the right ventricle, without a Lecompte maneuver. The posterior aspect of the pulmonary root is sutured to the superior edge of the

right ventriculotomy, using 6-0 polydioxanone running technique suture. Usually, this suture line connects about 40–50 % of the pulmonary root circumference, directly, to the right ventricular wall (Fig. 22.6a). The remainder of the right ventricular outflow tract reconstruction is completed, whenever possible, with an in situ autologous pericardial patch, maximizing RVOT potential for growth (Fig. 22.6b, c).

– Enlargement is elected based on measurement of the pulmonary annulus diameter. This diameter is evaluated preoperatively by echocardiogram or angiography and confirmed intraoperatively by calibration with Hegar dilator. In general, we do not enlarge when the pulmonary annulus Z-score is greater than –3 in tricuspid pulmonary valves. The enlargement decision is again reassessed after coming off of cardiopulmonary bypass, when we measure the right ventricular

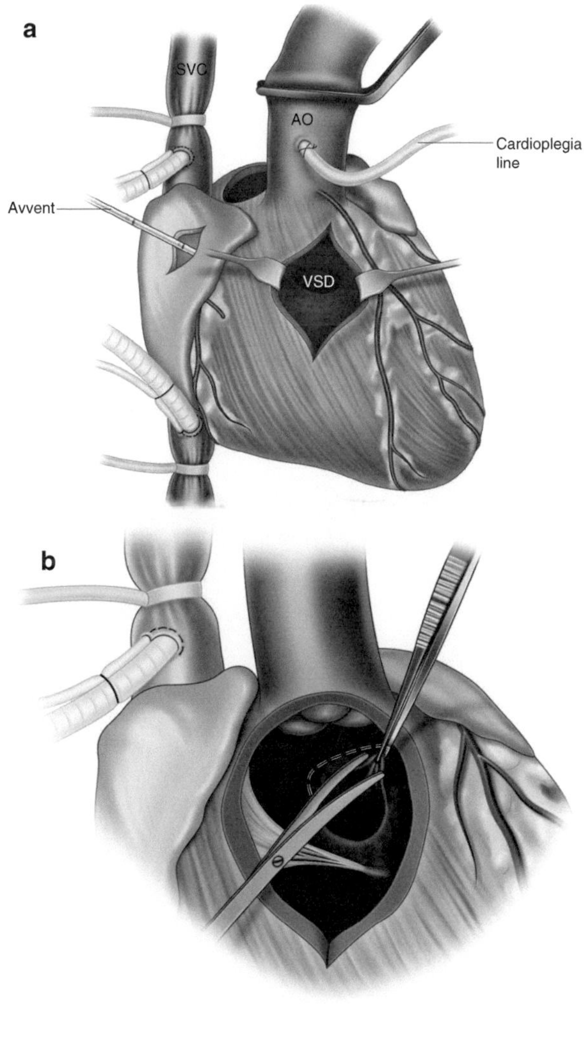

Fig. 22.3 Exposure of the ventricular septum by retraction of the ventriculotomy edges (**a**) and incisions for conal septal resection, which can be normal or extensive ressection (**b**). *Dashed line* indicates the incision site, *Ao* aorta, *VSD* ventricular septal defect, *PAH* pulmonary artery hole, *CS* conal septum, *PM* papillary muscle, and *LAV* left atrial vent

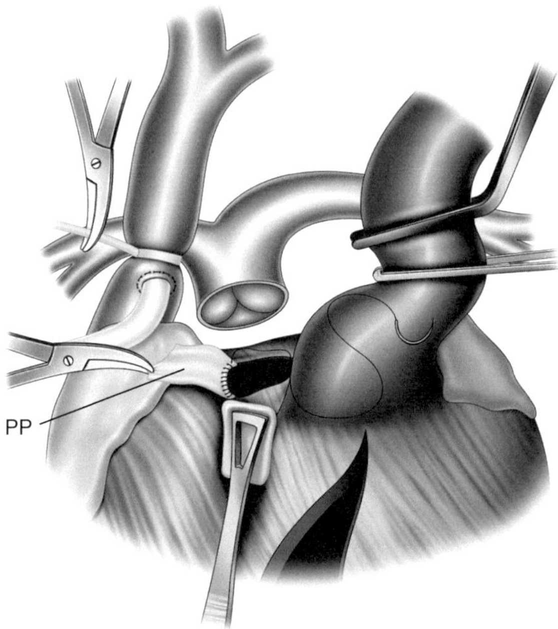

Fig. 22.4 Closure of the left ventricle orifice, resulting from pulmonary root removal, with glutaraldehyde treated autologous pericardial patch using polypropylene running technique suture. *PP* pericardial patch

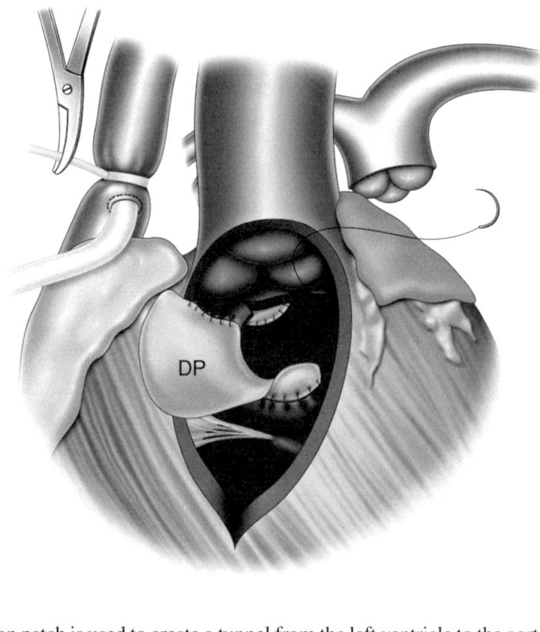

Fig. 22.5 A Dacron patch is used to create a tunnel from the left ventricle to the aorta. *DP* dacron patch

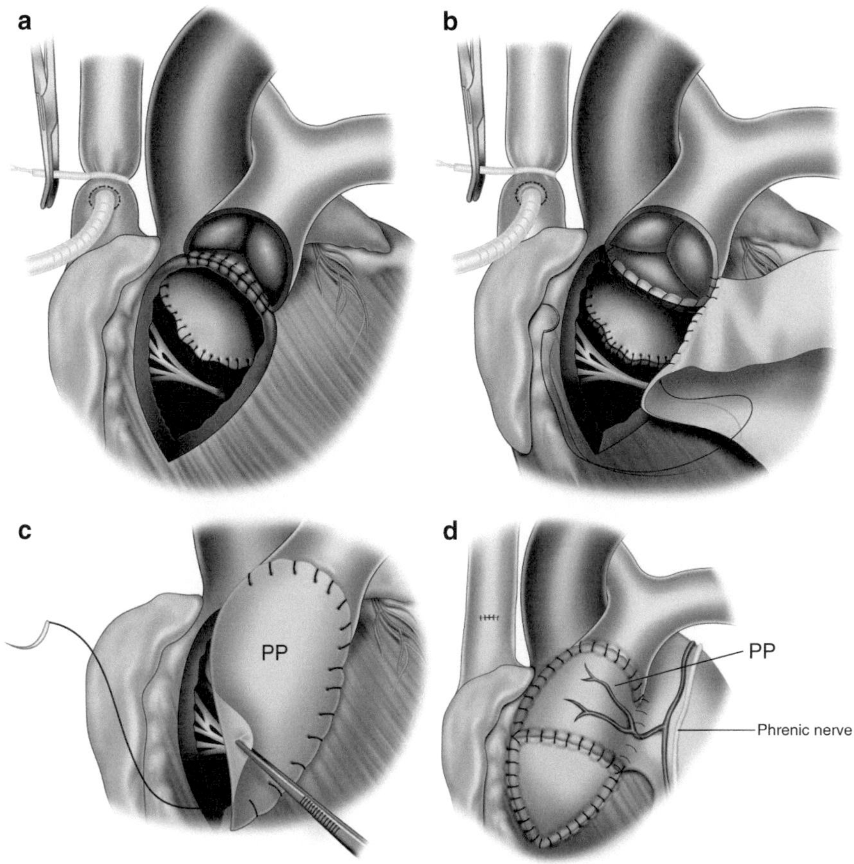

Fig. 22.6 Translocation of the pulmonary root and construction of a new right ventricular outflow tract: the pulmonary root is sutured to the right ventriculotomy with a running 6-0 polydioxanone suture (**a**) and the right ventricular outflow tract is completed using an in situ pericardial patch (**c**, **d**). *RV* right ventricle, *Ao* aorta, *PA* pulmonary artery, *PP* autologous pericardial patch, *PV* pulmonary valve, and *T* left ventricle-to-aorta tunnel

and pulmonary artery pressures. If the systolic gradient exceeds 35 mmHg, we go back on pump, remove one or two interrupted sutures from the anterior aspect of the autologous pericardium to pulmonary artery anastomosis, exposing the pulmonary artery valve at the anterior commissural site, and perform a small enlargement with a valved patch. In the majority of patients the decision to enlarge the pulmonary root is made preoperatively. The pulmonary valve enlargement is shown in Fig. 22.7a–c. Notice that the pulmonary circumference is augmented using the smallest patch possible just enough to prevent an important trans pulmonary valve gradient. Enlargement of the pulmonary root has been performed in approximately 40 % of our patients. We are more prone to enlarge bicuspid pulmonary valves.

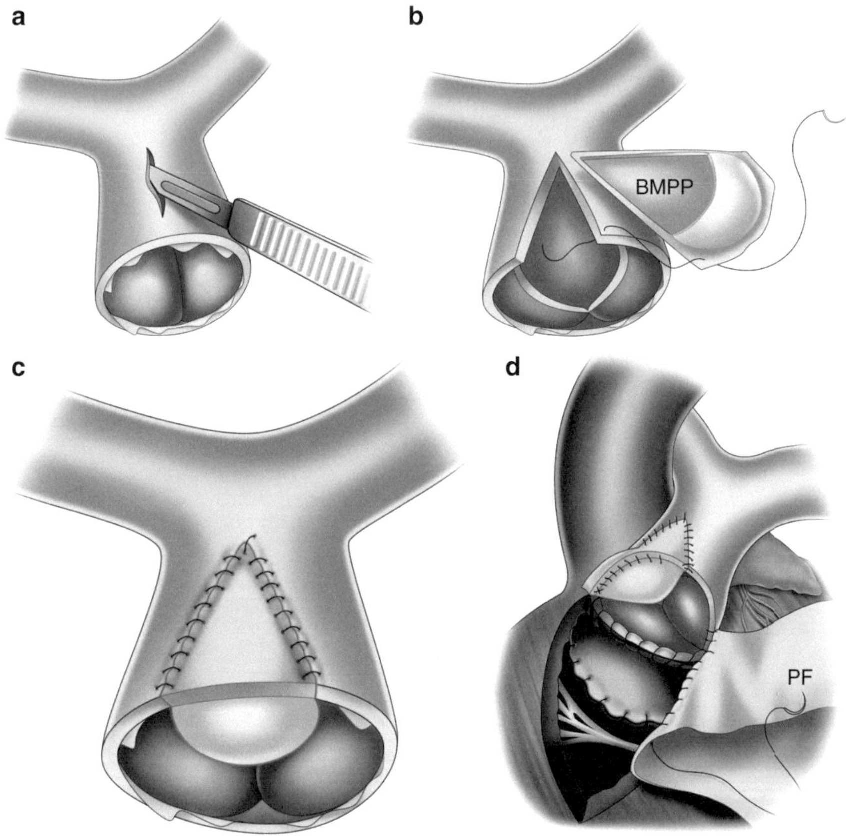

Fig. 22.7 Enlargement of the pulmonary root with a monocusp bovine pericardial patch (**a**–**c**) and completion of the right ventricle outflow tract with in situ pericardial flap. *BMPP* bovine monocusp pericardial patch, *PF* pericardial flap

– These are pre repair (Fig. 22.8a) and post repair (Fig. 22.8b) antero-posterior cross-section view of a heart with TGA, VSD and PS.

Outcomes

From April 1994 to December 2013 we have applied pulmonary valve translocation to 42 patients with TGA, VSD and PS. This is a sub group of our consecutive series of 61 patients presenting with complex congenital heart disease associated to malposition of the great arteries who were subjected pulmonary artery root translocation as part of the anatomical repair of their heart. The main diagnosis and mortality rate are shown in Table 22.1.

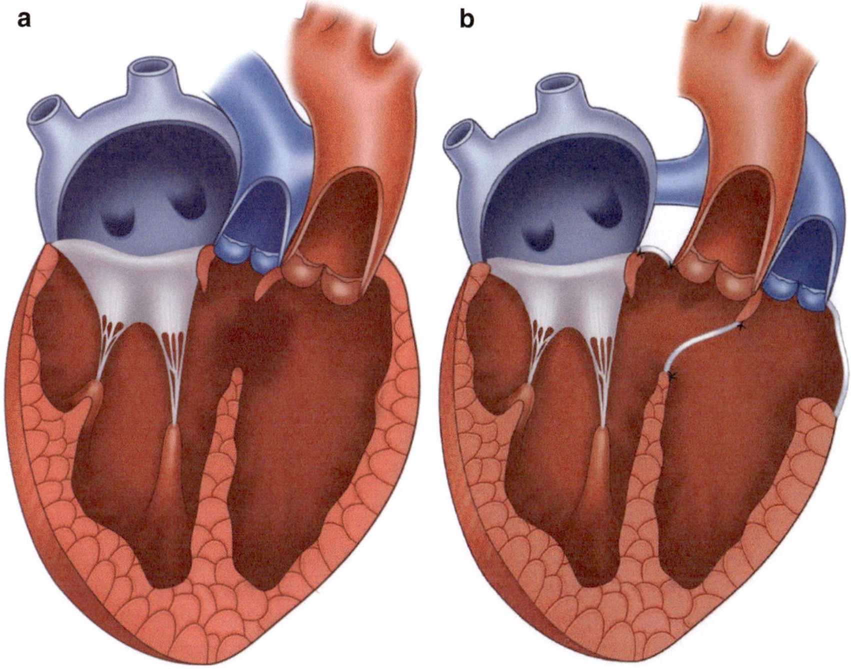

Fig. 22.8 Anteroposterior cross-section view of a heart with transposition of the great arteries, with ventricular septal defect and pulmonary stenosis: pre repair (**a**) and post repair (**b**)

Table 22.1 Pulmonary root translocation in malposition of great arteries

Diagnosis	Number of patients	Hospital mortality	Late mortality
TGA, VSD, PS	42	3 (7.1 %)	1 (2.8 %)
DORV, VSD, MPGA, PS	10	0	0
DORV, AVSD, MPGA, PS	2	0	0
CCTGA, VSD, PS	7	0	1 (14.3 %)
Total	61	3 (4.9 %)	2 (3.3 %)

Early Mortality

Regarding the early mortality after PRT, all three deaths occurred in patients with TGA, VSD, and PS who were operated on between 1994 and 2005. The first patient was an 8-year-old boy with a long history of cyanosis who died of heart failure, and the second patient was a 6-month-old boy who had a good hemodynamic result after the operation but died of gram-negative sepsis. The third patient was a 36-day-old baby who underwent surgery 1 day after being intubated and transfused owing to severe hypoxemia. He could not be weaned from cardiopulmonary bypass and died of multiple organ failure despite the use of cardiopulmonary support with extracorporeal membrane oxygenation for 3 days. After those deaths, we undertook a general revision of the operation in March 2005 and resolved to indicate the operation in clinically stable infants older than 2 months, performing modified Blalock-Taussig shunts to younger than 2 months with severe cyanosis, deferring the PRT, to be done electively at 4–6 months of age. Concerning the surgical technique, we adopted a strategy for the enlargement of the pulmonary root that was similar to that described for the repair of tetralogy of Fallot [6]. Also we began to cover all the enlarged pulmonary root anterior aspect with live autologous pericardium, as depicted in Fig. 22.7. This was done in order to optimize its growth potential. Thereafter, we have operated on 43 consecutive patients without any early or late deaths. The long-term follow-up has shown excellent clinical outcome.

Long Term Results

Two patients died in long term follow-up of all patients after PRT (Table 22.1). The first was a 2 year-old-boy, from the TGA, VSD and PS group, whose hospital discharge echocardiogram revealed a 45 mmHg RV-PA gradient that progressed to 70 mm after 2 months. He was scheduled to return to hospital for reintervention, but he died suddenly when running. The second was a 17 year-old-girl from the ccTGA with VSD and PS group, who was under treatment for ventricular arrhythmia but also died suddenly at the high school ward 5 years after her operation.

At follow-up, eight patients needed a total of ten reinterventions after the PRT. These reinterventions were required owing to residual VSD in three patients, LVOT obstruction (left ventricular–aortic tunnel stenosis) in one patient, RVOT aneurysm in two patients (one owing to endocarditis and one owing to in situ pericardial flap dilation), and RVOT obstruction (pulmonary stenosis) in three patients. All the three patients with RVOT obstruction were treated with percutaneous balloon dilation of the pulmonary valve, two of them had important reduction of the transpulmonary gradient mmHg and excellent outcome thereafter. The first patient of this series, who at the operation had her 3 mm valve connected to the RV complemented with the placement of a parallel RV-PA valved conduit, underwent pulmonary vale balloon dilation 13 years after PRT, reducing the right ventricular–pulmonary arterial gradient from 95 to 70 mmHg. A surgical approach was recommended, but the patient and her family declined surgery because she was asymptomatic. The patient who had endocarditis underwent homograft replacement of the pulmonary valve and, 5 years later, implantation of pericardial valve prosthesis. Therefore, only four patients required reinterventions owing to right ventricular outflow tract problems. In our study [7] published in 2012, involving our initial series of 44 patients, mean follow-up time of 72 ± 52.1 months it was shown that: the Kaplan-Meier survival was 92.8 % and reintervention-free survival was 82.9 % at 12 years. Repeat echocardiographic data showed nonlinear growth of the pulmonary root and good performance of the valve in the great majority of patients at 10 years.

Comments

The technique of pulmonary root translocation keeps the aorta untouched in its original anterior position, without any coronary artery manipulation. As a consequence, postoperative aortic valve dysfunction or coronary artery distortion is not expected after pulmonary root translocation. In our 19-year experience with this procedure, we have not observed these complications to date. The Lecompte maneuver is not useful in this operation, which leaves the aorta in its native position, because the aorta is already in a very anterior position in patients with TGA. After the Lecompte maneuver, the translocated pulmonary trunk would be very close to the sternum, increasing the risk of bleeding during a reintervention. Conversely, the elongation of the pulmonary artery owing to retention of its root allows anastomosis of the pulmonary artery to the right ventricle to be performed without tension. An autologous pericardial flap was used to complete the RVOT reconstruction, optimizing its potential for growth. This pericardial flap was limited to the anterior aspect of the pulmonary root, and a piece of glutaraldehyde treated autologous pericardium was added to complete the RVOT reconstruction. We used this composite patch technique rather than using a single flap of in situ pericardium in an effort to prevent aneurysmal dilation of the pericardial hood, which occurred in one case in this series. When enlargement of the pulmonary root circumference was needed, we augmented it with a small monocusp bovine pericardial patch, the size of which was just sufficient for preventing an elevated RV-PA pressure gradient. We hope that as the patient's own valve grows, using the smallest possible artificial patch will result in less pulmonary valve regurgitation. We found that pulmonary valve growth was less adequate in patients who underwent patch enlargement of the pulmonary root than in patients without enlargement. This was associated with a greater incidence (statistical tendency) of pulmonary regurgitation in those patients, indicating that it is important to preserve the pulmonary valve without enlargement whenever possible [7].

Left ventricular outflow tract obstruction, which is an important problem following the initial series of Rastelli operation [8, 9], has a low incidence after pulmonary root translocation. The explanation for this is that when harvesting the pulmonary root, some subvalvar myocardium is also removed, giving more room for the left ventricular outflow tract. Furthermore, partial resection of the conal septum favors the construction of an obstruction-free left ventricular outflow tract. This is in accordance with Lecompte and colleagues [10, 11], who addressed problems of LVOT obstruction related to the classic Rastelli operation by extensive conal septum resection, resulting in a wider left ventricular–aortic tunnel and decreasing the risk of subaortic stenosis. It is interesting to observe that some patients from our series, presented progressive improvement on the left ventricle to aorta alignment, as they grow.

In cases of CCTGA, the technique for pulmonary root harvesting in CCTGA is somewhat easier than in d-TGA cases because the pulmonary valve is usually more superficially located in CCTGA, maintaining continuity with the aortic valve but being far from the mitral valve. While in d-TGA, the pulmonary valve is closely related to the mitral valve (anterior leaflet) and aortic valve. However, the surgeon needs to be aware that the conduction axis is intimately related to the pulmonary valve anterior aspect in CCTGA, being necessary to make the incision very close to the pulmonary valve hinge line when harvesting the pulmonary root. This maneuver is important to prevent heart block.

The left ventricle-to-aorta alignment tends to be good after construction of the left ventricular outflow tract in CCTGA repair due to the anterior position of the left ventricle, which is in a similar anteroposterior plane as the aortic valve plane, facilitating repair of the ventriculoarterial discordance. Tateishe et al. [12] also reported this result when repairing CCTGA with pulmonary root translocation.

Regarding the atrial switch technique, some surgeons prefer to perform the Mustard operation to achieve atrioventricular concordance in CCTGA [7], because CCTGA patients usually present with a small right atrium, which makes difficult to obtain a properly sized atrial chambers with the Senning procedure. However, the Senning procedure can be used with the addition of some technical maneuvers such as: the pulmonary atrium enlargement with an autologous in situ pericardial flap and leaving the left atrial appendage incorporated in the systemic venous tunnel. This latter maneuver facilitates the correction of persistent left cava by, simply, connecting the left cava to the left atrial appendage, as we did in two patients of this series.

The patients who were referred for anatomical repair of CCTGA with VSD and LVOTO generally present with symptoms related to chronic hypoxemia, and some have previous BT shunt. Also, the majority of patients under the age of 3 years at the time of surgery had their pulmonary valve spared without patch enlargement, whereas all patients older than 3 years required monocusp pulmonary valve enlargement. This finding supports approaching these patients at a younger age, as our previous study [3] showed that patients that do not require patch enlargement of their pulmonary valve have better growth patterns and functional results of the pulmonary valve after pulmonary root translocation.

DORV patients with the VSD committed to the pulmonary artery can also be managed with PRT. As in CCTGA, the pulmonary root harvesting is easier than in patients with d-TGA. However, it poses some technical difficulties in case of coronary arteries anatomical variation. Per example, when the left anterior coronary artery (LAD) rises from the right coronary artery, the surgeon has to make the RV incision, the RV's pulmonary orifice patch closure and the RV-pulmonary artery anastomosis without compromising the LAD blood flow.

The PRT is indicated in patients with DORV, VSD, pulmonary RVOTO and malposition of the great arteries (VSD committed to pulmonary artery). Patients with the above lesions and anomaly of the systemic veins drainage and/or atrioventricular septal defect can either be approached with PRT as part of their heart malformations repair.

In addition, patients with DORV, VSD, and malposition of the great arteries can be approached with PRT if the coronary arteries anatomy is considered not adequate for the Jatene's arterial switch operation. In this situation, the PRT procedure may be preceded by pulmonary artery banding if the patient is a newborn in heart failure or an older child presenting with severe under-nutrition or with important elevation of the pulmonary vascular resistance.

The knowledge that DORV patients subjected to the switch procedure present with high incidence of aortic regurgitation in long term follow-up, supports the use of PRT in this group of patients.

Limitations for the Procedure

PRT has technical limitations in a subgroup of patients with the same diagnosis as in our series who have small or noncommitted VSDs or small or heavily trabeculated right ventricles. These conditions present difficulties for left ventricular–aortic tunnel construction. Furthermore, pulmonary atresia or very small and dysplastic pulmonary valves are contraindications for this technique.

Conclusions

PRT is a good surgical alternative for treatment of patients with TGA complexes, VSD, and PS with acceptable operative risk, high long-term survivals, and few reinterventions. Most patients had adequate pulmonary root growth and performance.

References

1. da Silva JP, Baumgratz JF, da Fonseca L. Pulmonary root translocation in transposition of great arteries repair. Ann Thorac Surg. 2000;69:643–5.
2. da Fonseca L, Baumgratz JF, Castro RM, Franchi SM, Vila JHA, Lopes LM, da Silva JP. Late results of pulmonary root translocation in the correction of transposition of the great arteries. Rev Bras Cir Cardiovasc. 2003;18(4):326–31.
3. Jaggers JJ, Cameron DE, Herlong JR, Ungerleider RM. Congenital heart surgery nomenclature and database project: transposition of the great. Ann Thorac Surg. 2000;69:S205–35.
4. Anderson RH, Becker AE, Freedom RM, et al. Sequential segmental analysis of congenital heart disease. Pediatr Cardiol. 1984;5:281.
5. Van Praagh R. Terminology of congenital heart disease: glossary and commentary. Circulation. 1977;56:139.
6. Kouchoukos NT, Blackstone EH, Doty DB, Hanley FL, Karp RB. Ventricular septal defect with pulmonary stenosis or atresia. In: Kouchoukos NT, Blackstone EH, Doty DB, Hanley FL, Karp RB, editors. Kirklin/Barratt-Boyes cardiac surgery: morphology, diagnostic criteria, natural history, techniques, results and indications, vol. 1. 3rd ed. Philadelphia: Elsevier Science; 2003. p. 946–1073.
7. da Silva JP, da Silva Lda F, Lopes LM, Moreira LF, Caneo LF, Franchi SM, Lianza AC, Baumgratz JF, Duarte JFM. Pulmonary root translocation in malposition of great arteries repair allows right ventricular outflow tract growth. J Thorac Cardiovasc Surg. 2012;143(6):1292–8.
8. Kreutzer C, De Vive J, Oppido G, Kreutzer J, Gauvreau K, Freed M, et al. Twenty-five–year experience with Rastelli repair for transposition of the great arteries. J Thorac Cardiovasc Surg. 2000;120:211–23.
9. Dearani JA, Danielson GK, Puga FJ, Mair DD, Schleck CD. Late results of the Rastelli operation for transposition of the great arteries. Semin Thorac Cardiovasc Surg Pediatr Card Surg Annu. 2001;4:3–15.
10. Lecompte Y, Zannini L, Hazan E, Jarreau MM, Bex JP, Tu TV, et al. Anatomic correction of transposition of the great arteries. J Thorac Cardiovasc Surg. 1981;82:629–31.
11. Raisky O, Vouhé PR. Pitfalls in repair of conotruncal anomalies. Semin Thorac Cardiovasc Surg Pediatr Card Surg Annu. 2013;16:7–12.
12. Tateishi A, Kasahara S, Kawabata T, et al. The effect of pulmonary root translocation on the left ventricular outflow tract. Ann Thorac Surg. 2013;96:1469–71.

Chapter 23
Bi-ventricular Repair of Double Outlet Right Ventricle

Francois Lacour-Gayet

Abstract Double outlet right ventricle (DORV) is a type of ventriculo-arterial connection where the great vessels arise entirely or predominantly from the right ventricle. The name DORV encloses a vast spectrum of congenital heart diseases with various clinical presentations and surgical treatment. Rarely a congenital heart disease has been the source of such controversial exchanges around the anatomical definitions and the optimal surgical techniques. The recent Functional Classification has greatly simplified the management of DORV in describing different functional types unified by a common clinical presentation and more importantly by a similar surgical management. The surgical repair of DORV-VSD type, DORV-Fallot and DORV-TGA (Taussig-Bing) is today performed with very low mortality. The surgical anatomy and the optimal surgical technique of DORV non-committed VSD and DORV-AVSD-Heterotaxy are still controversial. In presence of two viable ventricles, we believe that biventricular repair is the optimal solution. This chapter and Chaps. 15 and 24 describe in details biventricular repair of DORV.

Keywords Congenital heart disease • Double outlet right ventricle • Conotruncal anomaly • Cardiac surgery • Anatomical repair • Pathology • Echocardiography • Pediatrics

Introduction

DORV remains the source of many controversies in anatomical definition and surgical management. DORV, a typical conotruncal anomaly, is not a single disease but essentially a primitive form of ventriculo-arterial connection with great variations in anatomy, clinical presentation and surgical management. DORV is classically classified according to the relationship of the VSD with the great vessels, as defined by

F. Lacour-Gayet, MD
Department of Pediatric Cardiac Surgery, National Heart and Lung Institute,
Royal Brompton Hospital, Imperial College University, Sydney Street, London SW3 6NP, UK
e-mail: flacourgayet@mac.com

F. Lacour-Gayet et al. (eds.), *Surgery of Conotruncal Anomalies*,
DOI 10.1007/978-3-319-23057-3_23

Lev et al. [1]. The surgeons, in charge of patients with DORV, have adopted for their great majority a Functional Classification of DORV [2], which has clarified the surgical indications of this complex condition.

Surgical Anatomy of DORV

The surgical anatomy is focusing on specific morphological structures relevant to surgical technique.

Anatomical Definitions

DORV is a primitive (Chaps. 2, 3, and 39) form of ventriculo-arterial connection where the two great vessels arise entirely or predominantly from the right ventricle. This conotruncal anomaly presents with various cardiac "phenotypes" and frequent extra cardiac anomalies. DORV is characterized by a large spectrum of lesions depending on: – the location of the VSD, – the relationship of the VSD and the great vessels, – the presence of pulmonary outflow obstruction and – the size of the ventricles. The anatomical definition of DORV remains controversial. There is not one but several definitions of DORV currently used.

- Historically, it is A. Calhoun Witham [3] who coined in 1957 the term double outlet right ventricle and defined it as a "partial transposition complex" by opposition to complete TGA. This definition was later endorsed by Neufeld et al. [4, 5].
- Lev et al. [1] produced in 1972 the universally accepted anatomical definition of DORV, based on the relationship of the VSD with the great vessels.
- Richard Van Praagh defines DORV as a fibrous discontinuity between the mitral and aortic valves due to the persistence of a subaortic conus [6, 7]
- Robert H. Anderson established the popular "50 % rule" [8, 9], which states that a DORV is present when more than 50 % of both arterial valves are connected to the morphologically right ventricle.
- R. Sakata and Y. Lecompte [10] defines DORV as a malposition of the great vessels
- François Lacour-Gayet et al. [11–13] supports the "200 % rule". From a surgical standpoint, "complete DORV" have both arterial valves arising entirely from the morphologic right ventricle. Consequently, DORV can be called a "Transposition of the Aorta", a synonym of "Partial Transposition"; the first definition given by Witham [3]

Morphology of DORV

DORV is essentially a conal malformation. In the most typical forms, due to the persistence of a subaortic conus [6, 7], DORV is characterized by a double conus, formed by a normal subpulmonary conus and an abnormally present subaortic conus. The two conus are formed by a common inter-conal septum (conal/infundibular/outlet septum) and their lateral walls. The right lateral conal wall (subpulmonary conus for R. Van Praagh) is normally developed creating a muscular discontinuity between the tricuspid and the pulmonary valve (ventricular infundibular fold, VIF, for RH Anderson). The persistence of the left lateral conal wall (left VIF for RH Anderson) maintains the aorta entirely or partially inside the cephalhead part of the right ventricle, creating an additional subaortic infundibulum with muscular mitro-aortic discontinuity. The conal septum remains inside the right ventricular cavity instead of its normal position between the limbs of the trabecular septo marginalis (TSM). The position of the parietal band (crista supra ventricularis) is variable in DORV. In many instances it can be normally situated in contact with the septal band (TSM). Elsewhere, it can be fairly recognizable or even absent.

The conal septum could be malaligned anteriorly or posteriorly creating a subpulmonary stenosis or a subaortic obstruction. It can be absent or deficient. The left subaortic conus could be more or less developed, with a large or shallow mitro-aortic discontinuity.

The aorta is either: – in normal position, located posteriorly and to the right of the pulmonary artery or – side by side to the right or – located anteriorly and to the right of the PA in the most typical DORV. *The more anterior the aorta, the more complex form of DORV.* When associated with an atrio-ventricular discordance, the aorta is located to the left of the PA.

The VSD in DORV can be located above and in between the limbs of the TSM or below the posterior limb of the TSM. Rarely, it can be situated in the inlet or trabecular muscular septum. It can be absent. The VSD in "complete DORV" is the only outlet of the left ventricle. Any restriction of the VSD prior or following surgery will induce an LV obstruction. The name to give to this "hole" is controversial: – bulbo-ventricular foramen, AV canal type VSD, inlet muscular VSD for Van Praagh [6, 7] or – perimembranous VSD, interventricular communication for Anderson [8, 9] or – primary interventricular foramen for Van Mierop [14–16]. The main point is the location of the conduction tissue in the DORV non committed VSD as discussed further.

It is noticeable that the conal morphology is quite stable in the "complete" form of DORV with two infundibulum, the conal septum standing in the RV, distant from the Y of the TSM and 200 % of great vessels in the right ventricle. In "partial" forms, when the vessels do not arise entirely from the right ventricle, the subaortic conus and its left lateral can be deficient.

Lev-Bharati Classification

Four anatomic types are recognized in Lev and Bharati *anatomical classification* [1] based on the relationship of the VSD with the great vessels:

- DORV with subaortic VSD
- DORV with doubly committed VSD
- DORV with subpulmonary VSD (Taussig-Bing anomaly)
- DORV with uncommitted or remote VSD

Associated Lesions

Associated anomalies are frequent:

- *Ventricular hypoplasia* is the most frequent association. DORV is often a component of single functioning ventricle; a clear contra-indication to biventricular repair
- *Valvar or subvalvar pulmonary obstruction* is frequent; however it is rare in Taussig Bing. Pulmonary atresia is possible.
- A *restrictive VSD* is frequent and should be recognized before surgery. Following biventricular repair, a restricted VSD (diameter less than the aortic valve) will create a subaortic obstruction. The VSD was found restrictive in 27 % of all DORV and in 66 % of DORV-non-committed VSD [11–13, 17].
- *Coarctation and interrupted aortic arch* are associated with the Taussig Bing anomaly [18].
- *Subaortic obstruction* is due to a stenosis on the persitant subaortic conus/infundibulum and is seen in Taussig-Bing and in DORV-nc-VSD.
- A *complete atrioventricular septal defect with pulmonary stenosis and heterotaxy/isomerism* is a complex association. It could be associated with total abnormal pulmonary venous return (TAPVR) and intestinal malrotation [13]
- *Pulmonary atresia and pulmonary arteries branches stenoses* can be present.
- *Straddling AV valves* is a complex association and could be a contra-indication to bi-ventricular repair
- *Pulmonary hypertension* should be prevented and is evaluated in patients seen late
- *AV discordance* can be associated with DORV [9].
- Other *rare associations* include: situs inversus, ectopia cordis, etc…
- *Chromosomic anomalies* are present in 20 % of DORV.

Functional Classification

Due to the variety of anatomic forms and the absence of consensus on the definition, the Functional Classification was created to clarify the surgical indications. It was adopted together by the Society of Thoracic Surgeons (STS) [2], the European Association of Cardiothoracic Surgery (EACTS) and by the Association for European Pediatric Cardiology (AEPC). It is based on the relationship of the VSD with the great vessels and the presence of a pulmonary outflow obstruction. These factors allow describing different *functional types* unified by a similar clinical presentation and more importantly by a common surgical management.

The Functional Classification of DORV recognizes four types [2]. The author is adding DORV-CAVSD as a fifth type (Fig. 23.1).

1. DORV-VSD type (DORV subaortic VSD and DORV doubly committed VSD)
2. DORV-Fallot type
3. DORV-TGA type. Taussig-Bing
4. DORV remote VSD
5. DORV-CAVSD-PS-Heterotaxy

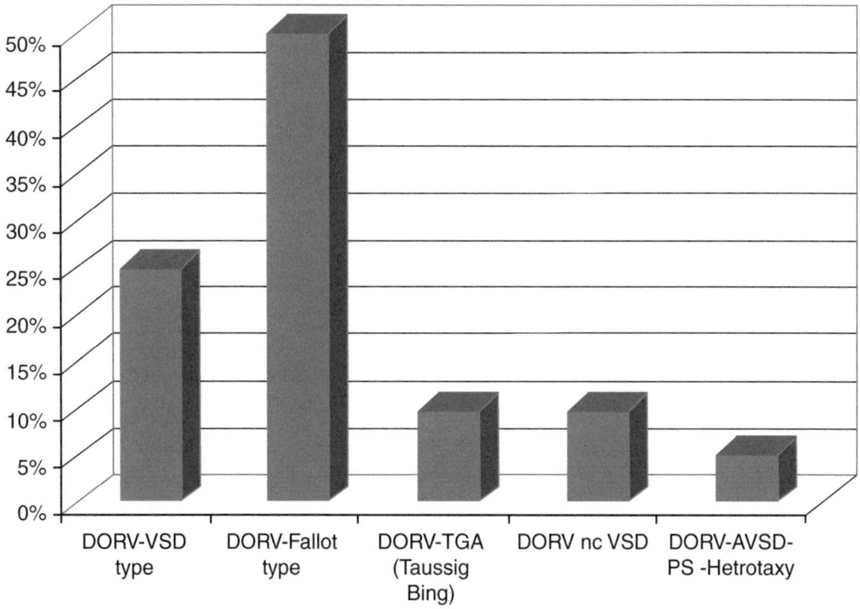

Fig. 23.1 The Functional Classification of DORV recognizes four types. The author is adding DORV-CAVSD as a fifth type. DORV non committed VSD and DORV-AVSD are complex DORV and require original and challenging surgical techniques, specific to this condition

DORV non committed VSD and DORV-AVSD are complex DORV and require original and challenging surgical techniques, specific to this condition.

DORV-VSD Types. They account for 25 % of DORV (Fig. 23.1) and Include Two Different Forms: DORV Subaortic VSD (Fig. 23.2) and DORV Doubly Committed VSD (Fig. 23.3)

DORV- Subaortic VSD (Fig. 23.2)

The VSD is located above and in between the limbs of the trabecula septo marginalis (TSM). There is no pulmonary stenosis. The clinical presentation is that of a VSD with large left-to-right shunt. The VSD can be restrictive [13, 17]. The aorta rarely arises entirely from the right ventricle. We considered this form as a "partial" DORV (not always 200 %).

DORV Doubly Committed VSD (Fig. 23.3)

This form seems the most infrequent one, around 3 %. When the VSD is doubly committed, the conal septum is absent or markedly deficient. Sometimes, the VSD

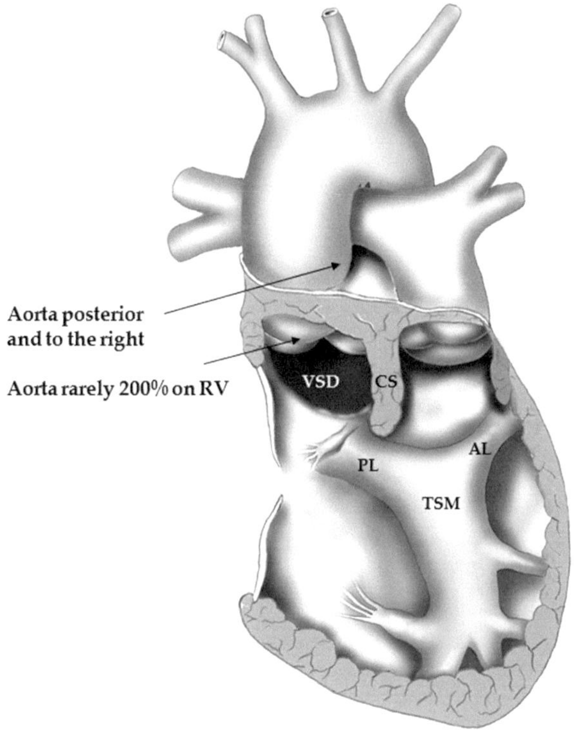

Fig. 23.2 DORV subaortic VSD. The VSD is subaortic, standing above the TSM. The aorta is in normal position posterior and to the right. It is not always arising entirely (200 %) from the right ventricle. The subaortic conus is rarely well developed (*VSD* ventricular septal defect, *TSM* trabecula septo marginalis/septal band, *AL* anterior limb, *PL* posterior limb)

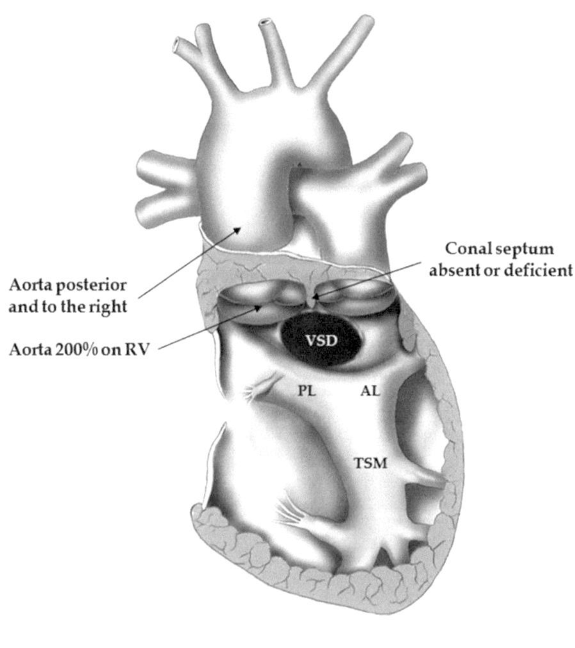

Fig. 23.3 DORV doubly committed VSD. The conal septum is absent or deficient. The VSD is located below the two arterial valves and above the TSM. The aorta is usually in normal position. Many times, the aorta is arising entirely (200 %) from the right ventricle (*VSD* ventricular septal defect, *TSM* trabecula septo marginalis/septal band, *AL* anterior limb, *PL* posterior limb, *CS* conal septum)

is located medially underneath the two orifices. Elsewhere, the VSD is located below the aorta or below the pulmonary, being a transitional form of DORV subaortic VSD or DORV-Taussig Bing. The aorta is most often entirely located inside the right ventricle, sitting side by side and to the right of the PA. A cyanosis could be present.

DORV-Fallot Type (*Fig. 23.4*)

In DORV-Fallot type, the VSD is subaortic and a pulmonary stenosis is constantly associated. With an occurrence around 50 %, it is the most common type. Patients with DORV-Fallot type present like a Tetralogy of Fallot. The degree of cyanosis depends on the severity of the pulmonary stenosis. The VSD can be restrictive in 20 % [17]. The aorta rarely arises entirely from the right ventricle. It is difficult to differentiate DORV-Fallot type from tetralogy of Fallot, and the diagnosis of DORV is frequently overestimated.

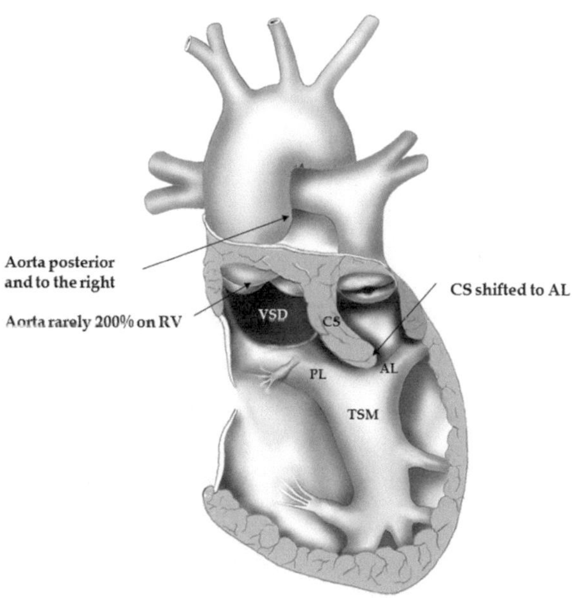

Fig. 23.4 DORV-Fallot. The VSD is subaortic, located above the TSM. The conal septum is shifted toward the anterior limb of the TSM, creating a pulmonary flow obstruction. The aorta is in normal position, posterior and to the right. It is not always arising entirely (<200 %) from the right ventricle. The subaortic conus is partially developed (*VSD* ventricular septal defect, *TSM* trabecula septo marginalis/septal band, *AL* anterior limb, *PL* posterior limb, *CS* conal septum)

A rare variant is DORV-Fallot with doubly committed VSD, where the conal septum is reduced or absent and the pulmonary annulus restrictive. It is similar to the Asian form of TOF.

DORV-TGA Type. Taussig-Bing (Fig. 23.5)

Taussig-Bing represents 10 % of DORV (see Chaps. 14 and 15). The clinical presentation is similar to patients with TGA-VSD. Aortic arch obstruction and subaortic obstruction are frequently associated. The great vessels are side by side, with the aorta on the right. The coronary arteries have usually a double looping pattern (Chaps. 14 and 15). The RV can be small but not really hypoplastic in neonates. The VSD is exceptionally restrictive. The aorta arises entirely from the right ventricle and the pulmonary artery arises more than 50 % from the left ventricle but rarely entirely. There are two conus and the conal septum is shifted toward the posterior limb of the TSM, creating potentially a subaortic obstruction (Fig. 23.5). It is often difficult to differentiate Taussig-Bing from TGA-VSD, depending on the limits chosen to anatomically

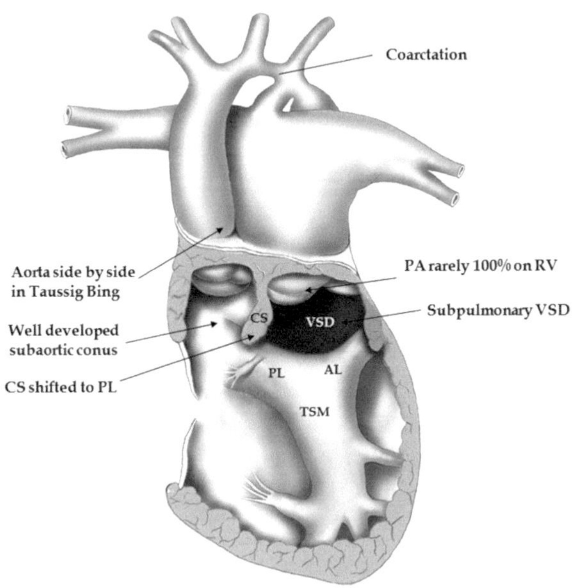

Fig. 23.5 DORV-TGA, Taussig Bing. The VSD is subpulmonary (Taussig Bing), located above the TSM. The conal septum is shifted toward the posterior limb of the TSM, creating potentially a subaortic obstruction. There is frequently a coarctation. The aorta is side by side and to the right of the pulmonary artery. The subaortic conus is well developed. The aorta is arising entirely from the right ventricle, while the PA arises most often only partially from the right ventricle [19]. In Taussig-Bing, there is a mitro-pulmonary discontinuity (*VSD* ventricular septal defect, *TSM* trabecula septo marginalis/septal band, *AL* anterior limb, *PL* posterior limb, *CS* conal septum)

separate the two ventricles; -either the axis of the muscular septum [6] or the interventricular communication [9]. The Taussig-Bing anomaly should have mitro-pulmonary discontinuity [19, 20], whereas the TGA-VSD have mitro-pulmonary continuity.

DORV-Non-committed VSD (Figs. 23.6 and 23.7)

This complex form of DORV, accounts for 10 % and presents with or without PS. Both great vessels arise entirely from the right ventricle (200 %) and this is the most typical form of "complete DORV", as shown on echocardiogram or angiogram (Fig. 23.6). The aorta stands anterior and to the right of the PA. The aorta is very remote from the VSD, by a distance described as "considerable" by Van Praagh et al. [6]. Belli et al. [21] arbitrarily defined DORV nc VSD, as a DORV where the

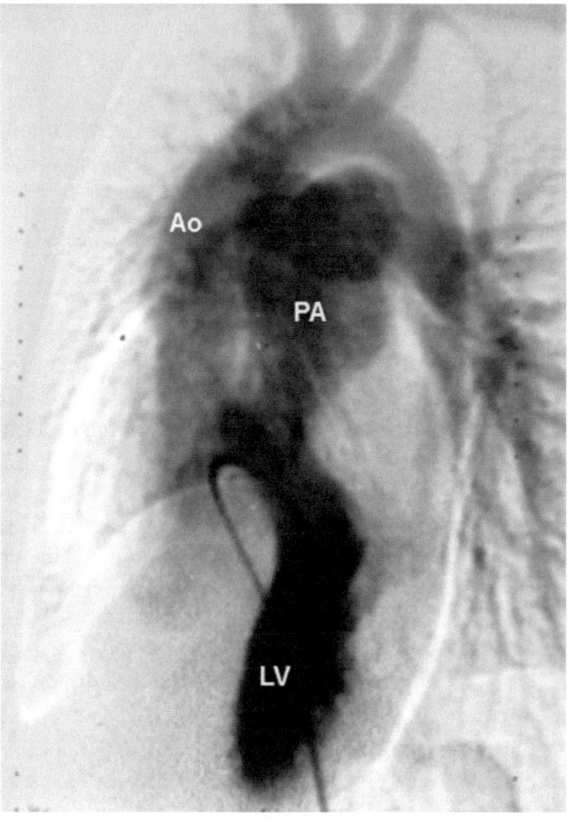

Fig. 23.6 DORV non-committed VSD angiogram. Notice that both great vessels arise 200 % from the right ventricle

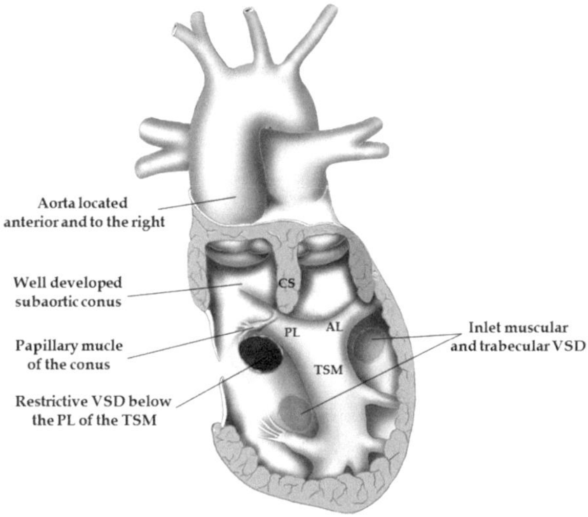

Fig. 23.7 DORV non committed VSD. The VSD is located below the PL of the TSM. It is frequently restrictive. The conal septum could be shifted toward the PL creating a potential subaortic obstruction or toward the AL (not represented on the figure) creating a pulmonary stenosis. The aorta is anterior and to the right. There is nearly constantly a mitro-pulmonary discontinuity. There are clearly two infundibuli with the subaortic conus and conus wall (left VIF for RH Anderson) being very well developed. In rare cases, the VSD can be located in the muscular or trabecular septum. Notice on this drawing that the papillary muscle of the conus is in the way of a tunnelization of the VSD to the aorta (*VSD* ventricular septal defect, *TSM* trabecula septo marginalis/septal band, *AL* anterior limb, *PL* posterior limb, *CS* conal septum, *VIH* ventriculo-infundibular fold)

distance between the superior edge of the VSD and any great vessel annulus is greater than the aortic valve diameter. The VSD is usually in contact with the tricuspid valve (Fig. 23.8) [8, 23]. It is rarely a truly inlet muscular or trabecular VSD (Fig. 23.6) [24]. The VSD is located below the posterior limb of the TSM; different from a Taussig Bing where the VSD is located above the posterior limb of the TSM [24]. In DORV nc VSD, *it is the aorta that is remote not the VSD*. In our experience, *the VSD was restrictive in nearly two third of the patients* [12, 13, 17]. The VSD has a natural tendency to close with time. The VSD can be absent with hypoplasia of the left ventricle [6], or obturated with time following a Fontan operation performed on DORV nc VSD [17, 25, 26]. A closing VSD can also be seen in the neonatal period requiring an urgent decompression of the left ventricle. There is usually an “inverted coronary anatomy” (see Chap. 14). There is *almost constantly a fibro-aortic discontinuity* as well as two well-developed infundibulum. The conal septum stands entirely in the right ventricle. It can be shifted toward the posterior limb of the TSM, potentially creating a subaortic obstruction.

Pulmonary outflow obstruction is present in one third of the cases. This form is different from a DORV-Fallot because the aorta is distant from the VSD by a longer distance, according to our definition [21]. The conal septum is shifted toward the anterior limb of the TSM, which opens up the subaortic infundibulum. Straddling AV valve and other association can be seen.

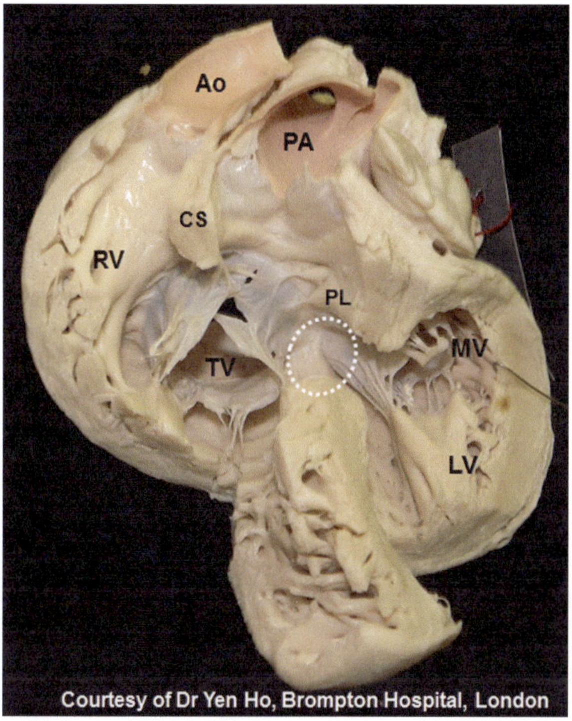

Fig. 23.8 DORV nc VSD Specimen. This specimen from the Morphologic Congenital Heart Disease Department of the Brompton Hospital, London is a "spectacular" DORV nc VSD. The ventricular septum was cut off and the two ventricles are well seen. The VSD is an oval in white. It is located below the TSM and remote from the two arterial valves. It is restrictive. Notice that it is impossible to baffle the VSD to the aorta due to the tricuspid valve and the conal septum. On the other hand, it is possible to tunnelize the VSD to the PA and add an arterial switch (see Fig. 23.11). Notice also that it is the aorta that is remote and not the VSD (*PL* posterior limb, *CS* conal septum, *RV* right ventricle, *LV* left ventricle, *TV* tricuspid valve, *MV* mitral valve) (Courtesy of Dr. Yen Ho, Brompton Hospital, London. Used with permission)

DORV-CAVSD-PS-Heterotaxy (*Figs. 23.9, 23.10, and 23.11*)

DORV-CAVSD is a complex form and accounts for 5 %. Pulmonary outflow obstruction is nearly constant. The clinical presentation is that of a Fallot-AVSD with cyanosis. The VSD has usually a large anterior component like in Rastelli type C (Figs. 23.9, 23.10, and 23.11) [22, 27–29]. The constant presence of heterotaxy makes this condition even more complex due to possible association with TAPVR and intestinal malrotation [13]. Both vessels arise entirely from the right ventricle (200 %) in this complete DORV. This is the best landmark between DORV-Fallot and AVSD-DORV which are difficult to differentiate. Another difference is the absence of Down's syndrome in DORV-AVSD in relation with the presence of isomerism [29]. The bi-ventricular repair of this complex form started 30 years ago [27] with Al Pacifico and is currently achieved by several centers [13, 22, 28–30] (See Chap. 26).

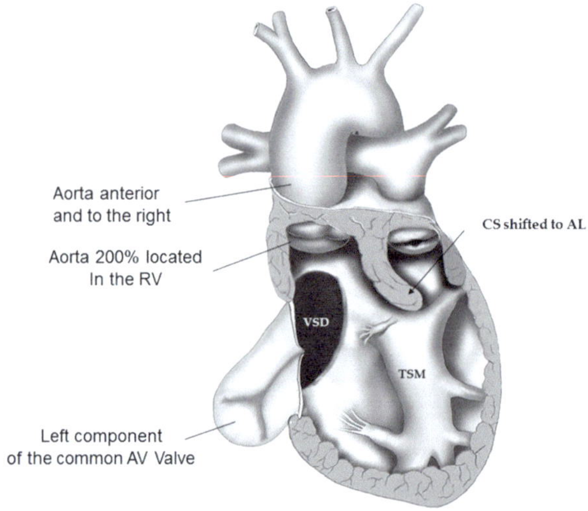

Fig. 23.9 DORV AVSD. The aorta is located anterior and to the right. The great vessels are 200 % on the RV. There is very frequently a pulmonary stenosis with anterior shifting of the conal septum. It is always a type C of Rastelli. The left AV valve is shown. The VSD has an anterior component toward the aorta. The subaortic conus is well developed. The tunnelization to the aorta is usually feasible (see Chap. 23) (*VSD* ventricular septal defect, *TSM* trabecula septo marginalis/septal band, *AL* anterior limb, *PL* posterior limb, *CS* conal septum)

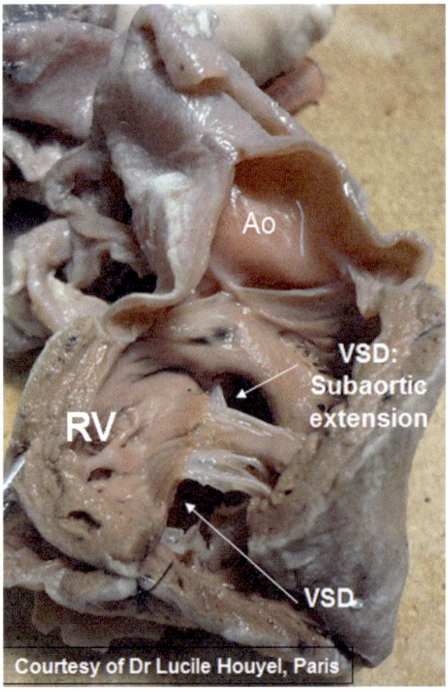

Fig. 23.10 DORV AVSD specimen. This specimen coming from Pathology Department of Marie Lannelongue Hospital, Paris shows clearly the anterior component of the VSD below the aorta (Used with the permission of Dr. Lucile Houyel, Paris) (*VSD* ventricular septal defect, *RV* right ventricle)

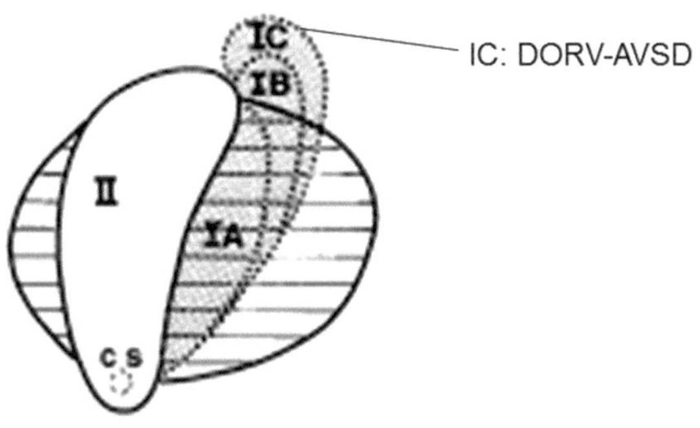

Fig. 23.11 Shape of the VSD in AVSD. *IA* VSD in complete AVSD, *IB* VSD in AVSD-Fallot, *IC* VSD in DORV-AVSD, *II* ostium primum, *CS* coronary sinus (From Kleinert and Mee [22], with permission)

Diagnosis-Imaging of DORV

Echocardiography

An accurate and comprehensive anatomical diagnosis is essential to define the DORV types and the surgical anatomy. *Echocardiography remains the optimal tool* to insure a complete inventory of the lesions. This is a complex evaluation, requiring an experienced operator. It could be useful for the surgeon to attend the exam. The echocardiogram needs to provide several specific information to guide the surgical indications.

The *dimension of the ventricles* will first orient towards a biventricular repair or single ventricle palliation. In borderline ventricular volumes, MRI is indicated.

The *alignment of the great vessels with the ventricular cavities* can be difficult to define. This is visualized with a sweep from the VSD to the great vessels. Depending upon the view-plane used for imaging, the arterial trunks may appear to be connected to different ventricles. It could be extremely difficult to delineate precisely the percentage of arterial valves overriding the right ventricle, even when the two vessels arise entirely from the right ventricle (200 %). The echocardiography could be misleading and the final anatomy ultimately confirmed during surgery. When present, a *mitro-aortic discontinuity* in long axis parasternal view is a major landmark for the diagnosis [6, 7]. In complex forms, the mitro-aortic discontinuity is usually large, whereas in simple forms like DORV-Fallot type or DORV-VSD-type, the mitro-aortic discontinuity could be shallow or absent. A *double infundibulum* is clearly seen in the most typical forms, with a long subaortic infundibulum, which can be narrowed. The other significant landmark in complex DORV is the *conal septum entirely located in the right ventricle*.

The *relationship and the distance between the VSD and the arterial trunks*. This allows deciding the type of the VSD re-routing; either to the aorta or to the pulmonary artery, and also defining DORV nc VSD type.

The diameter of the VSD in comparison with the diameter of the aortic annulus. When smaller than the aortic diameter, the VSD is to be enlarged.

The distance between the tricuspid and pulmonary valves [10, 31]. This space is the site of the baffle to be constructed to connect the VSD to the aorta. It is frequently occupied by the conal septum and the conal papillary muscle (Fig. 23.8).

The *coronary artery anatomy* is usually similar to a normal heart, with the right coronary artery arising from the left antero-lateral sinus and the common left trunk rising for the left postero-lateral sinus. This is the coronary pattern in Taussig Bing, named "inverted" in TGA (see Chaps. 15 and 16). Other coronary anomalies like left anterior descending crossing the infundibulum and single coronary can be seen by echocardiogram.

Cardiac association. Right ventricular outflow tract obstruction is the most frequent association. It can be either valvular and/or infundibular or atretic. *Other associations* are diagnosed: multiple VSD, aortic arch obstruction and subaortic obstruction, straddling AV valves, etc…

Catheterization-Angiography

Catheterization is rarely performed in simple forms. It is useful in complex forms (Fig. 23.6) to evaluate: systemic and pulmonary venous return, coronary anatomy, PA branches size and pulmonary vascular resistances in older patients.

CT Scan. MRI. 3D Echo

Magnetic resonance imaging, computed tomography, and three-dimensional echocardiography provide interesting imaging and *are required in complex forms*. MRI is needed to evaluate border line ventricular volumes.

3D Printing and 3D Computed Reconstruction

3D printing and 3D computed reconstruction based on CT scan [32] are under progress and may become the best tool to define the feasibility of rerouting the VSD to the great vessels in complex DORV.

Prenatal Diagnosis and Chromosomic Anomalies

DORV can be diagnosed by fetal echocardiography with a good degree of accuracy [33] when the two vessels arise from the right ventricle. DORV can be associated with chromosomic abnormalities. Di George-deletion 22q11 syndrome is frequent in patients with Taussig Bing. CHARGE syndrome and other rare chromosomic anomalies are possible. Trisomy 21 is exceptional in DORV-AVSD-heterotaxy. The occurrence of DORV during the embryologic development is related to a genetic dysfunction of the second heart field which regulates the conotruncal formation [34] (See Chaps. 2 and 36).

DORV Pre-operative Checklist

- Dimension of the ventricles
- Ventriculo-arterial alignment
- VSD-great vessels relationship and distance
- VSD diameter
- Distance tricuspid-pulmonary valves
- Great vessels relationship
- Coronary anatomy
- Associations:

  Pulmonary valvar- subvalvar stenosis, atresia
  Additional VSD
  Subaortic obstruction
  Coarctation, IAA
  ASD, PDA
  CAVSD
  Heterotaxy/Isomerism: LSVC, asplenia, azygos continuation
  TAPVR
  Straddling AV valves
  Intestinal malrotation
  Pulmonary hypertension
  Chromosomic anomaly
  Others; situs inversus, AV discordance, etc…

Surgical Techniques of DORV Biventricular Repair

Repair of DORV-VSD Type

DORV Subaortic VSD

Patients with *DORV-VSD and subaortic VSD* (Fig. 23.2) are treated by one stage repair in the first months of life. A prior PA banding is sometimes indicated and is contra-indicated if the VSD is restrictive. The operation is performed through the tricuspid valve. The VSD is found close to the aortic valve that stands partially and sometimes entirely in the right ventricle. A right ventriculotomy is rarely requested. The VSD can be restrictive requiring a ventral enlargement [17]. The patch is longer than usual to re-route the VSD to the aorta. It is secured using pledgeted separated stitches and continuous sutures.

DORV Doubly Committed VSD

In DORV doubly committed VSD (Fig. 23.3), a right ventriculotomy is needed. The VSD is infundibular. There conal septum is absent or deficient and the aortic and pulmonary annulus could be in continuity. The VSD baffle to the aorta needs to be sutured between the two annuli and should not be too large to avoid a subpulmonary obstruction. A patch enlargement of the ventriculotomy limits the risk of subpulmonary stenosis. When the tunnelization to the aorta is difficult, the tunnelization to the PA followed by arterial switch should be considered.

Repair of DORV-Fallot Type (Fig. 23.4)

Patients with DORV-Fallot type present like Tetralogy of Fallot. A Blalock-Taussig shunt is considered in the first months of life and is indicated in cases of abnormal coronary, severe PA branches hypoplasia and multiple VSD. The operation is sometimes conducted through the atrium, but a right ventriculotomy offers a better approach to both the aortic valve and the VSD borders. Dividing first the parietal band allows a good visualization of the aortic annulus. The VSD patch should be large enough to reach the anterior part of the aortic annulus that is overriding the right ventricle.

Repair of DORV-TGA Type (Taussig-Bing) (Fig. 23.5)

See Chap. 16

Repair of DORV-Non-committed VSD (Figs. 23.7, 23.8, and 23.12)

Biventricular repair of DORV-nc-VSD remains challenging and is performed only by a few centers [11–13, 21, 22, 24, 28, 30, 31] The VSD is restrictive in 60 % of the DORV-nc-VSD [13, 17] and need to be enlarged as shown below.

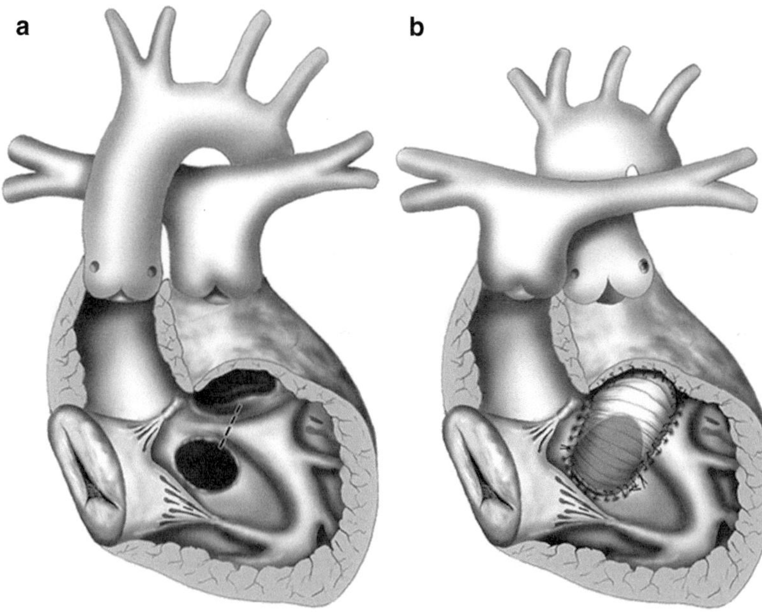

Fig. 23.12 DORV nc VSD, Tunnelization to the pulmonary artery + arterial switch. The VSD is frequently enlarged anteriorly and to the left (**a**). The repair includes a tunnelization to the pulmonary artery and an arterial switch procedure (**b**). Notice that the tunnel is quite short because the tunnel ends on the ostium infundibuli

Repair of DORV-nc-VSD Without Pulmonary Obstruction

A palliative PA banding is preferable due to the need of a significant intraventricular baffle. Depending on the anatomy, the VSD can be tunnelized either to the aorta or to the PA followed by an arterial switch.

Tunellisation of the VSD to the Aorta

This operation is undertaken when the child has reached 6–8 kg. If this technique seems logical, it is in fact quite challenging. In many instances, constructing a tunnel to the aorta requires to resect the conal septum and sacrifice part of the tricuspid valve and/or the papillary muscle of the conus (Fig. 23.8) [10, 24]. The aorta is transposed and always distant from the VSD. It requires a very long patch that could impair the LV function. In these cases, Barbero-Marcial et al. [24] has proposed a multiple patch with resection of the conal septum, reimplantation of the TV chordate on the patch and partial sacrifice of the tricuspid valve or the pulmonary artery.

It is our preference to tunnelize to the VSD to the aorta only when the baffle can be constructed without impairing the conal septum or the tricuspid and pulmonary valves [11–13]. The baffle is constructed through a double approach, through the tricuspid valve and a right ventriculotomy, using a patch of Goretex or bovine pericardium, sutured with separated pledgeted stitches and continuous suture. When the VSD size is less than the aortic annulus, the VSD is to be enlarged anteriorly as shown on Fig. 23.12.

Tunnelization of the VSD to the PA Followed by an Arterial Switch

This technique was described by the author in 2002 [11] (Fig. 23.12). When the aorta can't be tunnelized to the aorta (Fig. 23.8), it can most often be tunnelized to the PA. This condition is therefore treated like a Taussig-Bing anomaly by tunnelization to the PA, associated with an arterial switch. The only difference being a longer patch and the need to frequently enlarge the VSD. The patch is shorter than the baffling to the aorta because the baffle ends at the level of the ostium infundibuli. In two third of the cases, the VSD needs to be enlarged. The incision of the septum is carried out on the superior border of the VSD and should be large enough as to create a VSD larger than the aortic orifice. Our surgical experience following safe ventral enlargement of the VSD [11–13, 17], suggests that the conduction tissue is located on the inferior rim of the VSD. The conduction tissue could also be located on the superior border into the posterior limb of the TSM and the avoidance of AV block could be due to the early division of the bundle.

The patch is constructed with a triple approach, through the tricuspid valve, the right ventriculotomy and the aorta. The baffle is constructed with pledgeted sutures in the area of septal incision and by continuous sutures. An arterial switch follows. It requires dealing with inverted coronary arteries anatomy, implying to move the reconstructed pulmonary trunk toward the right PA branch (see Chaps. 15 and 16) if a Lecompte maneuver is performed.

Repair of DORV-nc-VSD with Pulmonary Obstruction

In all cases with pulmonary stenosis, *a palliative BT shunt* is preferable.

Tunnelization of the VSD to the Aorta and RVOT Reconstruction

Due to the anterior malalignement of the conal septum toward the pulmonary infundibulum, the space between the tricuspid and the pulmonary valve is often larger, authorizing a safer baffling to the aorta, particularly in pulmonary atresia. This technique of intraventricular repair (not to be confused with R.E.V) is the most adapted to DORV-nc-VSD with RVOTO, providing that the VSD can be safely baffled to the aorta without resection of the conal septum or sacrifice of the PA. The RVOT is simply reconstructed with a transannular patch enlargement or a RV to PA valved conduit in pulmonary atresia.

R.E.V. Operation and Rastelli Procedure

These techniques combined a tunnelization of the VSD to the aorta with an interruption of the pulmonary trunk associated with a RV to PA valved conduit (Rastelli) or a Lecompte maneuver (R.E.V.) [31]. A R.E.V procedure is indicated in patients with restrictive tricuspid- pulmonary valve space, when the resection of the conal septum cannot spare the pulmonary annulus. It includes a resection of the conal septum, the interruption of the PA trunk and a Lecompte maneuver with RV to PA reconstruction using a monocusp valve (see Chap. 20). The conal papillary muscle is frequently detached and reimplanted on the patch. As already mentioned earlier, we are not in favor of impacting on the tricuspid valve apparatus.

Tunnelization to the PA and Arterial Switch

In the rare forms where the pulmonary obstruction is limited to an infundibular stenosis, with a normal PA valve, a tunnelization to the PA with arterial switch could be theoretically performed associated with a patch enlargement of the infundibulum.

Double Root Translocation (see Chap. 21)

This complex operation previously described for TGA-VSD-PS [35, 36] has found indications [37, 38] (see Chap. 21), in DORV nc VSD-PS, where the tunnelization to the aorta is not possible. In DORV-nc-VSD, the two great vessels are entirely located in the RV and the translocation of the aorta on the PA annulus does not repair the DORV. The objective of the double root translocation is only to place the remote aorta, which will remain on the RV, in a position closer to the VSD. This very complex technique is an interesting solution which would need a longer follow up to be adopted in the armamentarium of DORV repair.

Repair of DORV-AVSD-PS-Heterotaxy

See Chap. 24.

Limitations of DORV Bi-ventricular Repair and Fontan Indication

This chapter is dedicated to bi-ventricular of DORV. It is clear that the surgical techniques described above are only indicated in selected patients.

Contra-indication to Biventricular Repair

There are several contra-indications:

- *Hypoplasia of one ventricle* is frequent [6–8]: it is the main contra-indication. Border line left or right ventricular cavities should be assessed by objective measurements of the end-diastolic LV and RV volumes using MRI.
- *Straddling AV valves*. Straddling type C is a contra-indication. It is defined as straddling chordae joining a papillary muscle or the parietal wall of the controlateral ventricle. Straddling A and B, when the straddling chordae are located on the edge or at some distance inside the contro-lateral ventricles, can be managed in moving the VSD baffle a few millimeters away [39].
- *Multiple VSD*. More than two associated VSD or an associated apical VSD contra-indicate two ventricles repair [13, 22]
- *Inlet muscular and trabecular VSDs* were described [8, 23, 24] in DORV nc VSD (Fig. 23.7). They are contra-indication to biventricular repair. We have not found such true inlet muscular or trabecular VSD in our series of bi-ventricular repair of DORV nc VSD [11–13].
- *Learning curve*. Bi-ventricular repair of simple forms (DORV-VSD, DORV-Fallot) and of Taussig Bing are routinely performed in most centers. Repair of complex forms is challenging and is considered too risky for many institutions not ready to engage in a learning curve.

Univentricular Repair in Complex DORV

Univentricular repair (Chap. 35) is clearly indicated in presence of the contra-indications listed above. In selected complex DORV with two viable ventricles, the optimal option is anatomical repair [13, 21, 22, 30]. Nevertheless, a Fontan procedure is still advocated by many centers because of the short term security offered by a Fontan undertaken on two ventricles. However, there are specific issues with the Fontan procedure in complex DORV.

In DORV nc VSD, the VSD is already small in 60 % and can become severely restricted with time. This dramatic complication of the Fontan procedure was described by the Boston group in eight patients in the follow up of Fontan undertaken in DORV nc VSD [25]. The VSD was totally closed in five patients and severely restrictive in three, with supra-systemic LV and compression of the right ventricle. One patient presented with an LV aneurysm. Attempts at surgical VSD enlargement or catheter-based procedures have resulted in almost constant recurrence. This recently reported complication is in favor of also performing a VSD enlargement at the time of the Fontan completion in complex DORV [17] (Chap. 35).

In DORV-AVSD-PS-heterotaxy, the association with a TAPVR is at risk for late pulmonary veins obstruction and pulmonary hypertension. A bi-ventricular circulation would be more suitable (see Chap. 24).

Heart transplantation may be contemplated in rare circumstances.

Outcomes

Mortality

The mortality reported in the literature depends on the anatomic types. In simple forms it is <5 % in DORV-VSD, 5–7 % in DORV Fallot [11] and 0–7 % in Taussig-Bing treated by arterial switch [18, 40].

The mortality is higher in complex forms. In DORV-nc-VSD, there are limited series as shown on Table 23.1. The average mortality, depending on series published, varies from 5 to 15 %. The recent introduction of the tunnelization to the pulmonary artery followed by arterial switch [11, 12, 38] is associated with a mortality of 6 % [13]. Multiple VSD is associated with significant higher mortality [13, 22].

In DORV-AVSD-PS-Heterotaxy, the mortality reported in recent publications is 5 % [13, 30].

Follow Up and Reoperation

The long term follow up in simple forms is equivalent to the surgical repair of respectively: VSD, Fallot and Taussig Bing. In complex forms, the midterm survival in is around 80–85 %. A recent large series from Fu Wai Hospital, Beijing [38] with 380 bi-ventricular repair of DORV, reports that in 67 DORV nc VSD (Table 23.1) the operative mortality was 10 % and the 5 years survival 85 %. Additional information on long term outcome is required.

Late subaortic obstruction at the level of the baffle tunnel and/or the VSD is the most frequent cause of reoperation [13, 38, 41–43] and varies from 5 to 35 % according to the series published. This complication was observed early in our experience and can be avoided by an appropriate enlargement of the VSD at the time of the repair [17, 42]. It is significantly more frequent in DORV nc VSD repair [38]. Intra-operative AV blocks have become seldom [17]. Late ventricular arrhythmias [22], pulmonary valve regurgitation, valved conduit failure, as well as aortic dilation require a life-long surveillance by paediatric and adult congenital cardiologists.

Table 23.1 Biventricular repair of DORV nc VSD

Sakata et al. [10]	Paris	Not given
S Kleinert, R Mee, et al. *JTCVS* (1997) [22]	Melbourne	12
E Belli, F Lacour-Gayet et al. [21]	Paris	23
M Barbero Marcial, et al. *JTCVS* (2000) [24]	Sao Paulo	17
J Artrip, F Lacour-Gayet et al. [13]	Denver	11
Li et al. [38]	Beijing	67

Bibliography

1. Lev M, Bharati S, Meng CCL, et al. A concept of double-outlet right ventricle. J Thorac Cardiovasc Surg. 1972;64:271–81.
2. Walters III HL, Mavroudis C, Lacour-Gayet F, et al. Congenital heart surgery nomenclature and database project: double outlet right ventricle. Ann Thorac Surg. 2000;69:S249–63, (suppl 4).
3. Witham AC. Double outlet right ventricle, a partial transposition complex. Am Heart J. 1957;53:928–39.
4. Neufeld HN, DuShane JW, Wood EH, Kirklin JW, Edwards JE. Origin of both great vessels from the right ventricle. I. Without pulmonary stenosis. Circulation. 1961;23:393–408.
5. Neufeld HN, DuShane JW, Edwards JE. Origin of both great vessels from the right ventricle. II. With pulmonary stenosis. Circulation. 1961;23:603–12.
6. Van Praagh S, Davidoff A, Van Praagh R. Double outlet right ventricle: anatomic types and developmental implications based on a study of 101 autopsied cases. Coeur. 1982;13:389–440.
7. Van Praagh R. Nomenclature and classification: morphologic and segmental approach to diagnosis. In: Moller JH, Hoffman JIE, editors. Pediatric cardiovascular medicine. New York: Churchill Livingstone; 2000. p. 275–88.
8. Becker AE, Anderson RH. Pathology of congenital heart disease. London: Butterworth; 1981. p. 297.
9. Mahle WT, Martinez R, Silverman N, Cohen MS, Anderson RH. Anatomy, echocardiography, and surgical approach to double outlet right ventricle. Cardiol Young. 2008;18 Suppl 3:39–51.
10. Sakata R, Lecompte Y, Batisse A, et al. Anatomical repair of anomalies of ventriculo-arterial connection associated with VSD. I. Criteria for surgical decision. J Thorac Cardiovasc Surg. 1988;95:90–5.
11. Lacour-Gayet F, Haun C, Ntalakoura K. Biventricular repair of DORV with non-committed ventricular septal defect (VSD) by VSD rerouting to the pulmonary artery and arterial switch. Eur J Cardiothorac Surg. 2002;21:1042–8.
12. Lacour-Gayet F. Biventricular repair of double outlet right ventricle with noncommitted ventricular septal defect. Semin Thorac Cardiovasc Surg Pediatr Card Surg Annu. 2002;5:163–72.
13. Artrip JH, Campbell DN, Lacour-Gayet F, et al. Biventricular repair in double outlet right ventricle: surgical results based on the STS-EACTS International Nomenclature Classification. Eur J Cardiothorac Surg. 2006;29:545–50.
14. Van Mierop LHS, Alley RD, Kausel HW, Stranahan A. Pathogenesis of transposition complexes. I. Embryology of the ventricles and great arteries. Am J Cardiol. 1963;12:216–25.
15. Van Mierop LHS, Wiglesworth FW. Pathogenesis of transposition complexes. II. Anomalies due to faulty transfer of the posterior great artery. Am J Cardiol. 1963;12:226–32.
16. Van Mierop LHS, Wiglesworth FW. Pathogenesis of transposition complexes. III. True transposition of the great vessels. Am J Cardiol. 1963;12:233–9.
17. Goldberg S, McCanta A, Lacour-Gayet F, et al. Implications of incising the ventricular septum in double outlet right ventricle and in the Ross-Konno operation. Eur J Cardiothorac Surg. 2009;35(4):589–93; discussion 593. Epub 9 Mar 2009.
18. Lacour-Gayet F, Serraf A, Galletti L, et al. Biventricular repair of conotruncal anomalies associated with aortic arch obstruction: 103 patients. Circulation. 1997;96:II-328–34.
19. Taussig HB, Bing RJ. Complete transposition of aorta and levoposition of pulmonary artery. Am Heart J. 1949;37:551–7.
20. Van Praagh R. What is the Taussig Bing malformation? Circulation. 1968;38:445–9.
21. Belli E, Lacour-Gayet F, Serraf A, et al. Double-outlet right ventricle with non-committed ventricular septal defect. Eur J Cardiothorac Surg. 1999;15:747–52.
22. Kleinert S, Sano T, Weintraub RG, Mee RBB, Karl TR, Wilkinson JL. Anatomic features and surgical strategies in double-outlet right ventricle. Circulation. 1997;96:1233–9.

23. Stellin G, Ho SY, Anderson RH, Zuberbuhler JR, Siewers RD. The surgical anatomy of double-outlet right ventricle with concordant atrioventricular connection and noncommitted ventricular septal defect. J Thorac Cardiovasc Surg. 1991;102(6):849–55.
24. Barbero-Marcial M, Tanamati C, Atik E, et al. Intraventricular repair of DORV with noncommitted VSD: advantages of multiple patches. J Thorac Cardiovasc Surg. 1999;118. 18. Freedom RM, Yoo ST. Double outlet right ventricle: pathology and angiocardiography. Semin Thorac Cardiovasc Surg Pediatr Card Surg Annu. 2000;3:3–19.
25. Meadows J, Pigula F, Lock J, Marshall A. Transcatheter creation and enlargement of ventricular septal defects for relief of ventricular hypertension. J Thorac Cardiovasc Surg. 2007;133:912–8.
26. Lacour-Gayet F. Management of older single functioning ventricles with outlet obstruction due to a restricted "VSD" in double inlet left ventricle and in complex double outlet right ventricle. Semin Thorac Cardiovasc Surg Pediatr Card Surg Annu. 2009:130–2.
27. Pacifico AD, Kirklin JX, Bargeron LM. Repair of complete atrioventricular canal associated with tetralogy of Fallot or double outlet right ventricle. Report of 10 patients. Ann Thorac Surg. 1980;29:351–6.
28. He GW, Mee RB. Complete atrioventricular canal associated with tetralogy of Fallot or double-outlet right ventricle and right ventricular outflow tract obstruction: a report of successful surgical treatment. Ann Thorac Surg. 1986;41(6):612–5.
29. Lacour-Gayet F, Bonnet N, Piot D, Serraf A, Sousa-Uva M, Belli E, Roussin R, Bruniaux J, Planché C. Surgical management of atrio ventricular septal defects with normal caryotype. Eur J Cardiothorac Surg. 1997;11(3):466–72.
30. Devaney EJ, Lee T, Gelehrter S, Hirsch JC, Ohye RG, Anderson RH, Bove EL. Biventricular repair of atrioventricular septal defect with common atrioventricular valve and double-outlet right ventricle. Ann Thorac Surg. 2010;89:537–43.
31. Rubay J, Lecompte Y, Batisse A, Durandy Y, Vouhe P, et al. Anatomic repair of anomalies of ventriculo-arterial connection. Eur J Cardiothorac Surg. 1988;2:305–11.
32. Chen SJ, Lin MT, Liu KL, Chang CI, Chen HY, Wang JK, Lee WJ, Tsang YM, Li YW. Usefulness of 3D reconstructed computed tomography imaging for double outlet right ventricle. J Formos Med Assoc. 2008;107(5):371–80.
33. Kim N, Friedberg MK, Silverman NH. Diagnosis and prognosis of fetuses with double outlet right ventricle. Prenat Diagn. 2006;26(8):740–5.
34. Waldo KL, Kumiski DH, Wallis KT, Stadt HA, Hutson MR, Platt DH, Kirby ML. Conotruncal myocardium arises from a secondary heart field. Development. 2001;128:3179–88.
35. Yamagishi M, Shuntoh K, Matsushita T, Fujiwara K, Shinkawa T, Miyazaki T, Kitamura N. Half-turned truncal switch operation for complete transposition of the great arteries with ventricular septal defect and pulmonary stenosis. J Thorac Cardiovasc Surg. 2003;125(4):966–8.
36. Mair R, Sames-Dolzer E, Vondrys D, Lechner E, Tulzer G. En bloc rotation of the truncus arteriosus – an option for anatomic repair of transposition of the great arteries, ventricular septal defect, and left ventricular outflow tract obstruction. J Thorac Cardiovasc Surg. 2006;131(3):740–1.
37. Hu S, Xie Y, Li S, Wang X, Yan F, Li Y, Hua Z, Li Y. Double-root translocation for double-outlet right ventricle with noncommitted ventricular septal defect or double-outlet right ventricle with subpulmonary ventricular septal defect associated with pulmonary stenosis: an optimized solution. Ann Thorac Surg. 2010;89:1360–5.
38. Li S, Ma K, Hu S, Hua Z, Yang K, Yan J, Chen Q. Surgical outcomes of 380 patients with Double Outlet Right Ventricle who underwent biventricular repair. J Thorac Cardiovasc Surg. 2014;148:817–24.
39. Serraf A, Nakamura T, Lacour-Gayet F, Piot D, Bruniaux J, Touchot A, Sousa-Uva M, Houyel L, Planche C. Surgical approaches for double-outlet right ventricle or transposition of the great arteries associated with straddling atrioventricular valves. J Thorac Cardiovasc Surg. 1996;111:527–35.

40. Lacour-Gayet F. Arterial switch operation with ventricular septal defect repair and aortic arch reconstruction. Semin Thorac Cardiovasc Surg. 2007;19:245–8.
41. Aoki M, Forbess JM, Jonas RA, Mayer Jr JE, Castaneda AR. Result of biventricular repair for double-outlet right ventricle. J Thorac Cardiovasc Surg. 1994;107:338–50.
42. Belli E, Lacour-Gayet F, Prodan S, Piot D, Losay J, Petit J, Bruniaux J, Planché C. Biventricular repair for double-outlet right ventricle. Results and long-term follow-up. Circulation. 1998;98(19 Suppl):II360–7.
43. Belli E, Lacour-Gayet F, Inamo J, Houyel L, Bruniaux J, Planché C. Surgical treatment of subaortic stenosis after biventricular repair of double-outlet right ventricle. J Thorac Cardiovasc Surg. 1996;112(6):1570–80.

Chapter 24
Biventricular Repair of Double Outlet Right Ventricle with Complete Atrioventricular Septal Defect

Ming-Sing Si, Richard G. Ohye, Jennifer C. Hirsch-Romano, and Edward L. Bove

Abstract The combination of double outlet right ventricle and complete atrioventricular septal defect (DORV-AVSD) is a rare congenital heart malformation. Double outlet right ventricle with complete atrioventricular septal defect is commonly associated with heterotaxy but is distinct from DORV as associated with tetralogy of Fallot. Biventricular repair of DORV-AVSD is challenging because it requires not only correction of the complete AVSD and DORV, but often also involves resection of the outlet portion of the ventricular septum to create an unobstructed left ventricular outflow tract as well as repair of the frequently associated systemic and pulmonary venous connection anomalies and right ventricular outflow tract obstruction. Because of this high degree of complexity, functional single ventricle palliation has been recommended as a treatment option for DORV-AVSD by some groups. However, biventricular repair in these patients, despite its complexity, can be accomplished with excellent results. Reoperation is common in this difficult group of patients, most commonly for conduit replacement. Reintervention for recurrent left ventricular outflow tract obstruction or atrioventricular valve stenosis or regurgitation is uncommon. We feel that biventricular repair of DORV-AVSD is the preferred treatment option, although further studies are needed to define long-term outcomes.

Keywords Double outlet right ventricle • Complete atrioventricular septal defect • Complete atrioventricular canal • Endocardial cushion defect • Biventricular repair

M.-S. Si, MD (✉) • R.G. Ohye, MD • J.C. Hirsch-Romano, MD, MS • E.L. Bove, MD
Section of Pediatric Cardiovascular Surgery, Department of Cardiac Surgery,
Michigan Congenital Heart Center, C.S. Mott Children's Hospital, University of Michigan,
Ann Arbor, MI 48109, USA
e-mail: mingsing@umich.edu; ohye@umich.edu; jhirsch@umich.edu; elbove@umich.edu

F. Lacour-Gayet et al. (eds.), *Surgery of Conotruncal Anomalies*,
DOI 10.1007/978-3-319-23057-3_24

Introduction

Atrioventricular septal defect (AVSD) and double outlet right ventricle (DORV) each have a 0.2 % prevalence amongst all live births [1]. Surgical management of these defects has improved over the past few decades such that low mortality and morbidity is expected of repair of major variations of these defects [2–6]. The combination of double outlet right ventricle and atrioventricular septal defect (DORV-AVSD) is rare. In a pathological series of over 500 AVSD specimens, 6.7 % also had DORV [7]. Despite its rare occurrence, DORV-AVSD is a challenging defect to repair and has seen an evolution to its management over the past few decades. It has been more than four decades since it had been postulated that DORV-AVSD could be repaired surgically by enlarging the ventricular septal defect and combining standard repairs for the other lesions [8]. Successful repair of DORV-AVSD was first reported in 1980 [9], but the mortality was high, especially in the presence of associated defects, such as pulmonary stenosis, heterotaxy or anomalous pulmonary venous connections [9]. Early reports, as well as some contemporary surgical series of DORV-AVSD, have combined this defect with the lesion TOF-AVSD [9–11]. The inclusion of TOF-AVSD with DORV-AVSD in early series is likely due to the rare incidence, as well as the similar technique that was used to approach both of these lesions surgically, as discussed later in this chapter. Because of this grouping, an in depth compilation of all series of DORV-AVSD is difficult. Other surgical series [6] define DORV-AVSD as only those patients where the great vessels are 200 % supported by the right ventricle (see Chap. 25). We recently described our experience with DORV-AVSD, which represents one of the largest series published to date [12]. We will refer to this cohort of patients extensively throughout the chapter as we discuss its anatomy and treatment. This chapter will review the anatomy of DORV-AVSD, historical aspects of treatment, our current surgical approach and contemporary results.

Anatomy

Double outlet right ventricle with AVSD is a combination of two lesions that, when considered in isolation, have well defined morphological features [13–16] (Fig. 24.1). Double outlet right ventricle is defined by the origin of the majority of both great vessels from the morphological right ventricle and the presence of a muscular subaortic infundibulum or conus. Importantly, this definition of DORV excludes the anatomy typical for tetralogy of Fallot, where aortic override of the right ventricle is less than or equal to 50 % and there is no muscular subaortic infundibulum. In DORV-AVSD, the main component of the VSD is of the inlet type. While there may be some outlet extension of the VSD, there is subaortic infundibular muscle which separates the defect from the aortic valve annulus. Therefore the VSD in DORV-AVSD can be considered to be remote and non-committed [12]. The

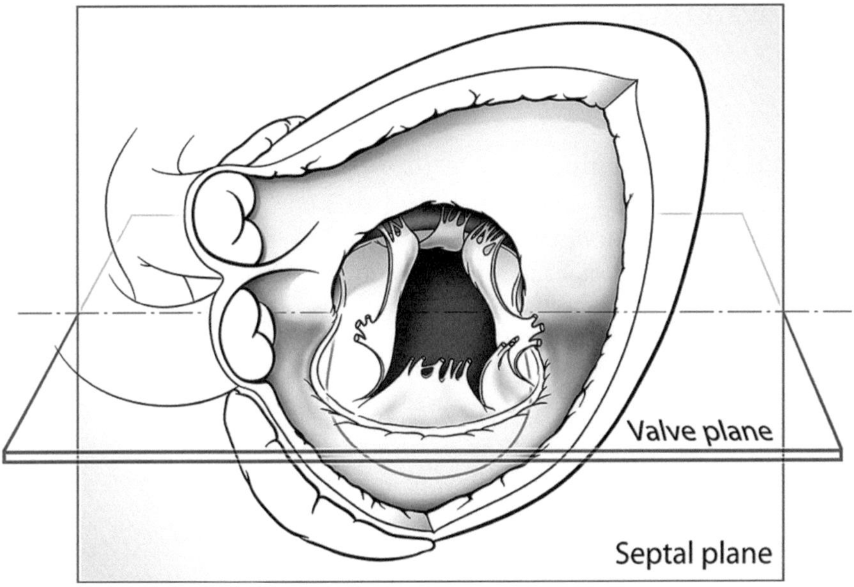

Fig. 24.1 Anatomy of DORV-AVSD with orthogonal atrioventricular valve and septal planes (Used with permission from Devaney et al. [12], with permission of Elsevier)

spatial relationship of the arterial trunks with one another can take any form as in isolated DORV: side by side as well as aorta anterior and to the right or left of the pulmonary artery (PA) [17]. In our series of DORV-AVSD patients, the great arteries were arranged in side-by-side fashion in 4 (with the aorta to the right), positioned with the aorta anteriorly and to the right in 6, and with the aorta anteriorly and to the left in 6 [12].

The definition of an AVSD is a common atrioventricular junction guarded by a common valve. These can be classified according to the Rastelli classification as A, B or C, which is based on the anatomy of the superior bridging leaflet. In our series, as well of those of others, nearly all patients had Rastelli type C [6, 12, 18]. Important atrioventricular valve regurgitation may also be present, and pulmonary stenosis occurred in the majority of our patients with DORV-AVSD [12].

Since DORV-AVSD is associated with heterotaxy syndrome, other cardiac lesions are common. Approximately two-thirds of our patients with heterotaxy had right atrial isomerism [6]. This diagnosis was made either preoperatively or intraoperatively using a number of criteria based on splenic anatomy, bronchopulmonary anatomy, venoatrial connections and morphology of the atrial appendages [19, 20]. Cardiac features of heterotaxy syndrome that may be found in association with DORV-AVSD include anomalous hepatic venous return, total anomalous pulmonary venous connection (TAPVC), interrupted inferior vena cava (IVC), bilateral superior vena cavae (SVC), partial anomalous pulmonary venous connection, common atrium, right aortic arch, and intestinal malrotation. These associated anomalous systemic and pulmonary venous connections further complicate the repair of

DORV-AVSD. Furthermore, none of the patients in our series of DORV-AVSD had trisomy 21.

Diagnosis and Imaging

The diagnosis of DORV-AVSD is made with transthoracic echocardiography. Essentially all anatomical features must be delineated prior to considering repair. These include venous connections, atrioventricular valve structure and function, right and left ventricular size and function, VSD anatomy, and great artery spatial relationship and position within the right ventricle. Cardiac magnetic resonance imaging can provide further anatomical details not adequately defined by echocardiography.

Checklist for Surgical Repair

The inherent complexity and the myriad of associated lesions that must be repaired during repair of DORV-AVSD makes a detailed, specific checklist for the surgeon important, as many physiologic and anatomic details need to be considered. Many of these specific details can be determined by transthoracic echocardiography and cardiac magnetic resonance imaging. Listed below are necessary issues that must be considered prior to embarking on a biventricular repair of DORV-AVSD.

1. Prior palliative operations: BT shunt or pulmonary artery band
2. Atrial inflow anomalies: systemic and hepatic venous anatomy
3. Ventricular size
4. Atrioventricular valve anatomy: mural leaflet size, papillary muscle anatomy.
5. Z scores for atrioventricular and semilunar valves
6. Associated anomalies: TAPVC, intestinal malrotation.

Surgical Approach

Our method of DORV-AVSD repair can be viewed as a 2-patch method of AVSD repair that has been modified to account for abnormalities in systemic and pulmonary venous connection as well as an absence of a contiguous left ventricular outflow tract (LVOT) that connects the left ventricle to the aorta. The septation of the common atrioventricular valve follows the two-patch method that we employ for isolated complete AVSD repair to allow for the creation of two competent, nonstenotic right and left atrioventricular valves [2]. However, modifications are made to the reconstruction of the atrial septum and shape as needed for anomalies of venous connection, as well as the contour and position of the VSD patch to account for the location of the aorta as it arises from the right ventricle. Further, pulmonary outflow obstruction may need to be addressed.

Biventricular repair of DORV-AVSD requires cardiopulmonary bypass, which is instituted via bicaval and ascending aortic cannulation with moderate hypothermia. Deep hypothermia with low-flow cardiopulmonary bypass or transient hypothermic circulatory arrest may be utilized during the repair of pulmonary venous connection anomalies to improve visualization. After cardioplegic arrest, a right-sided atriotomy is performed to provide access to the atria and common atrioventricular valve. In some anatomic varieties associated with heterotaxy, the approach to the internal cardiac structures may be more appropriate through a left-sided atriotomy.

Repair of the AVSD is then performed. The initial steps of the repair are identical to the ones used in the two-patch method for isolated complete AVSD [2]. The intracardiac anatomy is inspected, and special attention is first given to the atrioventricular valve coaptation points. The inlet component of the ventricular septal defect is then partially closed. A crescent shaped patch of polytetrafluoroethylene (PTFE) is fashioned and sewn to the crest of the defect. This is accomplished by first starting the suture line at the midpoint of the ventricular septum and corresponding posterior portion of the patch and continuing it inferiorly and posteriorly to the junction of the muscular ventricular septum and the annulus of the atrioventricular valve (Fig. 24.2). The entire anterior and superior half of the patch is left unsutured. Marking sutures are then placed in [1] the patch superiorly where it would join the atrioventricular valve annulus and [2] at the midpoint of the inlet component of the ventricular septal defect (Fig. 24.2).

At this point the repair proceeds in an identical manner to a complete AVSD repair. The corresponding portions of the superior and inferior bridging leaflets are secured to the crest of the patch. This is accomplished by placing a series of mattress sutures through the crest of the patch and then passing them through the hinge points of the atrioventricular valve. These sutures are left untied, as they will also be used to anchor the patch used to repair the atrial component of the defect. The zone of apposition between the left ventricular components of the superior and inferior bridging leaflets or "cleft" is then closed with fine interrupted sutures. Next the atrial septum is reconstructed using an autologous pericardial patch. In heterotaxy syndrome, associated bilateral SVC, separate hepatic vein and IVC connections, and anomalies of the pulmonary venous connection can make the reconstruction of the atrial septum challenging with a single patch. Thus, in these situations, separate pericardial patches may be required to fashion the complex baffle geometry without obstruction.

At this stage of the repair, the superior portion of the VSD remains unsutured and will be used to fashion the pathway between the left ventricle and the aortic valve. The next stage of the procedure is focused on the creation of an unobstructed left ventricular outflow tract (LVOT) and establishing RV to PA continuity, if needed. Accessing the subaortic region where the new LVOT will be constructed is best approached through a ventriculotomy (Fig. 24.3) made in the free wall of the right ventricle. The previously placed marking sutures are transposed from the atrium through the ventriculotomy.

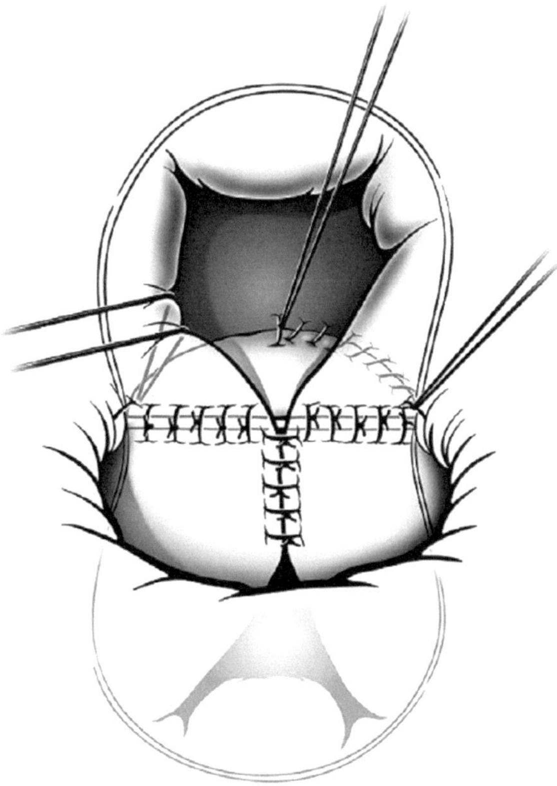

Fig. 24.2 Biventricular repair of DORV-AVSD starts with repair of complete AVSD component, leaving the superior portion of VSD patch unsutured (Used with permission from Devaney et al. [12], with permission of Elsevier)

Fig. 24.3 After the atrial septum is reconstructed, a right ventriculotomy is made to provide exposure to the muscular outlet septum and superior portion of VSD patch (Used with permission from Devaney et al. [12], with permission of Elsevier)

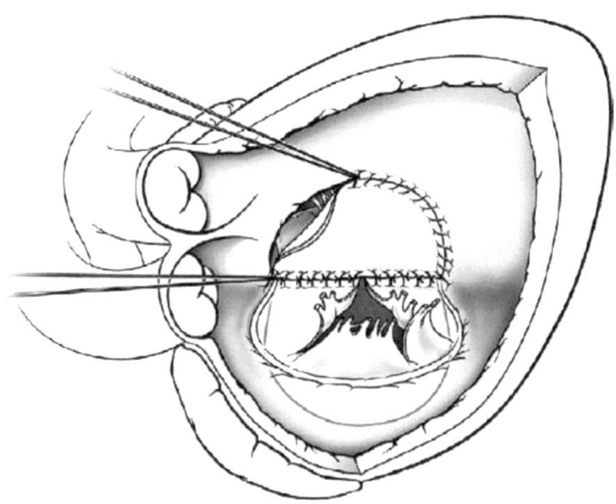

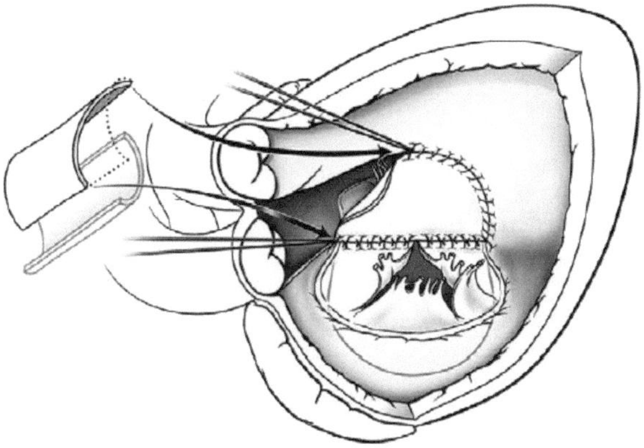

Fig. 24.4 The muscular outlet septum is resected from the superior portion of VSD patch to the aortic annulus and the left ventricular outflow tract is reconstructed with a PTFE patch (Used with permission from Devaney et al. [12], with permission of Elsevier)

The ventricular septal defect usually needs to be enlarged because it is generally confined primarily or entirely to the inlet septum, making it remote from the aortic valve. In our recent series, the VSD was enlarged in 11/16 patients [12]. Attempting to baffle such remote defects to the aortic valve without enlarging the ventricular septal defect is likely to result in obstruction of the left and right ventricular outflow tract as well as interference with the right atrioventricular valve apparatus. Enlarging the VSD in the direction of the subaortic region essentially shortens the LVOT, thus addressing the above pitfalls.

Enlarging the VSD is accomplished by resecting the muscular outlet or infundibular septum. This resection spans the region between the unsutured edge of the prosthetic patch/superior portion of the crest of the ventricular septum and the subvalvar area of the aortic valve (Fig. 24.4). Closure of the remaining portion of the ventricular septum to create an unobstructed LVOT is then undertaken. A second patch of PTFE is trimmed from a tube graft (Fig. 24.4), and then sutured to the free edge of the original patch. The suture lines are then carried superiorly along the edges of resected septum up to the aortic valve annulus (Fig. 24.5).

As a final step, the right ventricular outflow tract is reconstructed. In patients with pulmonary stenosis or atresia, division of septoparietal trabeculations in the right ventricular outflow tract is performed, or a conduit may be placed from the right ventricle to the pulmonary arteries. In our series of 16 patients, 13 received a conduit and one patient received a right ventricular outflow patch with a monocusp valve. Conduits used include bovine jugular venous xenografts, pulmonary allograft, aortic allograft and porcine heterograft.

After separation from cardiopulmonary bypass, the repair is assessed by direct pressure measurements to determine left and right ventricular outflow and, if necessary, atrial inflow gradients. Intraoperative transesophageal echocardiography is performed to assess the atrial and ventricular inflow and outflow pathways, atrioventricular valve stenosis and regurgitation and semilunar valve function.

Other reported series [6] of repair for DORV-AVSD have utilized an approach shared with the repair of TOF-AVSD. This method utilizes a single VSD patch that

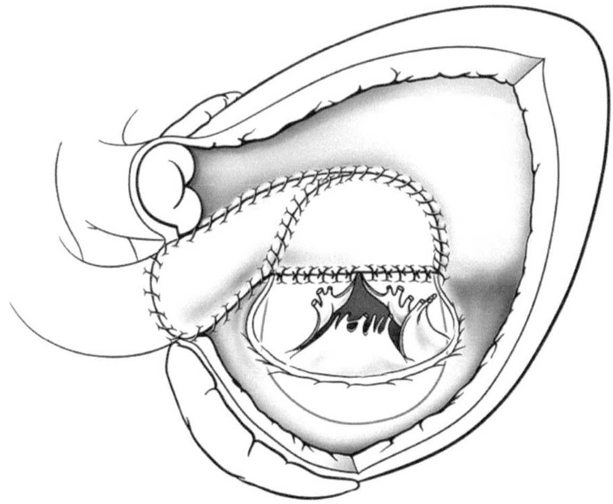

Fig. 24.5 Completed reconstruction of LVOT and complete AVSD with two separate PTFE patches. The right ventricular outflow tract is reconstructed with an outflow patch or valved conduit (Used with permission from Devaney et al. [12], with permission of Elsevier)

is comma-shaped with the wider end of the patch forming part of the LVOT [9, 21]. It has been recommended that the superior portion of the patch should be larger in cases where the aorta is located more rightward of the ventricular septum [21]. We view the repair of DORV-AVSD as being distinctly different from that for TOF-AVSD primarily because of the exclusive right ventricular origin of the aorta, with the aortic valve supported by a distinct muscular infundibulum. This anatomical arrangement makes redirecting the outflow from the left ventricle through the VSD to the aortic valve difficult and prone to obstruction. We and others feel that even when the communication opens toward the outlet region, it is frequently difficult to avoid obstruction of the newly created channel from the left ventricle without enlarging the VSD, also referred to as "VSD translocation" [22].

There have been a few early reports of a physiological repair of DORV-AVSD utilizing a double-switch procedure in which the morphologic right ventricle remains as the systemic ventricle and the morphological left ventricle remains connected to the pulmonary arteries via a conduit, although in the current era it is recognized that this arrangement is not preferable [9, 23]. Because of the risk LVOT obstruction and the complexity of biventricular repair, some groups have recommended a functional single ventricle palliation [24–27]. However, cautious enthusiasm for this strategy must be exercised because many patients may be poor candidates owing to pulmonary artery stenosis, pulmonary hypertension, pulmonary venous obstruction, atrioventricular valve insufficiency, as well as the well-recognized long-term complications of the Fontan procedure.

Results

We have recently summarized our contemporary experience at the University of Michigan C. S. Mott Children's Hospital Congenital Heart Center. In our series, 16 patients were described as having a biventricular repair of DORV-AVSD. The median age at the time of operation was 16 months. A complete repair was accomplished as the primary operation in only 6 patients. The remainder underwent at least one palliative procedure and/or repair of an associated lesion. Seven patients with inadequate pulmonary blood flow required a systemic-to pulmonary shunt. Three of these patients also underwent concomitant repair of total anomalous pulmonary venous connections. One patient underwent banding of the pulmonary trunk to restrict pulmonary blood flow. One patient who was previously shunted underwent a patch augmentation of the branch pulmonary arteries. Isolated repair of total anomalous pulmonary venous connection was performed in 2 patients. One patient who had undergone repair of infracardiac total anomalous pulmonary venous connection developed pulmonary venous stenosis which was addressed at the time of biventricular repair. In one patient, single ventricle palliation had been previously performed by means of a total cavopulmonary connection at another institution.

Biventricular repair was successfully accomplished in all 16 patients. The median cardiopulmonary bypass time was 242 min, with a median cross-clamp time of 158 min. Arrhythmias were common. Most of these were transient tachyarrhythmias with 8 patients having junctional ectopic tachycardia. Complete heart block requiring a permanent pacemaker developed postoperatively in 2 patients. One patient required ECMO postoperatively because of severe hypoxemia. Another patient had a prolonged recovery due to ventilator dependence and hydrocephalus. There were two deaths in our series. There was one early death that was secondary to pulmonary vascular obstructive disease and one late death secondary to complications related to renal failure.

Five patients had moderate atrioventricular valve insufficiency at discharge while no patient had stenosis. None had significant residual ventricular septal defects or left ventricular outflow tract obstruction. At a median follow-up of 66 months, all discharged patients were clinically well and in New York Heart Association class I or II heart failure.

Causes of reoperation in isolated DORV or CAVSD repair are shared in the biventricular repair DORV-CAVSD, and reoperation is not uncommon in these patients. In our series, six patients needed reoperation. A patient who initially received a pulmonary monocusp valve required a pulmonary valve replacement and atrioventricular valve repair 8 months after repair. Another patient required replacement of a left atrioventricular valve and pacemaker implantation 3 months after repair. Right ventricle to pulmonary artery conduit replacement was required in two patients. Another patient had a significant residual atrial septal defect from a patch dehiscence which required reoperation. The rate of reoperation in our series is not different from those that have been reported by other groups [11].

Three patients have at least moderate atrioventricular valve regurgitation. None have experienced obstruction of the left ventricular outflow tract. Total anomalous pulmonary venous connection was the only significant risk factor for mortality and significant morbidity in our series.

Because DORV-AVSD is such a rare lesion, the optimal surgical approach will be difficult to determine. Nevertheless, we feel that our results support biventricular repair, even in the presence of complex venous connections and a remote interventricular communication. Biventricular repair is associated with a significant rate of reoperation, particularly for replacement of the conduit, but this may ultimately provide long-term benefits when compared with single ventricle palliation. Formal clinical trials and collaborative investigative groups that provide a comprehensive comparison of these two approaches for DORV-AVSD are needed to evaluate long-term outcomes.

References

1. Zhao QM, Ma XJ, Jia B, Huang GY. Prevalence of congenital heart disease at live birth: an accurate assessment by echocardiographic screening. Acta Paediatr. 2013;102:397–402.
2. Suzuki T, Bove EL, Devaney EJ, et al. Results of definitive repair of complete atrioventricular septal defect in neonates and infants. Ann Thorac Surg. 2008;86:596–602.
3. Bradley TJ, Karamlou T, Kulik A, et al. Determinants of repair type, reintervention, and mortality in 393 children with double-outlet right ventricle. J Thorac Cardiovasc Surg. 2007;134: 967–73 e6.
4. Bakhtiary F, Takacs J, Cho MY, et al. Long-term results after repair of complete atrioventricular septal defect with two-patch technique. Ann Thorac Surg. 2010;89:1239–43.
5. Bogers AJ, Akkersdijk GP, de Jong PL, et al. Results of primary two-patch repair of complete atrioventricular septal defect. Eur J Cardiothorac Surg. 2000;18:473–9.
6. Artrip JH, Sauer H, Campbell DN, et al. Biventricular repair in double outlet right ventricle: surgical results based on the STS-EACTS International Nomenclature classification. Eur J Cardiothorac Surg. 2006;29:545–50.
7. Bharati S, Kirklin JW, McAllister Jr HA, Lev M. The surgical anatomy of common atrioventricular orifice associated with tetralogy of Fallot, double outlet right ventricle and complete regular transposition. Circulation. 1980;61:1142–9.
8. Sridaromont S, Feldt RH, Ritter DG, Davis GD, Mcgoon DC, Edwards JE. Double-outlet right ventricle associated with persistent common atrioventricular-canal. Circulation. 1975;52:933–42.
9. Pacifico AD, Kirklin JW, Bargeron Jr LM. Repair of complete atrioventricular canal associated with tetralogy of Fallot or double-outlet right ventricle: report of 10 patients. Ann Thorac Surg. 1980;29:351–6.
10. He GW, Mee RB. Complete atrioventricular canal associated with tetralogy of Fallot or double-outlet right ventricle and right ventricular outflow tract obstruction: a report of successful surgical treatment. Ann Thorac Surg. 1986;41:612–5.
11. Raju V, Burkhart HM, Rigelman Hedberg N, et al. Surgical strategy for atrioventricular septal defect and tetralogy of Fallot or double-outlet right ventricle. Ann Thorac Surg. 2013;95:2079–84; discussion 84–5.
12. Devaney EJ, Lee T, Gelehrter S, et al. Biventricular repair of atrioventricular septal defect with common atrioventricular valve and double-outlet right ventricle. Ann Thorac Surg. 2010;89: 537–42; discussion 42–3.
13. Anderson RH, Wessels A, Vettukattil JJ. Morphology and morphogenesis of atrioventricular septal defect with common atrioventricular junction. World J Pediatr Congenit Heart Surg. 2010;1:59–67.
14. Anderson RH, Ho SY, Falcao S, Daliento L, Rigby ML. The diagnostic features of atrioventricular septal defect with common atrioventricular junction. Cardiol Young. 1998;8:33–49.
15. Mahle WT, Martinez R, Silverman N, Cohen MS, Anderson RH. Anatomy, echocardiography, and surgical approach to double outlet right ventricle. Cardiol Young. 2008;18 Suppl 3: 39–51.
16. Anderson RH, Ho SY, Wilcox BR. The surgical anatomy of ventricular septal defect part IV: double outlet ventricle. J Card Surg. 1996;11:2–11.
17. Anderson RH, Becker AE, Wilcox BR, Macartney FJ, Wilkinson JL. Surgical anatomy of double-outlet right ventricle – a reappraisal. Am J Cardiol. 1983;52:555–9.

18. Ong J, Brizard CP, d'Udekem Y, et al. Repair of atrioventricular septal defect associated with tetralogy of Fallot or double-outlet right ventricle: 30 years of experience. Ann Thorac Surg. 2012;94:172–8.
19. Jacobs JP, Anderson RH, Weinberg PM, et al. The nomenclature, definition and classification of cardiac structures in the setting of heterotaxy. Cardiol Young. 2007;17 Suppl 2:1–28.
20. Anderson RH, Webb S, Brown NA. Defective lateralisation in children with congenitally malformed hearts. Cardiol Young. 1998;8:512–31.
21. Karl TR. Atrioventricular septal defect with tetralogy of Fallot or double-outlet right ventricle: surgical considerations. Semin Thorac Cardiovasc Surg. 1997;9:26–34.
22. Tchervenkov CI, Hill S, Del Duca D, Korkola S. Surgical repair of atrioventricular septal defect with common atrioventricular junction when associated with tetralogy of Fallot or double outlet right ventricle. Cardiol Young. 2006;16 Suppl 3:59–64.
23. Caffarena JM, Gomez-Ullate JM. Biventricular repair of complete atrioventricular canal, double-outlet right ventricle and common atrium using a modified double switch technique. A valid alternative to univentricular procedure. Interact Cardiovasc Thorac Surg. 2005;4:200–2.
24. Ruzmetov M, Rodefeld MD, Turrentine MW, Brown JW. Rational approach to surgical management of complex forms of double outlet right ventricle with modified Fontan operation. Congenit Heart Dis. 2008;3:397–403.
25. Russo P, Danielson GK, Puga FJ, McGoon DC, Humes R. Modified Fontan procedure for biventricular hearts with complex forms of double-outlet right ventricle. Circulation. 1988;78:III20–5.
26. Takeuchi K, McGowan Jr FX, Bacha EA, et al. Analysis of surgical outcome in complex double-outlet right ventricle with heterotaxy syndrome or complete atrioventricular canal defect. Ann Thorac Surg. 2006;82:146–52.
27. Aoki M, Forbess JM, Jonas RA, Mayer Jr JE, Castaneda AR. Result of biventricular repair for double-outlet right ventricle. J Thorac Cardiovasc Surg. 1994;107:338–49; discussion 49–50.

Chapter 25
Double Outlet Left Ventricle

Hiromi Kurosawa

Abstract Double outlet left ventricle (DOLV) is a rare congenital cardiac malformation in which both great arteries arise entirely or predominantly from the morphologic left ventricle.

Dextroposition of the posterior great artery causes double outlet right ventricle, while levoposition of the anterior great artery causes DOLV. Combination of dextroposition and levoposition results in conotruncal criss cross. There are two types of DOLV, normal great arteries (NGA) type and transposition of the great arteries (TGA) type. Most cases of DOLV require Rastelli operation.

Keywords Double outlet left ventricle • Double outlet right ventricle • Dextroposition • Levoposition • Conotruncal criss cross • Ventricular septal defect • Primary interventricular foramen • Secondary interventricular foramen

Double outlet left ventricle (DOLV) is a rare congenital cardiac malformation in which both great arteries arise entirely or predominantly from the morphologic left ventricle [1, 2].

Definition of DOLV

Definition of DOLV is "more than half of the great arteries originate from the left ventricle". This concept is similar to the definition of double outlet right ventricle (DORV) based on "50 % rule" [3, 4]. Degree of overriding of the great arteries to

H. Kurosawa, MD
Cardiovascular Surgery, Tokyo Women's Medical University,
1-7-12 Marunouchi Chiyodaku, Tokyo 100-0005, Japan

Sakakibara Sapia Tower Clinic, Tokyo, Japan

Jikei University, Tokyo, Japan
e-mail: hkurosawa@r6.dion.ne.jp

F. Lacour-Gayet et al. (eds.), *Surgery of Conotruncal Anomalies*,
DOI 10.1007/978-3-319-23057-3_25

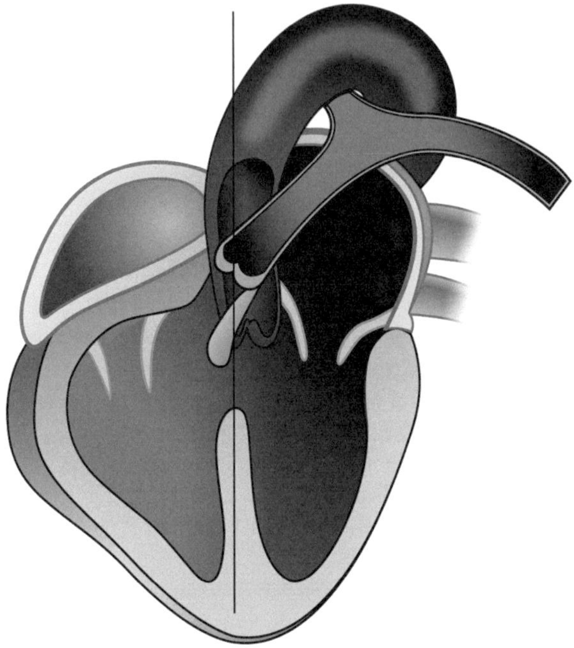

Fig. 25.1 Overriding Overriding on central line of ventricular septum. After contrast medium was applied on the surface of the ventricular septum and two wire rings were attached on the valves of the great arteries, X-ray photograph was taken with the ventricular septum in vertical position

the central line of the ventricular septum is a fundamental indicator of DORV and DOLV [5] (Fig. 25.1). Usual isolated VSD is the secondary interventricular foramen (S-IVF) and VSD of DORV is the primary interventricular foramen (P-IVF) [6–8], while VSD of "200 %" DOLV is the junction between the right ventricle and both great arteries (Fig. 25.2). Overriding can be measured by echocardiogram prior to the surgery, by surgeon's eye during the surgery and by morphologist's eye in the laboratory.

Morphology and Classification of DOLV

Morphogenesis of VA Connections

In early stage of the development of the normal heart, the common trunk of the great arteries originate from the primitive ventricle which will become the right ventricle. After the common trunk divides into two great arteries, the posterior aorta shifts to the left and eventually connects to the left ventricle which separates from the primitive ventricle. This is concordant ventriculo-arterial (VA) connection, i.e. normal great arteries (NGA). Lack of leftward shift of the posterior aorta results in dextroposition of the aorta which is NGA-DORV (Figs. 25.3 and 25.4). The leftward shift of the anterior great artery is levoposition. If usual leftward shift of the posterior aorta and levoposition of the anterior pulmonary artery concomitantly occurs, NGA-DOLV

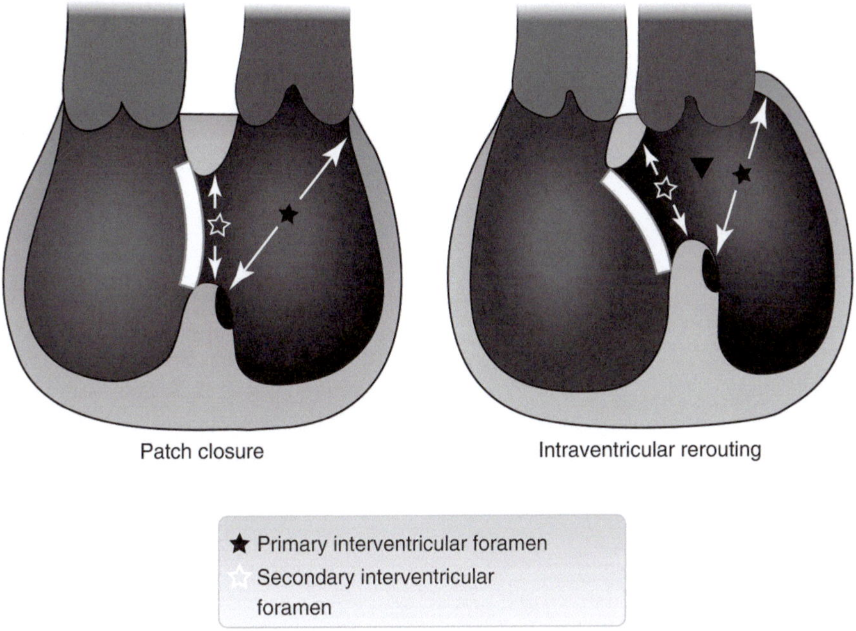

Fig. 25.2 VSD of DORV. Isolated usual VSD is secondary interventricular foramen (S-IVF=☆) and VSD of 200 % DORV is primary interventricular foramen (P-IVF=★). Patch closure of isolated VSD and intraventricular rerouting of DORV are same in terms of closure of S-IVF. Triangle space surrounded by P-IVF, S-IVF and overriding aorta/pulmonary trunk is cone of space beneath overriding aorta/pulmonary trunk (▼)

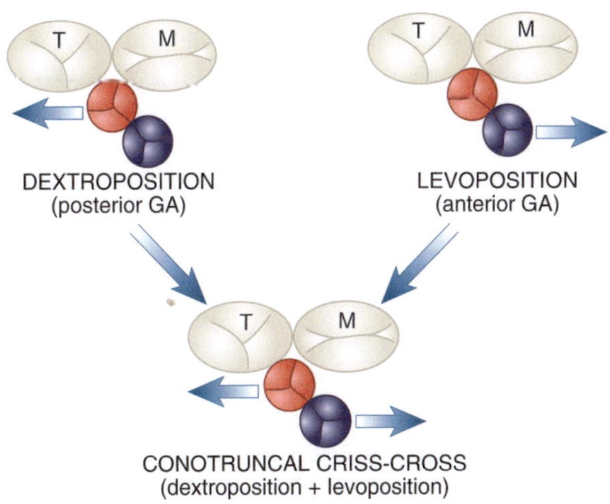

Fig. 25.3 Dextroposition, levoposition and conotruncal criss cross. Dextroposition occurs at the posterior great artery, i.e. lack of leftward shift, and levoposition occurs at the anterior great artery. Combination of dextroposition and levoposition is conotruncal criss cross

could appear (Figs. 25.3 and 25.5). Levoposition of the anterior great artery is rather more seldom than dextroposition of the posterior great artery. This is reason why DORV occasionally occurs, while DOLV is rare. If both dextroposition of the

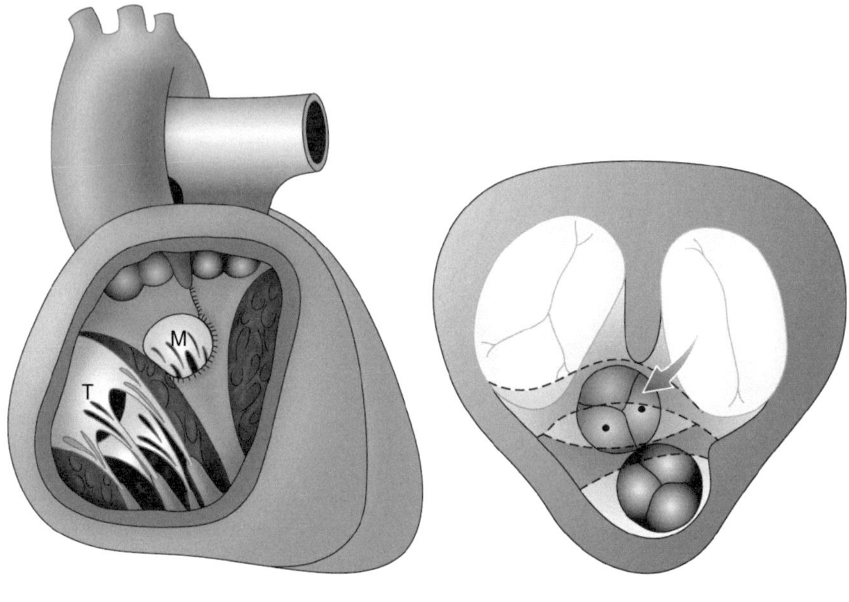

Fig. 25.4 NGA-DORV. Dextroposition of the posterior aorta causes NGA-DORV. *simple black arrow*: blood stream from left ventricle to aorta, *gray zone*: ventriculo-infundibular fold, *dark zone*: infundibular septum

posterior aorta and levoposition of the anterior pulmonary artery are moderate, NGA-DOBV (double outlet both ventricles) could appear (Figs. 25.3 and 25.6). If both dextroposition of the posterior aorta and levoposition of the anterior pulmonary artery completely occur at once, conotruncal criss cross (CCC) could appear. This combination is extremely rare, i.e. NGA-CCC. Incomplete form of NGA-CCC is thought as original Taussig-Bing [6–8] (Figs. 25.3 and 25.7) and complete form of NGA-CCC is thought as 'posterior' TGA [9, 10]. This classification is based on Van Mierop's concept [6–8, 11–13]. This concept is very useful from surgical viewpoint.

Characteristics of CCC are an infundibulum of the left ventricle which is a remnant of levoposed right ventricular infundibulum with anterior great artery, a dimple on the left ventricular septum which is a remnant of closed VSD, right posterior subarterial obstruction of the right ventricle and juxtaposition of atrial appendages [13].

If the posterior great artery is the pulmonary artery and the anterior great artery is the aorta, VA connection is discordant, i.e. transposition of the great arteries (TGA). Lack of leftward shift of the posterior pulmonary artery results in dextroposition of the pulmonary artery. This is TGA-DORV, i.e. false Taussig-Bing [7, 8, 11–13] (Figs. 25.3 and 25.8) Levoposition of the anterior aorta results in TGA-DOLV [14]. If both dextroposition of the posterior pulmonary artery and levoposition of the anterior aorta occur at once, conotruncal criss cross (CCC) may appear. This combination (TGA-CCC) is extremely rare [7, 8, 11–13], i.e. anatomically corrected

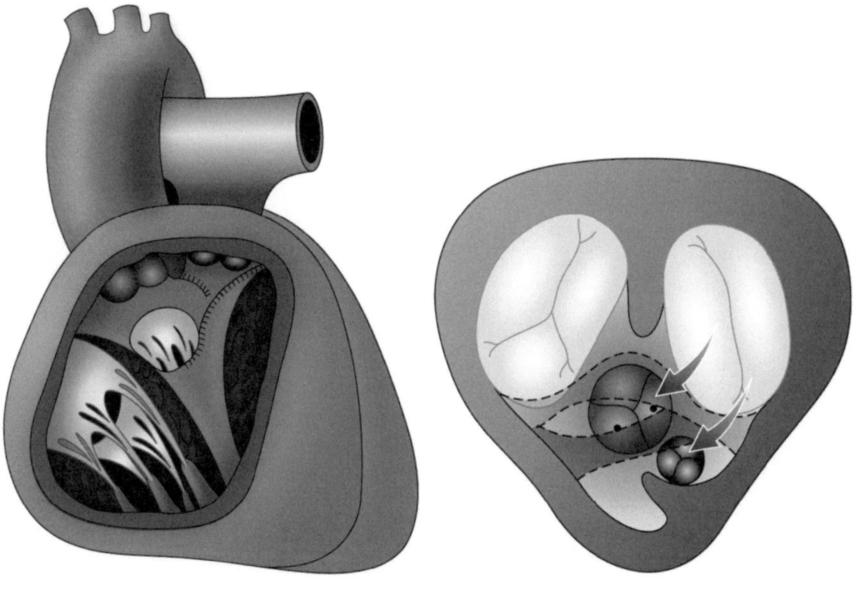

Fig. 25.5 NGA-DOLV. Levoposition of the anterior pulmonary artery causes NGA-DOLV. *simple black arrows*: blood stream from left ventricle to aorta and pulmonary artery, *gray zone*: ventriculo-infundibular fold, *dark zone*: infundibular septum

malposition of the great arteries (SDL: situs solitus, d-loop, l-transposition) [15–17] (Figs. 25.3 and 25.9) If levoposition of the anterior aorta is incomplete, the situation could be SDL-DORV [18].

Ventricular Septal Defect of DOLV

Ventricular septal defect (VSD) exists on the extension of the central line of the ventricular septum (Fig. 25.1). Usual VSD is the secondary interventricular foramen (S-IVF) and VSD of DORV is the primary interventricular foramen (P-IVF) [6–8, 12, 13] (Fig. 25.2). VSD of "200 %" DOLV is the junction between the right ventricle and both great arteries. VSD of "100 ~ 190 %"DOLV has overriding aorta/pulmonary trunk as superior rim of the defect (Fig. 25.5). This type of VSD divides the cone of space beneath overriding aorta/pulmonary trunk which consists of P-IVF, the junction between the right ventricle and both great arteries, and overriding aorta/pulmonary trunk. This situation occasionally causes double outlet both ventricles (DOBV) (Fig. 25.6).

Classic classification of DORV didn't distinguished P-IVF and S-IVF [19]. This is a reason that classic classification is rather obscurity.

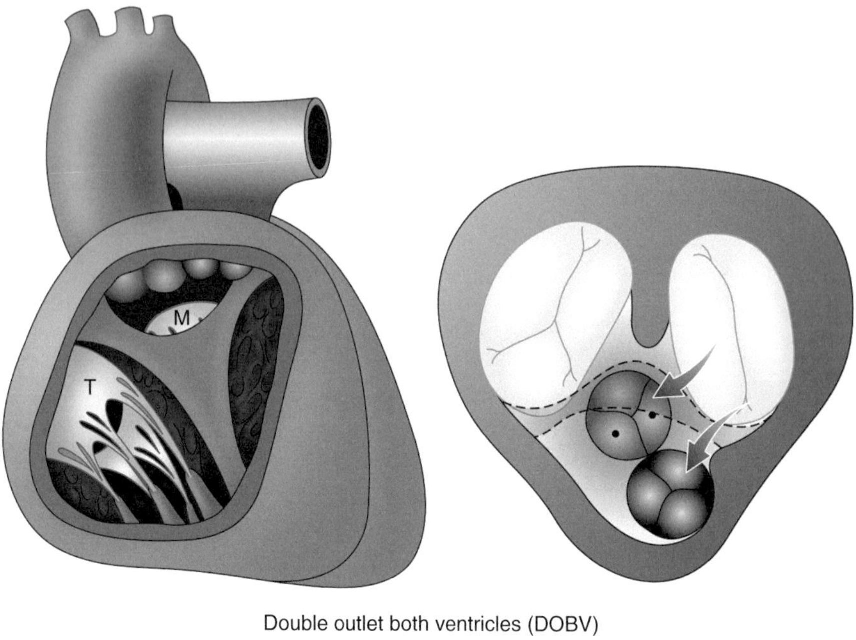

Fig. 25.6 NGA-DOBV. Partial dextroposition of the posterior aorta and partial levoposition of the anterior pulmonary artery cause NGA-DOBV. Infundibular septum is absent. *simple black arrows*: blood stream from left ventricle to aorta and pulmonary artery, *gray zone*: ventriculo-infundibular fold

VSD of DOLV is mostly outlet type, either perimembranous, muscular or subarterial.

Superior rim of VSD consists of variable structures such as hypoplastic/absent infundibular septum, the aorta, the pulmonary artery and ventriculo-infundibular fold. On the other hand, inferior rim of VSD is uniform in DORV, DOLV, DOBV and CCC. Inferior rim of VSD of DOLV usually have membranous flap with well developed trabecula septomarginalis or muscle bar separating VSD from the central fibrous body area. Therefore atrioventricular conduction bundle of DOLV is similar to that of tetralogy of Fallot, DORV and transposition of the great arteries [13, 20–22].

Closure of isolated VSD is simple patch closure of S-IVF, while intraventricular rerouting of DORV is an oblique patch closure of S-IVF [12, 13] (Fig. 25.3). VSD closure of DOLV is a closure of the junction of both great arteries and the right ventricle. DORV has either well developed or hypoplastic infundibular (outlet) septum, while DOLV and DOBV mostly have hypoplastic or absent infundibular septum (Figs. 25.5 and 25.6).

Classification of DOLV

DOLV is a sub-type of usual VA connections as DORV [23, 24].

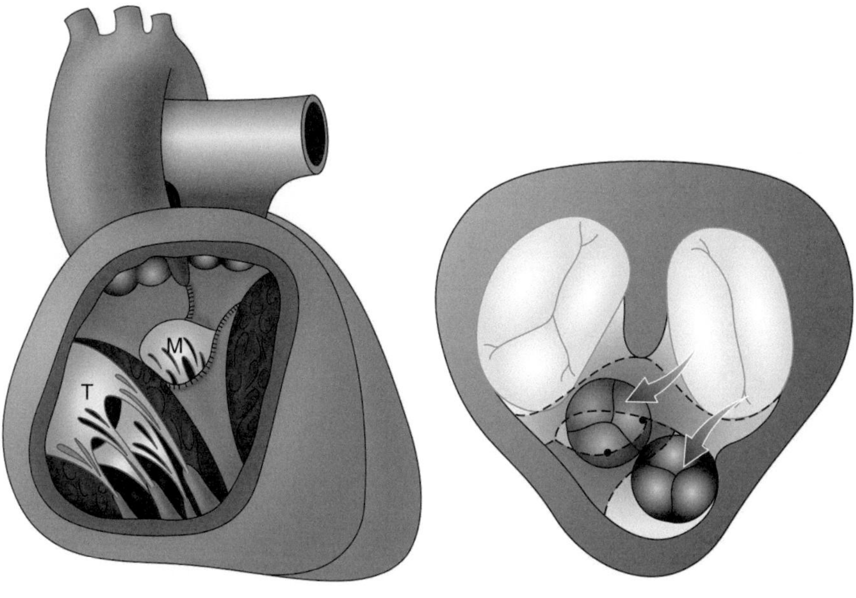

NGA-CCC (original Taussig-Bing)

Fig. 25.7 NGA-CCC. Combination of complete dextroposition of the posterior aorta and partial levoposition of the anterior pulmonary artery causes NGA-CCC-DORV, i.e. original Taussig-Bing. Combination of complete dextroposition of the posterior aorta and complete levoposition of the anterior pulmonary artery causes NGA-CCC, i.e. 'posterior' TGA. *simple black arrows*: blood stream from left ventricle to aorta and pulmonary artery, *gray zone*: ventriculo-infundibular fold, *dark zone*: infundibular septum

There are two VA connections, concordant (NGA) and discordant (TGA) in the setting of concordant atrioventricular (AV) connections.

In the setting of concordant AV and VA connection (NGA);

Dextroposition of the posterior aorta is NGA-DORV (Fig. 25.4).
Levoposition of the anterior pulmonary is NGA-DOLV [1] (Fig. 25.5).
Combination of partial dextroposition and levoposition is NGA-DOBV (Fig. 25.6).

Incomplete CCC is original Taussig-Bing [7, 8, 25] and complete CCC is posterior TGA [9, 10] (Fig. 25.7).

In the setting of concordant AV connection and discordant VA connection (TGA);

Dextroposition of the posterior pulmonary is TGA-DORV, i.e. false Taussig-Bing [6–8, 11–13] (Fig. 25.8).
Levoposition of the anterior aorta is TGA-DOLV [14].
Combination of partial dexroposition and levoposition is TGA-DOBV.
Incomplete CCC is SDL-DORV and complete CCC is anatomically corrected malposition of the great arteries [6–8, 11–13] (Fig. 25.9).

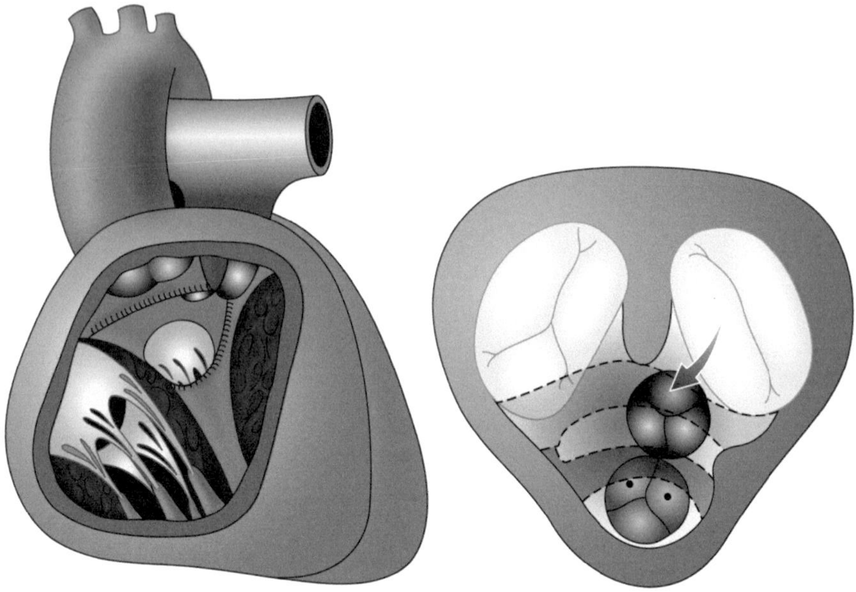

TGA-dextroposition(false Taussig-Bing)

Fig. 25.8 TGA-DORV. Dextroposition of the posterior pulmonary artery causes TGA-DORV, i.e. false Taussig-Bing. *simple black arrow*: blood stream from left ventricle to posterior pulmonary artery, *gray zone*: ventriculo-infundibular fold, *dark zone*: infundibular septum

Surgery of Abnormal VA Connections

Because of hypoplastic or absent infundibular septum, DOLV often has right or left ventricular outflow tract obstruction (RVOTO or LVOTO).

Biventricular repairs for the spectrum of DORV-DOLV are as following;

NGA-DORV with RVOTO: Right ventricular outflow tract reconstruction or Rastelli operation.
NGA-DORV with LVOTO: Yasui operation [26].
NGA-DOLV with/without RVOTO: Rastelli operation. (See case presentation)
NGA-DOLV with LVOTO: Yasui operation.
NGA-CCC: arterial switch operation (ASO) for 'posterior' TGA [9–11] and Kawashima operation [27] for original Taussig-Bing.
TGA-DORV with/without RVOTO: Rastelli operation/ASO.
TGA-DORV with LVOTO: Yasui operation.
TGA-DOLV with/without RVOTO: Rastelli operation.
TGA-DOLV with LVOTO: Yasui operation.
TGA-CCC with RVOTO: atrioventricular groove patch plasty [28].

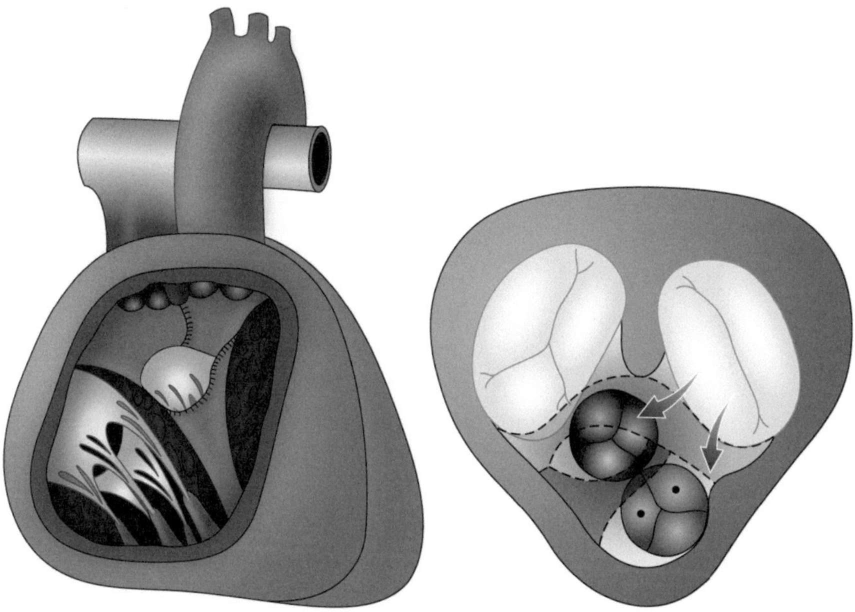

Fig. 25.9 TGA-CCC. Combination of dextroposition of the posterior pulmonary artery and levoposition of the anterior aorta causes TGA-CCC, i.e. anatomically corrected malposition of the great arteries. *simple black arrows*: blood stream from left ventricle to aorta and pulmonary artery, *gray zone*: ventriculo-infundibular fold, *dark zone*: infundibular septum

Either NGA-DOLV or TGA-DOLV could be repaired by pulmonary root translocation [1] or a modification of half turned truncal switch operation [29]. DOLV occasionally has right ventricular hypoplasia [2]. Patients with DOLV and functionally single-ventricle or AV valve atresia will require Fontan operation [1].

Case Presentation

One month-old girl. Preoperative diagnosis was complete TGA, subpulmonic infundibular muscular VSD, unusual coronary anatomy of Shaher type 9 of TGA which is same to normal coronary of NGA [30] and coarctation of the aorta. She underwent coarctectomy by subclavian flap and pulmonary artery banding in early infancy. Then, at the age of 1 month, she underwent intracardiac repair.

When the chest was opened, it was found that the aorta was right posterior and the pulmonary artery was left anterior which looked like normal relationship of the great arteries (Fig. 25.10). Coronary anatomy was seen basically normal pattern as in normal heart. However there was a groove between the right ventricle

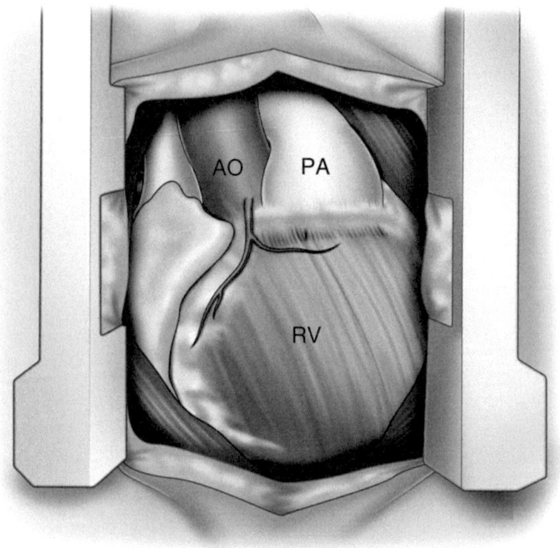

Fig. 25.10 NGA-DOLV before surgery. VA connection looks concordant, i.e. NGA. There is a groove between the right ventricle and the pulmonary artery. *Ao* aorta, *PA* pulmonary artery, *RV* right ventricle

and the pulmonary artery. Intraventricular anatomy was examined through a transverse ventriculotomy between a large conus branch and right ventricular branch of the right coronary artery. A shallow doubly committed subarterial VSD was found. The infundibular septum was absent. The right posterior aorta was overriding on the interventricular septum but mostly arising from the left ventricle. The left anterior pulmonary artery entirely arised from the left ventricle. The intracardiac anatomy was similar to Fig. 25.5 and VSD was similar to Fig. 25.6. The diagnosis was confirmed as NGA-DOLV. Intraventricular spiral rerouting from the left ventricle to the aorta behind the pulmonary artery was thought to cause subaortic narrowing. Intraventricular rerouting from the left ventricle to the pulmonary artery in front of the posterior aorta with arterial switch operation was also thought to cause neo-subpulmonic narrowing which required enlargement of neo-subpulmonic portion with interruption of a large coronary artery. Therefore Rastelli operation was eventually chosen. The junction between both great arteries and the right ventricle was closed using Gore-Tex patch. Inferior margin was a muscle bar separating doubly committed subarterial VSD from the central fibrous body area. Thus atrioventricular conduction bundle was anticipated beneath the muscle bar covered by posterior extension of the trabecula septomarginalis as in Tetralogy of Fallot [13, 20–22]. The pulmonary artery was transected. When the intraventricular anatomy was examined through the pulmonary valve, the pulmonary artery was found to arise entirely from the left ventricle. Proximal stump of the pulmonary artery was sutured. Autologous pericardial conduit with Gore-Tex monocusp was adopted for right ventricular outflow tract reconstruction to connect the right ventricle to the distal stump of the pulmonary artery (Fig. 25.11).

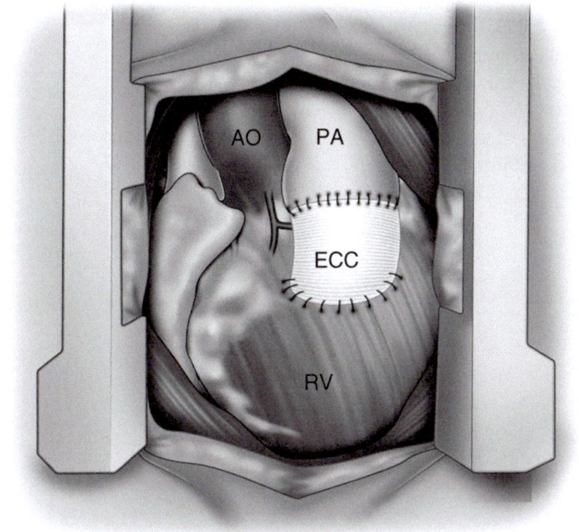

Fig. 25.11 Rastelli operation for NGA-DOLV. Rastelli operation was performed for NGA-DOLV. Autologous pericardial conduit with Gore-Tex monocusp was used. *Ao* aorta, *PA* pulmonary artery, *ECC* extracardiac conduit of autologous pericardium, *RV* right ventricle

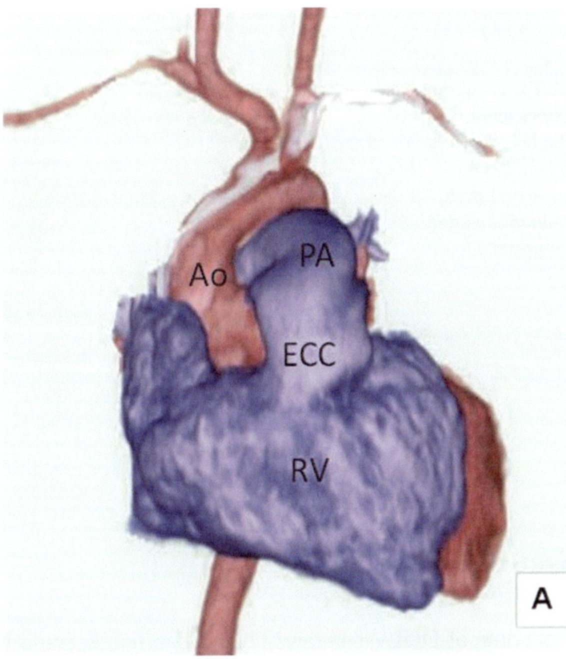

Fig. 25.12 Computer tomography 7 years after Rastelli operation. Autologous pericardial conduit is well adapted. *Ao* aorta, *PA* pulmonary artery, *ECC* extracardiac conduit of autologous pericardium, *RV* right ventricle

Six years after operation, right ventricular pressure was 31 mmHg and computer tomography revealed a good shape of concordant VA connection (Figs. 25.12 and 25.13). The proximal stump of the pulmonary artery entirely originated from the left ventricle (Figs. 25.13 and 25.14).

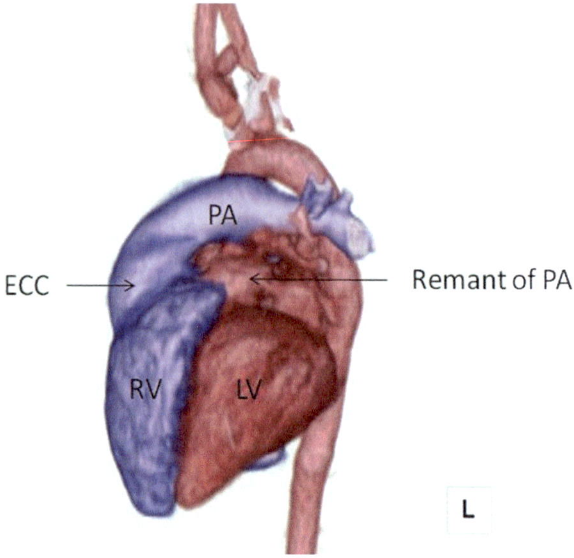

Fig. 25.13 Lateral view of Fig. 25.12. Concordant VA connection is well established. *PA* pulmonary artery, *ECC* extracardiac conduit of autologous pericardium, *RV* right ventricle, *LV* left ventricle

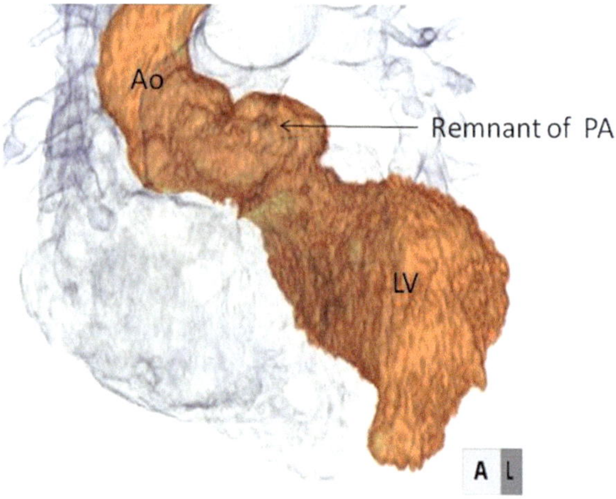

Fig. 25.14 Left ventricle-aorta of Figs. 25.12 and 25.13. The pulmonary artery entirely arises from the left ventricle. *Ao* aorta, Remnant of PA: closed proximal stump of the pulmonary artery, *LV* left ventricle

Outcomes

Outcome of DOLV has rarely been reported. It could be similar to that of Rastelli type operation for DORV and TGA. Obstruction of left ventricular outflow tract and/or right ventricular outflow tract may occur. Conduit replacement could be occasionally necessary.

References

1. Menon SC, Hagler DJ. Double-outlet left ventricle: diagnosis and management. Curr Treat Options Cardiovasc Med. 2008;10:448–52.
2. Imai-Compton C, Elmi M, Manlhiot C, Floh AA, Golding F, Williams WG, McCrindle BW. Characteristics and outcomes of double outlet left ventricle. Congenit Heart Dis. 2010; 5:532–6.
3. Wilcox BR, Ho SY, Macartney FJ, Becker AE, Gelis LM, Anderson RH. Surgical anatomy of double-outlet right ventricle with situs solitus and atrioventricular concordance. J Thorac Cardiovasc Surg. 1981;82:405–17.
4. Anderson RH, Becker AE, Wilcox BR, Macartney FJ, Wilkinson JL. Surgical anatomy of double-outlet right ventricle–a reappraisal. Am J Cardiol. 1983;52:555–9.
5. Hinkes P, Rosenquist GC, White Jr RI. Roentgenographic re-examination of the internal anatomy of the Taussig-Bing heart. Am Heart J. 1971;81:335–9.
6. Van Mierop LHS, Alley RD, Kausel HW, Stranahan A. Pathogenesis of transposition complexes. I. Embryology of the ventricles and great arteries. Am J Cardiol. 1963;12:216–25.
7. Van Mierop LHS, Wiglesworth FW. Pathogenesis of transposition complexes. II. Anomalies due to faulty transfer of the posterior great artery. Am J Cardiol. 1963;12:226–32.
8. Van Mierop LHS, Wiglesworth FW. Pathogenesis of transposition complexes. III. True transposition of the great vessels. Am J Cardiol. 1963;12:233–9.
9. Van Praagh R, Perez-Trevino C, Lopez-Cuellar M, Baker FW, Zuberbuhler JR, Quero M, Perez VM, Moreno F, Van Praagh S. Transposition of the great arteries with posterior aorta, anterior pulmonary artery, subpulmonary conus and fibrous continuity between aortic and atrioventricular valves. Am J Cardiol. 1971;28:621–31.
10. Wilkinson JL, Arnold R, Anderson RH, Acerete F. 'Posterior' transposition reconsidered. Br Heart J. 1975;37:757–66.
11. Kurosawa H, Van Mierop LH. Surgical anatomy of the infundibular septum in transposition of the great arteries with ventricular septal defect. J Thorac Cardiovasc Surg. 1986;91:123–32.
12. Kurosawa H. Double outlet right ventricle. J Jp Surgical Society. 2001;102:578–83.
13. Kurosawa H. Conduction system in cardiac surgery. Igakushoin (ISBN978-4-260-01504-2), Tokyo; 2013. p. 86–100, p. 101–120, p. 121–134, p. 135–141.
14. Vukomanovic V, Prijic S, Bjelakovic B. Double-outlet left ventricle with L-malposition of the great arteries and subpulmonary ventricular septal defect. Pediatr Cardiol. 2013;34:476–7.
15. Pernkopf E, Wirtinger W. Das Wesen der Transposition im Gebeiete des Herzens, ein Versuch der Erklarung auf ent wick lungsgeshichtlicher Grund large. Virchows Archiv Fur Pathologische Anatomie und Phisiologie. 1935;295:143.
16. Van Praagh R. Transposition of the great arteries. II. Transposition clarified. Am J Cardiol. 1971;28:739.
17. Kirklin JW, Pacifico AD, Bargeron Jr LM, Soto B. Cardiac repair in anatomically corrected malposition of the great arteries. Circulation. 1973;48:153–9.
18. Anderson RH. Anatomically corrected malposition and double outlet ventricle. World J Pediatr Congenit Heart Surg. 2013;4:457.
19. Neufeld HN, Dushane JW, Wood EH, Kirklin JW, Edwards JE. Origin of both great vessels from the right ventricle: I. Without pulmonary stenosis. Circulation. 1961;23:399–412.
20. Kurosawa H, Becker AE. Atrioventricular conduction in congenital heart disease. Surgical anatomy. Tokyo, Berlin, New York: Springer; 1987. p. 97–144, p. 145–173, p. 175–224.
21. Kurosawa H, Becker AE. Modification of the precise relationship of the atrioventricular conduction bundle to the margins of the ventricular septal defects by the trabecula septomarginalis. J Thorac Cardiovasc Surg. 1984;87:605–15.

22. Kurosawa H, Morita K, Yamagishi M, Shimizu S, Becker AE, Anderson RH. Conotruncal repair for tetralogy of Fallot: midterm results. J Thorac Cardiovasc Surg. 1998;115:351–60.
23. Kurosawa H, Gaynor JW, Jacobs JP, Jacobs ML, Elliot MJ, Lacour-Gayet F, Tchervenkov CI, Maruszewski B, Mavroudis C. Congenital heart surgery nomenclature and database project. Update and proposed data harvest. Jpn J Thorac Cardiovasc Surg. 2002;50:498–501.
24. Jacobs JP, Maruszewski B, Tchervenkov CI, Lacour-Gayet F, Jacobs ML, Clarke DR, Gaynor JW, Spray TL, Stellin G, Elliott MJ, Ebels T, Franklin RC, Beland MJ, Kurosawa H, Aiello VD, Colan SD, Krogmann ON, Weinberg P, Tobota Z, Dokholyan RS, Peterson ED, Mavroudis C. The current status and future directions of efforts to create a global database for the outcomes of therapy for congenital heart disease. Cardiol Young. 2005;15 Suppl 1:190–7.
25. Taussig H, Bing R. Complete transposition of the aorta and a levoposition of the pulmonary artery. clinical, physiological, and pathological findings. Am Heart J. 1949;37:551–9.
26. Yasui H, Kado H, Nakano E, Yonenaga K, Mitani A, Tomita Y, Iwao H, Yoshii K, Mizoguchi Y, Sunagawa H. Primary repair of interrupted aortic arch and severe aortic stenosis in neonates. J Thorac Cardiovasc Surg. 1987;93:539–45.
27. Kawashima Y, Fujita T, Miyamoto T, Manabe H. Intraventricular rerouting of blood for the correction of Taussig-Bing malformation. J Thorac Cardiovasc Surg. 1971;62:825–9.
28. Morita K, Kurosawa H, Koyanagi K, Nomura K, Uno Y, Naganuma H, Matsumura Y, Inoue T. Atrioventricular groove patch plasty for anatomically corrected malposition of the great arteries. J Thorac Cardiovasc Surg. 2001;122:872–8.
29. Yamagishi M, Shuntoh K, Matsushita T, Fujiwara K, Shinkawa T, Miyazaki T, Kitamura N. Half-turned truncal switch operation for complete transposition of the great arteries with ventricular septal defect and pulmonary stenosis. J Thorac Cardiovasc Surg. 2003;125:966–8.
30. Kurosawa H, Imai Y, Takanashi Y, Hoshino S, Sawatari K, Kawada M, Takao A. Infundibular septum and coronary anatomy in Jatene operation. J Thorac Cardiovac Surg. 1986;91: 572–83.

Chapter 26
Corrected TGA-VSD: The Double Switch Procedure

David J. Barron

Abstract Congenitally Corrected Transposition of the Great Arteries (ccTGA) is a rare, complex condition that is characterised by atrio-ventricular and ventriculo-arterial discordance. There are a great variety of associated defects, of which VSD is commonest. The VSD is usually perimembranous but is variable in size. Patients with large VSD may require early pulmonary artery (PA) banding to prevent congestive cardiac failure.

Management is not straightforward since the associated defects and morphological sub-types produce a variety of symptoms that present at varying ages. This is complicated by the unpredictable performance of the morphological right ventricle and tricuspid valve in the systemic circulation. If surgery is required; then the aim for most procedures is to repair any associated lesions and restore the morphological left ventricle to the systemic circulation. This is achieved with the so-called 'Double Switch' procedure that combines atrial inversion (the Senning or Mustard procedure) with an arterial switch. This is also referred to as 'anatomical repair' to differentiate it from procedures that only address the associated lesions and leave the morphologic right ventricle in the systemic circulation ('physiological repair').

Patients with restrictive VSDs may require preparatory PA banding to retrain the morphological LV to sustain the systemic circulation.

The double-switch procedures pose specific technical challenges which are discussed in detail, together with management strategies and related surgical options such as the 'one-and-a-half' type repair.

Keywords Congenitally corrected transposition • Double-switch • Pulmonary artery banding • Senning • Mustard • One-and-a-half repair

D.J. Barron, MD, FRCP, FRCS(CT)
Department of Paediatric Cardiac Surgery, Birmingham Children's Hospital,
Level 2 Ladywood House, Steelhouse Lane, Birmingham, West Midlands B4 6NH, UK
e-mail: david.barron@bch.nhs.uk

F. Lacour-Gayet et al. (eds.), *Surgery of Conotruncal Anomalies*,
DOI 10.1007/978-3-319-23057-3_26

Introduction

Congenitally corrected transposition of the great arteries (ccTGA) is part of the family of cono-truncal anomalies, characterised by atrio-ventricular (AV) and ventriculo-arterial (VA) discordance. Thus, physiologically the circulation is correct – with pulmonary venous blood being committed to the systemic circulation and systemic venous blood to the pulmonary circulation. However, the systemic ventricle is a morphological right ventricle (mRV), guarded by the tricuspid valve whereas the sub-pulmonary ventricle is a morphological left ventricle (mLV) guarded by the mitral valve.

It is a rare condition, accounting for 0.5 % of all congenital heart disease, but classification is complex due to the spectrum of morphological variants and associated cardiac anomalies that co-exist under the heading of ccTGA. This heterogeneity of anatomy and morphology is reflected in the variable and unpredictable way in which the condition can present clinically – from newborns with large VSD and arch obstruction requiring urgent surgical intervention, to adults with no associated lesions who can live a normal life without ever requiring treatment.

Between 80 and 85 % of cases will have some associated cardiac anomaly, the commonest being a VSD and these are summarised in Table 26.1. Although indications for surgery are usually related to these associated lesions, it must also be remembered that even 'isolated ccTGA' (i.e. ccTGA with no other associated cardiac anomalies) can also become symptomatic due to the unpredictable nature of the mRV in the systemic circulation. Progressive mRV failure and tricuspid regurgitation can lead to signs and symptoms of congestive cardiac failure at any age, and the inter-relationship of primary ventricular dysfunction leading to tricuspid regurgitation or of primary TV dysfunction leading to ventricular failure is a complex topic, each leading to a vicious circle of progressive circulatory failure [1, 2].

Table 26.1 Associated Lesions in ccTGA undergoing anatomical repair

Associated lesions/conditions	Frequency (%)
VSD	75–80
Dextrocardia	20–25
Mesocardia	10–15
Situs Inversus	5–7
DORV	5–7
Coarctation/arch hypoplasia	10–15
Ebsteinoid tricuspid valve	10–15
Bicuspid aortic valve	3
Abnormal mitral valve	3
Pre-operative heart block	15–20

There are considerable variations in the pattern of lesions seen based on geographical variation. The table reflects typical lesions seen in the Western hemisphere. In the Eastern hemisphere LVOTO with VSD is commoner with lower incidence of arch hypoplasia and Ebsteinoid tricuspid valve

Over 20 % of ccTGA are associated with abnormal position of the heart, most typically mesocardia with the ventricular mass sitting anteriorly and the atria more posteriorly; thus the AV-valves tend to sit more in the coronal plane (facing forward) than in the normal heart which carries important considerations in terms of surgical approach and access.

Surgical intervention in ccTGA was historically based on correcting the associated lesions, such as closing VSDs or repairing tricuspid regurgitation. Overall, results were disappointing as the fundamental issue of leaving the mRV as the systemic ventricle had not been addressed. The natural history of the condition remained unchanged with 50 % of patients in congestive heart failure by the age of 40 [3, 4]. This led to the concept of "anatomical repair" to restore the mLV to the systemic circulation, and the family of the "double switch" operations. In TGA-VSD without LVOTO, the operation combines switching the atrial pathways with the Mustard or Senning procedure associated with a VSD patch closure and an arterial switch. Any associated lesions must also be addressed as part of the repair. The concept of anatomical repair has transformed the outcome for symptomatic patients with ccTGA and has gained increasing popularity over the last 20 years. Selecting the appropriate timing for the procedure and a detailed understanding of the morphological variants is essential to achieving good outcomes. Many patients with ccTGA-VSD and no pulmonary stenosis require a pulmonary artery banding early in life to protect the lung vascular resistances allowing to delay the double switch operation.

Anatomy

The condition is defined by atrio-ventricular and ventriculo-arterial discordance. The aorta is usually anterior and to the left with the pulmonary trunk tucked in slightly posterior and to the right. The great vessels originate from a levo (leftward) looping of the primitive heart, hence the term l-TGA. Although the aorta is always anterior to the pulmonary root, the vessels tend to be more side-by-side when compared to their more antero-posterior arrangement typically found in d-TGA. Venous connections are usually normal. The landmarks of the right atrium are normal, but it leads into the mLV through a mitral valve. The left atrium leads through a tricuspid valve into the mRV.

The conduction system (Fig. 26.1) is very abnormal in ccTGA with anterior and superior displacement of the AV node in the atrial septum, adjacent to the mitral and pulmonary valves. This gives rise to a penetrating bundle that passes around the free wall of the left ventricle in a subendocardial position above the pulmonary valve orifice, just beneath the anterior part of the pulmonary valve annulus. The bundle then sweeps down onto the ventricular septum in the morphologic left ventricle, supplying a left bundle branch over the septal surface of the left ventricle and a penetrating right branch into the morphologic right ventricle [5]. The sinus node is in a normal position adjacent to the entrance of the superior vena cava into the right atrium (note reversion to normal conduction in the setting of situs inversus, see below).

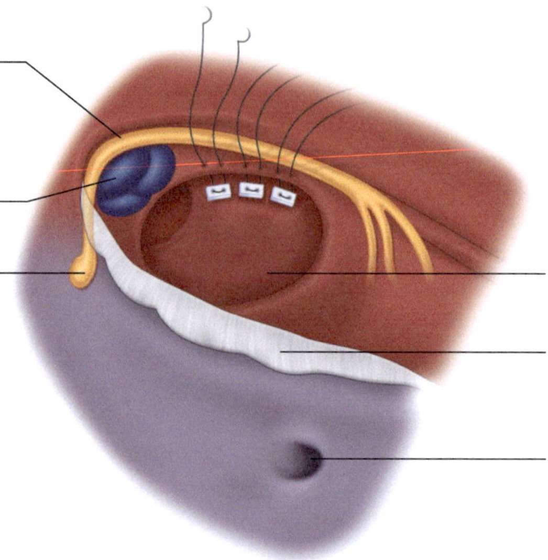

Fig. 26.1 Conduction tissue in ccTGA. Suture placement for VSD closure in ccTGA. The view is from the right atrium, looking through the mitral valve at a perimembranous VSD. The position of the conduction tissue is shown, passing along the supero-lateral aspect of the defect. Sutures in this area are placed from the morphological right ventricular side to avoid the bundle

The VSD is most commonly perimembranous outlet and variable in size. When there is associated LVOTO the VSD is large but occasionally can be committed more to the inlet, making it remote from the aorta. Coarctation, arch hypoplasia and, rarely, interruption can occur in the presence of a VSD and require neonatal intervention, typically with arch repair and PA band.

Unusual variants include AV discordance with DORV and left isomerism with l-TGA.

Imaging and Diagnosis

The majority of information can be obtained from transthoracic echocardiography and cardiac catheterisation. Most cases will need haemodynamic data from catheterisation, particularly if a pulmonary artery band has been placed. CT scan or cardiac MRI are not strictly necessary unless there is concern regarding the location of the VSD. Each component of the anatomy and physiology should be carefully assessed.

Abnormal cardiac position is common and can greatly influence access for components of the surgery. Normal situs with dextrocardia will make access to the atria difficult, impacting on the type of atrial switch technique. The angulation between the right atrium and ventricular mass tends to reduce the surface area of the free wall of the right atrium, which means less tissue available to create the baffles of the atrial switch. Left juxtaposition of the atrial appendages is a contra-indication to the Senning operation.

Situs inversus will occur in 5 % of cases and can be associated with dextrocardia or laevocardia. It must be remembered that situs inversus with ccTGA will restore normal 'right handed' topography to the conduction system of the heart so that the position of the AV node will be returned to the usual position in the triangle of Koch. Varying degrees of mesocardia are common – access to the atria is not impeded, but the position of the ventricular mass is such that AV valves tend to face forward, making it difficult to access them if they need to be repaired.

The *VSD* is usually a large sub-arterial perimembranous defect. The relationship of the VSD to the great vessels is assessed at echo or CT scan. It is variable in size and most commonly orientated towards the outlet. There may be accessory or reduplicated valvar tissue partially closing the defect which can lead to larger defects becoming restrictive or even closing over the first years of life. Multiple VSDs can occur and muscular VSDs can be easily missed if the focus is on a larger perimembranous defect.

The morphology of *the pulmonary valve* is usually normal. In situations where a PA band has been placed previously the valve must be carefully assessed on echo to look for any distortion or thickening of the leaflets in relation to the band. The sinuses can become quite dilated following a PA band and if the annulus is also dilated then the valve may be at risk of becoming regurgitant. The absence of LVOT obstruction is assessed by echocardiogram (including TOE). The reversal of pressures in the ventricles after the arterial switch will help to hold open out any aneurysmal septal tissue that is projecting into the LV outflow tract pre-operatively.

The coronary pattern is not usually an issue in ccTGA. The coronaries arise from the facing sinus of the aorta with the anterior coronary dividing to give an anterior descending and circumflex artery. The posterior coronary is the RCA which run directly backwards to reach the left atrio-ventricular grove. Pre-operative aortography should confirm the position of the coronaries, but they are usually managed in a standard fashion. Intramural coronary arteries do not appear to be common and have not been reported in surgical series.

Good function of the mLV is essential for the double-switch to be successful. Patients with ccTGA and large VSD have always had a mLV exposed to systemic pressures and its ability to support the systemic circulation is not usually in question. Patients who have required pulmonary artery banding prior to double switch most often have equal pressure between the two ventricles. The quality of the LV function is confirmed by echo. MRI can also be used to calculate LV mass index.

Abnormalities of the *tricuspid valve* are common, the most frequent being exaggerated offsetting of the AV valves with the apical displacement of the septal leaflet of the tricuspid valve. Extreme cases of this are referred to as 'Ebsteinoid' displacement of the valve – however, despite this displacement there is *not* usually any 'atrialisation' of the ventricular wall nor any failed delamination of the tricuspid valve leaflets, as seen in classical Ebstein's Most commonly the cause of the tricuspid valve regurgitation is the dilation of the systemic mRV with distortion of the annulus inherent to the septal origin of the anterior papillary muscle. Simple clefts in the anterior tricuspid leaflet have also been documented. Careful echo assessment is essential to establish whether any intervention on the valve should be considered at the time of surgery. Usually, excluding the valve from the systemic circulation is enough to restore competence in the majority of cases. In the rare cases, where an Ebsteinoid tricuspid valve is associated with some hypoplasia of the right ventricle a 1½ -type repair with hemi-Mustard and bidirectional Glenn could be considered.

The *mitral valve* is usually normal. Occasionally cleft in the anterior leaflet have been reported.

Systemic venous connections are usually normal. Bilateral SVC can occur, but with the usual drainage of the left SVC to the coronary sinus. Abnormal drainage of the hepatic veins can be present in atrial isomerism, indicating more a Mustard than a Senning operation.

The high incidence of *AV block* in ccTGA, that is around 30–40 %, is in relation with the abnormal pathway of the conduction tissue. The patients will either be born with complete heart block or develop block as part of the natural history. Any degree of pre-operative conduction delay pre-disposes to post-operative heart block and a 24 h ECG recording should be performed in all cases with evidence of any conduction anomaly.

DORV can be associated. *Coarctation and interrupted aortic arch* can be seen in neonates indicating two stage repair.

Pre-operative Check List

Situs and cardiac position
VSD location and size. Multiple VSDs
Coronary anomalies
Pulmonary valve morphology
Tricuspid valve morphology
Ventricular functions
Aortic arch obstruction
Association with DORV

Surgical Technique

PA Banding Palliation

Banding can be indicated for a variety of reasons. If the VSD is large then the band is necessary to balance the circulation and protect the lungs from over-circulation. In smaller VSDs (or intact septum) the band is necessary to train the mLV to become suitable for a subsequent double-switch. Banding also has a therapeutic role in splinting the ventricular septum and reducing the degree of tricuspid regurgitation.

We place the band via median sternotomy and float an mLV pressure line via a sheath in the right internal jugular vein. A limited opening is made in the pericardium and the main PA is carefully dissected so that the position of the branch PAs are clearly seen. The circumference of the main PA is measured and the band is initially fixed at half of the initial circumference. We use a 3 mm silastic impregnated nylon tape, but Goretex® can also be used. The band is placed immediately above the sinotubular junction. If there is a large VSD then we would alter the band to achieve a pressure of 1/3 systemic in the PAs distal to the band and confirm good position on epicardial echo to ensure there is no distortion of the pulmonary valve and ensure that the mLV function remains unchanged.

In smaller (restrictive) VSD or intact septum we alter the band to achieve 60–70 % systemic pressure in the mLV. Epicardial echo is helpful to assess mLV function and the septal positioning. The band should create some straightening of the ventricular septum and help reduce the degree of TR if it was ≥ moderate pre-operatively. If pressures do not reach this level then it can be incrementally tightened maintaining careful assessment of mLV function on echo. If function becomes impaired then the band must be loosened, accepting a lower pressure. The band should not be so tight that it causes R-L shunting at the VSD and desturation.

Once the band position is agreed it is secured with an additional stitch and then two 6/0 prolene sutures used o fix it to the adventia of the PA to aim to prevent it migrating distally over time.

Patients are monitored carefully on ICU for the next 24 h with the mLV line in situ to monitor for any subtle deterioration in mLV function. In cases of small VSD, particularly in older children, it may be necessary to loosen the band if the mLV will not tolerate it.

Double Switch Technique

The double switch, i.e., arterial and atrial switch, is indicated in ccTGA-VSD with normal LVOT dimensions and normal pulmonary valve. The atrial switch is either the Mustard or Senning techniques according to preference. The Senning is most commonly used option and is the technique described here; the Senning does not require any artificial material to create the intra-cardiac baffles and has generally had a better freedom from late arrhythmias and baffle obstructions in comparison to the Mustard.

It is difficult to define the optimal age for the double-switch because of the variability in associated lesions, age at presentation and associated symptoms. The majority of patients with ccTGA-VSD will have been initially palliated with PA band – the relative tightness of the band with somatic growth can become the indication for Double Switch. However, associated worsening of Tricuspid Regurgitation or the development of congenital heart block could equally be reasons to expedite the surgery. Typically, the surgery is carried at between 2 and 7 years of age.

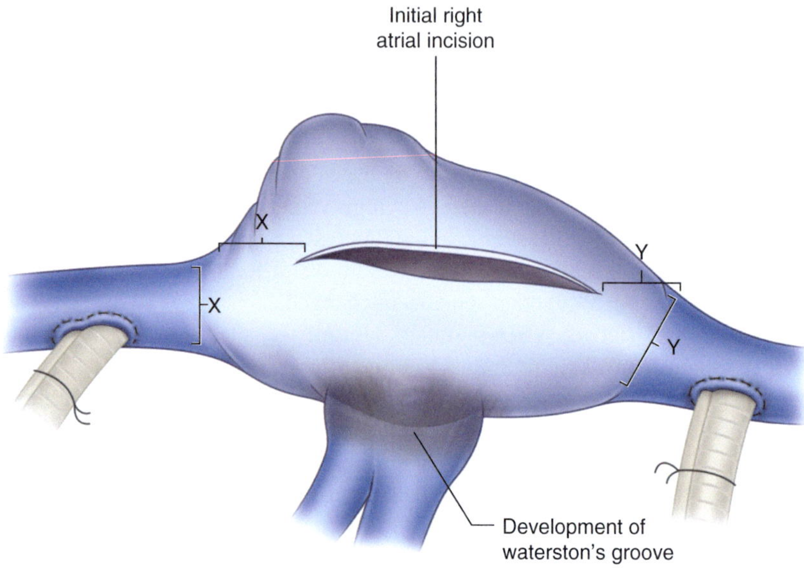

Fig. 26.2 Right Atrial landmarks for initial incisions. Note high SVC and low IVC cannulation. Waterston's groove has been developed as much as possible. The initial incision is made anterior and parallel to the crista terminalis. The incision stops short of the cavae by a distance roughly equal to the diameter of each vessel (X and Y)

Preparation The variability and complexity of anatomy in ccTGA requires extensive and careful pre-operative assessment, and each component of the repair needs to be carefully considered as outlined above. Many patients will have undergone previous PA banding and great attention must be placed on extensive and thorough dissection of all components of the heart free from any adhesions as complete mobility of the heart is essential to enable successful creation of both the venous and arterial pathways. The pulmonary artery and its branches must be fully mobilised and separated from the aorta, the cavae must be extensively mobilised, identifying the azygous vein superiorly and freeing up the IVC as inferiorly as possible onto the diaphragmatic surface.

Cardiopulmonary bypass is established with high aortic cannulation and bi-caval cannulation. Moderate hypothermia to 25 °C is used to ensure thorough cooling and allow for short periods of low flow or arrest in assessing the pathways. The SVC should be cannulated high (above the azygous vein if possible, snaring the azygous separately) and the IVC at the diaphragm as low as possible. It may be easier to cannulate the right atrial appendage initially (the pursestring can be used to site a left atrial pressure line at completion) to allow the heart to decompress and then cannulate the IVC with the heart collapsed. Waterston's groove should be developed as much as possible to facilitate the Senning (see Fig. 26.2). The aorta is cross-clamped and the heart arrested. We use cold crystalloid cardioplegia (St Thomas') given at 20–25 min intervals.

The initial incisions for the Senning are then made. The right atrial incision is as shown in Fig. 26.2, anterior and parallel to the crista terminalis. The incision stops short of the SVC and IVC junctions by a length approximately equal to the diameter

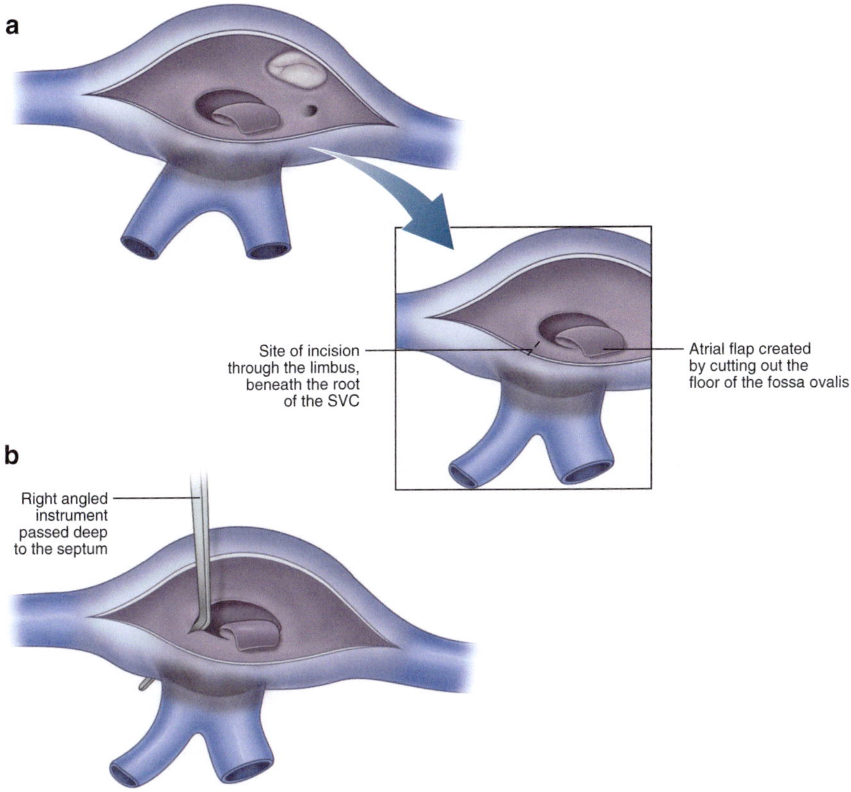

Fig. 26.3 View inside the Right Atrium. (**a**) The floor of the fossa ovalis is cut out to create a hinged flap based on the lateral wall. A further incision is then made across the limbus, beneath the root of the SVC as shown by the *dotted line*. (**b**) A right-angled instrument is then passed beneath this incision and will emerge through Waterston's groove. This opening is then extended inferiorly to create a wide opening into the left atrium

of the cavae. The atrial septal flap is then created, incising along the medial margin of the fossa ovalis and cutting back along the floor of the atrium inferiorly (Fig. 26.3a). Superiorly the incision aims back towards the lateral root of the SVC, crossing the limbus with a bold incision through full thickness of the muscular tissue below the SVC orifice. A right-angled instrument can then be passed under this incision which will emerge through the point where Waterston's groove was dissected out (Fig. 26.3b). Using this point as a guide, a long opening can be made into the left atrium through the thin tissue of Waterston's groove. This then frees up the atrial septal flap which is hinged against the lateral atrial wall. This flap does not need to be very large and we have not found it necessary to augment the flap with any additional material. The remainder of the Senning is completed at the end of the procedure and attention is now turned to the VSD closure.

VSD Closure In the double switch the VSD is usually perimembranous and closed with a patch using interrupted pledgetted sutures. We generally close the

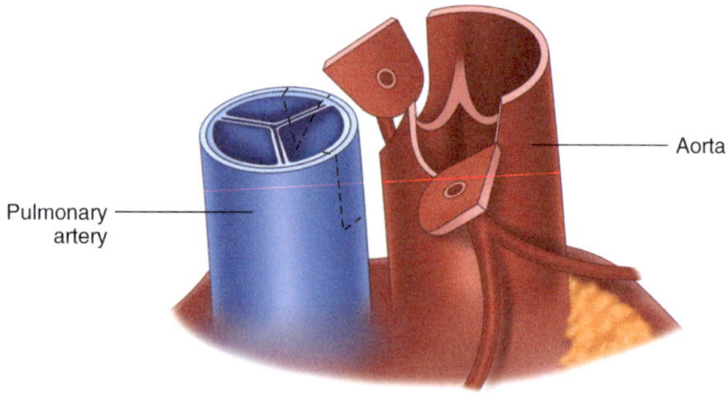

Fig. 26.4 The aorta is anterior and to the left of the pulmonary artery. Both vessels have been transected and the coronary buttons have been harvested from the facing sinuses of the aorta. The *dotted lines* show the typical incisions made into the pulmonary root to accommodate the coronary buttons

VSD transatrially, working through the mitral valve. The abnormal pathway of the conduction tissue dictates that the sutures should be placed from the right ventricular aspect superior-laterally to avoid the bundle, which passes down over this aspect of the VSD (see Fig. 26.1) [6]. An alternative is to close the VSD working through the aorta [21], after removing the coronary buttons – this allows for placement of all sutures on the right ventricular side but is only suitable if the VSD is relatively outlet perimambranous in orientation.

Arterial Switch The principles of coronary transfer are the similar as those in d-TGA but deal with a mirror image of the coronary arteries. However, the slightly more side-by-side nature of the great vessels requires attention. The leftward aorta is transected well above the sino-tubular junction. The coronaries arise from the facing sinuses and are taken out on generous buttons of aortic tissue and mobilised until they are free floating; this is particularly important with the anterior coronary which needs a little more distance to rotate than the posterior vessel. The defects in the aorta are repaired with a patch of autologous pericardium or pulmonary homograft leaving plenty of patch tissue sitting above the height of the transected root (see Fig. 26.4). The coronary buttons are then implanted into the neo-aorta facing sinuses. We tend to cut out a small V-incision for the posterior coronary and create a medially hinged trap-door for the anterior coronary (Fig. 26.5).

A decision then has to be made whether or not to perform a Lecompte manoeuvre. Generally, this is preferred but in older patients, when the pulmonary arteries are not so elastic and the great vessels are more side-by-side, then it may be better to leave the PAs behind the aorta. In either case, the generous patch used to repair the coronary defects aids reconstruction and allows for more flexibility, and it may be necessary to move the opening for the neo-PA leftwards to allow the vessels to sit comfortably (Fig. 26.6). If a Lecompte is not performed, an additional patch may have to be placed anteriorly to avoid distorting the circumflex coronary artery, immediately anterior to the neo-PA. Leaving a relatively long neo-PA (by transecting the aorta well above the sino-tubular junction) again allows for more flexibility in reconstruction.

Completion of the Senning The procedure is completed in three layers, creating a Y-shaped systemic venous channel, encircled by a C-shaped pulmonary venous channel. The first layer consists of the hinged septal flap created by the initial incisions. The flap is sewn into the left atrium, leaving only the left pulmonary veins

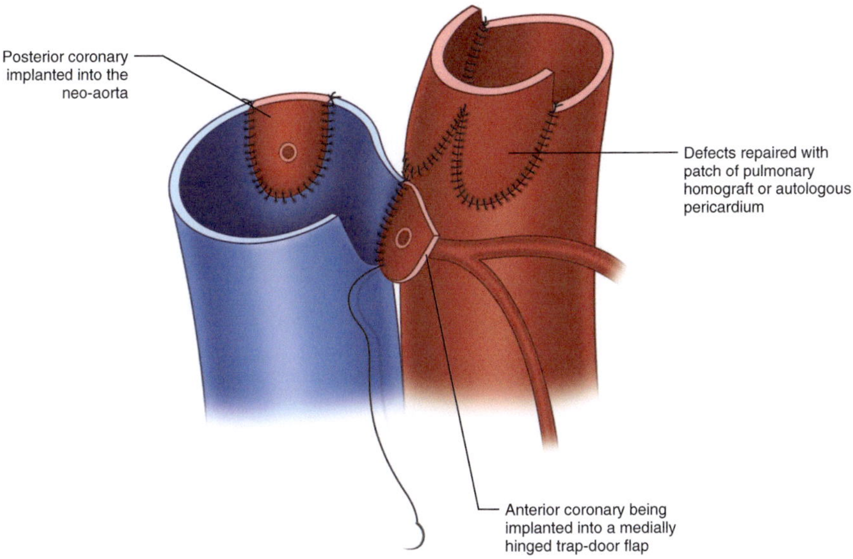

Fig. 26.5 Implantation of the coronary buttons. The posterior coronary has been completed and the anterior coronary is being implanted using a medially hinged trap-door technique

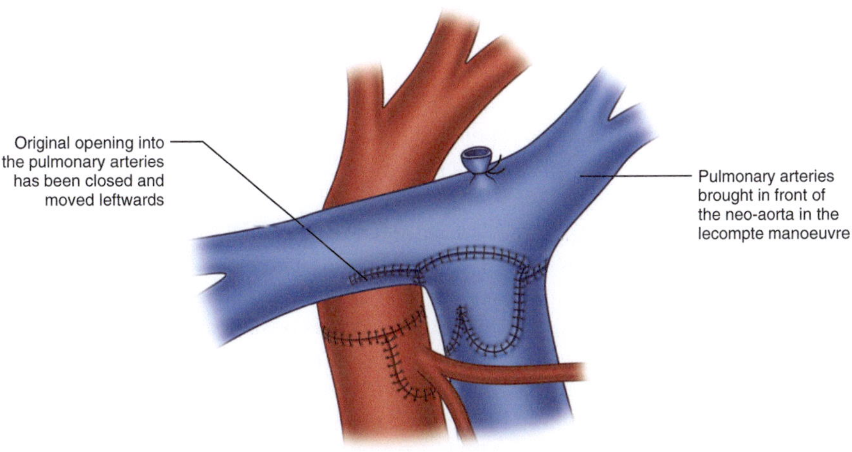

Fig. 26.6 The Lecompte manoeuvre has been performed. Due to the more side-by-side nature of the vessels it is sometimes better to close off the original opening into the pulmonary arteries and move this over to the left to allow the neo-PA to sit more comfortably

behind it. The base of the left atrial appendage is a useful landmark to start the suture line and the free edge of the flap is sutured here, then running superiorly across and up towards the root of the SVC (Fig. 26.7). It is important to keep this suture line posterior to allow volume above it for the SVC pathway to the tricuspid valve. In order to achieve this it is helpful to use 2/3 of the patch free edge for this superior half of the suture-line. The inferior half of the suture line gathers up the

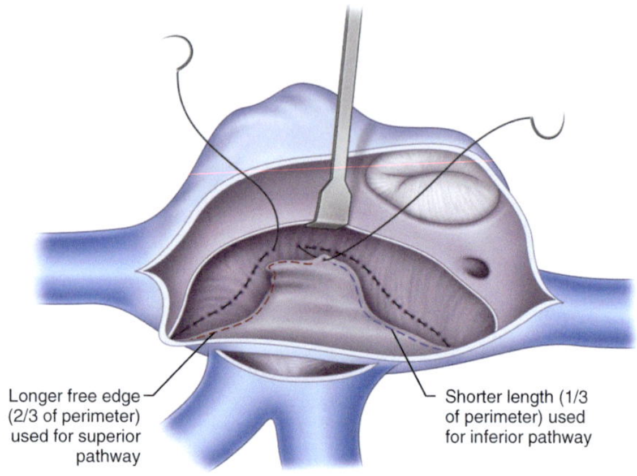

Fig. 26.7 Creation of the first layer of the Senning. The view is through the right atrium and the retractor is across the remnant of the inter-atrial septum. The suture-line starts at the root of the left atrial appendage. Approximately 2/3 of the flap free edge is used to create the superior half of the sutureline, this allows for a longer pathway creating more room above the flap for the SVC pathway. This leaves only 1/3 of the free edge for the inferior half, but the floor of the left atrium can be gathered up onto the patch as there is no risk of narrowing here

floor of the left atrium to the remaining free edge of the patch coming back towards the IVC (Fig. 26.7).

The second layer creates the systemic venous pathway. The lower free edge of the original right atrial incision is folded in to meet the remnant of the interatrial septum. Again it is easier to start at the midpoint and run the suture superiorly and inferiorly to create the SVC and IVC limbs. If there is good Eustachian valve then this can be used, sewing the atrial edge to the valve, leaving the IVC behind it and creating extra volume to the IVC pathway (hence the advantage of cannulating the IVC very low, below the level of the Eustachian valve (Fig. 26.8). Since the AV node is not in the triangle of Koch, the suture line can pass anterior to the coronary sinus (in contrast to the Senning in d-TGA where the suture line comes posteriorly, leaving the coronary sinus in the pulmonary venous atrium) and so incorporates the coronary sinus into the systemic venous channel. If necessary, the coronary sinus can be laid open into the floor of the left atrium to further enlarge the IVC pathway.

The third layer completes the pulmonary venous pathway by bringing the superior free wall of the original right atrial incision down onto the right pulmonary veins where the left atrium was opened through Waterston's groove. The flap needs a long free edge to ensure there is plenty of tissue draped across the outside of the SVC and IVC pathways – otherwise the suture line can cause external constriction (Fig. 26.9). If there is insufficient tissue for this to be achieved (as is commonly the case in mesocardia and dextrocardia since the surface area of the right atrium is reduced) then we frequently augment this layer with a patch of pulmonary homograft or autologous pericardium (Fig. 26.10) either for the complete layer or using the atrial flap to close off the inferior component around the IVC and then adding

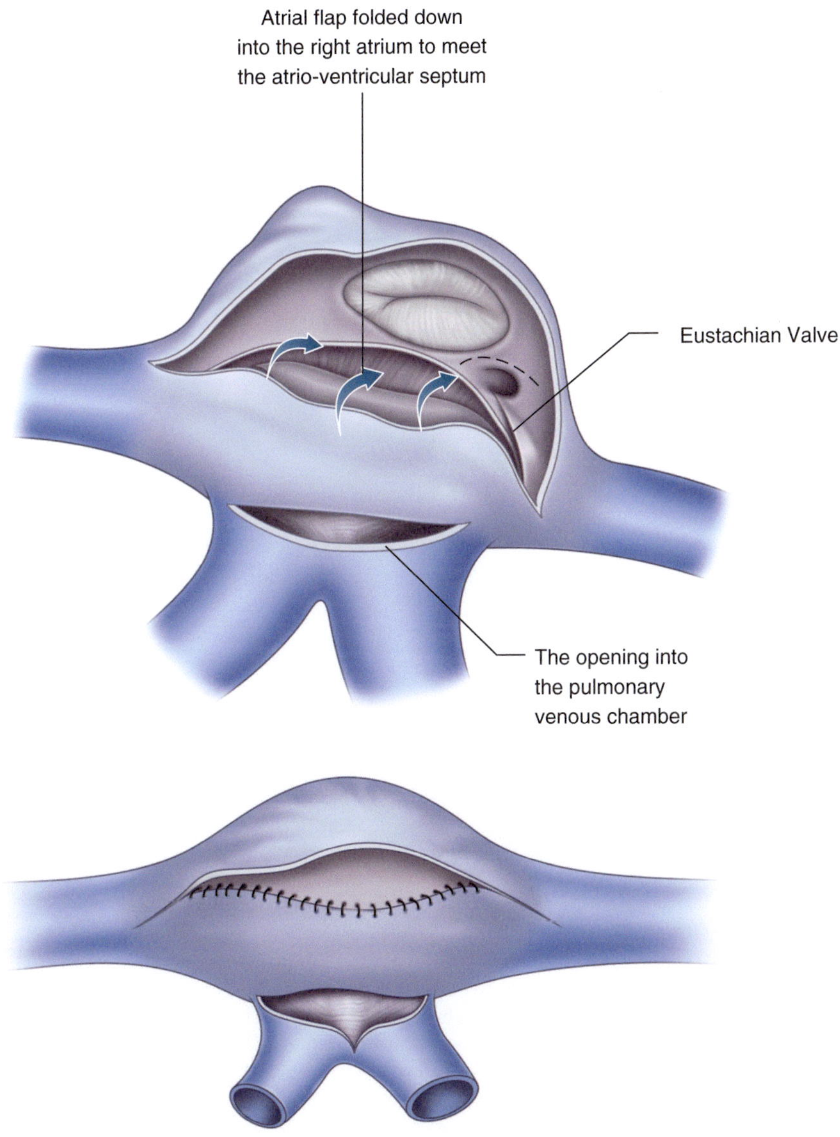

Fig. 26.8 Creation of the Systemic Venous Baffle. The right atrial free edge is rolled forward onto the remnant of the inter-atrial septum. The Eustachian valve can be used to attach the flap to inferiorly. The AV node is deviated antero-superiorly in ccTGA, away from the triangle of Koch. Thus, the coronary sinus can be incorporated into the systemic venous baffle without risking damage to the AV node (shown by the *dotted line*)

the patch to augment the superior part of the flap (Fig. 26.10). An alternative is to create a pericardial well, suturing the mobilised pericardium to follow the same suture-line (Shumacher technique) [7].

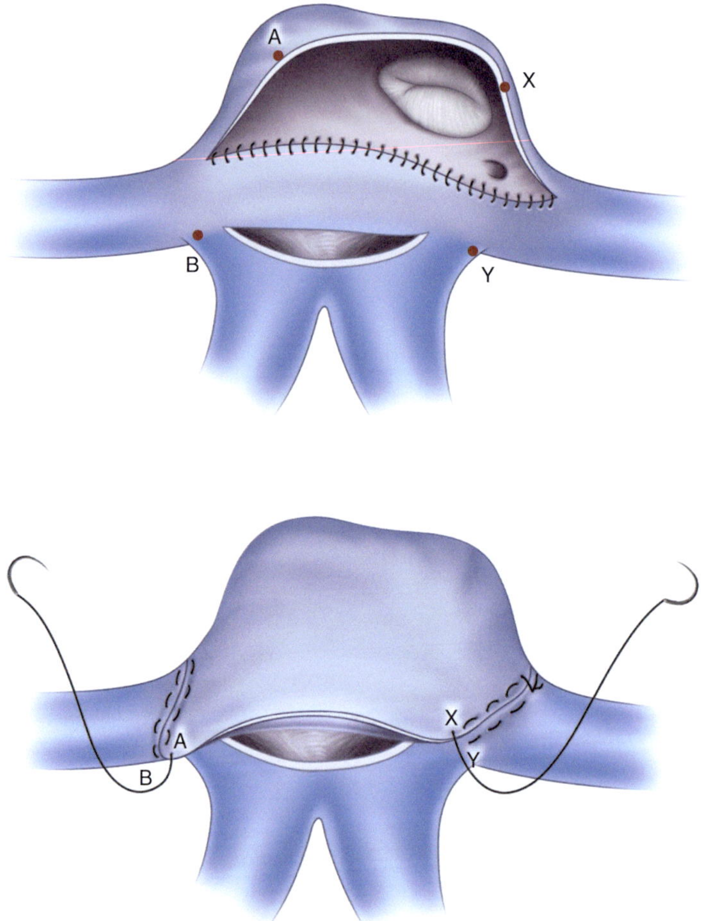

Fig. 26.9 Completion of the Senning, the outer layer that creates the pulmonary venous pathway. The superior free edge of the right atrium is brought down like the lid of a suitcase onto the opening into the pulmonary veins posteriorly. Point A must come to B and point X to Y in order to avoid externally compressing the systemic venous pathways

The atrial appendages have now 'swapped' and a left atrial pressure line is placed through the morphological right atrial appendage.

The One-and-a Half Repair An alternative technique to the complete atrial switch is to perform a bidirectional Glenn first, which simplifies the atrial switch. The atrial septum is excised and then a single patch is used to direct the IVC flow back to the tricuspid valve – sometimes referred to as a 'hemi-Mustard' procedure (Fig. 26.11).

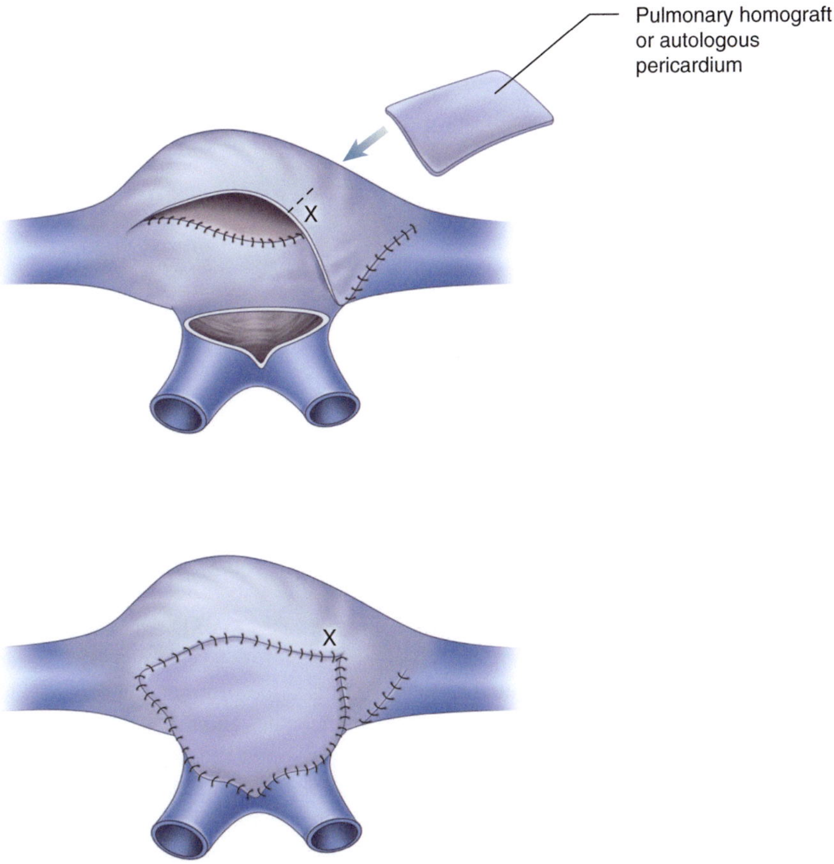

Fig. 26.10 Alternative method for the final layer of the Senning. Augmentation with a patch of pulmonary homograft or autologous pericardium. The inferior component of the layer has been completed using atrial tissue as in Fig. 26.9 but an augmentation patch has been used to give more volume to the pathway. A relieving incision can be made at point 'x' if the baffle is at risk of being narrowed here. A further alternative is to create a pericardial well with a Shumaker technique

A large, circular patch of Goretex® is used to baffle the IVC orifice across, over the ridge of the remnant of the inter-atrial septum and then around the margins of the tricuspid valve [8, 9]. It may be helpful to lay open the coronary sinus to provide additional volume to the pathway. This simplifies the atrial repair and can be particularly useful if there is concern over the size of the right ventricle. On the other hand, the PA pressures must be low to tolerate the Glenn and the anatomy will deny access to the atrium should subsequent pacing or ablation procedures be required in the future. There is also evidence that the functional capacity of the one-and-a-half circulation is not as good as that of true biventricular circulation.

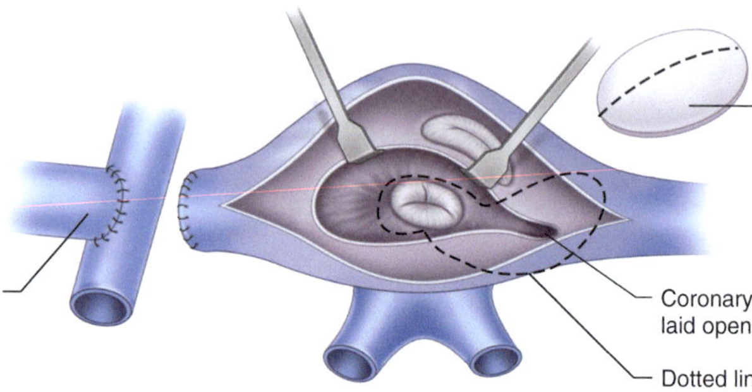

Fig. 26.11 The 'Hemi-Mustard' technique. A Bidirectional Glenn shunt has been performed and the atrial septum has been excised. A circular patch of Goretex® is used to baffle the IVC through to the tricuspid valve. The coronary sinus has been laid open to give extra volume to the pathway

Outcomes

Surgical outcomes for double-switch procedures in ccTGA-VSD are excellent with early mortality in the modern era of typically 1–5 % [10–21]. The wide range of clinical presentation and associated lesions requires some stratification according to complexity: highest risk procedures tend to be in neonates and infants who are clinically unstable and in heart failure pre-operatively, often requiring arch repair in addition to double switch. Mortality here is 8–15 % but in elective repairs in older children with well-preserved ventricular function the mortality approaches zero [15–21]. Most series report lower mortality amongst the Rastelli-Senning group compared to double switch as the former tend to be more elective procedures with no concerns over mLV function and no need for coronary transfer.

The commonest early complications are heart block (new pacemaker required in 5–10 %) and low cardiac output partly related to long bypass and cross-clamp times [10–15]. High SVC pressures with facial suffusion and pleural effusions can be seen, related to the dog-legged SVC Senning pathway, but tend to settle over 48–72 h, partly helped by natural decompression through the azygous vein. TOE is helpful is assessing the pathways post-operatively, but unless severe obstruction is seen these do not usually need surgical revision.

Longer term follow-up is now becoming available and survival is dramatically better than the natural history of symptomatic ccTGA managed conventionally (i.e. leaving the mRV as the systemic ventricle). In our series of 113 patients the survival was 94 % at 1 year, and 90 % at 4 and 9 years. Freedom from reoperation for all patients was 94 % at 1 year, 85 % at 5 years, and 76 % at 9 years [15]. There were no reoperations for tricuspid valve regurgitation and removing the tricuspid valve from the systemic circulation universally improved function. A recent study from Boston emphases the importance of assessing the tricuspid valve at time of surgery and even simple repairs of anatomically abnormal valves further improve the late tricuspid valve performance [16]. There is a spectrum of lesions that may require reintervention, including pulmonary artery augmentation in the Lecompte maneuver group, late aortic valve replacement and revision of baffle obstruction in the atrial pathway (the majority of which can be successfully treated with ballooning or stent placement). Baffle obstruction and late atrial tachycardias are commoner with the Mustard procedure which has contributed to the popularity of the Senning technique. Consequently, the freedom from re-intervention is strikingly similar in both the double-switch and Rastelli-Senning groups [15].

As longer follow-up results are reported there is a concern over the incidence of late mLV dysfunction, which occurs in 15–20 % of patients at 20 year post-op. This has been reported by several groups with similar findings [15, 17]. The aetiology appears to be multifactorial. Aortic regurgitation is specific to the double-switch group, in which the old pulmonary valve becomes the new aortic valve [12]. The use of a palliative PA banding is a risk factor for late aortic regurgitation as it is also in dTGA.

There is increasing interest in the fate of the mLV retrained by application of the pulmonary artery band, and the interaction with late LV dysfunction. The problem is that the relationship is by no means consistent [18, 19]. The Boston group have shown a greater risk of late mLV dysfunction in patients who were initially banded at >2 year of age whereas there was no incidence of late dysfunction in patients banded at <2 year [19]. This group of retrained morphologic left ventricles will certainly require careful follow-up. These findings have fuelled interest in the concept of early 'prophylactic' PA banding in symptomless infants [20], which might protect the mLV in these patients from late failure.

It has also been noted that LV dysfunction is also associated with a high incidence of patients requiring pacing and of patients who have a prolonged QRS interval [17]. There are several reported successes with resynchronization using biventricular LV and right ventricular pacing improving mLV function in these patients, with some individual cases of dramatic improvement [15, 17]. This may be of value in patients requiring pacemaker insertion after a double-switch procedure.

Despite these concerns, the outcomes of the double switch operation in ccTGA-VSD remain substantially better than both the natural history and for traditional physiological repair, with more than 75 % of patients sustaining good mLV function at 20 years. It is also important to note that the group of 'high risk' patients who present with severe cardiac failure have done particularly well with no incidence of late mLV failure [15].

References

1. Connelly M, Liu PP, Williams WG, et al. Congenitally corrected transposition of the great arteries in the adult: functional status and complications. J Am Coll Cardiol. 1996;27: 1238–43.
2. Graham Jr TP, Bernard YD, Mellen BG, et al. Long term outcome in congenitally corrected transposition of the great arteries. A multi-institutional study. J Am Coll Cardiol. 2000;36:255–61.
3. Sano T, Riesenfeld T, Karl TR, Wilkinson JL. Intermediate-term outcome after intracardiac repair of associated cardiac defects in patients with atrioventricular and ventriculoarterial discordance. Circulation. 1995;92:II272–8.
4. Yeh TJ, Connelly MS, Coles JG, et al. Atrioventricular discordance: results of repair in 127 patients. J Thorac Cardiovasc Surg. 1999;117:1190–203.

5. Anderson RH, Becker AE, Arnold R, Wilkinson JL. The conducting tissues in congenitally corrected transposition. Circulation. 1974;50:911–24.
6. De Leval MR, Basto P, Stark J, et al. Surgical technique to reduce the risks of heart block following closure of ventricular septal defect in atrioventricular discordance. J Thorac Cardiovasc Surg. 1979;78:515–26.
7. Shumacker Jr HB. A new operation for transposition of the great vessels. Surgery. 1961; 50:773–7.
8. Malhotra SP, Reddy VM, Qiu M, Pirolli TJ, Barboza L, Reinhartz O, Hanley FL. The hemi-Mustard/bidirectional Glenn atrial switch procedure in the double-switch operation for congenitally corrected transposition of the great arteries: rationale and midterm results. J Thorac Cardiovasc Surg. 2011;141(1):162–70.
9. Sojak V, Kuipers I, Koolbergen D, Rijlaarsdam M, Hruda J, Blom N, Hazekamp M. Mid-term results of bidirectional cavopulmonary anastomosis and hemi-Mustard procedure in anatomical correction of congenitally corrected transposition of the great arteries. Eur J Cardiothorac Surg. 2012;42(4):680–4.
10. Langley SM, Winlaw DS, Stumper O, et al. Midterm results after restoration of the morphologically left ventricle to the systemic circulation in patients with congenitally corrected transposition of the great arteries. J Thorac Cardiovasc Surg. 2003;125:1229–41.
11. Duncan BW, Mee RB, Mesia CI, Qureshi A, Rosenthal GL, Seshandi SG, Lane GK, Latson LA. Results of the Double Switch operation for congenitally corrected transposition of the great arteries. Eur J Cardiothorac Surg. 2003;24(1):11–9.
12. Karl TR, Weintraub RG, Brizard CP, et al. Senning plus arterial switch operation for discordant (congenitally corrected) transposition. Ann Thorac Surg. 1997;64:495–502.
13. Bove EL, Ohye RG, Devaney EJ, Kurosawa H, Shin'oka T, Ikeda A, Nakanishi T. Anatomic correction of congenitally corrected transposition and its close cousins. Cardiol Young. 2006;16:85–90.
14. Shin'oka T, Kurosawa H, Imai Y, Aoki M, Ishiyama M, Sakamoto T, et al. Outcomes of definitive surgical repair for congenitally corrected transposition of the great arteries or double outlet right ventricle with discordant atrioventricular connection: risk analyses in 189 patients. J Thorac Cardiovasc Surg. 2007;133:1318–28.
15. Murtuza B, Barron DJ, Stumper O, Stickley J, Eaton D, Jones TJ, Brawn WJ. Anatomic repair for congenitally corrected transposition of the great arteries: a single-institution 19-year experience. J Thorac Cardiovasc Surg. 2011;142(6):1348–57.
16. Myers PO, Bautista-Hernandez V, Baird CW, Emani SM, Marx GR, del Nido PJ. Tricuspid regurgitation or Ebsteinoid dysplasia of the tricuspid valve in congenitally corrected transposition: is valvuloplasty necessary at anatomic repair? J Thorac Cardiovasc Surg. 2014;147(2): 576–80.
17. Bautista-Hernandez V, Marx G, Gauvreau K, Mayer JE, Cecchin F, del Nido PJ. Determinants of left ventricular dysfunction after anatomic repair of congenitally corrected transposition of the great arteries. Ann Thorac Surg. 2006;82:2059–66.
18. Quinn DW, McGuirk SP, Metha C, Nightingale P, de Giovanni JV, Dhillon R, et al. The morphologic left ventricle that requires training by means of pulmonary artery banding before the double-switch procedure for congenitally corrected transposition of the great arteries is at risk of late dysfunction. J Thorac Cardiovasc Surg. 2008;135(5):1137–44:1144.e1–2.
19. Myers PO, del Nido PJ, Geva T, Bautista-Hernandez V, Chen P, Mayer Jr JE, Emani SM. Impact of age and duration of banding on left ventricular preparation before anatomic repair for congenitally corrected transposition of the great arteries. Ann Thorac Surg. 2013;96(2):603–10.
20. Metton O, Gaudin R, Ou P, Gerelli S, Mussa S, Sidi D, Vouhé P, Raisky O. Early prophylactic pulmonary artery banding in isolated congenitally corrected transposition of the great arteries. Eur J Cardiothorac Surg. 2010;38(6):728–34.
21. Ly M, Belli E, Leobon B, Kortas C, Grollmüss OE, Piot D, Planché C, Serraf A. Results of the double switch operation for congenitally corrected transposition of the great arteries. Eur J Cardiothorac Surg. 2009;35(5):879–83.

Chapter 27
Anatomic Correction of Corrected Transposition of the Great Arteries with Ventricular Septal Defect and Obstruction of the Left Ventricular Outflow Tract

Viktor Hraška and Peter Murín

Abstract The long-term outcome of patients with corrected transposition of the great arteries and associated lesions after physiologic repair is uncertain. Anatomic correction, utilizing the morphologic left ventricle as a systemic pumping chamber and the mitral valve as the systemic atrio-ventricular valve, is considered the preferred method, especially for patients with either tricuspid valve regurgitation, with Ebstein's malformation of the tricuspid valve, or with right ventricle dysfunction. Anatomic correction of corrected transposition of the great arteries with ventricular septal defect and left ventricular outflow tract obstruction represents a group of procedures in which the atrio-ventricular discordance is 'corrected' by an atrial switch, and ventriculo-arterial discordance is 'corrected' by the Rastelli procedure, by translocation of the aortic root, or by an arterial switch operation, depending on the underlying morphology and mechanism of the left ventricular outflow tract obstruction and/or morphology and position of the ventricular septal defect. These operations can be performed with minimal mortality and acceptable morbidity. In the mid-term, an excellent functional outcome can be achieved, which leads to normal ventricular function, with low incidence of complete heart block. However, the long-term functioning of the conduction system, the aortic valve, the intraventricular tunnel, the conduit, and the ventricles is variable and requires close surveillance. Prophylactic anatomic correction in patients without symptoms and a well-functioning tricuspid valve and right ventricle is not recommended.

Keywords Corrected transposition of the great arteries • Surgical repair • Anatomic correction • Senning operation • Rastelli operation • Aortic translocation procedure • Arterial switch procedure

---

V. Hraška, MD, PhD (✉) • P. Murín, MD
Department of Pediatric Cardiac Surgery, Asklepios Clinic Sankt Augustin, German Pediatric Heart Center, Arnold Jansen Str. 29, Sankt Augustin 53757, Germany
e-mail: v.hraska@asklepios.com; p.murin@asklepios.com

F. Lacour-Gayet et al. (eds.), *Surgery of Conotruncal Anomalies*,
DOI 10.1007/978-3-319-23057-3_27

Introduction

Congenitally corrected transposition of the great arteries (ccTGA) is a rare cardiac malformation, with double discordance, in which the two ventricles are connected inappropriately to the atria (atrioventricular (AV) discordance) and the great arteries are transposed (ventricular-arterial discordance). Thus, the systemic venous atrium (right atrium) is connected to the morphologically left ventricle (LV), and the pulmonary venous atrium (left atrium) is connected to the morphologically right ventricle (RV). The connection of the great arteries is also abnormal, with the aorta originating from the RV and the pulmonary artery (PA) from the LV [20]. Associated lesions such as left ventricular outflow tract obstruction (LVOTO), particularly in the presence of a ventricular septal defect (VSD), and tricuspid valve (TV) abnormalities are common findings occurring in about 40 % of patients [6]. Anatomic correction of ccTGA/VSD/LVOTO is designed to utilize the morphologically LV as the systemic pumping chamber and the mitral valve (MV) as the systemic AV valve. The operations fall into seven categories:

1. Temporary palliative procedures.
2. Anatomic correction utilizing a combination of the Senning and Rastelli operations.
3. Anatomic correction utilizing a combination of the Senning and ASO operations and resection of the LVOTO.
4. Anatomical correction utilizing a combination of the Senning and Rastelli operations and a Damus-Kay Stensel (DKS) anastomosis.
5. Anatomic correction utilizing a combination of the Senning operation and aortic translocation.
6. 1½ anatomic palliation utilizing a bidirectional cavo-pulmonary anastomosis (BDG) and a ½ Mustard with a Rastelli operation.
7. Implantation of a permanent pacemaker.

The long-term survival and functional benefits after anatomic correction have been demonstrated, particularly in patients with preoperative tricuspid valve regurgitation and right ventricle dysfunction [1, 12, 18, 19].

Anatomy

L-looping of the cardiac tube during embryonic development leads to an abnormal connection between the atrial, ventricular, and arterial segments of the developing heart. The malformation may occur in a situs solitus or in a situs inversus arrangement. In ccTGA situs solitus, the outflow tracts of the ventricles are most often in a parallel position, although other relationships do exist (criss-cross or inferosuperior position). The entire ventricular mass is frequently abnormally located within the thorax, the location ranging from levocardia (left-sided ventricular mass/apex), to mesocardia (central/midline ventricular mass/apex), or dextrocardia (right-sided ventricular mass/apex). The right-sided, morphologically LV gives rise to the pulmonary trunk, and there is almost always fibrous continuity between the leaflets of the pulmonary and mitral valves. The subpulmonary LVOT is wedged between the MV and the interventricular septum. A hemodynamically significant obstruction of the outflow tract of the morphologically LV is a common finding, occurring in about 40 % of patients, particularly in the presence of a VSD [5, 6]. Apart from pulmonary atresia, the mechanism of the obstruction is multifactorial, the factors including valvar stenosis, annular hypoplasia and a variety of subpulmonary obstructions (muscular tunnel-like obstruction, membranous stenosis, aneurysmal dilation of the fibrous tissue derived from the interventricular component of the membranous septum, or accessory tissue from atrioventricular valves etc.). The right-sided morphological MV is supported by posteromedial and anterolateral papillary muscles. Overriding and/or straddling of the MV are seen in combination with a double outlet from the RV.

The left-sided morphological RV empties into the aorta, which is supported by a complete infundibulum. The aorta is typically located anterior and to the left, relative to the pulmonary trunk. The left-sided morphological TV is frequently dysplastic. This abnormality is described as an Ebstein-like deformity with short, thick chordae tethering the valve, but unlike Ebstein's anomaly, apical displacement of the septal leaflet, with failure of delamination, is rare. Clinically, a significant insufficiency of the valve is seen in up to 40 % of adults with ccTGA. The TV may also override and straddle causing hypoplasia of the left-sided morphological RV [5, 13].

Ventricular Septal Defect

A VSD is detected in at least 50 % of the patients. Due to the wedged position of the subpulmonary outflow tract in the morphologically LV, there is gross malalignment between the atrial septum and the inlet part of the ventricular septum [10]. If this malalignment gap is not filled, a perimembranous ventricular septal defect develops. Such perimembranous defects occupy a subpulmonary position, extending posteriorly and inferiorly towards the crux of the heart. The defect opens primarily into the inlet of the morphologically LV; the posterior margin is therefore formed by an extensive area of fibrous continuity between the leaflets of the pulmonary, mitral, and tricuspid valves. In rare instances, the defect can be subpulmonary but with exclusively muscular rims. If there is pulmonary atresia or subpulmonary obstruction, the malalignment gap is not so prominent, and usually a large nonrestrictive conoventricular defect, naturally committed to the aorta, is found. Defects can also be found in a doubly-committed position, with absence of the septal component of the infundibulum [5].

Conduction System

In situs solitus, the wedging of the pulmonary valve between the septum and the MV diverts the atrial septum away from the ventricular septum, making penetration of the atrioventricular bundle, which originates from the regular atrioventricular node, impossible. Instead, the atrioventricular conduction axis originates from a second (anterior) anomalously located atrioventricular node lodged between the annulus of the MV and the superior and anterior aspect of the limbus of the fossa ovalis. After penetrating the fibrous trigone (pulmonary to mitral fibrous continuity), the conduction bundle runs superficially underneath the pulmonary valve, and then descends along the anterior septal surface of the subpulmonary outflow tract before diverging into the bundle branches. The cord-like right bundle branch extends towards the left to reach the morphologically RV, and a fan-like left bundle branch cascades down the smooth LV septal surface. When there is a perimembranous VSD (type II), the conduction system travels along the anterosuperior margin of the defect [2]. However, the variability of the conduction system is probably significant. If there is minimal or no wedging of the pulmonary artery (severe LVOTO, double outlet from the RV or pulmonary atresia), better septal alignment is achieved. Then both the regular and the anterior nodes (dual atrioventricular nodes) can give rise to penetrating bundles, producing a sling of conduction tissues [10]. From a surgical perspective, the close relationship between the non-branching bundle and the pulmonary valvar orifice complicates either closure, or enlargement of the VSD, and relief of the LVOTO.

In situs inversus, there is no septal malalignment and the atrioventricular conduction axis originates from a posterior atrioventricular node to follow a conventional path along the posteroinferior margin of the ventricular septal defect.

Coronaries

The Leiden convention is used to describe the origin of the coronary arteries. The ventricular topology determines the epicardial distribution of the arteries. In situs solitus, the right-sided coronary artery is therefore a morphologically left coronary artery, with a short main stem dividing into the anterior descending and circumflex coronary arteries. The circumflex artery encircles the mitral orifice, and anterior descending artery labels the position of the ventricular septum. The left-sided coronary artery is a morphologically right coronary artery. It has infundibular and marginal branches, while encircling the left-sided tricuspid orifice. In situs inversus, the epicardial arrangement of the coronary arteries is completely mirror-imaged [5]. The usual coronary artery pattern in situs solitus and situs inversus are labeled as: (1 R; 2 AD, Cx) and (1 AD, Cx; 2 R) respectively [13].

Diagnosis and Imaging

Clinical Signs and Symptoms

Clinical presentation reflects the degree of LVOTO, the function of the TV, and problems with the conduction system.

1. In the most extreme forms, neonates and infants present with severe cyanosis and with a ductus arteriosus-dependent (PDA) pulmonary circulation.
2. Patients with congestive heart failure are found at the other end of the spectrum.
3. The majority of patients with well-balanced circulation may be asymptomatic.
4. The possibility of complete heart block must be considered, even in infants.

Chest X-ray

Chest radiography may reveal typical features of ccTGA.

1. There may be dextrocardia, mesocardia or levocardia in situs solitus or inversus.
2. The great vessels tend to be parallel, with placement of the aorta on the left in situs solitus; thus there is a prominent left upper heart border, lacking a PA knob.
3. The pulmonary vascular signs reflect the degree of the LVOTO and the function of the TV and RV.

Echocardiography

Echocardiography is the mainstay of evaluation in ccTGA, providing comprehensive diagnostic and hemodynamic information.

1. The details of the VSD should be clarified. The size and relationship of the VSD towards the aorta should be determined, with regard to the construction of intraventricular tunnel (IVT). Multiple VSD's should be ruled out.
2. The morphology and mechanism of the LVOTO and the degree of obstruction should be determined. The subpulmonary area and position of the MV should be visible. The size of the pulmonary annulus and the morphology and function of the pulmonary valve should be shown.
3. The main and proximal branches of the PA's should be shown.
4. Additional sources of pulmonary blood flow (major aorto-pulmonary collaterals, PDA, modified Blalock-Taussig (MBT) shunt) should be determined.
5. The morphology and function of the TV should be determined. Straddling or overriding of the TV should be ruled out. The relationship between the TV and the VSD, as well as a possible high subaortic attachment of the TV, which makes construction of the IVT very difficult, should be clarified.
6. The morphology and function of the MV should be determined. Straddling or overriding of the MV should be ruled out.
7. The morphology of any accessory tissue from the MV, which can obstruct the LVOT, should be clarified.

8. The position and function of the aortic valve should be determined. The length of the subaortic infundibulum and the relationship of the aorta to the TV and VSD should be clarified.
9. The spatial relationship of the great arteries should be defined.
10. The origins of the right and left coronary arteries from the aorta and the point at which they branch should be determined.
11. The normal systemic and pulmonary venous connections should be defined. A left superior vena cava (LSVC) should be ruled out. The entrance of the inferior vena cava (IVC) or hepatic veins should be defined.
12. The morphology and function of the LV and RV should be determined.

Cardiac Catherization

Cardiac catheterization should be considered if additional anatomic or functional information are needed.

1. In patients with pulmonary atresia, the origin of the pulmonary blood flow should be determined. If there is a PDA, stenting should be considered. If there are major aorto-pulmonary collaterals, their origin and course should be clarified.
2. If an MBT shunt has already been placed, the architecture of the PA's should be shown. Eventually, if the shunt is stenotic, stenting may be considered.
3. If the coronary anatomy is uncertain, a coronary angiography might be helpful.
4. In late presenters with pulmonary overcirculation, evaluation of pulmonary resistance and its reactivity may be helpful.
5. The systemic and pulmonary venous anomalies should be evaluated.
6. Multiple VSD's may be seen better in an angiography.
7. Electrophysiological studies may be useful if there is suspicion of a conduction sling with a restrictive and/or remote VSD, which would require enlargement of the VSD.

Additional Diagnostic Studies

Computer tomography and magnetic resonance imaging (MRI) are valuable noninvasive tools for comprehensive preoperative and postoperative evaluation of the morphology and hemodynamics of patients with ccTGA/VSD/LVOTO.

A cardiac MRI provides precise information on the LVOTO, right ventricular outflow (RVOT), the morphology and function of both ventricles, the position and function of the AV valves, the relationship of the great arteries, the architecture of the PA's, and the systemic and pulmonary venous anatomy. As opposed to computer tomography, obtaining a cardiac MRI of newborns and infants may require intubation, which limits the applicability of this method.

Checklist Prior to Surgery

Situs and Cardiac Position
VSD (size, location, relationship to the aorta, multiple VSD's)
Pulmonary valve morphology and function (stenosis, regurgitation, atresia, annulus diameter, gradient)
PA architecture and position of BT shunt or stented PDA (branch stenosis, distortions…)
LVOTO morphology
Tricuspid valve morphology (Ebstein like, straddling, accessory tissue)
Mitral valve morphology (cleft, straddling, accessory tissue)
Aortic valve morphology and function
Coronary artery anatomy
Ventricular function and volume
Systemic and pulmonary venous anatomy
MAPCAs
AV block, arrhythmias

Decision-Making and Management Strategy

Decision-Making

The indications for, and the timing of the operation depend on the clinical state and age of the patients. In ccTGA/VSD/LVOTO the LV is trained for systemic function. Provided both ventricles are balanced and properly developed, the type of operation is determined by the underlying anatomy of the LVOT and/or the morphology of the VSD, as well as the function of the AV valves.

1. Development of cyanosis requires either placement of an MBT shunt or stenting of the PDA. One may also consider a BDG.
2. The definitive operation is usually performed between the 1st and 2nd year of life.
3. A Senning/Rastelli procedure is indicated if there is no resectable LVOTO, and there is a committed and nonrestrictive VSD. Resectable LVOTO includes membranous stenosis, aneurysmal dilation of the fibrous tissue derived from the interventricular component of the membranous septum, or accessory tissue from atrioventricular valves, or stenotic.
4. If there is any concern with regard to the size of the RV, a one and a half ventricle repair may be considered. Usually, the first step is a BDG anastomosis and final repair, which includes a ½ Mustard operation and the Rastelli procedure, is performed at the age of about 1–2 years.
5. If there is a smaller VSD, which would require enlargement, and the LVOT is only stenotic but not atretic, apart from the Senning/Rastelli procedure, one could consider creation of a DKS anastomosis (Chap. 30). Under these

circumstances, there is no need to enlarge the VSD; therefore, the risk of acquired heart block is minimal.

6. A Senning procedure with aortic translocation is indicated if there is no resectable severe LVOTO and the creation of a straight IVT baffling the LV to the aorta is impossible due to an inlet and/or restrictive VSD.
7. The double switch procedure is indicated if there is a surgically resectable LVOTO and the LV is properly trained for systemic function. A primary double switch with unrestrictive VSD is usually performed between 3 and 6 months of age.
8. If there is no TV regurgitation or RV dysfunction, and the pulmonary circulation is "protected" by pulmonary stenosis, while circulation is appropriately balanced one should wait for clear clinical deterioration before surgery is indicated surgery.

Medical Management

The medical management of a symptomatic child is devoted principally to preparation for surgery. Congestive heart failure is treated by decongestive therapy (diuretics, inotropics, lusitropics, afterload reduction drugs); progressive cyanosis requires prostaglandin infusions and subsequently, either stenting of the PDA or a shunt procedure. Abrupt complete heart block requires pacemaker implantation. In general, prophylaxis for bacterial endocarditis should be provided.

Surgical Management

The operation takes time, therefore proper planning is crucial. A standard cardiopulmonary bypass is instituted with direct venous cannulation. Cannulation of the inominate vein is preferable. In order to facilitate completion of the Senning operation, the superior vena cava right atrial pericardial reflection is preserved, and the superior aspect of the right pulmonary artery and vein is left intact [13]. The azygos vein is preserved as it can provide an important runoff for the SVC. The aorta is cannulated as high as possible. Myocardial protection is provided by crystalloid antegrade cardioplegia. At first, the Senning part of the operation is completed, followed by the Rastelli component or aortic translocation. If there is doubt with regard to the feasibility of constructing an IVT, one should check the position of the VSD, the AV valves and the aorta through the MV, and open the aorta first, before proceeding with the Senning procedure.

Modified Senning Operation

The technique in a modified Senning procedure differs from the original concept [7] as it is adapted to the specific atrial morphology of the ccTGA with underdevelopment of the free right atrial wall, especially in situs solitus with mesocardia or dextrocardia, or in situs inversus with levocardia. There are no technical differences between the operation for situs solitus and situs inversus [13].

Specific steps of the operation in situs solitus:

1. The right atrium is opened and the interatrial septum is completely excised (Fig. 27.1).
2. An ablation of the cavo-mitral isthmus may be considered (Fig. 27.2).
3. The posterior wall of the systemic baffle is developed with a patch (Fig. 27.3).
4. A large incision is made at the entrance point of the right pulmonary veins.
5. The anterior wall of the systemic venous baffle is developed (Fig. 27.4)
6. The pulmonary venous atrium is completed (Fig. 27.5).

Modified ½ Mustard Operation

The goal of the procedure is rerouting of the IVC with a baffle to the contralateral TV [13, 16].

Specific steps of the operation

1. The interatrial septum is completely excised.
2. The inferior vena cava entrance is baffled to the TV, keeping the coronary sinus in a venous tunnel (Fig. 27.6).

Arterial Switch Operation

The technique of the arterial switch operation in ccTGA is elaborated in Chap. 28 Part of this strategy is resection of the LVOTO [13].

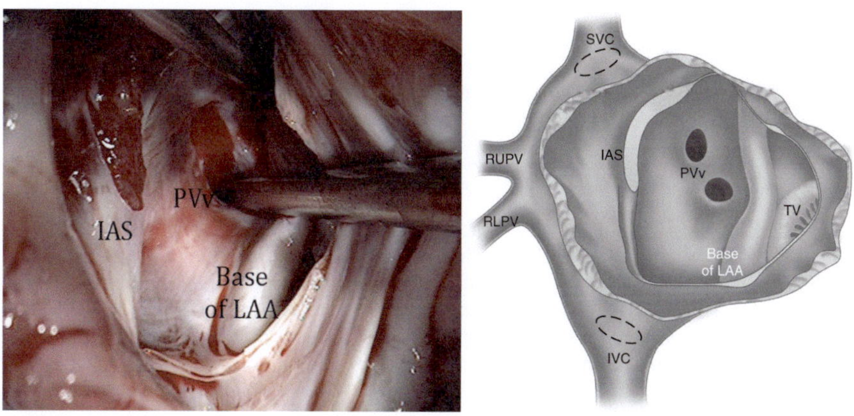

Fig. 27.1 The right atrium is opened in an oblique manner, aiming toward the medial aspect of the inferior vena cava—right atrial junction, but close to the atrio-ventricular groove. The idea is to develop and preserve as large a flap of free anterior wall of the right atrium as possible for the systemic venous baffle. The interatrial septum is completely excised, including superior limb of fossa ovalis under the superior vena cava- right atrial junction. The suckers are placed into the left pulmonary veins. *IAS* interatrial septum, *IVC* inferior vena cava, *LAA* left atrial appendage, *PVv* pulmonary veins, *RLPV* right lower pulmonary vein, *RUPV* right upper pulmonary vein, *SVC* superior vena cava, *TV* tricuspid valve

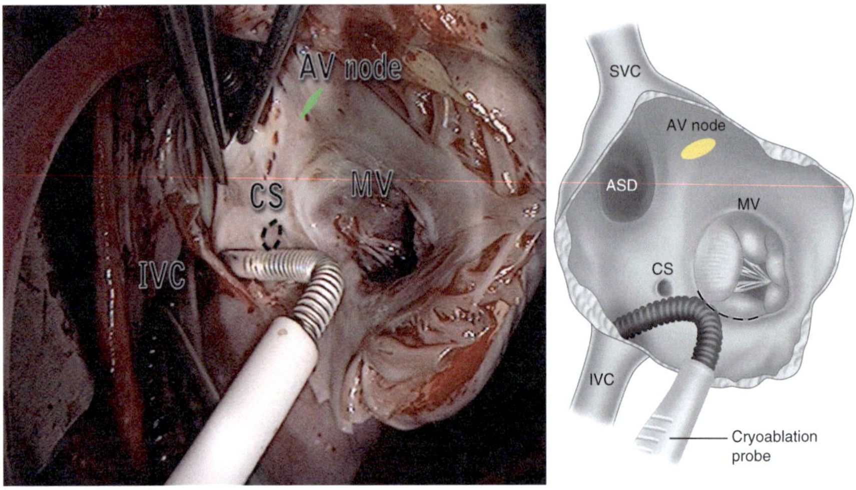

Fig. 27.2 As a part of preventive anti-arrhythmic surgery, a cryo ablation of cavo-mitral isthmus should be considered. *ASD* atrial septal defect, *AV node* atrioventricular node, *CS* coronary sinus, *IVC* inferior vena cava, *MV* mitral valve, *SVC* superior vena cava

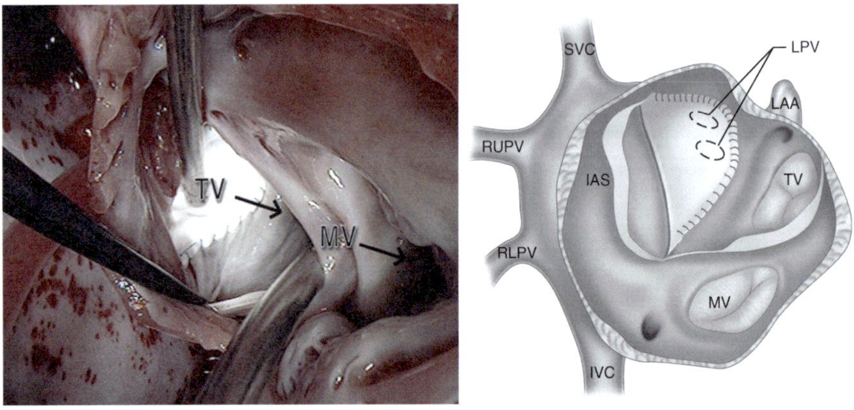

Fig. 27.3 The posterior wall of the systemic baffle is developed with a trapezoid-shaped Goretex patch (Gore©), which is sutured anterior to the left-sided pulmonary veins and posterior to the base of the left atrial appendage. The patch should be seated as low as possible beneath the superior vena cava – right atrial junction (area of resected limbus of the fossa ovalis) to prevent obstruction. On the picture the tricuspid valve is not seen, instead the sucker is placed into the tricuspid valve. *IAS* interatrial septum, *IVC* inferior vena cava, *LAA* left atrial appendage, *LPV* left pulmonary veins, *MV* mitral valve, *RUPV* right upper pulmonary vein, *RPLV* right lower pulmonary vein, *SVC* superior vena cava, *TV* tricuspid valve

Rastelli Operation

The technique does not differ from a Rastelli correction of a complete TGA with LVOTO [4, 13].

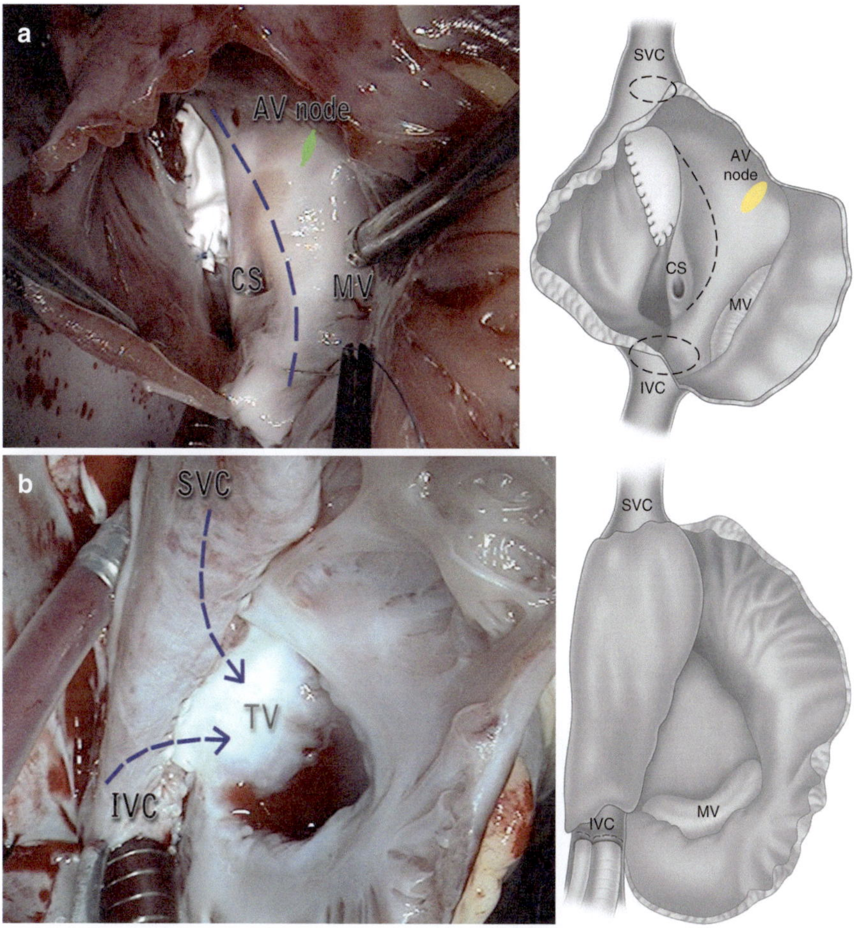

Fig. 27.4 The anterior wall of the systemic venous baffle is developed by suturing the right atrial free wall to the edge of the excised atrial septum between the mitral and tricuspid valves. Preferably, the coronary sinus is kept in the systemic venous atrium so that it is approachable for future electrophysiological studies. However, in situs solitus it is better to run the suture line behind the coronary sinus to avoid a 'normal' (inferior) position of the atrio-ventricular node and the conduction system. The tricuspid valve is "hidden behind" the remnant of the inter-atrial septum (**a**, **b**). *AV node* atrioventricular node, *CS* coronary sinus, *IVC* inferior vena cava, *MV* mitral valve, *SVC* superior vena cava, *TV* tricuspid valve

Specific steps of the operation

1. The VSD is exposed through an oblique ventriculotomy of the RV (Fig. 27.7).
2. The intracardiac anatomy is evaluated. In particular, the relationship between the TV and the VSD and the aorta must be clarified. If the VSD is not of a sufficient size, it needs to be enlarged. To avoid the conduction system, the enlargement should be performed towards the apex in situs solitus, and in situs inversus the

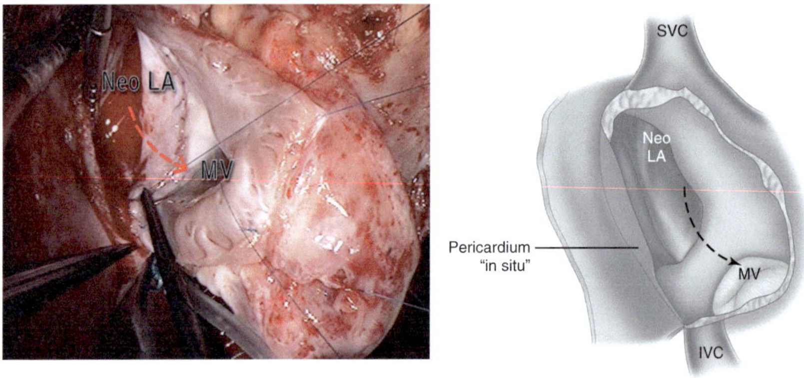

Fig. 27.5 For completion of the pulmonary venous atrium, the in situ pericardium is utilized (Shumaker modification). The suture line commences between the pericardial wall and the pericardial reflection, which was left intact around the anterior aspect of superior vena cava – right atrium junction. The suture line is kept superior and away from the sinus node. Another suture line is commenced at the very inferior end of the anterior lip of the incised right pulmonary veins and pericardium. The suture line swings anterior, reaching the remnant of the right atrial wall. Adequate capacity of the left atrial chamber is created, preserving the optimal position of the mitral valve. One should stay away from the phrenic nerve. *IVC* inferior vena cava, *MV* mitral valve, *Neo LA* neo-left atrium, *SVC* superior vena cava

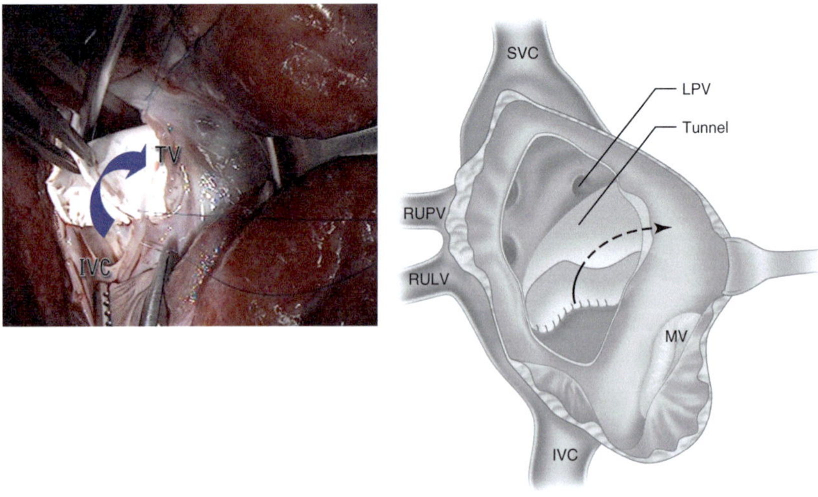

Fig. 27.6 The inferior vena cava entrance is connected to the tricuspid valve annulus using an appropriately shaped and longitudinally opened Gore-Tex prosthesis (Gore©) or other material. The coronary sinus is incorporated into the baffle. The tricuspid valve is "hidden behind" the remnant of partially excised inter-atrial septum. *IVC* inferior vena cava, *LPV* left pulmonary veins, *RUPV* right upper pulmonary vein, *RPLV* right lower pulmonary vein, *SVC* superior vena cava, *TV* tricuspid valve

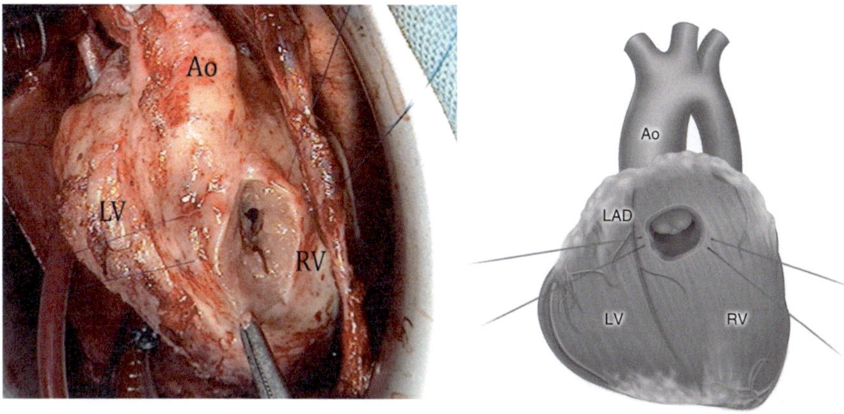

Fig. 27.7 Ventriculotomy of the right ventricle is positioned leftward, while avoiding the aortic valve and coronaries. The picture shows ventriculotomy only. The egress from the right ventricle must be cored out to avoid obstruction. *Ao* aorta, *LV* left ventricle, *RV* right ventricle

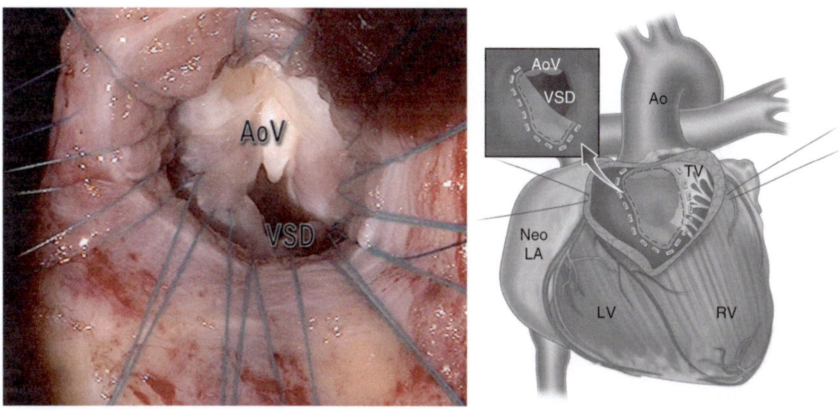

Fig. 27.8 Working through the right ventriculotomy, pledgeted sutures are placed in the right ventricular aspect of the septum starting at the junction of the tricuspid valve and the inferior aspect of the ventricular septal defect. There are marked trabeculae and infundibular folds that support the aortic valve. It is important to stay close to the aortic annulus to avoid residual defects. The remaining sutures should be placed on the anterior aspect of the ventricular septal defect. An oversized patch is trimmed, the patch is secured with interrupted sutures, and construction of the baffle is completed. *Ao* aorta, *AoV* aortic valve, *LV* left ventricle, *RV* right ventricle, *TV* tricuspid valve, *VSD* ventricular septal defect

VSD should be enlarged anteriorally. Partial resection of the subaortic infundibulum might also provide better alignment of the VSD with the aorta.

3. An IVT is created through the RV (Fig. 27.8).
4. Any possible entrapment of the TV by the sutures or patch must be ruled out. If there is doubt about the geometry of the tunnel, the aorta is opened and the baffle is checked from inside, looking through the aortic valve.

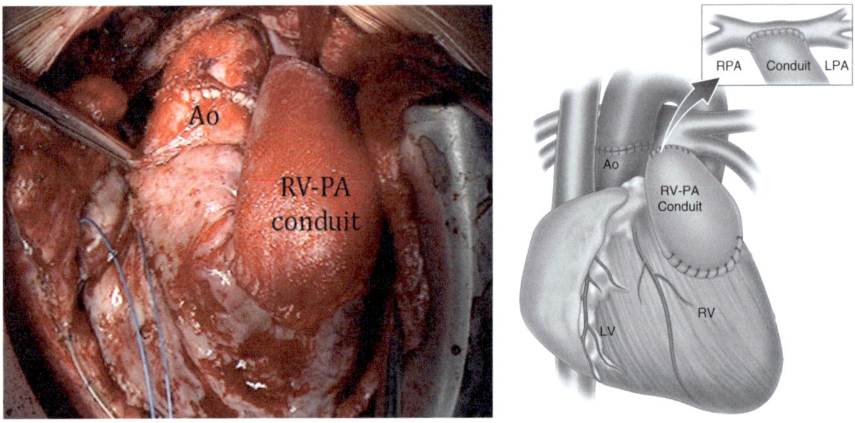

Fig. 27.9 While still on the aortic cross clamp, the pulmonary artery trunk is cut off, the cardiac end is oversewn, and both pulmonary arteries are controlled by clips. The confluence of both pulmonary arteries is widely opened. The distal anastomosis of the conduit to the pulmonary arteries is oblique. If distal anastomosis is sufficiently beveled, kinking of the left pulmonary artery is very unlikely (see insert). After finishing the distal anastomosis aortic cross clamp is released, the conduit is routed under the aorta to the left side, to avoid sternal compression. This is possible even in situs inversus. The conduit is shortened and directly anastomosed to the right ventriculotomy. The conduit valve is located in the distal part of the conduit, avoiding potential compression. *Ao* aorta, *LPA* left pulmonary artery, *LV* left ventricle, *RV-PA conduit* right-ventricle-to-pulmonary artery conduit, *RPA* right pulmonary artery, *RV* right ventricle

5. A connection between the RV and the PA's is provided by a valved conduit of adequate size, appropriate to the age and size of the patient (Fig. 27.9).

Aortic Translocation

The technique of aortic translocation in ccTGA is very similar to that in a complete TGA operation (see Chap. 22) ([11]; Weyand et al. 2010; [13]). However, the technique of coronary artery detachment is always used.

Outcomes

Historically, patients with ccTGA and associated lesions were managed by physiological correction in which the RV was preserved as a systemic pumping chamber, while the associated lesions were repaired. The long-term outcomes of patients after physiologic corrections have clearly demonstrated that the TV and RV function is the Achilles heel of the physiology of ccTGA [11, 19]. Anatomic correction, utilizing the LV as the systemic pumping chamber and the MV as the systemic AV valve, has therefore been proposed, in the hope that it might serve patients better in the long run. At present, the mid-term outcomes after anatomical correction are encouraging. However, the long-term outcomes show that anatomical correction has only a slight advantage over other types of surgical treatment. Long-term survival and functional benefits after anatomic correction were particularly demonstrated in patients with preoperative TV regurgitation [19]. All types of procedures for ccTGA/VSD/LVOTO are safe and have an acceptable degree of morbidity for such complex procedures. The early mortality rate is between 0 and 10 %, and mid-term survival benefits are between 70 and 100 % at 10 years of follow-up. An event-free survival rate of between 70 and 85 % at 10 years has been reported. Reinterventions or redos are related to obstructions of the systemic and venous Senning baffles, to obstructions of the IVT, to aortic or MV regurgitation, to residual VSD's, a failed conduit, or to the need for pacemaker implantation [1, 3, 8, 12, 18, 19].

Deterioration of LV function after anatomical correction of ccTGA/VSD/LVOTO is significantly less prominent than after a double switch procedure. Freedom from LV dysfunction or heart transplant is between 0 and 15 % at 10 years of follow-up [1, 18]. The negative impact of complete heart block, progressive aortic regurgitation, and IVT obstruction on the long-term function of the LV are well documented [3, 18]. On the other hand, universal improvement in the function of the RV and TV occurs when they are exposed to the lower pressures in the pulmonary circulation after anatomic correction. Even in the presence of dysplasia of the TV, with severe preoperative regurgitation, concomitant TV repair is only rarely needed at the time of the anatomic correction [12]. Any patient with ccTGA is at risk of complete heart block, even without surgery, and it has been estimated to affect approximately 2 % of patients per year after diagnosis. Surgically acquired heart block is related to resection of the LVOTO or to closure and/or enlargement of the VSD. The incidence of surgically acquired heart block is between 5 and 20 %, with freedom from pacemaker implantation being 70–80 % at 15 years [3, 12, 18]. There are several specific issues related to the different types of procedure.

Issues Related to the Senning Procedure

Historically, a significant incidence of systemic and pulmonary venous tunnel obstruction has been reported after the Senning operation. Moreover, late development of atrial arrhythmias can be up to 50 % at 10 years of follow-up, with the risk of sudden death [7]. Currently, with the technical aspect of the modified Senning procedure well-accomplished, the incidence of tunnel obstructions is less than 10 %. Furthermore, the modified technique has the potential to provide adequate capacity of the pulmonary venous atrium, to preserve optimal geometry of the MV, to minimize damage to the sinus node and to make the coronary sinus accessible for electrophysiological studies or intervention [13]. Preventive ablation of the cavomitral isthmus might decrease the incidence of atrial re-entrant tachycardia [9]. The modified Senning is highly reproducible and applicable, regardless of the situs and position of the apex of the heart [12, 13].

Issues Related to the 1½ Mustard Procedure

This strategy, which technically simplifies the atrial switch operation, may decrease the risk of sinus arrhythmias and prolong conduit survival due to decreased flow secondary to the BDG [16]. The main drawbacks are the long-term moderate elevation of the SVC pressure, the need for a competent pulmonary valve, the inability to use transvenous access for pacing, and the impaired functional capacity of patients [15].

Issues Related to the Rastelli Procedure

Conduit reoperations are unavoidable; however, the risk of reoperation is minimal. Construction of an obstruction-free and straight IVT is essential for preserving the LV function. There are several morphological scenarios which could prohibit creation of an obstruction-free tunnel.

1. The VSD is committed but borderline in size.
   (a) An enlargement of the VSD is necessary
      (i) In situs solitus, one should guide the direction of the enlargement of the restrictive VSD based on the anticipated position of the AV node, with respect to the degree of misalignment between the interventricular and atrial septum. Unless there is no conduction sling, an anterior position of the conduction system is expected in situs solitus, and the VSD is enlarged towards the apex. Otherwise, an electrophysiological study might be helpful in planning the enlargement of the VSD.
      (ii) In situs inversus, anterior enlargement of the VSD is performed.
   (b) In specific cases with a patent LVOT a DKS anastomosis should be considered in order to minimize the risk of acquired heart block, thus providing two systemic outflows (Chap. 30)
   (c) If there is no TV regurgitation, one might consider the conventional Rastelli operation (VSD closure and LV to PA conduit). The survival benefit has been reported to be close to 80 % at 30 years of follow-up [19].
2. There is a non-committed VSD or significant straddling of the atrio-ventricular valve.
   Under these circumstances, consideration should be given either to conversion to the Fontan procedure, or in suitable patients, to a combination of a Senning operation and the aortic translocation procedure [12, 14].

Issues Related to the Aortic Translocation Procedure

Aortic translocation in ccTGA with a complex LVOTO is a challenging procedure that should only be considered if the anatomy is inadequate for an IVT as part of a Rastelli operation (Weyand et al. 2010). The specific issue is the risk of damaging the conduction system during the division of the outlet septum in situs solitus. Partial division of the muscular outlet septum does not result in complete heart block; however, care should be taken when suturing the patch around the septal defect so as not to injure the conduction tissue [17]. The position of the conduction system in situs inversus allows the risk-free transection of the outlet septum. Other issue is related to coronary transfer. Apart from the risk of coronary ischemia, any coronary transfer is related to a higher risk of aortic regurgitation. Usually, aortic regurgitation is apparent immediately after surgery, confirming the importance of the technical aspects of aortic root transfer [12, 13]. Experience with the aortic translocation technique combined with a Senning procedure is very limited. Excellent short term results with regard to functional outcomes and low incidence of heart block in situs solitus and inversus have been reported [12, 17].

Summary

1. Anatomic correction of ccTGA/VSD/LVOTO can be performed with minimal mortality and acceptable morbidity.
2. In the mid-term, an excellent functional outcome can be achieved, which leads to normal ventricular function, with minimal incidence of complete heart block.
3. The treatment option should be individualized on the basis of the morphology of the LVOTO and the size and position of the VSD and the AV valves.
4. In order to minimize the recognized morbidity associated with the different procedures, one might consider:

   (a) Simplification of the required palliation e.g., avoiding shunting by stent placement.
   (b) Using a modified Senning procedure, which is applicable regardless of situs and age.
   (c) Performing a preventive cavo-mitral isthmus ablation.
   (d) Guiding the direction of the enlargement of the restrictive VSD, based on the anticipated position of the AV node with respect to the degree of misalignment between the interventricular and atrial septum.
   (e) DKS anastomosis can be performed if the LVOTO is patent, to minimize the possible risk of complete heart block associated with VSD surgery.
   (f) Using the aortic translocation procedure if the VSD is uncommitted.

5. The long-term functioning of the conduction system, the aortic valve, the intraventricular tunnels, the conduits, and the ventricles is variable, and close surveillance is required.

References

1. Alghamdi AA, Van Arsdell GS. Physiological versus anatomic repair of congenitally corrected transposition of the great arteries: meta-analysis of individual patient data. Ann Thorac Surg. 2006;81:1529–35.
2. Anderson RH, Arnold R, Wilkinson JL. The conduction tissue in congenitally corrected transposition. Lancet. 1973;1:1286–7.
3. Bautista-Hernandez V, Marx GR, Gauvreau K, et al. Determinants of left ventricular dysfunction after anatomic repair of congenitally corrected transposition of the great arteries. Ann Thorac Surg. 2006;82:2059–65.
4. Brawn WJ, Barron DJ. Technical aspects of the Rastelli and atrial switch procedure for congenitally corrected transposition of the great arteries with ventricular septal defect and pulmonary stenosis or atresia: results of therapy. Semin Thorac Cardiovasc Surg Pediatr Card Surg Annu. 2003;6:4–8.
5. Brawn WJ, Jones TJJ, Anderson RH, et al. Congenitally corrected transposition. In: Anderson RH, Becker EJ, Penny D, Redington AD, Rigby ML, Wernowski G, editors. Pediatric cardiology. 3rd ed. Churchill Livingston; Elsevier Philadelphia, PA, 2010. p. 818–35.
6. Del Nido PJ, Hraska V, Mayer Jr JE. Corrected transposition of the great arteries. In: Kaiser LR, Kron IL, Spray TL, editors. Mastery of cardiothoracic surgery. Philadelphia: Lippincott-Raven Publishers; 1998. p. 800–4.
7. Dodge-Khatami A, Kadner A, Berger F, et al. In the footsteps of senning: lessons learned from atrial repair of transposition of the great arteries. Ann Thorac Surg. 2005;79:1433–44.
8. Gaies MG, Goldberg CS, Ohye RG, et al. Early and intermediate outcome after anatomic repair of congenitally corrected transposition of the great arteries. Ann Thorac Surg. 2009;88:1952–60.
9. Chan DP, Van Hare GF, Mackall JA, et al. Importance of atrial flutter isthmus in postoperative intra-atrial reentrant tachycardia. Circulation. 2000;102:1283–9.
10. Hosseinpour AR, McCarthy KP, Griselli M, et al. Congenitally corrected transposition: size of the pulmonary trunk and septal malalignment. Ann Thorac Surg. 2004;77:2163–6.
11. Hraska V, Duncan BW, Mayer JE, et al. Long-term outcome of surgically treated patients with corrected transposition of the great arteries. J Thorac Cardiovasc Surg. 2005;129:182–91.
12. Hraska V, Mattes A, Haun C, et al. Functional outcome of anatomical correction of the great arteries. Eur J Cardiothorac Surg. 2011;40:1227–34.
13. Hraska V, Murin P. Surgical management of congenital heart disease I: complex transposition of great arteries right and left ventricular outflow tract obstruction, Ebstein's Anomaly. A Video Manual. Heidelberg: Springer; 2012.
14. Jacobs ML, Pelletier G, Wearden PD, et al. The role of Fontan's procedure and aortic translocation in the surgical management of patients with discordant atrioventricular connections, interventricular communication, and pulmonary stenosis or atresia. Cardiol Young. 2006;16:97–102.
15. Raisky O, Gaudin R. Anatomic repair for congenitally corrected transposition of the great arteries: easier is better? Eur J Cardiothorac Surg. 2012;42:685–6.
16. Malhotra SP, Reddy VM, Qiu M, et al. The hemi-Mustard/bidirectional Glenn atrial switch procedure in the double-switch operation for congenitally corrected transposition of the great arteries: rationale and midterm results. J Thorac Cardiovasc Surg. 2011;141:162–70.
17. Morell VO, Jacobs JP, Quintessenza JA. Aortic translocation in the management of transposition of the great arteries with ventricular septal defect and pulmonary stenosis: results and follow-up. Ann Thorac Surg. 2005;79:2089–92.

18. Murtuza B, Barron DJ, Stumper O, et al. Anatomic repair for congenitally corrected transposition of the great arteries: a single-institution 19 years experience. J Thorac Cardiovasc Surg. 2011;142:1348–57.
19. Shin'oka T, Kurosawa H, Imai Y, et al. Outcomes of definitive surgical repair for congenitally corrected transposition of the great arteries or double outlet right ventricle with discordant atrioventricular connections: risk analyses in 189 patients. J Thorac Cardiovasc Surg. 2007;133:1318–28.
20. Wilkinson JL, Cochrane AD, Karl TR. Congenital Heart Surgery Nomenclature and Database Project: corrected (discordant) transposition of the great arteries (and related malformations). Ann Thorac Surg. 2000;69:S77–82.

Chapter 28
Corrected TGA-VSD-LVOTO: Rastelli + Atrial Switch + Damus-Kaye-Stansel Operation

Takaya Hoashi, Koji Kagisaki, Toshikatsu Yagihara, and Hajime Ichikawa

Abstract Atrial switch combined with Rastelli operation for ccTGA, VSD, and left ventricular outflow tract obstruction (LVOTO) is a technically challenging operation. Especially for patients with pulmonary stenosis and a restrictive VSD, additional procedures to baffle the LV to the aortic valve through the VSD are required to avoid systemic ventricular outflow tract obstruction (SVOTO) and permanent pacemaker implantation. From 1987 to 2012, 47 patients with ccTGA, VSD, and LVOTO underwent anatomic repair. Of 20 patients with pulmonary stenosis, 11 patients had a restrictive VSD and required additional procedures during the intraventricular rerouting, including VSD enlargement in 2 patients, combined VSD enlargement and Damus-Kaye-Stansel (DKS) anastomosis in 2 other patients, and only DKS anastomosis in 7 patients. An actuarial survival rate at 20 years was 70.3 %. No mortality has been observed in the consecutive 21 patients since 1997. During the mean follow-up period of 11.6 ± 7.3 years, no patients required reoperation for SVOTO. All patients who underwent a Senning procedure for atrial switch procedure, including patients with apicocaval juxtaposition, were free from caval obstruction. Surgical heart block occurred in only 1 patient who concomitantly underwent VSD enlargement. No patients developed complete heart block.

Keywords Congenitally corrected transposition of great arteries • Senning operation • Rastelli operation • Damus-Kaye-Stansel anastomosis • Anatomical repair • Left ventricular outflow tract obstruction • VSD enlargement

T. Hoashi, MD, PhD (✉) • K. Kagisaki, MD • T. Yagihara, MD, PhD
H. Ichikawa, MD, PhD
Department of Pediatric Cardiovascular Surgery,
National Cerebral and Cardiovascular Center, 5-7-1, Fujishirodai,
Suita, Osaka, Japan
e-mail: thoashi@surg1.med.osaka-u.ac.jp; kagisaki@hsp.ncvc.go.jp;
toshikatsu66@hotmail.com; ichikawa@hsp.ncvc.go.jp

F. Lacour-Gayet et al. (eds.), *Surgery of Conotruncal Anomalies*,
DOI 10.1007/978-3-319-23057-3_28

Background

Atrial switch combined with Rastelli operation for congenitally corrected transposition of the great arteries (ccTGA) and left ventricular outflow tract obstruction (LVOTO) is a technically challenging operation. It is known to have a risk of surgical heart block, post-operative systemic ventricular outflow tract obstruction (SVOTO), and necessary reoperation for right ventricular outflow tract obstruction [1–4]. Mainly for patients with pulmonary stenosis and a restrictive ventricular septal defect (VSD), additional procedures to the Rastelli procedure were required to avoid SVOTO and permanent pacemaker implantation. VSD enlargement was most commonly employed to overcome this issue, however, VSD enlargement toward the postero-inferior direction was somehow limited and still posed a risk for late SVOTO as well as for septal penetrating branch artery injury. In addition, the posterior atrioventricular node sometimes coexists under the presence of concomitant pulmonary stenosis even in patients with {S, L, L} configuration, which indicates VSD enlargement as a risk of surgical heart block [5, 6].

Additional Dams-Kaye-Stansel (DKS) anastomosis was indicated originally for the treatment of patients with Taussig-Bing anomaly and LVOTO requiring Rastelli-type intra-ventricular rerouting at our center [7]. We applied this technique concomitantly with VSD enlargement first, then shifted to perform DKS without VSD enlargement. This technical modification is also suggested for patients with non-restrictive VSDs that are not located in the subaortic area [5, 8, 9].

In the following section, we introduce a surgical technique including DKS anastomosis concomitant with intra-ventricular rerouting as a part of Senning-Rastelli operation for ccTGA, VSD, and pulmonary stenosis. This procedure is not possible in presence of pulmonary atresia.

Anatomic Classification

For intra-ventricular rerouting without systemic ventricular outflow tract obstruction, the size and location of the VSD must be in consideration for anatomic repair. In this anatomical group, restrictive VSD is frequently coexisted with pulmonary stenosis cases. VSD usually locates at sub-aortic area, but some cases with atrio-ventricular discordance and double outlet right ventricle have sub-pulmonic or remote type VSD. The restrictive VSD or not restrictive but remotely located VSD are usually thought to be contraindications for anatomic repair, however, both of them could often be managed by the concomitant DKS anastomosis [9]. The attachment of subvalvular structures of morphological tricuspid valve on the intra-ventricular route would also be the contraindication for anatomic repair.

Typically, the anterior atrioventricular node is believed to form in patients with [S, L, L] segmental diagnosis, and the posterior atrioventricular node in patients with [I, D, D] segmental diagnosis, however, the posterior atrioventricular node sometimes coexists under the presence of concomitant pulmonary stenosis or atresia, moreover, we experienced anterior atrioventricular node remained in patients with [I, D, D] segmental diagnosis and mild pulmonary stenosis [10].

Diagnosis-Imaging

The preoperative evaluation of the VSD size and location is essential for intra-ventricular rerouting as a part of Senning-Rastelli operation (Fig. 28.1). Chordal attachment of the tricuspid valve onto the anticipated intra-ventricular route should also be evaluated.

The primary diagnosis was confirmed by 2D echocardiography. The atrial situs, atrio-ventricular relationship, ventricular looping, ventriculo-arterial relationship, and the presence of a VSD and pulmonary stenosis were examined first. Further examination was conducted to detect mitral regurgitation, the presence of muscular VSDs, major aorto-pulmonary collateral arteries, and other additional abnormalities. Then, the necessity of a systemic-to-pulmonary shunt, balloon atrial septostomy,

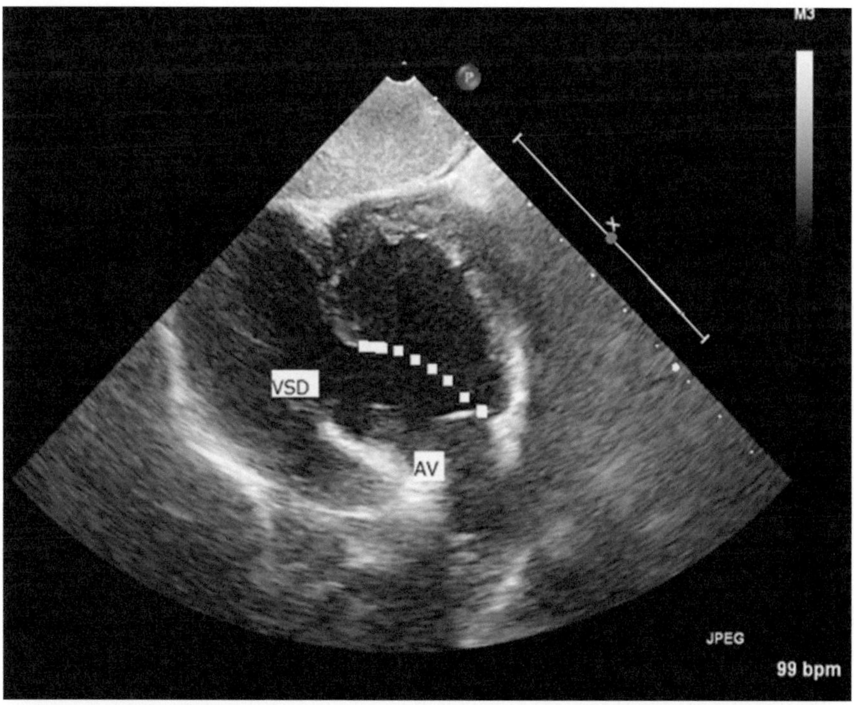

Fig. 28.1 The evaluation of the intra-ventricular route (*dotted line*) by 2D echocardiography. The size of the ventricular septal defect (*VSD*) is large, but remote from the aortic valve (*AV*). This indicates the necessity of the additional DKS

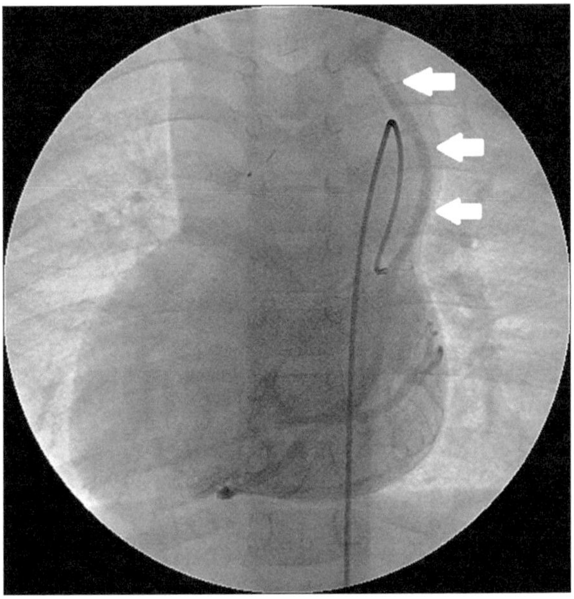

Fig. 28.2 A coronary venous drainage anomaly is frequently associated with ccTGA. Late phase image of left coronary angiography detected coronary sinus atresia. The *white arrow* indicates a drainage vein to the innominate vein

or pulmonary artery plasty with unifocalization, was determined as the preparative operation for anatomical repair to develop the ventricles and PA.

A cardiac catheter examination and angiography provided more detailed information concerning the ventricular volume, end-diastolic pressure, forms of vena cavae connection to the right atrium, and coronary arterial origin and venous drainage (Fig. 28.2). Particularly, ventriculography provided much information concerning how to design the intra-ventricular route, and the course of the right ventricle-to-pulmonary artery (RV-PA) connection.

Two- or three-dimensional computed tomography is also helpful to confirm the shape and form of the heart and vessels, as well as the relationship of the heart to the surrounding structures, like the sternum, chest wall, and airway tract (Fig. 28.3).

Electro-physiologic study using the CARTO system (Biosense-Webster, a Johnson & Johnson Company) combined with ventriculography is useful to detect the exact location of atrioventricular conduction (Fig. 28.4) [10].

Check List

LVEDV of more than 100 % the normal size
RVEDV of more than 120 % the normal size
VSD size and location, chordal attachment of TV
Location of atrioventricular conduction identified by EPS study
Origin of coronary arteries
Coronary venous drainage
TR
MR

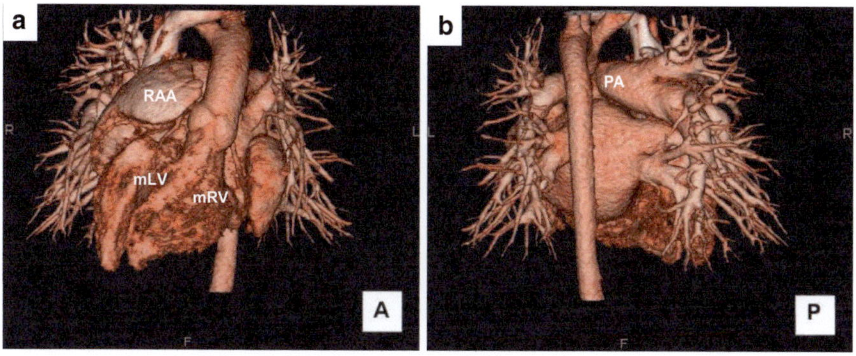

Fig. 28.3 3D image of the patient with Dextrocardia, ccTGA, VSD, and LVOTO. (**a**) antro-posterior view. (**b**) postero-anterior view. *mRV* morphological right ventricle, *mLV* morphological left ventricle, *RAA* right atrial appendage, *PA* pulmonary artery

Surgical Techniques

Following sternotomy, a piece of autologous pericardium is harvested for construction of the posterior wall of the RV-PA connection. For DKS anastomosis, ascending aorta should be fully dissected to the proximal aortic arch. If present, the previously placed systemic-to-pulmonary shunt should be dissected. For establishment of cardiopulmonary bypass, the ascending aortic cannula should be placed in a high position to make DKS anastomosis easier. Bicaval venous cannulae are then directly inserted. The venting cannula is inserted through the left atrial appendage at first, and then moved to the LV through the right atrial appendage, which will eventually become a part of the functional left atrium after the atrial switch procedure. The cardio-pulmonary bypass is run under mild hypothermia, and cold blood cardioplegia is administered through the aortic root and repeated every 30-min.

Procedures for Senning Atrial Switch

The morphological right atrial incision was initiated at the appendage, then obliquely downward to the anterior of the sinus node, toward the crista terminaris. This incision was continued along the crista terminaris, then obliquely upward toward the anterior aspect of the inferior vena cava to the right atrial junction. After the dissection of the intra-atrial groove, the anterior aspect of the right pulmonary vein at the left atrial junction was incised transversely (Fig. 28.5). Then, the anterior edge of the septum secundum was longitudinally incised and extended toward the right superior/upper pulmonary vein and the right inferior/lower pulmonary vein to create the trapezoid-shaped atrial septal flap. At this moment, the coronary sinus was cut back to drain the coronary venous blood to the functional right atrium later

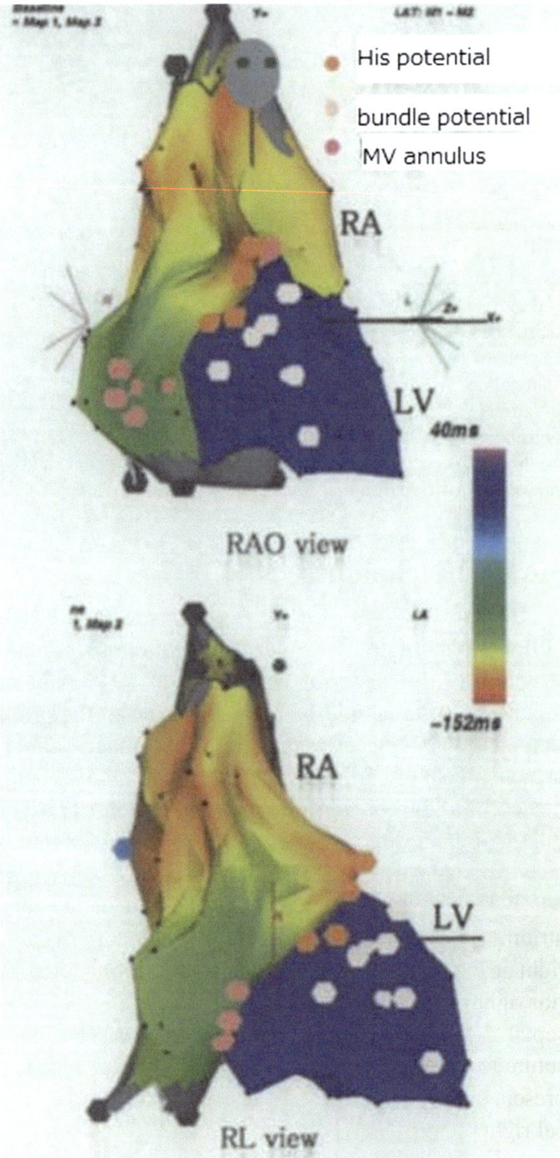

Fig. 28.4 Right atrium and left ventricle mapping with the CARTO system to detect His bundle potentials in patients with {I, D, D} ccTGA, mild pulmonary stenosis, and ventricular septal defects [10]

(Fig. 28.6). If the atrial septal flap is small, it is augmented by a fresh autologous pericardial patch.

The suture was initiated to anastomose the atrial septal flap. After fixation of both superior and inferior edges, the flap is fixed above, the left pulmonary veins (Fig. 28.7). Then, the flap was completely attached to the posterior wall of the morphological left atrium, to cover the left pulmonary venous orifices. Next, the posterior atrial flap is anastomosed to the posterior wall of the morphological right

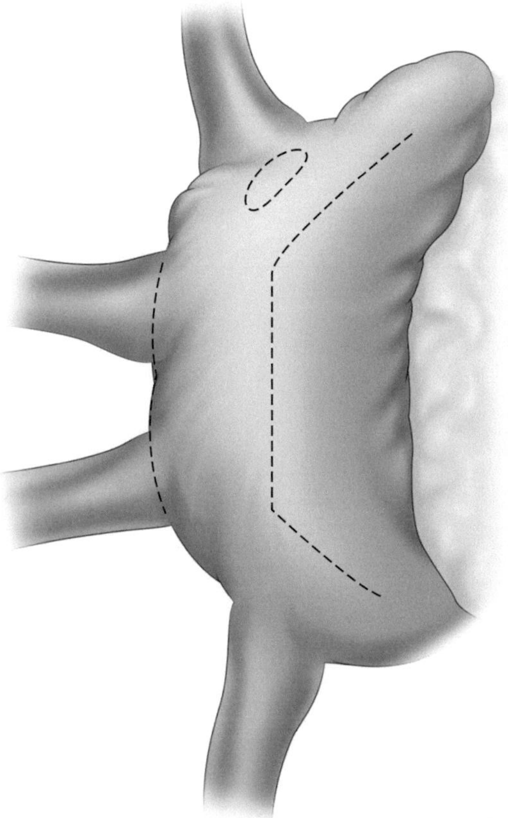

Fig. 28.5 The morphological right atrial incision was initiated at the appendage, then obliquely downward to the anterior of the sinus node, toward the crista terminaris. This incision was continued along the crista terminaris, then obliquely upward toward the anterior aspect of the inferior vena cava to the right atrial junction. The anterior aspect of the right pulmonary vein at the left atrial junction was incised transversely after the dissection of the intra-atrial groove

atrium to drain the caval blood flow to the tricuspid valve through the functional right atrium. Continuous sutures from both superior and inferior edges of the posterior right atrial flap is placed toward the superior rim of the created secundum atrial septal defect, and then along with it. For the anastomosis of the inferior edge, a suture should be initially made on the edge of the Eustachian valve if the valve is present and well developed. Thebesian veins directly draining into the morphological right atrium should also be covered by the flap as much as possible to attenuate post-operative cyanosis (Fig. 28.8). Before finishing the anastomosis, Hegar dilarors are inserted into both vena cavae to test their exact inner diameter.

The anterior right atrial flap was finally anastomosed onto the outer surface of the posterior atrial flap and stretched to the right pulmonary venous orifices in order to create the functional pulmonary veins channel. The superior edge of the flap was obliquely sutured down to the orifice of the right upper pulmonary vein, away from the inferior sinus node (Fig. 28.9). To prevent superior vena caval obstruction, the stitches between the SVC and the atrial flap tissue should be of equal distance. At pulmonary venous orifices, interrupted sutures were selected to prevent narrowing

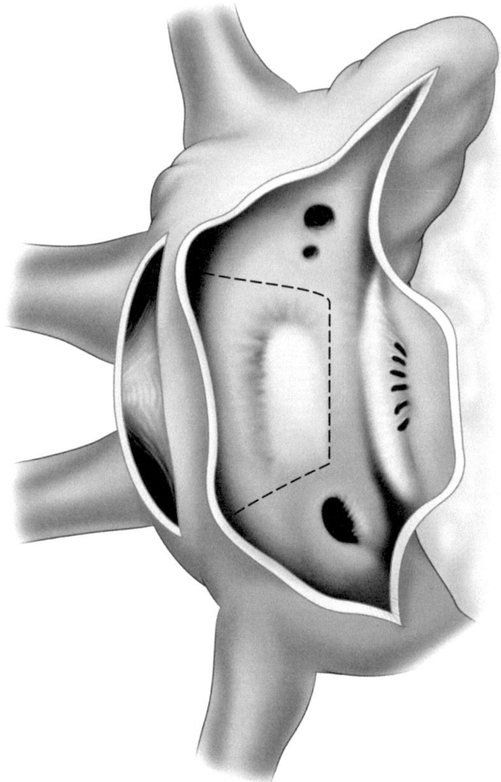

Fig. 28.6 The anterior edge of the septum secundum was longitudinally incised and extended toward the right superior/upper pulmonary vein and the right inferior/lower pulmonary vein to create the trapezoid-shaped atrial septal flap. At this moment, the coronary sinus was cut back to drain the coronary venous blood to the functional right atrium later

of the pulmonary venous pathway. Suture line of the anterior atrial flap could be extended to additional incision (A), or patch augmentation by prosthetic materials should be considered (B) (Fig. 28.10a, b).

Procedures for Left Ventricular Outflow Tract: Intra-ventricular Rerouting

An intra-ventricular baffle from the morphological left ventricle to the aortic valve through the VSD (intra-ventricular rerouting) was created with a patch made by a knitted Dacron vascular graft. Through the infundibular incision of the morphological right ventricle, intra-cardiac anatomy was examined. The length of the right ventriculotomy was set to permit a Hegar of the normal calculated pulmonary valve diameter plus 2–4 mm. An oversized incision should be avoided to preserve the right ventricular function.

Even if a VSD is remote from the subaortic area, the conal septum resection should be limited onto the right ventricular side, not to injure the conduction system. The VSD should be enlarged towards poster-inferior in patients with {S, L, L} configuration, or superior-anterior in patients with {I, D, D} (Fig. 28.11a, b).

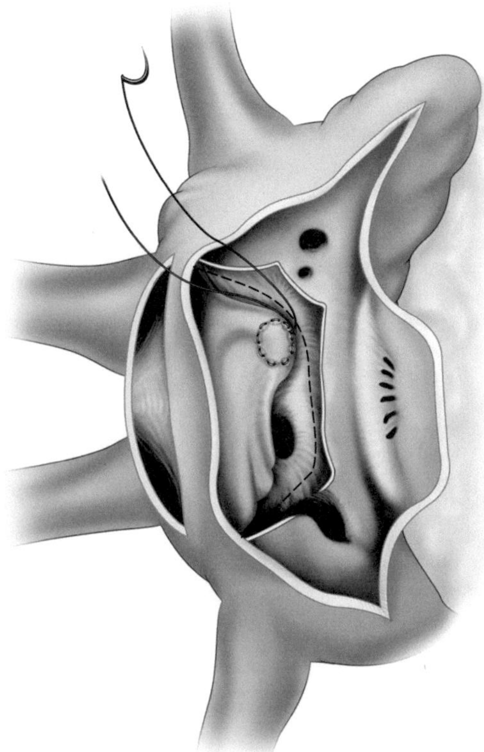

Fig. 28.7 After fixation of both superior and inferior edges of the flap, the left apexes were fixed to the left superior/upper pulmonary vein and the left inferior/lower pulmonary vein

Pledgeted mattress stitches were placed on the right ventricular side from the junction between the tricuspid valve and inferior rim of the VSD first, then upward around the aortic valve in a clockwise fashion. Then, the stitches were subsequently placed in the counter-clockwise direction. Around the septal leaflet of the tricuspid valve, 2 or 3 stitches were placed from the morphological left atrial side (Fig. 28.12). Care should be taken to place fine stitches around the ventriculo- infundibular fold to avoid a residual leak. The patch should have should have a round or oval shape to reconstruct a redundant intra-ventricular VSD to aorta baffle.

Procedures for Left Ventricular Outflow Tract: Additional DKS Anastomosis

DKS in a side-by-side fashion without additional patch materials is our standard maneuver. After intra-ventricular rerouting, both the pulmonary arterial trunk and ascending aorta are transected at the same level, just below the pulmonary arterial bifurcation. At that time, the intra-ventricular rerouting patch is inspected from the inside the aortic valve, and the intended baffle redundancy is assessed. Then, the facing walls of both the proximal great arteries are partially sewn together above the sino-tubular junction to

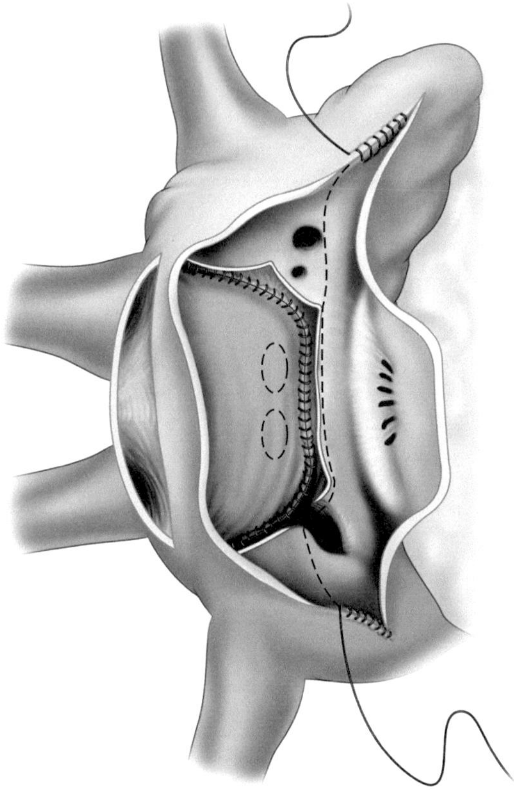

Fig. 28.8 The posterior atrial flap was anastomosed to the posterior wall of the morphological right atrium to drain the caval blood flow to the tricuspid valve through the functional right atrium. Continuous sutures from both superior and inferior edges were placed toward the superior rim of the created secundum atrial septal defect, and then made across it. For an anastomosis from the inferior edge, a suture should be initially made on the edge of the Eustachian valve if the valve is present and well developed. Thebesian veins directly draining into the morphological right atrium should also be covered by the flap as much as possible to attenuate post-operative cyanosis

create a neo-aortic double root and a double outlet left ventricle, the double root is then anastomosed to the distal end of the ascending aorta with continuous sutures (Fig. 28.13).

Procedures for Right Ventricular Outflow Tract

After removal of the aortic croos clamp, The RV-PA continuity is achieved under beating heart using our original technique [11]. A trimmed, fresh auto-pericardial patch was anastomosed proximally to the posterior half of the right ventriculotomy, and distally to the pulmonary arterial bifurcation. The remaining anterior section was covered by a handmade monocusp ePTFE patch (Fig. 28.14).

Outcomes

From 1987 to 2012, a total of 47 patients with ccTGA-VSD-LVOTO, including 27 pulmonary atresia and 20 pulmonary stenosis, underwent an anatomical repair. A follow-up was completed on 100 % of the patients and the mean follow-up period

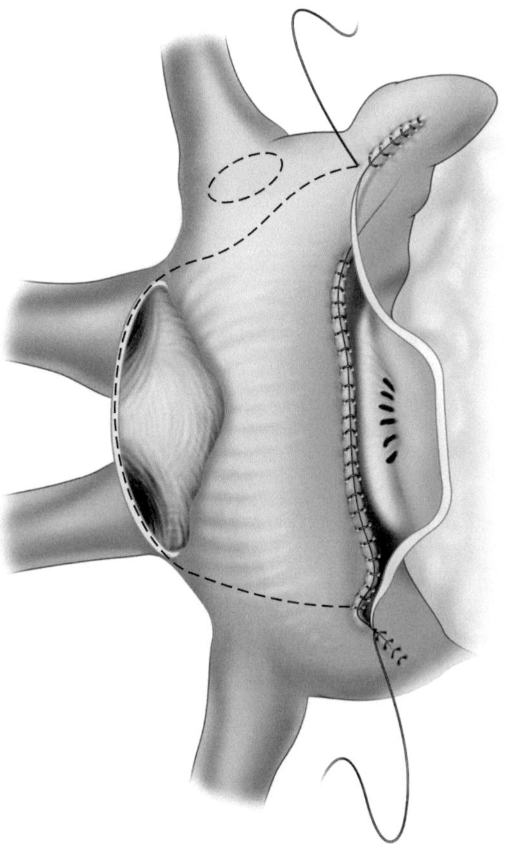

Fig. 28.9 The anterior atrial flap was finally anastomosed onto the outer surface of the posterior atrial flap and stretched to the right pulmonary venous orifices in order to create the functional left atrium. The superior edge of the flap was obliquely sutured down to the orifice of the right upper pulmonary vein, away from the inferior sinus node

was 11.6±7.3 years (max 23.7 years). An actuarial survival rate at 20 years was 70.3 %. There were 5 hospital deaths and 7 late deaths, and no mortalities have been observed in the consecutive 21 patients since 1997.

In the 20 patients with pulmonary stenosis, amenable to an associated Damus-Kaye-Stansel procedure, the VSD diameter ranged from 46 to 158 % of the normal aortic valve diameter. Of those, 11 patients had a restrictive VSD and required additional procedures at the intra-ventricular rerouting, including VSD enlargement in 2 patients, combined VSD enlargement and DKS anastomosis in 2 other patients, and only DKS anastomosis in 7 patients. All 9 patients undergoing concomitant DKS anastomosis showed that the total VSD and LVOT areas were larger than the normal aortic valve area [9]. No patients required reoperation for systemic LVOT obstruction during the follow-up period.

Since 2002, Mustard procedure was no longer performed and all 16 patients have undergone a Senning procedure as atrial switch procedure. Freedom from re-intervention for post-operative caval obstruction at 20 years was 74.8 %. All patients who developed post-operative caval obstruction had undergone a Mustard operation; and all patients undergoing Senning operation were free from caval obstruction.

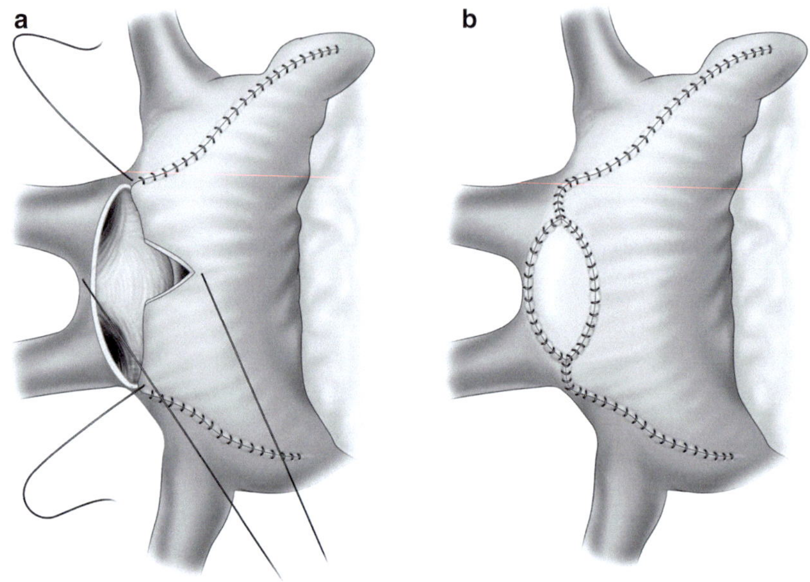

Fig. 28.10 At pulmonary venous orifices, interrupted sutures were selected that did not distort or narrow the pulmonary venous pathway. Suture line of the anterior atrial flap could be extended to additional incision (**a**), or patch augmentation by prosthetic materials was considered (**b**)

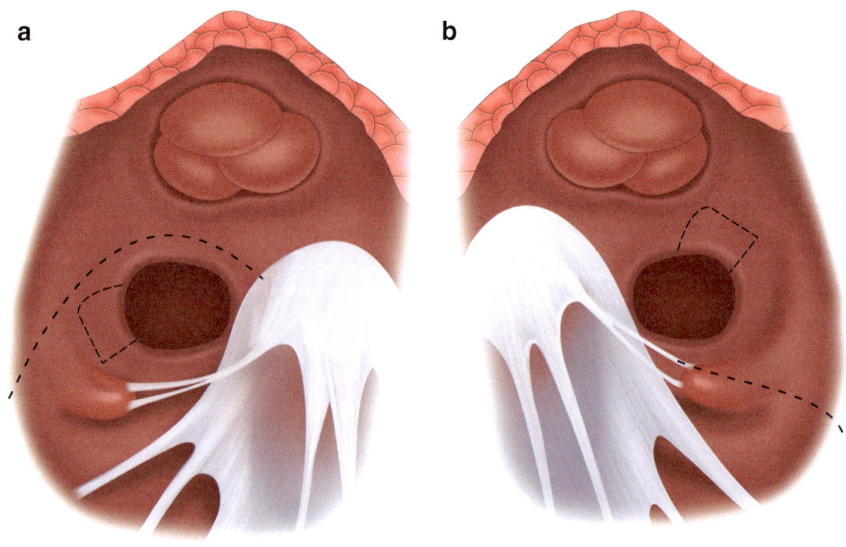

Fig. 28.11 VSD should be enlarged towards poster-inferior in patients with {S, L, L} configuration (**a**), or superior-anterior in patients with {I, D, D} (**b**). *Dotted white line* indicated the conduction running

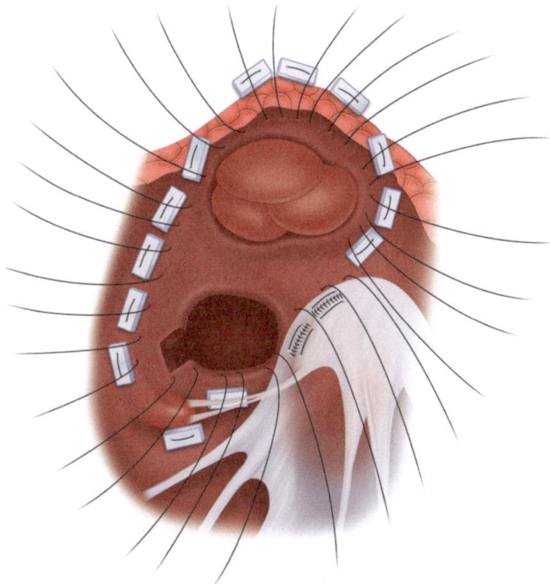

Fig. 28.12 Pledgeted mattress stitches were placed on the right ventricular side from the junction between the tricuspid valve and inferior rim of the VSD first, then upward to around the aortic valve in a clockwise fashion. Then, the stitches were subsequently placed in the counter-clockwise direction. Around the septal leaflet of the tricuspid valve, 2 or 3 stitches were placed from the morphological left atrial side

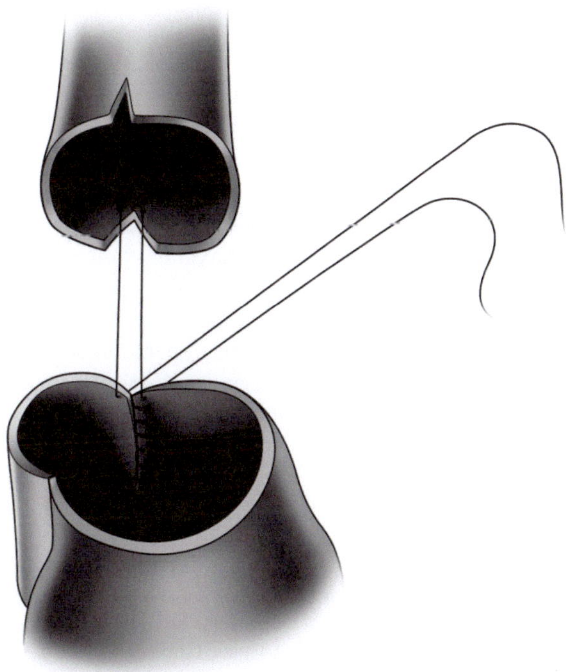

Fig. 28.13 Then, both of the walls facing the proximal great arteries were partially sewn together above the sino-tubular junction to create a neo-aortic route, which was anastomosed to the distal end of the ascending aorta with continuous sutures

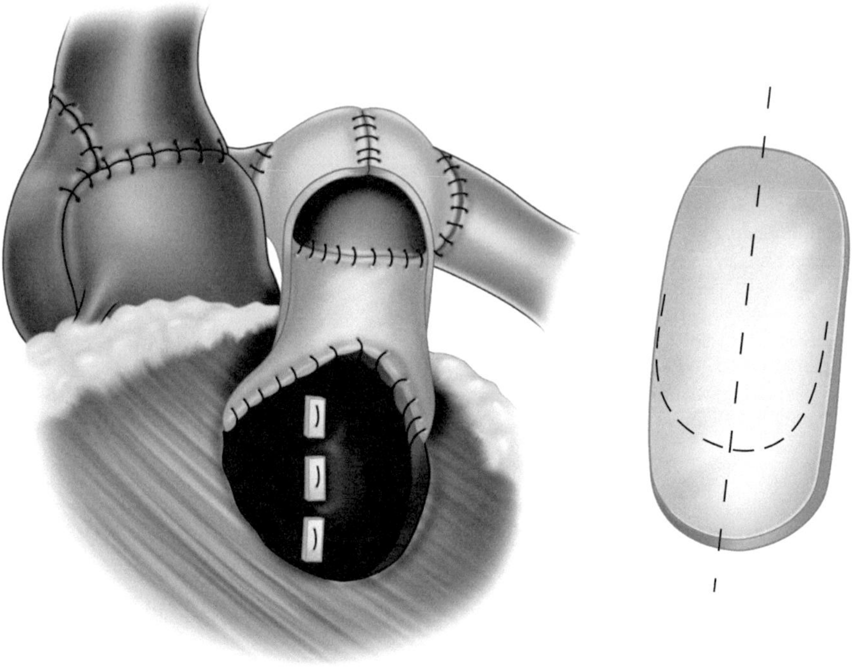

Fig. 28.14 A trimmed, fresh auto-pericardial patch was anastomosed to the posterior half of the right ventriculotomy, and then the opposite side of the patch was anastomosed to the whole circumference of the pulmonary arterial bifurcation. The remaining anterior section was covered by a handmade monocusped ePTFE patch

Freedom from reoperation for the right ventricular outflow tract at 20 years was 52.6 %. Recently, 14 patients undergoing our original RVOT reconstruction did not necessitate reoperation during a maximum follow-up of 15 years.

Freedom from permanent pacemaker implantation at 20 years was 92.9 %. One patient who underwent VSD enlargement developed surgical heart block, and 2 patients who underwent the Senning operation developed late sick sinus syndrome and necessitated permanent pacemaker implantation.

References

1. Shin'oka T, Kurosawa H, Imai Y, Aoki M, Ishiyama M, Sakamoto T, Miyamoto S, Hobo K, Ichihara Y. Outcomes of definitive surgical repair for congenitally corrected transposition of the great arteries or double outlet right ventricle with discordant atrioventricular connections: risk analyses in 189 patients. J Thorac Cardiovasc Surg. 2007;133:1318–28,1328.e1.
2. Murtuza B, Barron DJ, Stumper O, Stickley J, Eaton D, Jones TJ, Brawn WJ. Anatomic repair for congenitally corrected transposition of the great arteries: a single-institution 19-year experience. J Thorac Cardiovasc Surg. 2011;142:1348–57.

3. Gaies MG, Goldberg CS, Ohye RG, Devaney EJ, Hirsch JC, Bove EL. Early and intermediate outcome after anatomic repair of congenitally corrected transposition of the great arteries. Ann Thorac Surg. 2009;88:1952–60.
4. Ilbawi MN, DeLeon SY, Backer CL, Duffy CE, Muster AJ, Zales VR, Paul MH, Idriss FS. An alternative approach to the surgical management of physiologically corrected transposition with ventricular septal defect and pulmonary stenosis or atresia. J Thorac Cardiovasc Surg. 1990;100:410–5.
5. Yagihara T, Kishimoto H, Isobe F, Yamamoto F, Nishigaki K, Matsuki O, Uemura H, Kamiya T, Kawashima Y. Double switch operation in cardiac anomalies with atrioventricular and ventriculoarterial discordance. J Thorac Cardiovasc Surg. 1994;107:351–8.
6. Hosseinpour AR, McCarthy KP, Griselli M, Sethia B, Ho SY. Congenitally corrected transposition: size of the pulmonary trunk and septal malalignment. Ann Thorac Surg. 2004;77:2163–6.
7. Kawashima Y, Matsuda H, Taniguchi K, Kobayashi J. Additional aortopulmonary anastomosis for subaortic obstruction in the Rastelli-type repair for the Taussig-Bing malformation. Ann Thorac Surg. 1987;44:662–4.
8. Koh M, Yagihara T, Uemura H, Kagisaki K, Hagino I, Ishizaka T, Kitamura S. Intermediate results of double-switch operations for atrioventricular discordance. Ann Thorac Surg. 2006; 81:671–7.
9. Hoashi T, Kagisaki K, Miyazaki A, Kurosaki K, Shiraishi I, Yagihara T, Ichikawa H. Anatomic repair for corrected transposition with left ventricular outflow tract obstruction. Ann Thorac Surg. 2013;96:611–20.
10. Miyazaki A, Kagisaki K, Kurita T, Yamada O. Corrected transposition of the great arteries involving situs inversus {I, D, D} and mild pulmonary stenosis: conduction system identified during preoperative investigations for a double-switch operation. Pediatr Cardiol. 2009; 30:516–9.
11. Oda T, Hoashi T, Kagisaki K, Shiraishi I, Yagihara T, Ichikawa H. Alternative to pulmonary allograft for reconstruction of right ventricular outflow tract in small patients undergoing the Ross procedure. Eur J Cardiothorac Surg. 2012;42:226–32.

Chapter 29
Physiologic Repair of Congenitally Corrected Transposition of the Great Arteries

Sameh M. Said and Joseph A. Dearani

Abstract Surgery for congenitally corrected transposition of the great arteries (ccTGA) has evolved overtime. Anatomical repair of ccTGA is now performed with quite satisfactory outcomes in children. The double switch operation has become the preferred surgical procedure in selected cases. Nevertheless, a number of patients with ccTGA still require physiological repair due to complex cardiac associations or impaired systemic ventricular function. This chapter outlines the mechanisms of right ventricular failure in ccTGA. Several "old techniques of repair" were abandoned. The introduction of PA banding has reduced the occurrence of tricuspid regurgitation and has allowed, in some cases, anatomical repair after proper LV retraining. The indications for TV repair and replacement, the place of the Fontan operation or heart transplantation are discussed. The decision to proceed with physiologic versus anatomic repair and the timing of operation is individualized.

Keywords ccTGA • Physiologic repair • Anatomical repair • Double switch • LV retraining • PA banding • Cardiac surgery • Complex CHD

Introduction

Background

In congenitally corrected Transposition of Great Arteries (cc-TGA), there is "double discordance," which involves the presence of both atrioventricular (AV) discordance (ventricular inversion) and ventriculoarterial (VA) discordance. It is a rare defect,

S.M. Said, MD
Department of Cardiovascular Surgery, Mayo Clinic, Rochester, MN, USA

J.A. Dearani, MD (✉)
Department of Cardiovascular Surgery, Mayo Clinic,
200 First Street, SW, Rochester, MN 55905, USA
e-mail: jdearani@mayo.edu

F. Lacour-Gayet et al. (eds.), *Surgery of Conotruncal Anomalies*,
DOI 10.1007/978-3-319-23057-3_29

seen in approximately 0.5 % of patients with congenital heart defects [1]. Anatomical repair of ccTGA is now performed with quite satisfactory outcomes and is becoming the preferred surgical procedure in selected cases. Nevertheless, a number of patients with ccTGA still require physiological repair due to complex cardiac associations or impaired systemic ventricular function

Anatomy

Situs There is usually a normal situs solitus arrangement, with the ventricular apex pointing to the left side (Fig. 29.1a) but mesocardia (Fig. 29.1b) and dextrocardia (Fig. 29.1c) can occur in up to 20 % of cases [2]. Situs inversus can occur in about 5 % of cases.

Aorta Characteristically, the aorta is anterior and to the left side (Fig. 29.2) of the more posteriorly positioned pulmonary artery (PA) – hence the older term "L-transposition." However, the aorta can be more anterior to the PA and can occasionally be on the right side. The ascending aorta is often quite short.

Ventricular mass There is malposition of the ventricular mass so that it comes to lie in front of the atrial mass that can make intracardiac surgical access difficult. With extreme malposition of the ventricular mass, there is usually severe pulmonary stenosis (PS) or pulmonary atresia in association with a large ventricular septal defect (VSD). Also, the morphologic left ventricle (LV) is usually to the right and slightly inferior to the morphologic right ventricle (RV); however, this can show great variability [3].

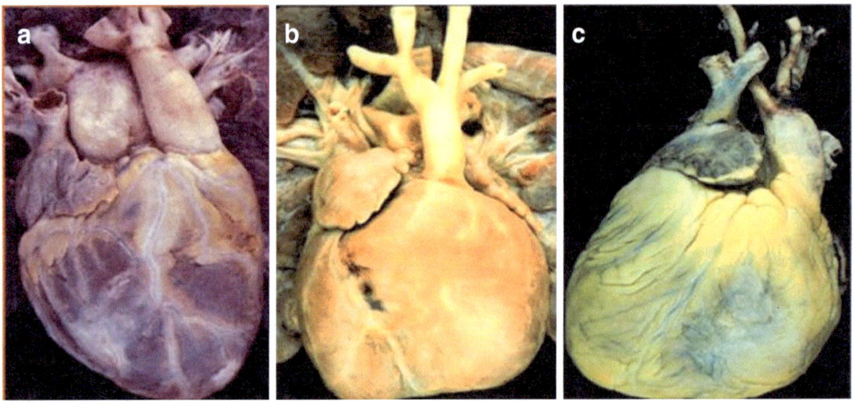

Fig. 29.1 (**a–c**) In congenitally-corrected Transposition of Great Arteries (cc-TGA), there is double discordance which entails the presence of both atrioventricular (AV) (ventricular inversion) and ventriculoarterial (VA) discordance. In the usual situs solitus arrangement, the ventricular apex usually points to the left side (patient **a**); mesocardia (**b**) and dextrocardia (**c**) can occur in up to 20 % of cases

Ventricular Septal Defect VSD occurs in about 70 % of cases [2]. It is usually of the perimembranous type but there can be multiple defects. If it is associated with severe PS or pulmonary atresia, the VSD is usually of the subaortic type, large and extending from the perimembranous area to reach beneath the aortic valve.

Pulmonary outflow tract obstruction Pulmonary outflow tract (morphologic left ventricular outflow tract) obstruction occurs in up to 50 % of cases [4]. This obstruction may be caused by accessory tissue around the VSD, which can balloon into the pulmonary valve, by accessory tissue tags from either the mitral or tricuspid valve that prolapses into the outflow tract (Fig. 29.3), by straddling of either the mitral or tricuspid valve (Fig. 29.4), or the pulmonary valve itself may be stenotic.

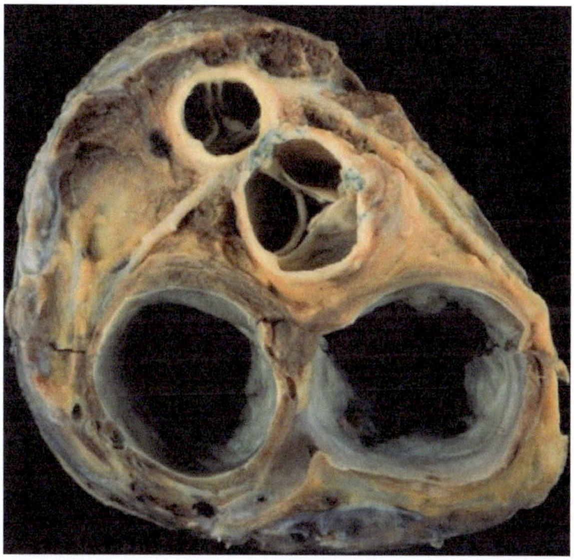

Fig. 29.2 In cc-TGA, the aorta is anterior and leftward of the more posteriorly positioned pulmonary artery – hence the older term "L-transposition."

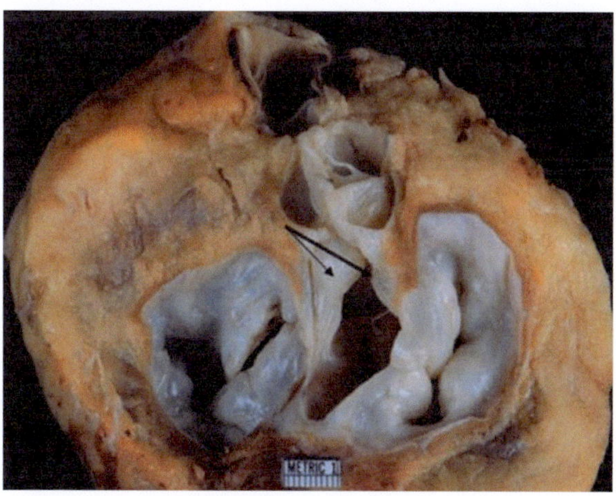

Fig. 29.3 Accessory tissue tags (*black arrows*) from the mitral valve prolapsing into the pulmonary outflow tract causing obstruction to the systemic outflow

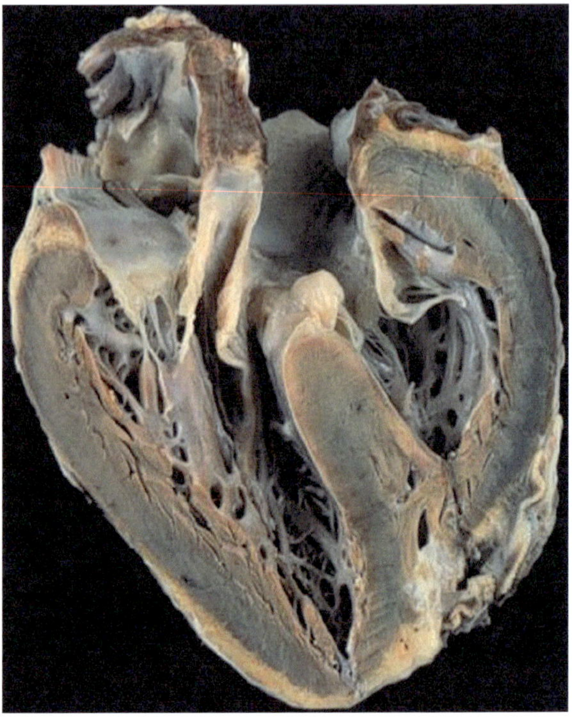

Fig. 29.4 Major atrioventricular valve straddling in cc-TGA. Note the presence of atrioventricular leaflet tissue on both sides of the VSD. This has been a contraindication to perform the double-switch operation

Mitral and Tricuspid Valves The mitral valve (MV) is usually normal but occasionally, a cleft or zone of apposition in the septal component may be noted [5]. The tricuspid valve (TV) may be intrinsically normal, but it can become progressively regurgitant over time secondary to dilatation of the RV and the tricuspid annulus.

More commonly, the TV is dysplastic, which predisposes to valvular regurgitation. Also, a double orifice TV, abnormal septal clefts, and marked annular dilatation have also been reported. The Ebsteinoid displacement (Fig. 29.5) of the TV into the morphologic RV is different from the classic right-sided Ebstein malformation in that there is a lack of atrialization of the RV free wall. The atrioventricular annulus has mild or no dilatation, the anterior leaflet is usually not sail-like and the right ventricle is small or normal in size. In addition, when functioning at lower pulmonary pressures after a double-switch procedure, the tricuspid regurgitation is markedly reduced; i.e., it is not a low-pressure regurgitant valve but tends to be a high-pressure regurgitant valve [6].

Coronary arteries In general, the coronary artery ostia face the corresponding sinuses of the pulmonary valve. The coronary arteries have a mirror image circulation (Fig. 29.6).

Conduction system abnormalities The sinus node is positioned in its normal location but the overall anatomical situation precludes normal conduction because the AV conduction tissue is profoundly abnormal. The normal AV node cannot give rise

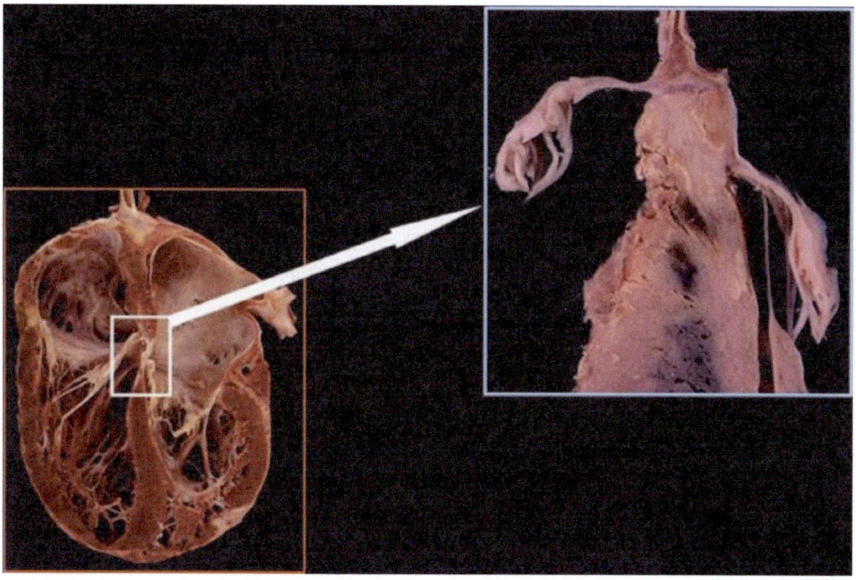

Fig. 29.5 Ebsteinoid displacement of the tricuspid valve (TV) (*Inset*) in cc-TGA. This is different from the typical right-sided Ebstein TV. Importantly, there is little if any atrialization of the RV free wall in cc-TGA

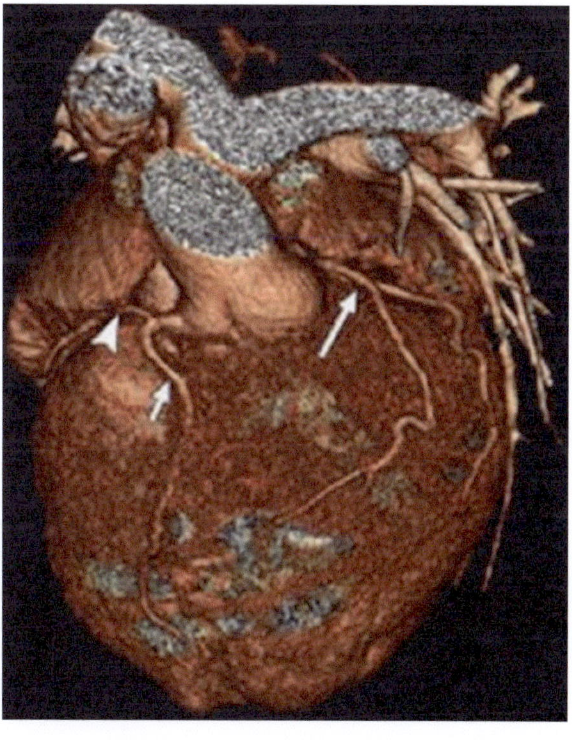

Fig. 29.6 The coronary artery ostia face the corresponding sinuses of the pulmonary valve most commonly. The coronary arteries have a mirror image circulation. *Arrowhead* points to circumflex coronary artery, *short arrow* points to LAD, and the *long arrow* points to RCA

to the penetrating AV bundle. An anomalous second AV node is the functional AV conduction system in many patients, generally located beneath the opening of the right atrial appendage at the lateral margin between the pulmonic valve and the MV; thus, the node has an anterior position. It gives rise to the AV conduction bundle, which penetrates into the left anterior LV wall at the base of the pulmonary valve and then runs onto the septum of the morphologic LV to pass anterior and superior of the ventricular septal defect, when present. This accessory node is not always present and may be hypoplastic or nonfunctional. Complete heart block occurs spontaneously in 30 % of patients and may be present at birth or develop at a rate of 2 % per year. Other conduction disturbances described include sick sinus syndrome, atrial flutter, re-entrant AV tachycardia due to an accessory pathway along the tricuspid valve annulus, and ventricular tachycardia [7].

Pathophysiology

During embryological development, left-handed looping of the heart tube results in AV discordance and the aorto-pulmonary septum fails to rotate 180°, resulting in VA discordance. Blood flows in an effective sequence, hence the name "corrected"; however, the RV supports the systemic circulation in this disorder. Venous blood returns from the body into the right atrium before passing through the mitral valve into a morphological LV. Blood then enters the lungs via the pulmonic valve into the main pulmonary artery. Pulmonary venous blood returns to the left atrium and then passes through the tricuspid valve into the morphological RV, exiting to the aorta through the aortic valve.

Diagnosis and Imaging

Echocardiography (transthoracic and transesophageal) can accurately make the diagnosis of cc-TGA and can show the important intracardiac morphology. Cardiac catheterization is used selectively and may be helpful in the following situations: (1) before surgical intervention to confirm the morphology of the ventricular septum, since there may be multiple VSDs, (2) outline the pulmonary arterial tree when previous surgery has been performed to place a pulmonary artery band, or to create a systemic-to-pulmonary artery shunt, (3) delineate coronary artery anatomy if an anatomic repair (double switch) is being considered, (4) hemodynamic assessment to measure the morphologic LV pressure when a pulmonary artery band has been placed, and (5) examine pulmonary artery pressures and resistance.

CT scan and MRI provide remarkable imaging. 3D reconstruction is becoming a popular method to evaluate the feasibility of bi-ventricular repair.

Surgical Option

The ability of the morphologic RV and TV to provide lifelong support of the systemic circulation is uncertain, even if associated lesions are mild or absent. For this reason, the double switch operation has been advocated by some for the treatment of cc-TGA. It has been suggested that the morphologic LV could be restored to the systemic circulation by redirecting the systemic and pulmonary venous returns via an atrial switch procedure (Mustard or Senning) and then performing an arterial switch if the pulmonary valve and LV outflow tract were unobstructed, or a Rastelli-type procedure (Fig. 29.7) with rerouting of the VSD to the aorta if there is systemic outflow tract obstruction [8]. Several groups have reported successful outcome with the double switch procedures, showing that the morphologic LV could be restored to the systemic circulation [9].

Although the concept of anatomic repair with double discordance is appealing, the following four issues determine the suitability for anatomic repair and ensure satisfactory outcome following anatomic correction: (1) suitability of the morphologic LV for handling the systemic afterload, (2) existence of ventricular hypoplasia of different degrees, (3) routability of the VSD, and (4) atrial size and suitability for rerouting. Our current strategy is illustrated in (Fig. 29.8).

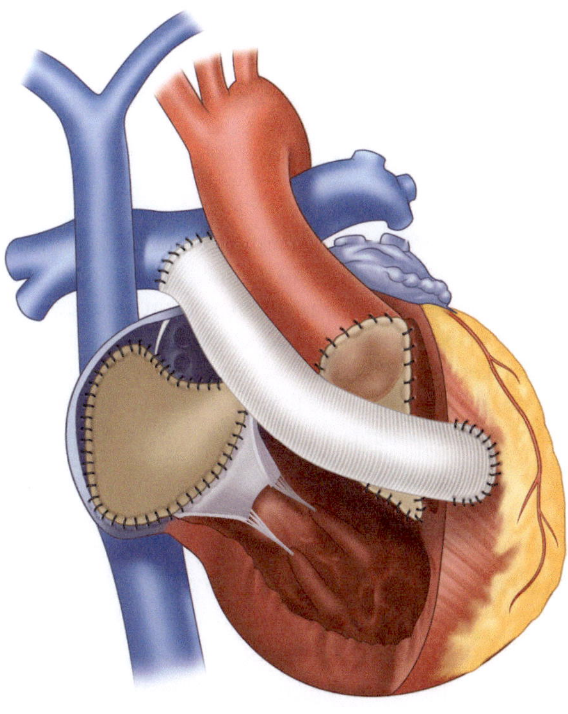

Fig. 29.7 Mustard atrial switch in combination with Rastelli procedure in the presence of systemic outflow tract obstruction in cc-TGA

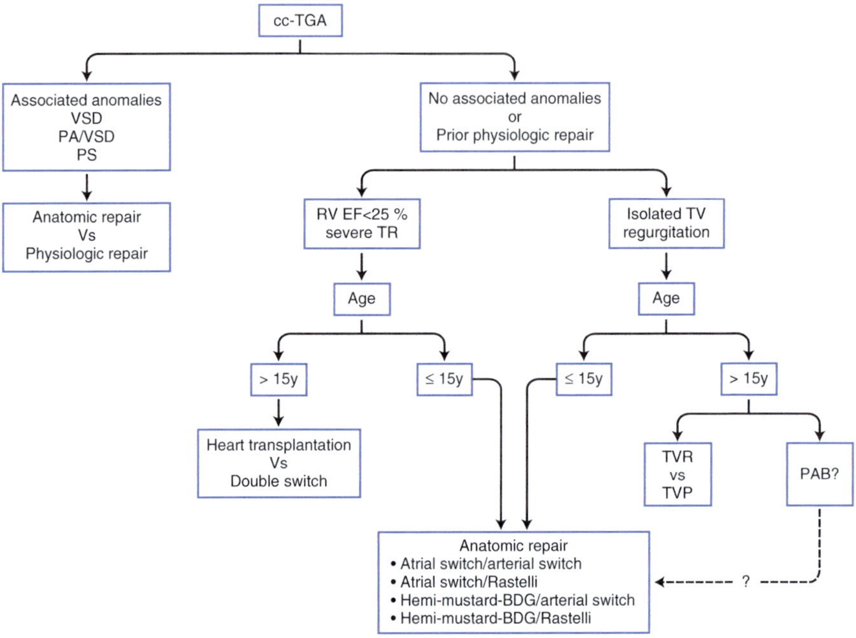

Fig. 29.8 Our preferred algorithm for the various surgical options in cc-TGA

Complications of Anatomic Repair

Complete Heart Block

If closure of VSD is done through the left-sided aortic valve or through a morphological right ventriculotomy the incidence of complete heart block should be low. Nevertheless, spontaneous complete heart block can occur in up to 30 % of patients with or without surgery. In general, caution is advised when placing a transvenous pacemaker system in a recent Senning or Mustard systemic venous baffle because of increased risk of baffle thrombosis. In addition, a transvenous pacemaker should be avoided in patients with residual intracardiac shunts because of potential paradoxical embolism.

Systemic Venous Baffle Obstruction

A gradient as low as 3–4 mmHg can result in important symptoms. Most commonly the SVC is the site of obstruction. This often manifests as persistent pleural effusions. The head and face may appear engorged and there may be prominent veins on the anterior chest wall and shoulders. This complication of the double switch could be minimized by a rigorous surgical technique of Senning or Mustard and by intra-operative TEE assessment of the systemic venous baffle pathways.

Pulmonary Venous Baffle Obstruction

If the right upper and lower pulmonary veins are positioned one in front of the other, this can result in a narrow pulmonary venous pathway where the pulmonary venous return passes around the systemic venous baffle to get to the TV. Furthermore, TEE can be misleading because of compression of the posterior wall of the pulmonary venous chamber by the TEE probe within the esophagus. It is usually possible to pass a left atrial pressure catheter that has been inserted through the original right atrial appendage across the "knee" of the pulmonary venous pathway and to obtain a pullback pressure measurement. A gradient greater than 4–5 mmHg is usually significant and consideration should be given to baffle revision.

Residual VSD

The absolute pulmonary artery pressure as well as any step-up between the right atrial oxygen saturation and pulmonary artery saturation will help to determine the functional significance of any residual VSD identified by echocardiography.

Physiological Repair

Surgical Options for Tricuspid Valve Regurgitation

Surgical options include: (1) TV repair, (2) TV replacement, (3) bidirectional cavo-pulmonary shunt, and (4) pulmonary artery banding. In addition to the morphological RV's inherent vulnerability to progressive dysfunction and failure, it has a complex relationship with the tricuspid annulus and function of the tricuspid valve resulting in systemic AV valve regurgitation. Whether the inciting event is the RV failure or severe systemic AV valve regurgitation, the "chicken or the egg," has been on ongoing controversy. In general, however, it appears that primary RV failure, while uncommon, is a frequent sequela to systemic AV valve regurgitation [10]. Thus, when systemic ventricular function deteriorates, AV valve regurgitation should be considered the cause until another etiology can be provided. Surgery should be considered before significant systemic ventricular dysfunction occurs. Unfortunately, late referral to surgery is common because of the absence of significant symptoms even in the presence of severe AV valve regurgitation. In the Mayo Clinic series of

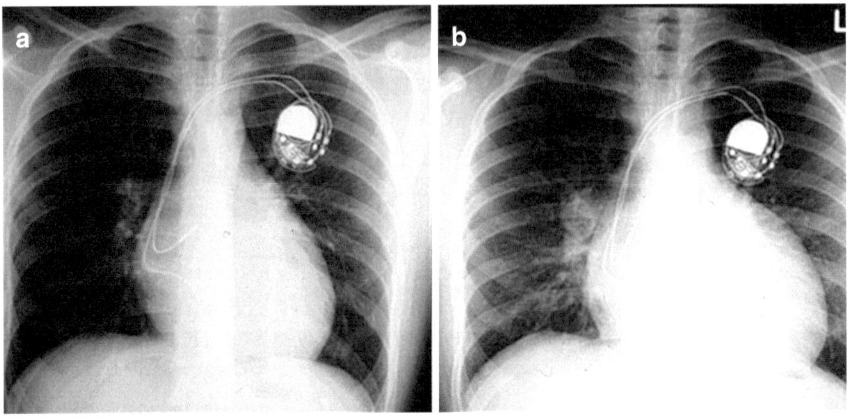

Fig. 29.9 (**a**, **b**) Chest x-ray of a 16 year-old-boy with cc-TGA early after implantation of an endocardial pacemaker (**a**). Implantation of an endocardial pacemaker for heart block may precipitate deterioration in systemic ventricular function and worsen atrioventricular valve regurgitation due to alteration of the ventricular septum, inducing "septal shift" and failure of tricuspid valve coaptation. In this patient, the increased cardiothoracic ratio noted in (**b**) occurred after the initiation of permanent pacing. In addition, the systemic atrioventricular valve regurgitation increased from mild to moderate and the ejection fraction decreased from 50 to 40 %

44 patients aged 20–79 years with no prior cardiac surgery, 26 patients (59 %) were referred with severe AV valve regurgitation. Of the 30 patients who needed systemic AV valve replacement, 16 were referred late with clinical ventricular dysfunction for more than 6 months. The mean preoperative ejection fraction was 39 %, which would be considered unacceptably late in patients with normal ventricular anatomy and severe mitral regurgitation. Although there was no early mortality, four patients ultimately needed late cardiac transplantation for poor systemic ventricular function, and the only marker for poor survival was a poor preoperative ejection fraction [11].

The following factors may predispose to progressive or severe TV regurgitation: age, associated lesions causing volume overload, e.g., VSD, systemic-to-pulmonary artery shunts, Ebstein malformation of the systemic AV valve, myocardial ischemia, and intracardiac surgical procedures. Because complete heart block is common, it should be noted that implantation of an *endocardial pacemaker* may also precipitate deterioration in systemic ventricular function and worsening AV valve regurgitation, because of the change in septal activation resulting in septal "shift", secondary dilatation of the systemic AV annulus with failure of TV coaptation and subsequent regurgitation [12] (Fig. 29.9a, b).

TV Replacement in ccTGA

TV replacement should be considered in relatively early stage when the RV function is still preserved [13]. The TV is approached through the right atrium with a transeptal approach, or through a standard left atriotomy or through the roof of the left atrium.

Surgical Techniques of TV Repair

Several techniques can be performed to repair the systemic AV valve in the setting of cc-TGA. These include: (1) edge-to-edge repair, (2) annuloplasty techniques, either suture or ringed annuloplasty, (3) patch augmentation to improve the surface area of coaptation by increasing the leaflet height, (4) artificial chordae, (5) modified Sebening stitch and (4) other principles of tricuspid repair used for Ebstein malformation can be applied to the systemic AV valve as well [14].

Pulmonary Artery Banding (PAB)

The principle of PAB is to maintain a conditioned ("prepared") morphologic LV, and to shift the interventricular septum partially towards the morphologic RV. This septal shift improves the geometry of the systemic tricuspid valve in shortening the anterior papillary muscle which results in improved anterior leaflet coaptation and less TV regurgitation. This mimics cc-TGA with pulmonary stenosis, which is known to have better outcome than simple cc-TGA [15, 16]. Recently, early PAB strategy has been applied by Metton et al. [17] to infant ccTGA with intact ventricular septum: – to retrain the functional morphologic LV for later systemic work and – to improve the TV coaptation. This strategy produces partial septal shift towards the morphologic RV, which further improves TV coaptation and reduces regurgitation [16, 18]. The PAB had no direct effect on morphologic RV function; in fact, the reduction in TV regurgitation may prevent morphologic RV dilatation and later dysfunction.

The challenge with pulmonary artery banding is to create an adequate gradient, not too tight or too loose; knowing that the gradient is influenced by systemic and pulmonary vascular resistances, heart contractility, FiO_2 and mechanical ventilation.

Techniques of PAB have been described [19]. The Trusler Formula [20] involves sizing the band according to the specific cardiac anatomy and setting the initial length of the band based on the patient's weight. Trusler formula mandates that the band circumference should be 20 + 1 mm/kg of body weight for simple defects with no intracardiac mixing lesions; however, it should be 24 + 1 mm/kg body weight in the presence of intracardiac mixing [21].

The following goals should be achieved with banding: (a) systolic blood pressure increase by 10–20 mmHg, (b) distal pulmonary artery pressure should be less than 50 % of aortic systolic blood pressure (2-ventricle repair) and lowest possible pressure that maintains an acceptable oxygen saturation. Target oxygen saturations are 80–85 % for single ventricle and 95 % for a two-ventricle repair. While the technical aspects of PAB are not complex, the procedure can be associated with significant ventricular dysfunction, even with minor changes in band tightness. Placement of the PAB is done with TEE guidance to watch for ventricular septal shift. Importantly, ventricular function can rapidly deteriorate even when the band appears to be in an ideal position resulting in hypotension and cyanosis. In general, the band is tightened and released on multiple occasions to allow the ventricle to adapt to the increased ventricular pressure. The postoperative ICU care of these critically ill patients requires constant adjustment of inotropic and ventilator support for a successful outcome. The use of a remotely adjustable band [22] that allows more gradual adaptation can be helpful.

The Failing Systemic Morphologic Right Ventricle

Mechanisms of Failure

A retrospective multi-institutional study clearly demonstrated an increasing incidence of systemic ventricular dysfunction and clinical congestive heart failure with advancing age. Even in patients with cc-TGA and no significant associated lesions, more than one third had congestive heart failure by the fifth decade. In patients with significant associated defects and prior open-heart surgery, two thirds of patients had congestive heart failure by the age of 45 years [23]. Some of the theories behind earlier heart failure that may include:

Bulging of the Interventricular Septum

Suboptimal function of the systemic RV at rest or with exercise is well established. Coexistence of abnormalities of the left-sided TV structure and function also predisposes the patient with cc-TGA to more rapid clinical deterioration. The development of RV failure can occur primarily, without previous surgical intervention and is usually associated with dysplasia of the TV, causing tricuspid regurgitation. RV failure may also occur secondarily after conventional repair (physiologic repair) of associated cardiac defects such as VSD or relief of PS or atresia when the RV remains in the systemic circulation. The deterioration in RV function associated with TV regurgitation may also develop insidiously over many years without associated cardiac anomalies. When associated with dysplasia or Ebsteinoid malformation of the TV, the deterioration may be rapid. Once tricuspid regurgitation has developed, the volume load of the RV, accentuated by any shunts or VSD, can cause further TV annular dilatation, creating more regurgitation, and worsening RV dysfunction and heart failure. The development of morphologic RV failure without previous surgical intervention is almost always associated with dysplasia of the TV. RV dilatation, in association with volume loading from tricuspid regurgitation, displaces the ventricular septum into the morphologic LV that leads to displacement of the septal components of the TV, which accentuates the regurgitation. In secondary morphologic RV failure following conventional closure of VSD or relief of PS, the fall in the morphologic LV pressure and realignment of the septum toward the pulmonary ventricle can have the same effect by creating tricuspid regurgitation. This is thought to be the mechanism of the development of tricuspid regurgitation and

RV failure, which is supported by the observation that, pulmonary artery banding to train the morphologic LV reduces tricuspid regurgitation by realignment of the ventricular septum [24]. If this is the mechanism of morphologic RV failure, then tricuspid regurgitation and RV failure can be expected to occur after conventional repair.

Role of Ischemia

The RV working as a systemic ventricle at systemic pressures with the resultant hypertrophy of the myocardium may not have sufficient coronary blood flow. This results in ischemia of the RV myocardium, which, in addition to volume loading secondary to tricuspid regurgitation, may also be a contributing factor in RV failure [25, 26].

Surgical Options

Bidirectional Cavopulmonary Anastomosis

The presence of the bidirectional cavopulmonary shunt may prolong the time to reoperation for pulmonary ventricle-PA conduit dysfunction and it simplifies baffle construction for the atrial switch procedure.

Fontan Procedure

If a decision is made following the right atriotomy that it will not be possible to baffle the VSD to the aorta, then a modified Fontan can be performed. This assumes that there are no other significant risk factors to establish a Fontan circulation. Our preference for modified Fontan is a total cavopulmonary connection with bidirectional cavopulmonary shunt and an extracardiac conduit with selective application of a fenestration. No incisions are made in either ventricle.

Use of Ventricular-Assist Devices (Fig. 29.10)

Use of a left ventricular assist device (LVAD) as a bridge to transplantation in transplant candidates with a deteriorating cardiac condition has become a common strategy [27]. The LVAD's inflow cannula is usually placed in the dilated systemic RV. In the presence of aortic valve regurgitation, LVAD implantation is more challenging, because the aortic regurgitation causes a major loss of pump stroke volume to the LV. This can be managed by suturing the nodules of Arantius together ("Park stitch"), or alternatively by valve excision and annulus closure with Dacron, or pericardium.

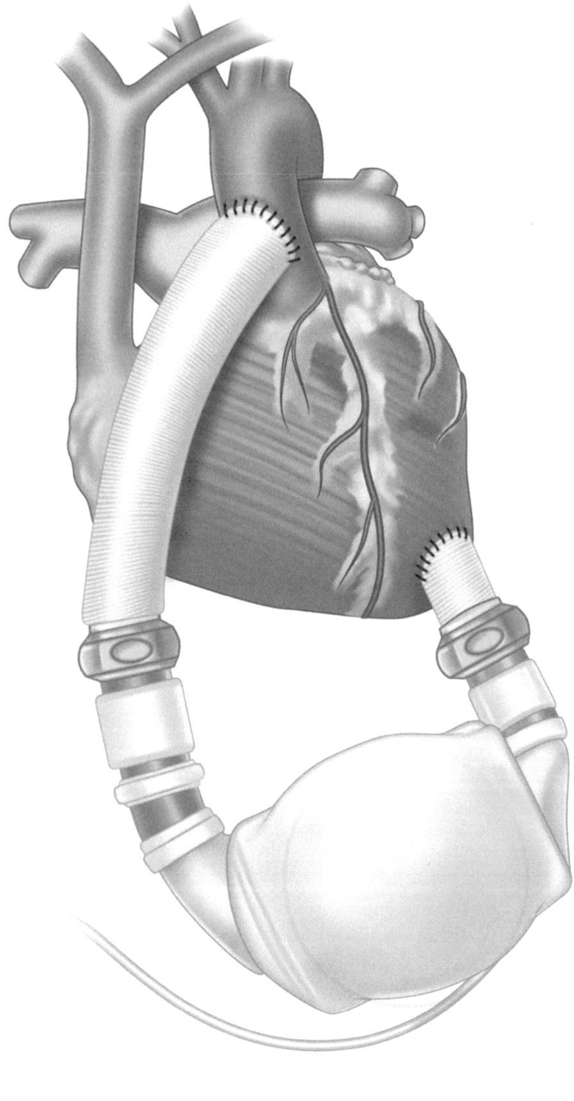

Fig. 29.10 Use of left ventricular-assist device (LVAD) to support the failing systemic ventricle. The LVAD's inflow cannula is normally placed in the dilated LV. However, cannula placement in patients with cc-TGA will be implanted in the morphologic right (systemic) ventricle

Heart Transplantation

According to the Registry of the International Society for Heart and Lung Transplantation in 2007, only 3.2 % of heart transplantations were performed for congenital heart disease in the adult population. Because of the abnormal alignment of the great arteries in cc-TGA, heart transplantation requires technical modifications. Reitz et al. at Stanford University Medical Center first reported successful heart transplantation for cc-TGA in 1982. Since then, only a few cases have been reported in the literature. During removal of the donor heart, the aortic arch and pulmonary arteries are harvested to provide sufficient tissue. During the implantation, minor clockwise rotation of the donor heart may be required and is acceptable [28].

Physiological Repair of ccTGA-VSD

The goal of the surgery is to close the VSD. This physiologic procedure was routinely performed in the past before the introduction of the double switch operation by Imai in 1997. A PA banding palliation is performed in early infancy and the operation is undertaken around 18 months. The presence of the PA banding maintains an elevated pressure in the subpulmonary left ventricle and prevent the occurrence of a systemic TV regurgitation. The VSD patch closure follows the same technique described in Chap. 29. The major risk is the AV block that is avoided in suturing the VSD on the right side of the septum. The VSD could be approached in three different way: through the mitral valve, through the aortic valve or through a right ventriculotomy. This operation is complicated in the long term by a high rate of late systemic TV regurgitation due to the bulging of the septum from right to left, following the drop in the pulmonary afterload.

Physiologic Repair of ccTGA-VSD-LVOTO with VSD Patch Closure and LV to PA Conduit

The physiologic repair is to close the VSD and correct the pulmonary stenosis in placing a LV to PA valved conduit; as the pulmonary annulus can't be divided due to the presence of the conduction bundle very close to the pulmonary annulus (in situs solitus). One danger is to damage the antero-lateral papillary muscle of the mitral valve in implanting the conduit. This operation has been progressively abandoned because of high rate of late TV regurgitation due to the pressure drop in the left ventricle. Some centers have recommended keeping the PA banding in place (see below). Another reason is the difficulty created by the very anterior position of the conduit behind the sternum, with a high risk of compression.

Physiologic Repair of ccTGA-VSD-LVOTO with VSD Patch Closure Only

This physiological repair option is appealing because in maintaining a high pressure in the LV, the interventricular septum could remain flat preventing a TV regurgitation in the long term. At the same time, the LV structure could sustain a systemic pressure. No publications are so far available with this technique to our knowledge.

Outcomes

Outcomes of Physiologic Repair

Hraska et al. [28] reported the long-term outcome of "classic surgical repair" of 123 patients with cc-TGA between 1963 and 1996. On the basis of the surgical approach, patients were placed in one of two categories: patients who underwent only palliative procedures and patients who underwent intracardiac repair. Patients who underwent intracardiac repair had either a 2-ventricle repair or a Fontan-type operation. Patients with a 2-ventricle type of repair were further subdivided according to the type of operation into three groups: VSD operation, tricuspid valve replacement (TVR) or repair, or other. The 1-, 5-, 10-, and 15-year survivals after the operation were 84 %, 75 %, 68 %, and 61 %, respectively. The authors identified the following: (1) Risk factors for mortality included subvalvular pulmonary stenosis, Ebstein malformation of TV, right ventricular end diastolic pressure >17 mmHg, preoperative RV dysfunction, complete heart block after the operation. (2) Predictors for right ventricular dysfunction including Ebstein malformation of TV, TV replacement, and complete heart block after the operation. (3) Predictors for tricuspid valve dysfunction included Ebstein malformation of TV, preoperative RV dysfunction, RV end diastolic pressure > 17 mm Hg (before the operation), operative group other than Fontan. The authors concluded that the long-term outcome of patients with cc-TGA after a classic surgical approach was not satisfactory. The poorest outcome was seen in patients who required tricuspid valve replacement either at their initial operation or later during follow-up. The alternative surgical approaches, such as the double-switch, Senning-Rastelli, or Fontan procedures, are likely to have better long-term results, especially in the highest risk groups (Fig. 29.11).

In the meta-analysis by Alghamdi and colleagues [29], the authors reviewed the results of 11 non-randomized studies involving 124 patients. Anatomic repair (Rastelli type) was performed in 69 patients, double switch was performed in 25 patients and 30 patients underwent physiologic repair. The age of included patients at time of surgery ranged from 0.25 to 55 years. Early mortality was significantly lower in the anatomic repair group type. The Rastelli group had better survival compared to others, which may be explained by the absence of coronary transfer in Rastelli, and lower incidence of heart block and systemic atrioventricular valve regurgitation that were noticed in these patients compared to others. However this meta-analysis did not answer the question of which patients may benefit from one surgical approach versus the other.

Outcomes of Systemic Atrioventricular Valve Surgery

Systemic AV valve replacement is relatively common in the adult age group. Surgery can be accomplished with low early mortality in experienced centers, particularly when systemic ventricular function is preserved. The outcome of 40 patients aged

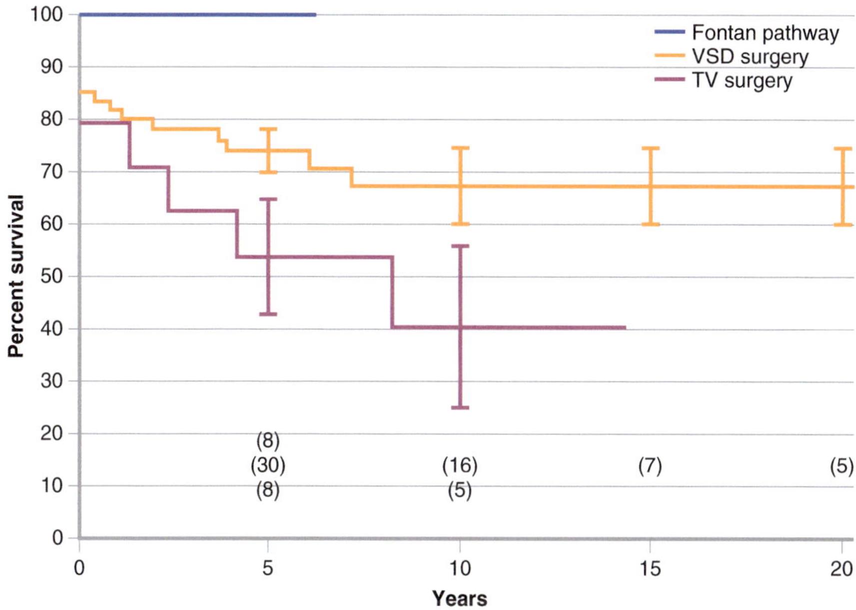

Fig. 29.11 Late survival for the following operative groups: Fontan pathway (*dotted line*; n =17), VSD surgery (*solid line*; n=76), and TV surgery (*dashed line*; n =14). Numbers of patients at risk are in parentheses. *Error bars* indicate 70 % confidence limits. *TV* tricuspid valve, *VSD* ventricular septal defect

5 months to 70 years who underwent systemic AV valve replacement at the Mayo Clinic between 1964 and 1993 were reported [30]. Of these 40 patients, 36 had severe regurgitation, and 29 (72.5 %) had associated cardiac anomalies. The preoperative ejection fraction ranged from 20 to 60 % (mean, 48 %). The early mortality in this high-risk group was 10 %; some of these operations occurred in the early era and prior to the use of cardioplegia. In the current era, early mortality has been reduced to <3 %. Late survival was 78 % at 5 years and 61 % at 10 years. The cause of death in all 12 patients in this series was systemic ventricular failure, an outcome that emphasizes the need for earlier operation, before the development of significant systemic ventricular dysfunction. Functional status improved in the 28 survivors, with 27 patients in NYHA functional class I or II. Survivorship correlated with a preoperative ejection fraction >44 %.

Rutledge et al. [31] reported a pediatric series of 121 patients seen at Texas Children's Hospital between 1952 and 1999 with a median age at diagnosis of 1 month. Asymptomatic patients had isolated cc-TGA, a small VSD, or mild pulmonary stenosis, or they were hemodynamically well balanced with a VSD and pulmonary stenosis. In contrast, patients with heart failure had a large VSD, a VSD with mild pulmonary stenosis, or a regurgitant systemic AV valve. Those with cyanosis had a VSD with either pulmonary stenosis or pulmonary atresia. At a median follow-up of 9.3 years, the 5-, 10-, and 20-year survival rates were 92 %, 91 %, and

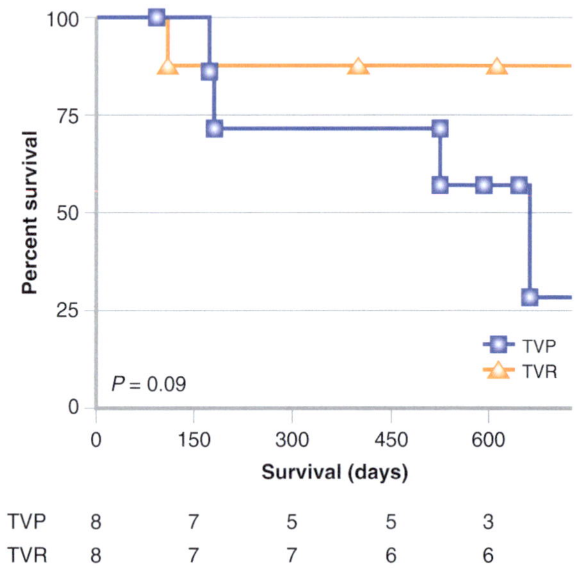

Fig. 29.12 Survival curves for the composite end point of death or recurrent tricuspid regurgitation. A trend toward less favorable survival characteristics for patients who underwent tricuspid valvuloplasty was observed, although it was not statistically significant. *TVP* tricuspid valvuloplasty, *TVR* tricuspid valve replacement

75 %, respectively. There were 20 deaths (16.5 %) at a median age of 13.2 years and five cardiac transplants (4 %). Surgery was performed in 86 patients with an operative mortality of 2.5 %. Biventricular repair was performed in 47 patients and varied according to the underlying cardiac anatomy. Risk factors for mortality included older age at biventricular repair, moderate or severe systemic AV valve regurgitation, and poor RV function. In this study, as in others, most patients undergoing surgical repair had worsening systemic AV valve regurgitation to a moderate or severe degree. Implicated factors include the "insult" of cardiopulmonary bypass leading to annular dilatation [32], annular distortion caused by VSD closure [33], changes in the position of the ventricular septum, and annular dilatation after relief of pulmonary stenosis [34, 35]. In addition, poor tolerance of the systemic AV valve to systemic pressure after VSD closure is possible because afterload is increased, and postoperative complete AV block may compound the adverse hemodynamics. The observation of progressive systemic AV valve regurgitation after operative intervention has prompted some authors to recommend systemic AV valve replacement at the time of intracardiac repair if the systemic AV valve regurgitation is moderate or more at the time of surgery [26].

Scherptong et al. [36] reported the outcome of 16 adult patients who underwent tricuspid valvuloplasty or replacement in the period 1999–2008. Three patients died 109, 180, and 659 days after surgery, respectively; the first patient after TV replacement (TVR) and the latter 2 after tricuspid valvuloplasty (TVP). Overall, tricuspid valve function improved and functional class improved; however, RV function remained unchanged. Follow-up of patients ranged from 92 to 3101 days after operation, with a 1-year survival rate of 86.7 %. Kaplan-Meier curves (Fig. 29.12) for the composite end point of death or recurrent severe tricuspid regurgitation demonstrated no significant difference in survival between TV replacement vs. repair

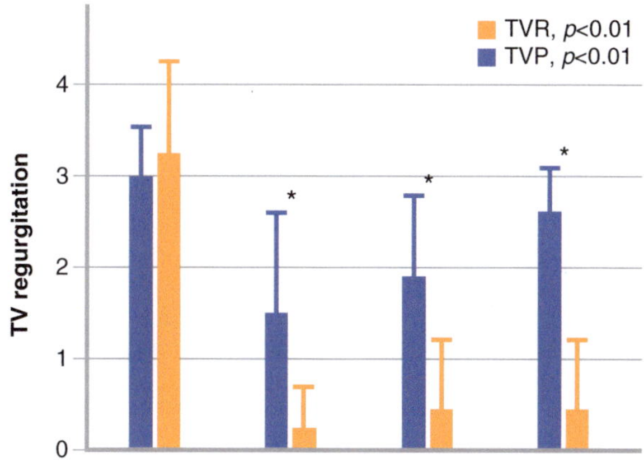

Fig. 29.13 Follow-up of tricuspid regurgitation. Significant improvement of tricuspid valve function was observed both after tricuspid valve replacement and after tricuspid valve repair. After tricuspid repair however, the improvement was less prominent, and recurrent tricuspid regurgitation was observed frequently. *TVP* tricuspid valvuloplasty, *TVR* tricuspid valve replacement

(p=0.09); however, recurrent moderate or more tricuspid valve regurgitation was observed frequently (37 %) in patients who underwent tricuspid valvuloplasty (Fig. 29.13).

Follow Up and Conclusion

All patients, unoperated and operated, should have periodic evaluation by a specialist in congenital heart disease. The evaluation should include a detailed imaging study by echocardiography and/or magnetic resonance imaging (MRI). Declining systemic ventricular function should prompt a search for worsening AV valve regurgitation. Exercise testing facilitates detection of subtle deterioration in "asymptomatic" patients and allows exercise guidelines to be prescribed and also helps with the timing of operation. Symptoms or signs of arrhythmia warrant detailed investigation and a review of underlying hemodynamic abnormalities. The decision to proceed with physiologic versus anatomic repair and the timing of operation is individualized. Most patients require endocarditis prophylaxis unless they have no valvular dysfunction, outflow obstruction, or VSD [37].

References

1. Ferencz C, Rubin JD, McCarter RJ, et al. Congenital heart disease: prevalence at live birth. The Baltimore-Washington infant study. Am J Epidemiol. 1985;121:31–6.
2. Losekoot TG, Becker AE. Discordant atrioventricular connexion and congenitally corrected transposition. In: Anderson RH, MacCartney FJ, Shinebourne EA, Tynan A, editors. Paediatric cardiology. Edinburgh: Churchill Livingstone; 1987. p. 867–88.
3. Becker AE, Anderson RH. Atrioventricular discordance in pathology of congenital heart disease. London: Butterworth; 1981. p. 225–40.

4. Freedom RM, Benson LN, Smallhorn JF. Congenitally transposition of the great arteries. In: Moller JH, Neal WA, editors. Fetal, neonatal and infantcardiac disease. Norwalk: Appleton and Lange; 1989. p. 555–70.
5. Langley SM, Winlaw DS, Stumper O, et al. Midterm results after restoration of the morphologically left ventricle to the systemic circulation in patients with congenitally corrected transposition of the great arteries. J Thorac Cardiovasc Surg. 2003;125:1229–41.
6. Anderson KR, Danielson GK, McGoon DW, et al. Ebstein's anomaly of the left-sided tricuspid valve. Pathological anatomy of the valvular malformation. Circulation. 1978;58:87–91.
7. Anderson RH, Becker AE, Arnold R, et al. The conducting tissues in congenitally corrected transposition. Circulation. 1974;50:911–23.
8. De Leval MR, Basto P, Stark J, et al. Surgical technique to reduce the risks of heart block following closure of ventricular septal defect in atrioventricular discordance. J Thorac Cardiovasc Surg. 1979;78:515–26.
9. Imai Y. Double-switch operation for congenitally corrected transposition. Adv Card Surg. 1997;9:65–86.
10. Prieto LR, Hordof AJ, Secic M, et al. Progressive tricuspid valve disease in patients with congenitally corrected transposition of the great arteries. Circulation. 1998;98:997–1005.
11. Beauchesne LM, Warnes CA, Connolly HM, et al. Outcome of the unoperated adult who presents with congenitally corrected transposition of the great arteries. J Am Coll Cardiol. 2002;40:285–90.
12. Warnes CA. The adult with congenital heart disease: born to be bad? J Am Coll Cardiol. 2005;46:1–8.
13. Mongeon FP, Connolly HM, Dearani JA, Li Z, Warnes CA. Congenitally corrected transposition of the great arteries ventricular function at the time of systemic atrioventricular valve replacement predicts long-term ventricular function. J Am Coll Cardiol. 2011;57:2008–17.
14. Dearani JA, Said SM, Burkhart HM, Pike RB, O'Leary PW, Cetta F. Strategies for tricuspid re-repair in Ebstein malformation using the cone technique. Ann Thorac Surg. 2013;96(1):202–8.
15. Hraska V, Duncan B, Mayer Jr JE, et al. Long-term outcome of surgically treated patients with corrected transposition of the great arteries. J Thorac Cardiovasc Surg. 2005;129:182–91.
16. Termignon JL, Leca F, Vouhe PR, et al. "Classic" repair of congenitally corrected transposition and ventricular septal defect. Ann Thorac Surg. 1996;62:199–206.
17. Metton O, Gaudin R, Ou P, et al. Early prophylactic pulmonary artery banding in isolated congenitally corrected transposition of the great arteries. Eur J Cardiothorac Surg. 2010;38(6): 728–34.
18. Jahangiri M, Redington AN, Elliott MJ, et al. A case for anatomic correction in atrioventricular discordance? Effects of surgery on tricuspid valve function. J Thorac Cardiovasc Surg. 2001;121:1040–5.
19. Baslaim G. Modification of Trusler's formula for the pulmonary artery banding. Heart Lung Circ. 2009;18(5):353–7.
20. Albus RA, Trusler GA, Izukawa T, Williams W. Pulmonary artery banding. J Thorac Cardiovasc Surg. 1984;88:645–53.
21. Trusler GA, Mustard WT. A method of banding the pulmonary artery for large isolated ventricular septal defect with and without transposition of the great arteries. Ann Thorac Surg. 1972;13:351–5.
22. Corno AF, Bonnet D, Sekarski N, Sidi D, Vouhé P, von Segesser LK. Remote control of pulmonary blood flow: initial clinical experience. J Thorac Cardiovasc Surg. 2003;126(6): 1775–80.
23. Graham Jr TP, Bernard YD, Mellen BG, et al. Long-term outcome in congenitally corrected transposition of the great arteries: a multi-institutional study. J Am Coll Cardiol. 2000;36: 255–61.
24. Acar P, Sidi D, Bonnet D, et al. Maintaining tricuspid valve competence in double discordance: a challenge for the pediatric cardiologist. Heart. 1998;80:479–83.
25. Tulevski II, Zijta FM, Smeijers AS, et al. Regional and global right ventricular dysfunction in asymptomatic or minimally symptomatic patients with congenitally corrected transposition. Cardiol Young. 2004;14:168–73.

26. Espinola-Zavaleta N, Erick AE, Attie F, et al. Right ventricular function and ventricular perfusion defects in adults with congenitally corrected transposition: correlation of echocardiography and nuclear medicine. Cardiol Young. 2004;14:174–81.
27. Gregoric ID, Kosir R, Smart FW, et al. Left ventricular assist device implantation in a patient with congenitally corrected transposition of the great arteries. Tex Heart Inst J. 2005;32:567–9.
28. Sue SH, Wei J, Chuang YC, et al. Cardiac transplantation for congenitally corrected transposition of the great arteries: a case report. Transplant Proc. 2008;40(8):2844–5.
29. Alghamdi AA, McCrindle BW, Van Arsdell GS. Physiologic versus anatomic repair of congenitally corrected transposition of the great arteries: meta-analysis of individual patient data. Ann Thorac Surg. 2006;81:1529–35.
30. Van Son JA, Danielson GK, Huhta JC, et al. Late results of systemic atrioventricular valve replacement in corrected transposition. J Thorac Cardiovasc Surg. 1995;109:642–52.
31. Rutledge JM, Nihill MR, Fraser CD, et al. Outcome of 121 patients with congenitally corrected transposition of the great arteries. Pediatr Cardiol. 2002;23:137–45.
32. Lundstrom U, Bull C, Wyse RK, et al. The natural and "unnatural" history of congenitally corrected transposition. Am J Cardiol. 1990;65:1222–9.
33. Metcalfe J, Somerville J. Surgical repair of lesions associated with corrected transposition: late results. Br Heart J. 1983;50:476–82.
34. McGrath LB, Kirklin JW, Blackstone EH, et al. Death and other events after cardiac repair in discordant atrioventricular connection. J Thorac Cardiovasc Surg. 1985;90:711–28.
35. Sano T, Riesenfeld T, Karl TR, et al. Intermediate-term outcome after intracardiac repair of associated cardiac defects in patients with atrioventricular and ventriculoarterial discordance. Circulation. 1995;92(9 suppl):II-272–8.
36. Scherptong RW, Vliegen HW, Winter MM, et al. Tricuspid valve surgery in adults with a dysfunctional systemic right ventricle: repair or replace? Circulation. 2009;119:1467–72.
37. Warnes CA. Transposition of the great arteries. Circulation. 2006;114:2699–709.

Chapter 30
Anatomically Corrected Malposition of the Great Arteries

Richard Van Praagh, Andrew D.G. Van Praagh, and Francois Lacour-Gayet

Abstract Anatomically corrected malposition (ACM) of the great arteries is a rare anomaly of the conotruncus (infundibulum and great arteries) and of the ventricles. Although very malpositioned, the great arteries nonetheless arise above the morphologically appropriate ventricles, aorta (Ao) above the morphologically left ventricle (LV), and pulmonary artery (PA) above the morphologically right ventricle (RV). How is this possible? Because the ventricles loop in one direction, and the great arteries twist in the opposite direction. For example, the ventricles loop in one direction, say to the right, forming a ventricular D-loop, and the infundibuloarterial cardiovascular segment twists to the left, resulting in L-malposition of the great arteries. This is how the commonest form of ACM is formed; the resulting segmental anatomy is situs solitus of the viscera and atria, *D*-loop ventricles, and *L*-malposition of the great arteries, i.e., ACM {S,D,L}. There is atrioventricular (AV) concordance and ventriculoarterial (VA) concordance (but very different from normally related great arteries). Although there is always VA concordance in ACM, by definition, there can be AV discordance, as for example in ACM {S,L,D} and in ACM {I,D,L}. In terms of segmental anatomy, there are six anatomic types of ACM. Associated malformation are often clinically, hemodynamically, and surgically important. Surgical repair of ACM is rarely reported, with some publications limited to the repair of associated lesions in the {S,D,L} form with atrio-ventricular concordance. In the presence of AV discordance ({S,L,D} and {I,D,L}), the condition presents with a transposition physiology. It could be anatomically and

R. Van Praagh, MD, FACC, FAHA, AM(Hon), DrMedHC
Professor of Pathology Emeritus, Harvard Medical School, Boston, MA 02115, USA

Departments of Pathology, Cardiology, and Cardiac Surgery, Boston Children's Hospital, 300 Longwood Avenue, Boston, MA 02115, USA

A.D.G. Van Praagh, PhD
Preclinical Imaging Department of Bruker, Biospin Corporation, Billerica, MA, USA

F. Lacour-Gayet, MD (✉)
Department of Pediatric Cardiac Surgery, National Heart and Lung Institute,
Royal Brompton Hospital, Imperial College University, Sydney Street, London SW3 6NP, UK
e-mail: flacourgayet@mac.com

F. Lacour-Gayet et al. (eds.), *Surgery of Conotruncal Anomalies*,
DOI 10.1007/978-3-319-23057-3_30

physiologically corrected by an atrial switch operation undertaken in the first month of life, or later following LV retraining. A Senning or a Mustard procedure could be considered and would be challenging because of the frequent association of left juxtaposition of the atrial appendages.

Keywords Anatomically corrected transposition of the great arteries • Congenital Heart Disease • Pathology • Cardiac Surgery • Conotruncal Anomaly • AV discordance • Left juxtaposition of atrial appendages

Introduction

Anatomically corrected malposition (ACM) of the great arteries is a rare type of conotruncal malformation in which the great arteries are malpositioned, but nonetheless arise above the anatomically correct ventricles: the malpositioned aorta (Ao) above the morphologically left ventricle (LV), and the malpositioned pulmonary artery (PA) above the morphologically right ventricle (RV) [1, 2]. In 1971 it was suggested that these anomalies be called anatomically corrected *malposition* of the great arteries [3], rather than anatomically corrected *transposition* — which was the prior name of these malformations [2], in the interests of anatomic accuracy. In ACM, transposition of the great arteries is not present, by definition [1, 3].

The surgery of this very rare conotruncal anomaly addresses the atrio-ventricular discordance, and the associated lesions.

Anatomy

Definition of Anatomically Corrected Malposition

ACM is a rare conotruncal anomaly in which *the ventricles loop in one direction, and the great arteries twist in the opposite direction, and there is ventriculo-arterial concordance.* Depending on the visceroatrial situs and on the looping of the ventricles, there are six anatomical types.

ACM {S,D,L}

ACM {S,D,L} Fig. 30.1, top row, leftmost diagram) is anatomically corrected malposition (ACM) of the great arteries with situs solitus of the viscera and atria {*S*,-,-}, D-loop ventricles {S,*D*,-}, and L-malposition of the great arteries {S,D,*L*}. Braces { } mean “the set of.” As the anatomy of the segmental situs set suggests — {*S*,*D*,L}, there is atrioventricular (AV) concordance (associated malformations permitting).

As the designation ACM indicates – *ACM* {S,D,L}, there is ventriculoarterial (VA) concordance. As the segmental anatomy indicates – ACM {S,*D,L*}, the ventricles have looped to the right (D-loop), but the great arteries have twisted to the left (L-malposition).

This is characteristic of ACM: *the ventricles loop in one direction, and the great arteries twist in the opposite direction.* Indeed, these opposite VA torsions make possible ACM. Associated malformations in ACM {S,D,L} can be numerous and severe, as will be seen. The subarterial infundibulum or conus arteriosus can be subaortic (only), or bilateral (subaortic and subpulmonary).

VA concordance is characteristic of ACM. There are two different anatomic types of VA concordance: 1- with normally related great arteries (solitus and inversus isomers), and 2- with ACM.

ACM {S,D,L} has AV concordance and VA concordance. Hence the systemic venous and pulmonary venous circulations are potentially normal physiologically, unless the potentially normal physiology is vitiated by associated malformations – which often is the case.

ACM {S,L,D}

ACM {S,L,D} (Fig. 30.1, top row, diagram second from the left) has visceroatrial situs solitus, L-loop ventricles, and D-malposition of the great arteries. The segmental anatomy – {S,L,D} – indicates AV discordance. The presence of ACM indicates VA concordance, by definition. The presence of one intersegmental discordance (at the AV level) indicates that this type of ACM is physiologically uncorrected. Hence, an atrial switch procedure (Senning or Mustard) might well merit consideration therapeutically. One would not want to perform an arterial switch procedure because VA concordance is present. Associated malformations should be searched for carefully and managed appropriately.

Note also that in ACM {S,L,D}, the ventricles have looped to the *left*, and the great arteries have twisted to the *right.* Opposite ventriculo-arterial torsions are why ACM is so rare. Usually, the direction of ventricular looping and the direction of great arterial twisting are the same – both to the right, as in TGA {S,D,D}, or both to the left, as in TGA {S,L,L}. Usually, the embryonic ventriculo-infundibulo-arterial loop resembles the letter C, convex to the right, as in TGA {S,D,D}. In TGA {S,L,L}, this embryonic loop resembles a "backwards" C, convex to the left. But in ACM, the embryonic loop has two opposite convexities, like the letter S, or like a backwards letter S.

The two opposite torsions of the embryonic heart tube in ACM explain not only why ACM is so rare, but also how it is possible for very malpositioned great arteries to originate nonetheless above the morphologically appropriate ventricles: Ao above the LV, and PA above the RV. Although there is VA concordance, the great arteries are not normally related in ACM (Fig. 30.1). Typically, the aortic valve is anterior to the pulmonary valve, and the aortic valve is widely separated from the mitral valve because of the presence of a subaortic muscular conus. As ACM

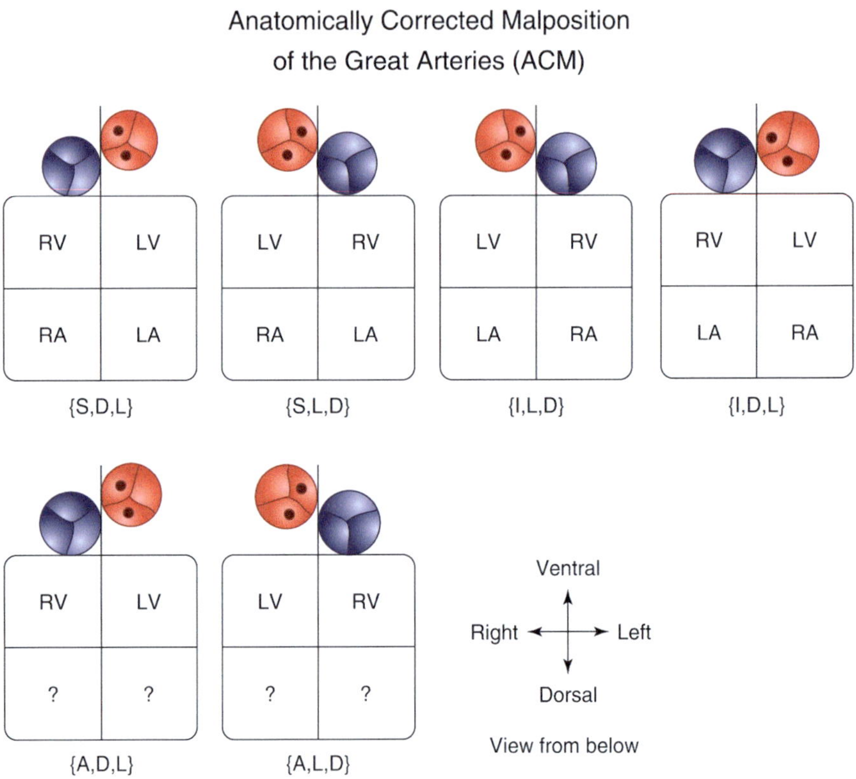
Anatomically Corrected Malposition
of the Great Arteries (ACM)
RV
LV
RA
LA
{S,D,L}
LV
RV
RA
LA
{S,L,D}
LV
RV
LA
RA
{I,L,D}
RV
LV
LA
RA
{I,D,L}
RV
LV
?
?
{A,D,L}
LV
RV
?
?
{A,L,D}
Ventral
Right
Left
Dorsal
View from below

Fig. 30.1 Types of anatomically corrected malposition of the great arteries (*ACM*). The diagrams are viewed from the front and below, similar to a subxiphoid two-dimensional echocardiogram: anterior (ventral), towards the *top* of the page; posterior (dorsal), towards the *bottom* of the page; right side of the hearts toward the viewer's left hand; and left side of the hearts towards the viewer's right hand. **Anatomically corrected** malposition of the great arteries means that despite their malposition, the great arteries nonetheless arise above the *anatomically correct* ventricles: aortic valve, indicated by the two coronary ostia above the morphologically left ventricle (*LV*); and pulmonary valve, indicate by no coronary ostia above the morphologically right ventricle (*RV*). **ACM {S,D,L}** (leftmost diagram, *top row*) indicates that viscera and atria are in situs solitus: {**S**,-,-}. The morphologically right atrium (*RA*) lies to the right and is right-handed, and the morphologically left atrium (*LA*) is to the left and is left-handed. A ventricular D-loop is present: {S,**D**,-}. The RV is right-sided and right-handed, and the LV is left-sided and left-handed. L-malposition of the great arteries is present: {S,D,**L**}. The aortic valve is left-sided and usually somewhat anterior relative to the pulmonary valve. There is atrioventricular (AV) concordance and ventriculoarterial (VA) concordance. In ACM, the VA concordance is very different from that of normally related great arteries (NRGA). With NRGA, there is aortic valve-to-mitral valve direct fibrous continuity. But with ACM, there typically is aortic valve-to-mitral valve wide separation because of the presence of subaortic conal musculature. **Braces {}** are mathematical symbols meaning "the set of". The elements of the segmental anatomic set are separated by commas, as in ACM {S,D,L}. The foregoing is standard mathematical set notation. Parentheses () or brackets [] are not used. **ACM {S,L,D}** (diagram second from the left, *top row*) means anatomically corrected malposition of the great arteries with situs solitus of the viscera and atria, discordant L-loop ventricles, and concordant D-malposition of the great arteries. There is *physiologic uncorrection* of the systemic and pulmonary venous circulations because there is one intersegmental discordance (of the AV alignments). Although there is VA concordance, it is very different from the VA concordance with normally related great arteries (NRGA). **There are two anatomic types of VA concordance: (1) with NRGA (solitus and inversus), and (2) with ACM. ACM {I,L,D}** (third diagram from the left, *top row*) denotes ACM with visceroatrial situs inversus, concordant ventricular L-loop, and concordant D-malposition of the great arteries. **ACM {I,D,L}** (rightmost diagram, *top row*) means ACM with visceroatrial situs inversus, discordant D-loop ventricles, and concordant L-malposition of the great arteries. Whenever there is AV discordance with ACM, the circulations are physiologically uncorrected, suggesting that an atrial switch procedure (Senning or Mustard) might be helpful therapeutically, depending also on the associated malformations that often coexist. **Note that in ACM, the ventricles have looped in one direction, and the infundibuloarterial segment (the conotruncus) has twisted in the opposite direction.** ACM rarely can also occur in the **heterotaxy syndromes with congenital asplenia or polysplenia and with visceroatrial situs ambiguus**. [Note: *ambiguus* is correct Latin spelling; *ambiguous* is correct English spelling.] When the viscera and atria are in situs ambiguus, the basic type of situs (solitus, or inversus) may be uncertain or unknown. Question marks (??) indicate that the situs of the atria (the pattern of anatomic organization) is uncertain or unknown (undiagnosed). The concept of atrial level *isomerism* (bilaterally right, or bilaterally left) is an error. Instead, we say that the atrial situs is unknown: ? means unknown, or situs ambiguus in Latin. **When the atrial situs is unknown, the diagnoses of AV concordance and AV discordance cannot be made. ACM {A,D,L}** (left diagram, *bottom row*) means that there is visceroatrial situs ambiguus, D-loop ventricles, and concordant L-malposition of the great arteries. **ACM {A,L,D}** (right diagram, *bottom row*) means that there is visceroatrial situs ambiguus, L-loop ventricles, and concordant D-malposition of the great arteries.

illustrates, VA concordance is not synonymous with normally related great arteries (solitus, and inversus).

ACM also occurs in patients with visceroatrial situs inversus (Fig. 30.1).

ACM {I,L,D}

ACM {I,L,D} has situs inversus of the viscera and atria, a concordant ventricular L-loop, and concordant D-malposition of the great arteries (Fig. 30.1, top row, third diagram from the left). If the absence of associated malformations permits, ACM {I,L,D} is both anatomically corrected and physiologically corrected. ACM {I,L,D} is a mirror-image of ACM {S,D,L} (Fig. 30.1).

ACM {I,D,L} [4]

ACM {I,D,L} [4] (Fig. 30.1, top row, rightmost diagram) has AV discordance, meaning that this anomaly is physiologically uncorrected. This, in turn, suggests that such a patient might benefit from a surgical atrial switch procedure (Senning or Mustard).

ACM has also been reported in the heterotaxy syndromes with visceroatrial situs ambiguus and asplenia [5] or polysplenia [6]. We have not seen such cases ourselves. AV concordance and/or AV discordance cannot be diagnosed when ACM is associated with the heterotaxy syndromes of asplenia or polysplenia with visceroatrial situs ambiguus – because the anatomic type of atrial situs is uncertain or unknown (Fig. 30.1, bottom row, *ACM {A,D,L}* and *ACM {A,L,D}*).

ACM {A,D,L}

ACM {A,D,L} (Fig. 30.1, bottom row, left diagram) has visceroatrial situs ambiguus (uncertain or unknown type of situs), with D-loop ventricles, and L-malposition of the great arteries. Because the anatomic type of visceroatrial situs is undiagnosed, the AV alignments cannot be described as concordant or as discordant.

ACM {A,L,D}

ACM {A,L,D} (Fig. 30.1, bottom row, right diagram) has visceroatrial situs ambiguus, L-loop ventricles, and D-malposition of the great arteries.

Associated Malformations

In ACM, associated malformations often are very important clinically and surgically. For example, **Case 1** of the Van Praaghs [2] was a 2 year and 20 day old girl with ACM **{S,D,L}** who also had (Fig. 30.2) dextrocardia, tricuspid atresia, a large secundum atrial septal defect, left-sided juxtaposition of the atrial appendages, a small conoventricular type of ventricular septal defect (VSD), and pulmonary valvar stenosis (PS) with a bicuspid and bicommissural pulmonary valve. The presence of tricuspid atresia, a small VSD (subpulmonary stenosis), and valvar PS (Fig. 30.2) vitiated the potential physiologic correction of the circulations suggested by the segmental anatomy ACM {S,D,L} (Fig. 30.1).

Note also that the subarterial infundibulum, which is mostly subaortic, is located mainly above the *left* ventricle. This observation emphasizes the basic point that the subarterial infundibulum or conus arteriosus is *not* an intrinsic, inseparable part of the RV. Instead, the infundibulum belongs with the great arteries, i.e., the conotruncus, The subarterial conus arteriosus is how the great arteries connect with the underlying ventricles, ventricular septum, and atrioventricular canal. This is why the conus can override the ventricular septum to any degree: because the subarterial conus or infundibulum is really *not* part of the RV (Fig. 30.2).

Case 2 of the Van Praaghs [2] was a girl who died at 4 weeks and 3 days of age. Autopsy revealed ACM **{S,D,L}** (Fig. 30.3) with very similar associated malformations: left-sided juxtaposition of the atrial appendages, secundum atrial septal defect, a conoventricular type of ventricular septal defect, mild hypoplasia of the right ventricle, a bilateral conus (subaortic and subpulmonary), the subaortic part of the conus mostly above the left ventricle (Fig. 30.3c), and pulmonary atresia (Fig. 30.3d).

Case 3 [2] (Fig. 30.4) was a 4 week and 5 day old boy with ACM **{S,L,D}** (Fig. 30.1 top row, second diagram from the left). Associated malformations included a conoventricular type of ventricular septal defect, preductal coarctation of the aorta, and a patent ductus arteriosus (Fig. 30.4). The conus was bilateral; the subaortic part of the conus was above the left ventricle, and the subpulmonary part was above the right ventricle (Fig. 30.4).

In 1975, Van Praagh and colleagues [7] published two autopsy-proved cases of ACM {S,D,L} with a muscular *subaortic conus only*. Their previously reported cases of ACM had all had a bilateral conus [2]. These observations proved that ACM can occur both with a suboartic conus (only) and with a bilateral (subaortic and subpulmonary) conus.

Surgery of Anatomically Corrected Malposition

Anatomically corrected malposition of great arteries (ACM) is a rare form of conotruncal anomaly in which the great arteries arise above the anatomically correct ventricles but have abnormal spatial relationship. First documented convincingly with photographs by Richard and Stella Van Praagh in 1967 [2] and later in 1975 [7], this rare condition is frequently misdiagnosed as congenitally corrected TGA. There are six forms of ACM as shown in Fig. 30.1, depending on the viscero-atrial situs (solitus, inversus, or ambiguus) and the presence of an atrio-ventricular discordance. A left juxtaposition of the atrial appendages is frequent and could modify the surgical techniques.

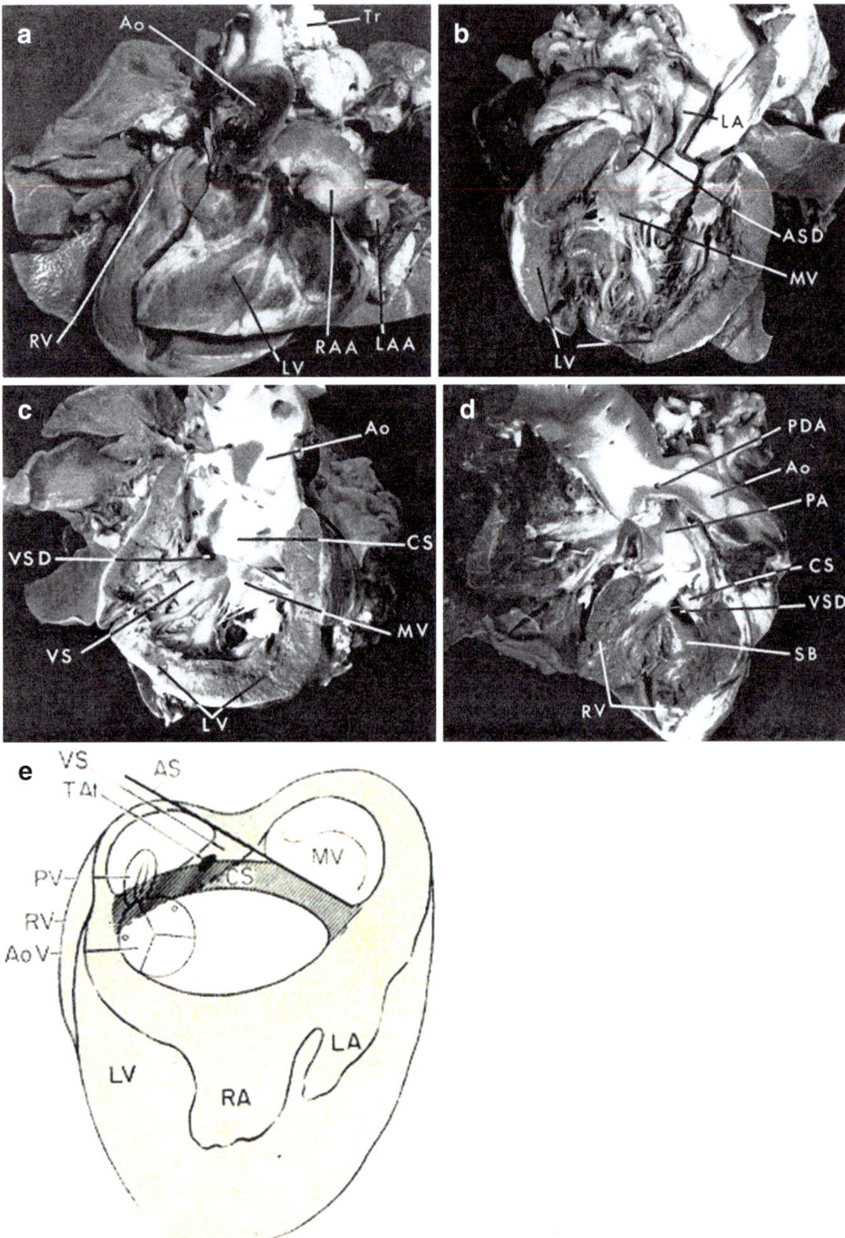
a
Ao
Tr
RV
LV
RAA
LAA
b
LA
ASD
MV
LV
c
Ao
CS
VSD
MV
VS
LV
d
PDA
Ao
PA
CS
VSD
SB
RV
e
VS
AS
TAI
MV
CS
PV
RV
AoV
LA
LV
RA

Surgery of ACM with AV Concordance (ACM-AVC)

A review of the literature indicates that the surgical results are satisfactory in patients with atrioventricular concordance {S,D,L} (Fig. 30.5), where the surgery in these forms is limited to the repair of the associated lesions. Several publications report successful correction of the {S,D,L} form: VSD repair [9, 10, 15]: relief of LVOT obstruction [8, 11] and others. Hypoplasia of one ventricle is frequent and would indicate a Fontan procedure.

Surgery of ACM with AV Discordance (ACM-AVD)

On the contrary, there are no publications to our knowledge on surgical repair of ACM with AV discordance {S,L,D}, {I, D,L} (Fig. 30.1). In the situs solitus form *{S,L,D}* (Fig. 30.1, top row, second from the left) (Fig. 30.5), the ventricles have looped to the left resulting in AV discordance with ventricular inversion, while the ventriculoarterial (VA) alignments are concordant. The situs inversus form {I,D,L} is the mirror-image of {S,L,D}. In ACM-AVD, the physiology and hemodynamics are similar to a transposition of the great arteries, because there is one intersegmental discordance at the AV level. The ventricles are "transposed". The systemic circulation is delivered by a morphologically left ventricle (LV), while the pulmonary circulation depends on a morphologically right ventricle (RV). This anomaly is not compatible with life unless a communication is present at the level of the great vessels (PDA), the interatrial septum (ASD), or the interventricular septum (VSD).

The ACM-AVD with intact ventricular septum could only survive the newborn period if managed like a transposition with intact septum and benefit from Prostaglandin infusion and/or Rashkind septostomy. Those with ACM-AVD with VSD will survive and are at risk for PHT.

An atrial switch operation (Senning or Mustard) would correct both the anatomy and the physiology, by placing: – the right atrium in continuity with the right ven-

Fig. 30.2 ACM {S,D,L} in a 2 year and 20 day old girl. (**a**). External anteroposterior view. (**b**). Opened left atrium (*LA*) and left ventricular (*LV*) inflow tract. (**c**). Opened LV outflow tract to L-malposed aorta (*Ao*). (**d**) Opened small right ventricle (*RV*) to malposed pulmonary artery (*PA*). (**e**) Geometric diagram of the heart, viewed from above. Associated malformations include: tricuspid atresia (*TAt*); left-sided juxtaposition of the atrial appendages; (*RAA*), right atrial appendage; (*LAA*), left atrial appendage; dextrocardia; secundum type of atrial septal defect (*ASD*); normally formed mitral valve (*MV*); prominent subaortic conal septal (*CS*) musculature above the LV, conal musculature widely separating aortic valve (*AoV*) above from MV below; small conoventricular type of ventricular septal defect (*VSD*) between conal septum (*CS*) above and the ventricular septum (*VS*) and septal band (*SB*) below; the smallness of the VSD contributes to the subpulmonary stenosis; the stenotic pulmonary valve (PV) is bicuspid and bicommissural. The associated malformations vitiated the potential physiologic correction of the circulations of this segmental set or combination, ACM {S,D,L} (Reproduced with permission from Van Praagh and Van Praagh [2])

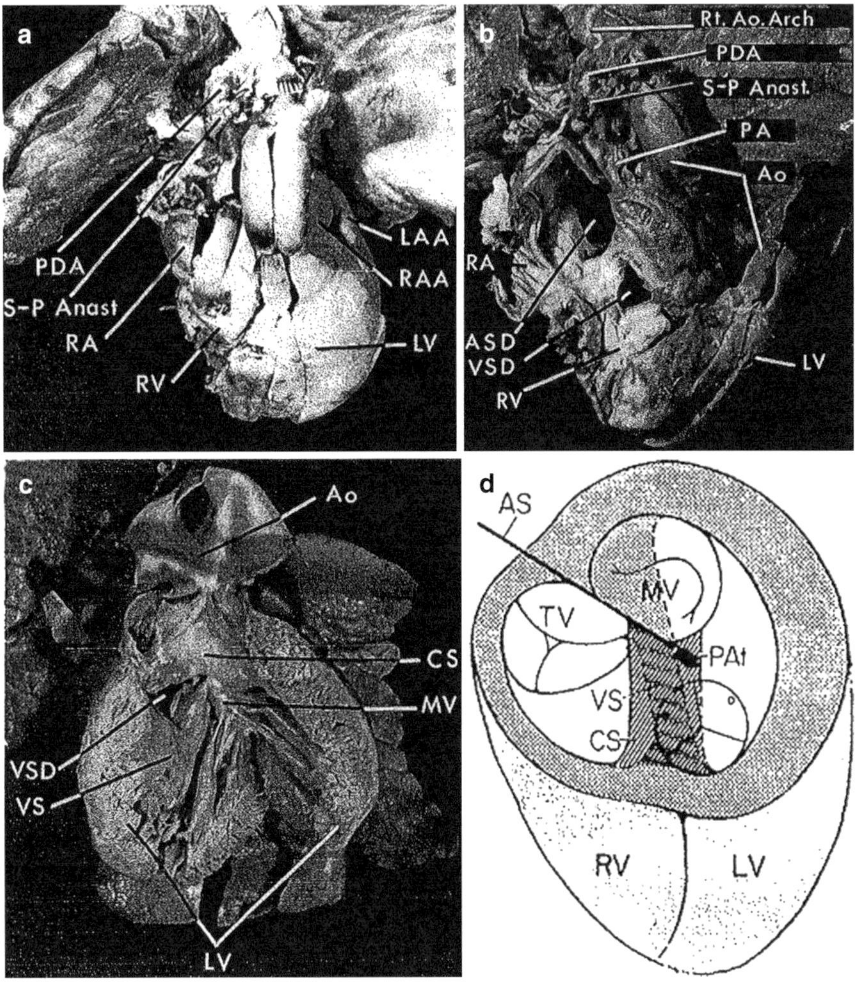

Fig. 30.3 **ACM {S,D,L}** in a 4 week and 3 day old girl. (**a**) Ventral view of the heart and lungs. (**b**) Opened right atrium (*RA*) and right ventricle (*RV*). (**c**) Opened left ventricle (*LV*) and L-malposed aorta (*Ao*). (**d**) Geometric heart diagram, viewed from above. Abbreviations as in Fig. 30.2, except for: *PAt* pulmonary outflow tract atresia, *PDA* patent ductus arteriosus, *Rt Ao arch* right aortic arch, *S-P Anast* subclavian pulmonary anastomosis. Associated malformations included: a large secundum type of atrial septal defect (*ASD*); a moderate sized conoventricular type of ventricular septal defect (*VSD*); conus arteriosus musculature (*CS*) that is located largely above the LV and that prevents aortic valve – mitral valve (*MV*) direct fibrous continuity; and pulmonary atresia (*PAt*) that was the most important associated anomaly (Reproduced with permission from Van Praagh and Van Praagh [2])

tricle and the pulmonary artery, – and the left atrium in continuity with the left ventricle and the aorta. However, the atrial switch in ACM-AVD with intact ventricular septum would need to be performed in the month of life when the LV has kept its capability to sustain a systemic pressure, or later following LV retraining.

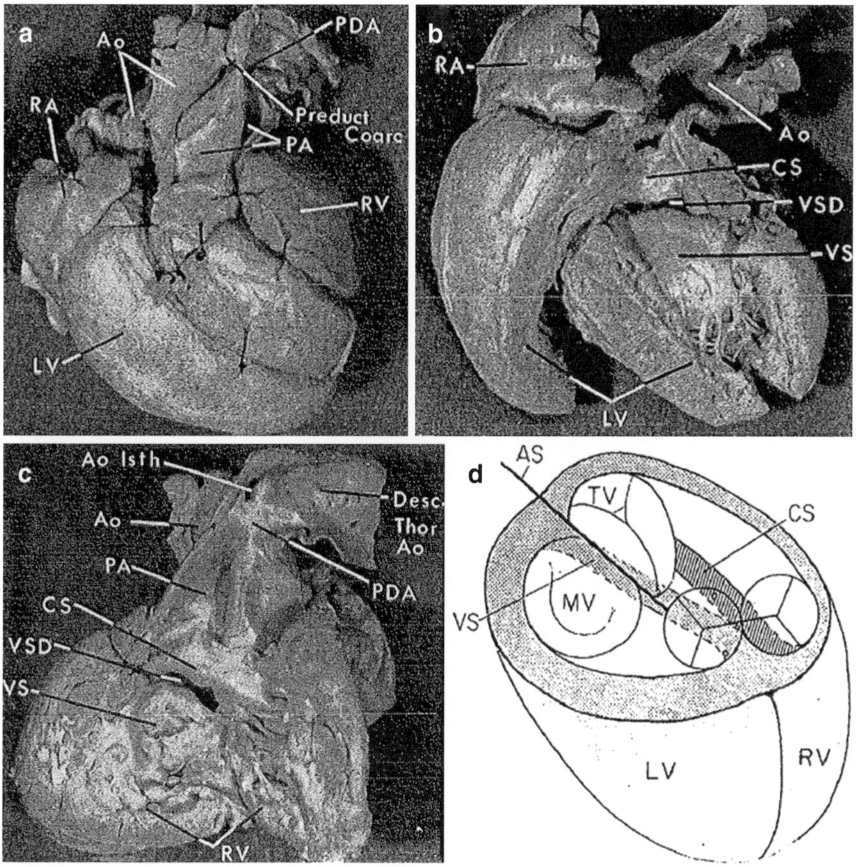

Fig. 30.4 **ACM {S,L,D}** in a 4 week and 5 day old boy who died of congestive heart failure. (**a**). Anterior (ventral) view of the heart specimen. (**b**). View of the opened right-sided left ventricle (*LV*) and of the narrowed right-sided D-malposed aorta (Ao). (**c**). The opened left-sided morphologically right ventricle (*RV*) and the opened widely patent outflow tract to the pulmonary artery (*PA*) and the PDA. Note the small lumen of the aortic isthmus (*Ao Isth*), indicating the presence of a preductual coarctation of the aorta (**a**, *Preduct Coarc*). (**d**). Geometric diagram of the heart, as seen from above. Abbreviations as previously, except for: (*Desc Thor Ao*), descending thoracic aorta. The conus arteriosus was bilateral, both subaortic (**b**) and subpulmonary (**c**). The aortic outflow was narrowed (**b**) and the ascending aorta was hypoplastic compared with the main pulmonary artery (**a**). Preductal coartation of the aorta was present (**a**), with narrowing of the aortic isthmus (*Ao Isth*). The ductus arteriosus was patent (*PDA*) in **a** and **c**. Aortic outflow tract stenosis, preductal coarctation of the aorta, a widely patent pulmonary outflow tract, and a patent ductus arteriosus together explain why this patient died of congestive heart failure at 4 5/7 weeks of age (Reproduced with permission from Van Praagh and Van Praagh [2].)

The frequent association of left juxtaposition of the atrial appendages complicates the atrial switch procedure because of the small size of the right atrium. The Senning procedure would be challenging and would need an enlargement of the pulmonary venous channel (the “knee” of the Senning) using a flap of autologous

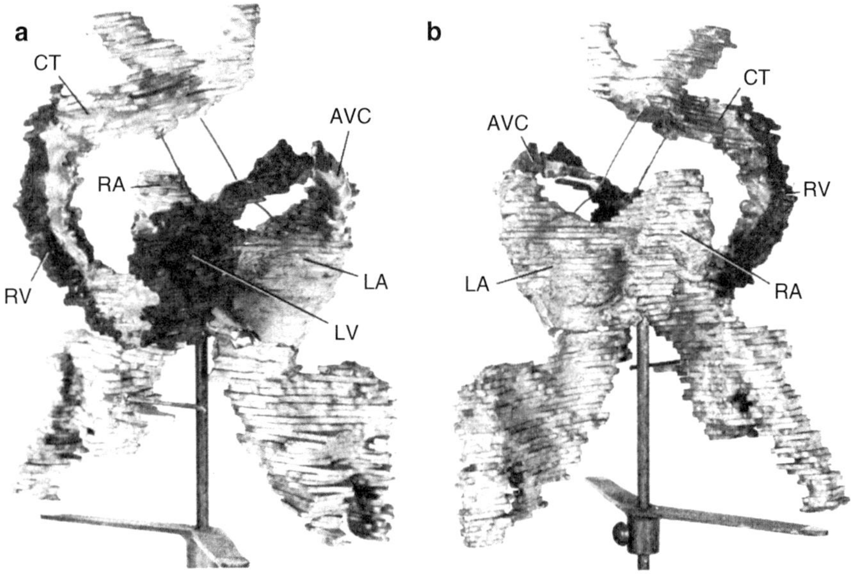

Fig. 30.5 A reconstruction of the cardiac lumen of Carnegie human embryo 470, Streeter's horizon 11, 17 pairs of somites, 4.3 mm crown-rump length, estimated age since ovulation 23 days. The spatial relations of left juxtaposition of the atrial appendages (LJAA) are present. The developing morphologically right ventricle (*RV*) and the conotruncus (*CT*) both lie to the right of the morphologically right atrium (*RA*) and the morphologically left atrium (*LA*). (**a**). Anterior (ventral) view. (**b**). Posterior (dorsal) view. *Other abbreviations:* (*AVC*), atrioventricular canal; (*LV*), morphologically left ventricle. (Reproduced with permission from Melhuish and Van Praagh [14])

pericardium, as described by Ake Senning [12]. A Mustard procedure undertaken in the first months of life would be the preferred technique as reported by Leonard Bailey in TGA [13].

Comment

ACM is presented at length in the literature, with more than 50 publications[1]. We will discuss the differential diagnosis and present some lessons learned concerning conotruncal anomalies, focusing on the morphology of ACM.

[1] Additional references may be accessed at PubMed using a keyword search of: anatomically corrected malposition of the great arteries

Differential Diagnosis

Isolated Infundibulo-Arterial Inversion {S,D,I}

Liske et al. in 2006 accurately reported a very rare case of isolated infundibulo-arterial inversion {S,D,I}. In this patient, there may have been aortic-mitral fibrous continuity. If so, the great arteries were inverted normally related; i.e., isolated infundibulo-arterial inversion would have been present as the authors stated.

Tsuchida et al. in 1989 reported two patients that they diagnosed as having ACM {S,D,L}. However, in these two patients, there definitely was aortic-mitral fibrous continuity. Consequently, inverted normally related great arteries were present; hence, the correct diagnosis in these two patients was isolated infundibulo-arterial inversion {S,D,*I*}. Anatomically corrected malposition {S,D,*L*} was not present – because the great arteries were inverted normally related (not malpositioned). However, it should be added that isolated infundibulo-arterial inversion {S,D,I} and anatomically corrected malposition {S,D,L} may be very similar or identical *physiologically*, because both have AV and VA concordance. However, the associated malformations in these two anatomically different anomalies may well prove to be distinctive and different. Foran et al. discovered and described isolated infundibulo-arterial inversion {S,D,I}, that was also afflicted with inverted tetralogy of Fallot, in 1988.

To *summarize the point,* isolated infundibuloarterial inversion {S,D,I} should be distinguished diagnostically from ACM {S,D,L}. *The subarterial infundibulum or conus arteriosus should be described with care in routine medical and surgical reports, including the presence or absence of aortic-mitral continuity.*

Double-Outlet Right Ventricle with L-Malposition of the Great Arteries

Anderson et al. accurately described double-outlet right ventricle with L-malposition of the great arteries in 1975. **DORV {S,D,L}** also should be distinguished with care in the differential diagnosis of ACM {S,D,L}.

Awasthy et al. presented a patient with DORV {S,D,L} in 2013. They thought that their patient had DORV {S,D,L} and ACM {S,D,L}. In terms of differential diagnosis, their patient posed the questions: DORV and ACM? Or DORV or ACM? The right answer is DORV or ACM, because the VA alignments are different in DORV and ACM. Their patient had DORV, not ACM. The segmental anatomic set {S,D,L} occurs with a variety of different VA alignments including TGA {S,D,L}, DORV {S,D,L}, and ACM {S,D,L}. Left juxtaposition of the atrial appendages (LJAA) may also coexist. These were the real points of Anderson et al. and of Awasthy et al., and they are entirely correct.

Left Juxtaposition of the Atrial Appendages (LJAA) and ACM

What does left juxtaposition of the atrial appendages (LJAA) have to do with ACM? LJAA is present in both of the aforementioned patients with D-loop ventricles (Figs. 30.2a and 30.3a). In patients with visceroatrial situs solitus and concordant D-loop ventricles, LJAA *indicates abnormal, incomplete D-loop formation.*

LJAA is normal at the early D-loop stage in the human embryo. In a reconstruction of the cardiac lumen of Carnegie human embryo 470, at Streeter's horizon 11 with an estimated age since ovulation of 23 *days*, 17 pairs of somites, and a crown-rump length of 4.3 mm, the morphologically right atrium (RA) and the morphologically left atrium (LA) both lie to the left of the developing morphologically right ventricle (RV) and the conotruncus (CT) (Fig. 30.6).

Soon, however, within about 4 days, this normal early left-sided juxtaposition of the atria and their developing appendages is "cured" by continuing normal development of the bulboventricular D-loop. In a reconstruction of the bulboventricular lumen and the atria of Carnegie human embryo 836 at Streeter's horizon 13, with an estimated age since ovulation of *27 days,* the conotruncus (CT) now passes in front of the RA and is located between the RA and the LA (Please see Fig. 30.2 in ref. [8]). Thus, the normal early LJAA of the human embryo at 23 days of age (Fig. 30.6) is normally "cured" by continuing leftward movement of the bulboventricular D-loop by about 27 days of age in utero (Fig. 30.7).

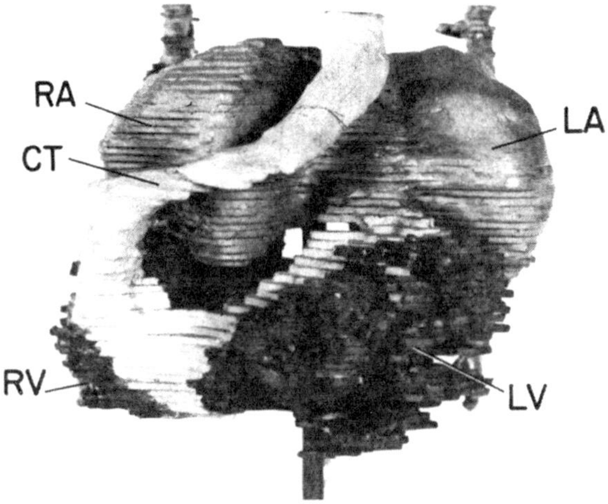

Fig. 30.6 Model of the cardiac lumen of Carnegie human embryo 836, horizon 13, 4 mm crown-rump length, estimated age since ovulation is 27 days. The spatial relations of left-sided juxtaposition of the atrial appendages have disappeared. Now the conotruncus (CT) runs between the RA and the LA. A. Anterior (ventral) view. Abbreviations as in Fig. 30.5. (Reproduced with permission from Melhuish and Van Praagh [14])

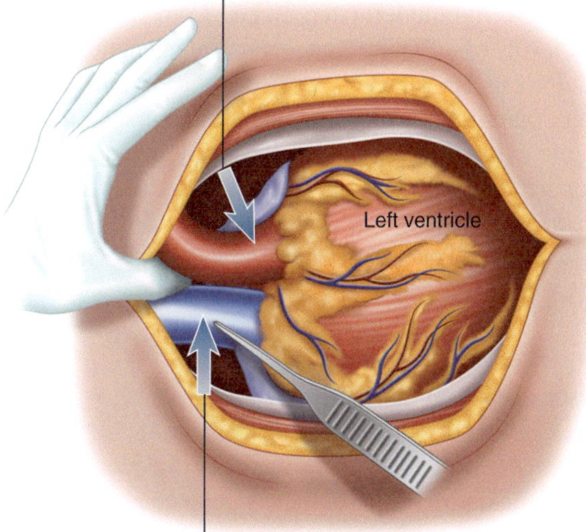

Fig. 30.7 Anatomically Corrected Malposition of the great arteries. {S,D,L} form. Notice the L malposition of aorta with ventriculo-arterial concordance (Reproduced with permission from Sridhar et al. [8])

It is helpful to understand that LJAA has nothing primarily to do with the atrial appendages themselves. The atria and their appendages are relatively fixed in position. But the bulboventricular loop is a professional contortionist. The postnatal presence of LJAA (Figs. 30.2 and 30.3) indicates that the morphogenetic movement of the bulboventricular loop has been abnormal and subnormal, such that the great arteries have not been carried far enough leftward so that they lie between the atrial appendages. Instead, the great arteries remain to the right of both atrial appendages, in their "starting position". Thus, the atrial appendages serve as markers of the abnormal and subnormal morphogenetic movement of the bulboventricular D-loop. The abnormal morphogenetic movement of the bulboventricular D-loop, that is the essence of ACM, is also indicated by the opposite torsions of the ventricles relative to the infundibulo-arterial segment (the conotruncus) (Fig. 30.1). LJAA, (Figs. 30.2 and 30.3) and the S-shaped or reverse S-shaped torsions of the bulboventricular loop (Fig. 30.1) both tell the same story: very abnormal development of the whole bulboventricular loop.

ACM is more than a conotruncal (infundibuloarterial) anomaly. The ventricles are also involved. This is also why so-called associated malformations are so prominent and so important in ACM.

Ventricular looping is a "two-step dance":

With D-looping, first you loop to the right. Then you swing to the left.
With L-looping, first you loop to the left. Then you swing to the right.

In other words, with *D-loop formation*, first the straight heart tube loops to the right (step 1), resulting in dextrocardia (Fig. 30.2a). Then the heart swings horizontally from right to left (step 2), i.e., from dextrocardia, through mesocardia, to normal levocardia. If step 2 of this morphogenetic dance occurs subnormally, then the results can be persistent dextrocardia or mesocardia. Persistent levocardia may occur (abnormal in visceroatrial situs inversus). RJAA may also occur, if both great arteries remain to the left of the atrial appendages. So, a subnormal step 2 of the looping "dance" results in both left-sided and right-sided JAA..

Juxtaposition of the appendages is bulboventricular-loop-dependent. With a D-loop, LJAA occurs because the *leftward* swing was subnormal. With an L-loop, *RJAA* occurs because the *rightward* swing was subnormal.

Associated Anomalies

Dextrocardia and mesocardia are also frequent with ACM, further evidence that in ACM, the entire bulboventricular loop can be malpositioned (Fig. 30.2).

ACM has also been reported in association with the heterotaxy syndromes that have visceroatrial situs ambiguus with asplenia [15], *or polysplenia* [9]; this we have not seen personally. However, ACM in situs ambiguus is included in Fig. 30.1, bottom row.

Although ACM with tetralogy of Fallot has been reported, we think that this is an error. TOF is closely related to normally related great arteries and has aortic-mitral fibrous continuity. In contrast, ACM typically has aortic-mitral discontinuity or wide separation because of the presence of a muscular subaortic conus. However, ACM can have a subaortic VSD with pulmonary outflow tract stenosis that resembles TOF *physiologically.*

ACM has been reported with a bilaterally absent conus by Loya, Desai, and Sharma in 1991 and by Aziz and Patel in 2013. These are noteworthy findings by excellent observers. We have not seen ACM with aortic-mitral fibrous continuity and with pulmonary-tricuspid fibrous continuity, i.e., with a bilaterally absent conus.

Right-sided juxtaposition of the atrial appendages (RJAA) has been reported in association with ACM {I,L,D} (Fig. 30.1). RJAA is a mirror-image of what happens to produce LJAA.

Evolution of the Infundibuloarterial Segment

A little comparative anatomy is helpful in understanding the mammalian conus arteriosus. In sharks, the conus arteriosus musculature extends from the heart all the way cephalad to the aortic (gill) arches. In sharks, the coronary arteries arise from aortic (branchial) arches 2–4. As vertebrates evolved from fish to amphibians, to reptiles, to birds, and to mammals, the conus arteriosus musculature receded to a subsemilunar location and the coronary arteries descended into the sinuses of

Valsalva. The ascending aorta thus became fibroelastic; it was no longer "muscle bound", i.e., encased in conus arteriosus musculature. The arterial trunk, that ascends from the heart, evolved in birds and mammals into the fibroelastic ascending aorta and main pulmonary artery. No longer muscle bound, the fibroelastic great arteries could *untwist normally* between the heart below and the aortic arch and pulmonary artery bifurcation above. That's what the great arteries are doing, both normally and abnormally — *untwisting*. The amount of untwisting performed by the great arteries equals (in degrees) the difference between the semilunar interrelationship proximally (which is highly *variable*), and the aortic arch — pulmonary artery bifurcation relationship distally (which is *fixed* by the aortic arch 4 — pulmonary arch 6 interrelationship). *Distally*, the aorta is always anterior (ventral) and superior (cephalad), and the pulmonary artery is always posterior (dorsal) and inferior (caudad) — as long as both great arteries are present and normal. *Proximally* at the semilunar valves, the aorto-pulmonary interrelationship is highly variable (normal, or abnormal).

With normally related great arteries, the ascending aorta (Ao) and the main pulmonary artery (PA) have much more untwisting to do (approximately 150° of leftward untwisting) than do the Ao and PA *with abnormally related great arteries, such as ACM* (often only about 30 or 40° of untwisting).

Normally, the aortic valve (AoV) typically is posterior relative to the pulmonary valve (PV) which is anterior. But distally, the aortic arch is always anterior relative to the pulmonary artery bifurcation which is posterior.

But *abnormally, such as with ACM*, both proximally (at the semilunar valves) and distally (at the aortic arch - pulmonary artery bifurcation), the Ao is anterior, and the PA is posterior. Hence, abnormally (such as with ACM), the great arteries have much less untwisting to do between the semilunar valves and the aortic arch – PA bifurcation.

The untwisting of the great arteries equals (in degrees) the difference between the AoV — PV interrelationship proximally and the aortic arch — PA *bifurcation relationship distally.*

Both interrelationships can be measured relative to the sagittal plane. Or, the distal aortic arch — PA bifurcation relationship can be regarded as zero degrees rotation. The degree of untwisting of the great arteries can be measured using elementary plane geometry. An accurate understanding of the *conal connector* is important. Anatomically, that is what this whole book is mostly about.

References

1. Van Praagh R. The story of anatomically corrected malposition of the great arteries. Chest. 1976;69:2.
2. Van Praagh R, Van Praagh S. Anatomically corrected transposition of the great arteries. Br Heart J. 1967;29:112.
3. Van Praagh R, Pérez-Treviño C, López-Cuellar M, Baker FW, Zuberbuhler JR, Quero M, Pérez VM, Moreno F, Van Praagh S. Transposition of the great arteries with posterior aorta,

anterior pulmonary artery, subpulmonary conus, and fibrous continuity between aortic and atrioventricular valves. Am J Cardiol. 1971;28:621.
4. Anderson RH, Arnold R, Jones RS. D-bulboventricular loop with L-transposition in situs inversus. Circulation. 1972;46:173.
5. Freedom RM, Harrington DP. Anatomically corrected malposition of the great arteries. Report of two cases, one with congenital asplenia; frequent association with juxtaposition of atrial appendages. Br Heart J. 1974;36:207–15.
6. Salazar J, López C, Felipe J, Ibarra F, Garcia M, Alonso-Lej F. Anatomically corrected malposition of the great arteries in situs ambiguus with polysplenia. Pediatr Cardiol. 1985;6:53–5.
7. Van Praagh R, Durnin RE, Jockin H, Wagner HR, Korns M, Garabedian H, Ando M, Calder AL. Anatomically corrected malposition of the great arteries {S, D, L}. Circulation. 1975;51:20.
8. Sridhar A, Subramanyan R, Verma S, Abraham S. Anatomically corrected malposition of great arteries. Ann Pediatr Cardiol. 2010;3(2):187–9.
9. Miyamura H, Tsuchida S, Matsukawa T, Eguchi S, Takeuchi Y. Surgical experience with anatomically corrected malposition of the great arteries without subpulmonary conus. Chest. 1982;82(1):115–7.
10. Tsuchida K, Fujiwara T, Ishihara S, Kurosawa H, Imai Y. Intracardiac repair in anatomically corrected malposition of the great arteries (SDL): report on 2 successful repair. Nihon Kyobu Geka Gakkai Zasshi. 1989;37(4):760–5.
11. Colli AM, de Leval M, Somerville J. Anatomically corrected malposition of the great arteries: diagnostic difficulties and surgical repair of associated lesions. Am J Cardiol. 1985;55(11): 1367–72.
12. Senning A. Correction of the transposition of the great arteries. Ann Surg. 1975;182:287–92.
13. Alonso de Begona J, Kawauchi M, Fullerton D, Razzouk AJ, Gundry SR, Bailey LL. The Mustard procedure for correction of simple transposition of the great arteries before 1 month of age. J Thorac Cardiovasc Surg. 1992;104(5):1218–24.
14. Melhuish BPP, Van Praagh R. Juxtaposition of the atrial appendages, a sign of severe cyanotic congenital heart disease. Br Heart J. 1968;30:269.
15. Rittenhouse EA, Tenckhoff L, Kawabori I, Mansfield PB, Hall DG, Brown JW, King H. Surgical repair of anatomically corrected malposition of the great arteries. Ann Thorac Surg. 1986;42(2):220–8.

Chapter 31
Truncus Arteriosus

Michael O. Murphy and Thomas L. Spray

Abstract Truncus arteriosus is a cono-truncal abnormality characterised by a single or common arterial trunk that gives origin to the coronary, pulmonary and brachiocephalic vessels. It is almost invariably associated with a ventricular septal defect below the solitary truncal valve. Presentation can occur by ante-natal scan or post-natal clinical features of pulmonary over circulation and volume overload. Associated cardiac lesions of truncal valve incompetence or interrupted aortic arch can result in surgery that is more challenging and needing to be preformed in the early neonatal period. With experience most centres are performing single stage neonatal repair of all types of truncus arteriosus. Repair is comprised of separating the pulmonary vessels from the common arterial trunk, closure of the ventricular septal defect and establishment of right ventricular to pulmonary artery continuity with a valved or valveless conduit. Severe truncal valve regurgitation can be repaired with leaflet resection or commisuroplasty, while repair of the interrupted arch is often augmented by pulmonary artery homograft to deal with any size mis-match. Choice of conduit will often dictate need for re-operation at a later date and some surgeons prefer to perform a valveless autologous repair to increase the time from initial repair to right ventricular to pulmonary artery re-intervention.

Keywords Truncus arteriosus • Common arterial trunk • Neonates • Congenital heart surgery • Complex CHD

Introduction

Truncus Arteriosus or Common Arterial Trunk is one of the family of cono-truncal anomalies and is characterised by a single arterial trunk arising from the base of the heart providing origins to the coronary, pulmonary and brachiocephalic arteries. It comprises less than 1 % of congenital heart disease and in almost all cases there is

---

M.O. Murphy, MA, MD, MRCP, FRCS
Department of Congenital Cardiac Surgery, Guy's and St. Thomas' Hospital, London, UK

T.L. Spray, MD (✉)
Division of Cardiothoracic Surgery, Department of Cardiothoracic Surgery,
The Children's Hospital of Philadelphia, Philadelphia, PA, USA
e-mail: spray@email.chop.edu

F. Lacour-Gayet et al. (eds.), *Surgery of Conotruncal Anomalies*,
DOI 10.1007/978-3-319-23057-3_31

a large ventricular septal defect under the solitary truncal valve, with virtual absence of the conal septum. The solitary semilunar valve of truncus arteriosus can be comprised of anything from one to six leaflets and though the leaflets are commonly thickened and dysplastic, with consequent regurgitation, it is rare for a truncal valve to be structurally stenotic.

In common with other cono-truncal defects, TA has an association with maternal diabetes [1] and is often associated with chromosome 22q11 deletion or Di George's syndrome [2]. Higher rates of familial recurrence are seen in common arterial trunk [3, 4] than in other congenital cardiac lesions. Truncus Arteriosus is likely the consequence of mal-septation of the conotruncus, due to failure of aortico-pulmonary septum to develop fully with consequent absence of the subpulmonary infundibulum and partial or complete absence of pulmonary valve tissue.

Studies of patients with truncus arteriosus, in the era prior to intervention, show a dismal natural history with less than one in ten surviving past infancy [5–7]. This attrition is due to haemodynamic instability in the neonatal period or accelerated pulmonary vascular disease in infancy. Initial attempts to intervene by bilateral pulmonary artery banding had very poor outcomes and this approach has been rendered all but obsolete by the improved short- and long-term outcomes of primary complete repair.

Experience with complete repair, in the 60s and 70s, was in the most part limited to older infants and children without irreversible pulmonary vascular disease [6, 8–12]. It was clear from these early series that operating on patients without pulmonary vascular disease was key to achieving good short- and long-term outcomes. It was also appreciated that infants with truncus arteriosus seemed to develop pulmonary hypertension at an earlier stage than with other congenital cardiac lesions with increased pulmonary blood flow [13].

It was with this understanding, that some centres in the 80s moved toward repair in early infancy, with dramatic improvements in operative outcomes and late survival reported [14]. This striking success stimulated most major centres to operate on truncus in early infancy [4, 15–24].

The haemodynamic instability of truncus arteriosus, associated in a proportion of patients with sudden death, lead to a number of centres performing truncus arteriosus repair in the neonatal period in almost all cases [25–34].

With growing experience and improved techniques, even the challenging issue of co-existing interrupted arch or significant truncal vale regurgitation seem to have been negated as causes of increased mortality [28, 29, 31]. The repaired common arterial trunk has introduced a new natural history to the condition characterised by excellent development, survival and ventricular function but still impacted by the consequences of the genetic burden of 22q11 deletion in many cases, impaired exercise capacity and re-intervention for truncal valve regurgitation, conduit dysfunction or branch pulmonary artery stenosis [35]. Though cases and series of delayed or two-stage repair are still reported, early primary single stage repair represent current best practice.

Anatomy & Physiology

Anatomy

A patent foramen ovale is almost always present, though a true oval fossa defect occurs in about 10 %. There is mitral to truncal continuity in almost all cases. The ventricular septal defect is usually found in arms of septal band. In the majority of cases it has a muscular inferior rim, protecting conduction system. The remainder have the tricuspid to aortic continuity of a peri-membranous defect where the conduction tissue passing along the inferior edge, on the left side of the defect.

The truncal valve is tricuspid in over half cases, bicuspid in a quarter and quadricuspid in 10–15 %. Occasionally the truncal valve has one, five or even six distinct leaflets. The valve can be dysplastic with one or two thickened, poorly formed leaflets resulting in significant truncal valve incompetence in 4–35 % of cases [4, 14–26, 28–34, 36, 37]. Though physiological stenosis due to volume overload and a hyper-dynamic circulation is common, it is unusual for there to be structural stenosis through the truncal valve.

The aortic arch is often left sided but can be right sided with mirror image branching in over a third of cases. Severe aortic coarctation or interrupted (see Chap. 35) occurs in 6–26 % of cases [4, 14–26, 28–34, 36, 37] and very occasionally double aortic arch can occur. Interruption is usually just beyond the left carotid or less frequently beyond the left subclavian, with both interrupted aortic arch and right aortic arch frequently associated with an aberrant subclavian artery. Apart from cases of interruption or discontinuous pulmonary arteries there is usually no ductal tissue. The proximal truncal root is frequently dilated and tapers down distal to the pulmonary artery take off. This may be related to the incorporation of elements of both the aortic and pulmonary trunk but may also be related to the fact that the truncal root has to accommodate all of the pulmonary and systemic blood flow until it is repaired. As with isolated interrupted aortic arch, the ascending aorta is often hypoplastic relative to the proximal pulmonary trunk and duct, in interrupted aortic arch with truncus arteriosus.

Although the coronaries are often normal, it is not unusual for one or both ostia to be abnormally positioned. Left dominant systems are more common and there can often be a branch of the right coronary crossing in front of the right ventricle as an infundibular or even anterior descending branch. Importantly, there have been a number of reports of coronaries with an intra-mural coarse in truncus arteriosus [15, 22, 37].

Uncommon associations with Truncus Arteriosus include the single ventricle physiologies associated, tricuspid atresia, atrioventricular septal defects and left ventricular hypoplasia with the truncal valve mostly over the right ventricle. Commonly associated lesions such as right aortic arch, aberrant subclavian, ovale fossa defects, unroofed coronary sinus, partial or total anomalous venous return, left superior vena cava and coronary artery abnormalities once appreciated, probably do elevate the risk of repair.

The connection of the pulmonary arteries to the common arterial trunk is variable and forms the basis for the classification systems (Fig. 31.1). Though hemi-

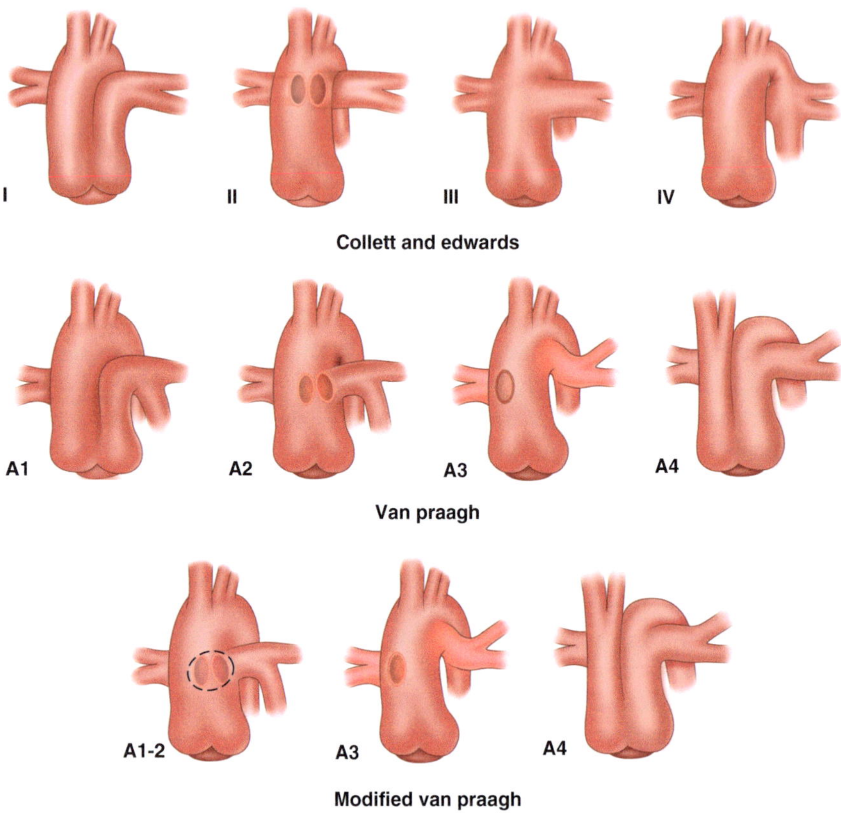

Fig. 31.1 Classification systems for Truncus Arteriosus. The two classical classification systems for truncus arteriosus and the newer modified Van Praagh System

and pseudo-truncus are not regarded as part of the spectrum of common arterial trunk, non-confluent pulmonary arteries feeding off the aortic arch or via a patent duct are part of truncus arteriosus.

Classification Systems

In the original numerical classification of Collett and Edwards [38], the pulmonary arteries arising from a discrete pulmonary trunk, usually on the left posterolateral aspect of the common arterial trunk is ascribed as type I, while when the arteries take separate but adjacent origins from the common arterial trunk, near the truncal valve, is described as type II. When the origins of the pulmonary arteries are distinct from each other, often quite a distance from the truncal valve, this is described as type III. Type IV or pseudo truncus and hemi-truncus are no longer considered variants of Truncus Arteriosus and should be viewed as variants of Tetralogy of Fallot with pulmonary atresia and aortic origin of a pulmonary artery, respectively.

The alphanumerical system of the Van Praagh's [39] designates the pulmonary arteries arising from a pulmonary trunk as type A1, while not distinguishing between type II and III with both being regarded as separate origins of the pulmonary arteries from the truncus or type A2. Type A3 serves to describe the not infrequent situation where one pulmonary artery arises from the trunk with the other arising from another part of the arterial tree, while type A4 describes another common variant, that being common arterial trunk with associated interrupted aortic arch. This system also takes into account the presence or absence of a ventricular septal defect with lesion type B1-4 representing the identical lesion but without a ventricular septal defect.

The Collett and Edwards system remains popular but fails to account for the important subgroups of arch or ductal origin of a pulmonary artery or co-existent interruption with associated hypoplasia of the aortic segment. The Van Praagh system can be complicated to apply and serves to describe accurately a situation that rarely occurs, where the ventricular septal defect is highly restrictive or non-existent with possible single ventricle physiology. Newer systems based on modifications of the Van Praagh system have also been proposed [40, 41] but truncus arteriosus promises to continue to be a lesion that is variable enough to be difficult to classify.

Physiology

Truncus arteriosus is a completely ad mixing lesion, with left to right shunting at atrial, ventricular and arterial levels and because the pulmonary arteries come directly off the common arterial trunk, the pulmonary vasculature is exposed to not only systolic ejection but also the diastolic flow from the systemic arterial system. In most cases, there is streaming of blood preferentially from the right ventricle to the pulmonary arteries and from the left ventricle to the aorta [5, 42] such that the degree of cyanosis at birth is predominantly a reflection of the pulmonary vascular resistance, which seems to drop earlier in Truncus Arteriosus than in other neonatal lesions [13]. The onset of tachypnoea and dyspnoea can be important signs of congestive cardiac failure.

Once the pulmonary vascular resistance starts to drop the saturations tend to increase as excessive pulmonary blood flow in systole and diastole flood the lungs, causing poor diastolic perfusion and volume over load of the heart, both of which can compromise coronary flow. The haemodynamic condition is made even more tenuous in the setting of truncal valve regurgitation, leading to a situation where there is massive volume overload of the ventricles, huge flows through the truncal valve and coronary diastolic perfusion may be even further impaired. It is not surprising that necrotising enterocolitis has a high incidence in neonates with Truncus Arteriosus [43].

Imaging and Diagnosis

Truncus Arteriosus is increasingly diagnosed at fetal scan with the characteristic single arterial valve overlying a large ventricular septal defect with absence of an arterial duct, though it can sometimes difficult to differentiate Truncus Arteriosus from Tetralogy of Fallot with pulmonary atresia. Though it is a cyanotic lesion, the degree of cyanosis is often mild due to pulmonary overcirculation, particularly as the pulmonary vascular resistance drops. Often times the neonate is born with a well balance circulation with neither cyanosis nor over-circulation due to the high pulmonary vascular resistance.

The diagnosis should be made in the first few hours of life if not antenatally detected.

Focussed post-natal transthoracic echo will establish or confirm the diagnosis in most cases and will add helpful information such as systemic and pulmonary venous anatomy, confirm the presence of two adequate ventricles and atrio-ventricular valves, number of truncal leaflets, presence and degree of regurgitation through valve, coronary anatomy and morphology of the pulmonary arteries. Doppler signal through pulmonary veins and degree of chamber dilation will indicate the degree of pulmonary over circulation and there may be reversal of flow in the descending aorta in the setting of severe pulmonary over circulation or significant truncal valve incompetence. It is important to confirm that the ventricular septal defect is unrestrictive and solitary.

Chest X-ray, arterial blood gas analysis, peripheral saturations and physical examinations can also help with assessment of perfusion status and the degree of congestive cardiac failure. Cardiac catheterisation is seldom needed in the neonatal period but may be worthwhile in infants and children with delayed presentation to delineate the pulmonary vascular resistance. Cardiac MRI has also been increasingly used pre-operatively and can be useful to delineate morphology, as well as to calculate pulmonary vascular resistance.

Medical management is limited to stabilisation of cardiac failure, maintenance of ductal patency in interruption or where a duct supplies a pulmonary artery. It is not infrequent for neonates to be ventilated prior to surgery. When intubated, hypoventilation can achieve permissive hypercapnoea to lessen pulmonary over circulation. Drugs that cause tachycardia or increase myocardial workload should be avoided. Attention should be paid to the possible diagnosis of DiGeorge syndrome or 22q11 deletion as affected patients can have facial anomalies, hypocalcaemia and immunodeficiency. Blood should be irradiated to prevent possible graft versus host disease.

Pre-operative Checklist

By the time the patient comes to surgery, a clear and complete diagnosis should be available.

- Pulmonary arteries morphology, stenosis: Type A1, A2 (frequently 1.5), A3
- Morphology of the truncal valve
- Truncal valve regurgitation
- Location and diameter of the VSD
- Dextroposition of the truncal valve
- Absence of IAA
- Presence of thymus gland, Di George syndrome, hypocalcaemia
- Irradiated blood, if needed

Surgical Technique

General Principles

Palliation with bilateral pulmonary artery banding for Truncus Arteriosus has become all but obsolete as primary repair in infancy became the standard of care in almost all congenital centres. The principal of Truncus Arteriosus repair include separating the pulmonary and systemic circulations, closing the ventricular defect and establishing right ventricular to pulmonary artery. The variability and complexity of anatomy in Truncus Arteriosus requires extensive and careful pre-operative assessment, and each component of the repair needs to be carefully considered prior to surgery

Pre-operatively, it is important not to increase myocardial demand in this tenuous haemodynamics state where myocardial ischaemia can be an issue. Manoeuvres such as keeping the haematocrit high, avoiding tachycardia and ventilating to balance the circulation, can minimise the risk of cardiovascular collapse. Administration of intravenous fluid and chronotropic drugs to increase the blood pressure should be avoided.

The presence of thymic tissue should be noted after sternotomy and a pericardial patch is harvested should it be required as part of the repair. The pulmonary arteries are dissected out completely to establish the type of connection to the trunk and the relationship of the pulmonary arties to the frequently abnormal coronary ostia. Both pulmonary arteries, even in the presence of a disconnected artery, are encircled with tourniquets, snaring the right pulmonary artery if haemodynamic instability occurs. The head and neck vessels are similarly dissected out and encircled with tourniquets if the aorta arch is interrupted.

Cardiopulmonary Bypass

Cardiopulmonary bypass is established with high aortic cannulation to allow for enough space to safely excise the pulmonary arteries and standard bi-caval cannulation, though many centres still perform the entire repair during one period of circulatory arrest utilising single venous cannulation (Fig. 31.2a). Moderate hypothermia is used to ensure thorough cooling and allow for short periods of low flow or arrest in carrying out the repair. Both pulmonary arteries are snared on bypass to prevent flooding of the lungs and to facilitate antegrade cardioplegia after cross clamping.

The aorta is cross-clamped as high as possible and the heart arrested with cold antegrade cardioplegia. This will often give an idea of the true degree of truncal valve insufficiency and in the presence of significant truncal incompetence, supplementary cardioplegia by direct coronary delivery or retrograde cardioplegia is necessary. Good myocardial protection can be challenging but is essential in these patients where repair often requires over one hour of myocardial ischaemia.

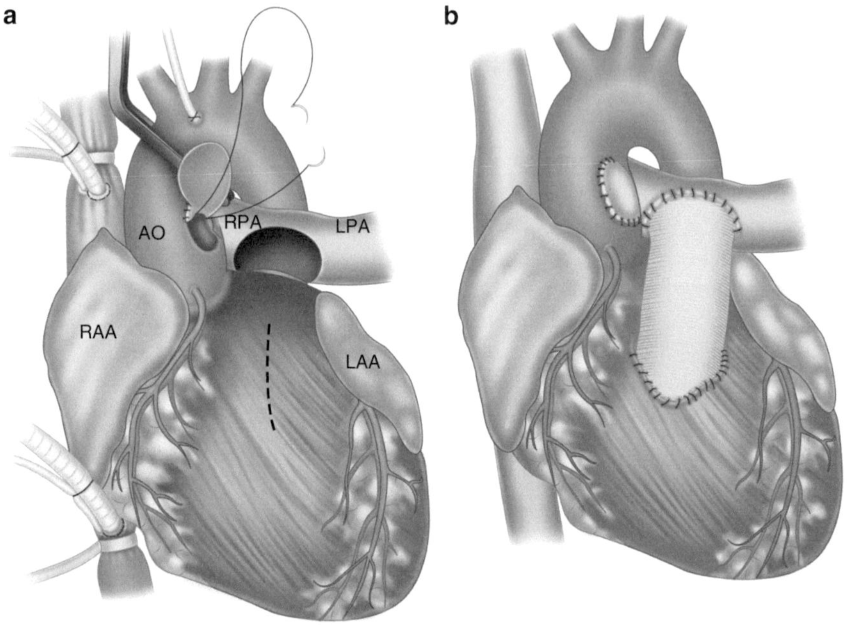

Fig. 31.2 Traditional repair of Truncus Arteriosus. After cardioplegic arrest the pulmonary arteries have been excised from the truncal root and the defect has been repaired using a patch (**a**). Alternatively the truncal root can be transected with excision of the pulmonary arteries. This allows reconstruction of the root in a symmetrical fashion. The dotted line represents the location of the right ventriculotomy, which is used to expose the ventricular septal defect (**b**). After closure of the ventricular septal defect, a valved conduit establishes right ventricular to pulmonary artery continuity

Oblique right atriotomy allows venting of the left heart through the inter-atrial communication if present, though this can be similarly achieved by cannualtion of the right superior pulmonary vein with a left ventricular vent. This latter technique can be particularly useful where a significant period of cooling is planned and there is more than mild truncal regurgitation.

Separating the Pulmonary and Systemic Circulation

The truncus is carefully inspected for the location of the coronary arteries ostia and the pulmonary arteries. The common arterial trunk is incised above the pulmonary arteries and the origins of both pulmonary arteries and left main coronary artery inspected, prior to excision of the pulmonary arteries from the trunk with a cuff of arterial wall. The truncal defect can be closed primarily, but it may be preferable to patch the defect to avoid distorting the neon-aorta, and decrease that chance of bleeding in an area (Fig. 31.2a). Bleeding where the pulmonary arteries have been excised is extremely difficult to access after separation form bypass and is often adjacent to the left main stem.

In situations where the truncal valve is to be repaired it may be preferable to transecting the trunk just above the commissures of the valve, again taking care not to injure the coronary origins (Fig. 31.4a). This incision offers unrivalled access to the truncal valve for repair allowing for resection of the sinus and leaflet, and also facilitates symmetrical reconstruction of any mismatch between the repaired trunk and the ascending aorta, tailoring this anastomosis can provide improved support to the commissures, improving competence of the valve and minimising any root distortion.

Ventricular Septal Defect Closure

In the Truncus Arteriosus the ventricular septal defect often has a muscular inferior rim but can also be peri-membranous. This can be closed via the right ventriculotomy or the right atrium using interrupted or continuous suture to a prosthetic patch. When the VSD is peri-membranous care should be taken inferiorly not to injure the conduction tissue. It is of importance to close the defect with a patch that is at least as large as the truncal valve annulus to avoid narrowing the left ventricular outflow tract.

Establish Right Ventricular to Pulmonary Artery Continuity

A valved conduit is the optimal technique to establish a competence right ventricular to pulmonary artery connection (Fig. 31.2b), in a condition where post-operative pulmonary vascular crises and right ventricular dysfunction are common and elevated pulmonary vascular resistances are a concern. In type A3, a non-confluent pulmonary artery, coming for a patent ductus or the aortic arch, is snared on bypass and resected at the same time as the other pulmonary artery and unfocalised as continuity is established between the right ventricle and the pulmonary arteries, often facilitated by using a patch of homograft tissue.

When available, small aortic homografts provide durable pulmonary valve competence, have a good length of curved artery to reach over the ventricular mass to the pulmonary vessels and allow for construction of the ventricular hood with the anterior leaflet of the mitral valve. Small pulmonary or bi-cuspidised aortic or pulmonary homografts provide a satisfactory alternative, though when these are large they may require wide opening of the left pleural cavity to achieve safe chest closure. Use of synthetic grafts containing xenografts and bovine jugular valved conduits (Contegra) have also been described. Direct connection of the pulmonary artery to the ventriculotomy with anterior patching with pericardium is also an option and may be particularly useful in very small neonates where homograft options may be limited. Non-valved conduits should be considered with great caution in the setting of significant truncal valve regurgitation, particularly if this is not to be addressed, as having two regurgitant arterial valves is invariably associated with very poor post-operative outcomes. A number of reports have described the use

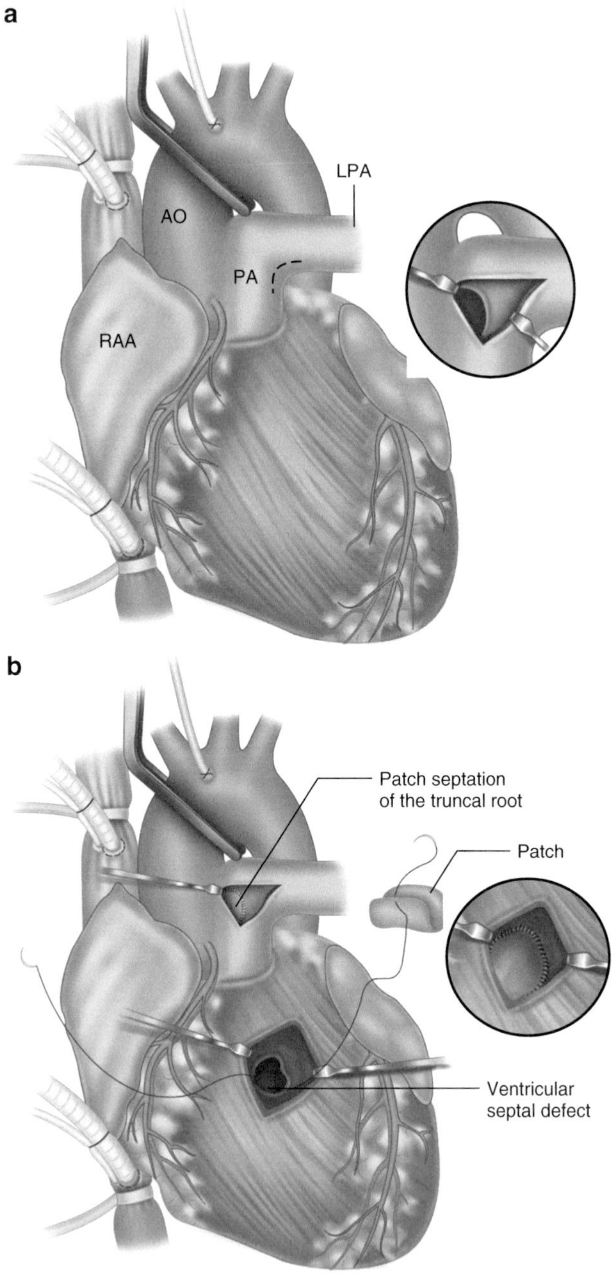

Fig. 31.3 Alternative repair of Truncus Arteriosus. A hockey-stick incision in the truncus root extends onto the left main pulmonary artery exposing the right pulmonary artery orifice superiorly (**a**). Extension of the incision allows access to the truncal valve in case of repair. The defect within the trunk is patch closed taking care not to injure or incorporate the right pulmonary artery orifice and the ventricular septal defect is patch closed through the ventriculotomy (**b**) Right ventricle to pulmonary artery continuity is established with a valved conduit or the back wall is filled in with pericardium or appendage and the anterior wall reconstructed with a monocusp of homograft or pericardium

of the Lecompte manoeuvre in a small number of patients with particular morphologies of Truncus Arteriosus in order to prevent pulmonary artery distortion.

Alternative Technique

An alternative to the traditional technique described, centres on using autologous tissue rather than allografts or heterografts to reconstruct the outflow tract and is most suited to the cases where the pulmonary arteries come off a pulmonary trunk or are close together coming off the truncus close to the truncal valve. In other morphologies the autologous method is less useful. As described first by Barbero-Marcial [44], the technique involves a limited incision over the pulmonary arteries often extending into the left pulmonary artery (Fig. 31.3a). The area between the truncus proper and the pulmonary arteries is patched closed and if there is a significant distance between the pulmonary artery incision and the right ventriculotomy (Fig. 31.3b) the defect is patched with autologous tissue such as pericardium, atrial appendage or is left unpatched, with the epicardium serving as the back wall. The front wall is patched with a monocusp of homograft tissue, pericardium or synthetic material. The purported advantages of this technique are that it allows growth of native tissue with time to decrease the need for re-intervention. Even in valved connections using the mono-cusp technique, long standing pulmonary incompetence is guaranteed.

Truncal Valve Repair

As previously mentioned, truncal transection above the commissures can greatly facilitate repair, though this can be achieved via the traditional incision. The technique of repair will in most cases be dictated by the valve itself. Quadricuspid valves with a single small prolapsing valve will benefit from resection of this leaflet and the adjacent truncal wall, with root reconstruction (Fig. 31.4b–d). This can involve resecting and then re-implanting a coronary button. An alternative technique where resection is not feasible involves suturing the proposing leaflet to one or more adjacent leaflets (Fig. 31.4e). Either technique can be re-enforced with sub-commissural sutures. When the root has been transected, tailored anastomosis to the frequently smaller ascending aorta can provide additional commissural support and will minimise root distortion.

Interrupted Aortic Arch (See Chap. 35)

Post-operative Care

Patients who have had truncus arteriosus repair are at high risk for pulmonary hypertensive crisis, particularly if this is carried out after the neonatal period, when some pulmonary vascular disease may already be established. Acidosis and hypercarbia should be avoided in the post operative period and many centres use

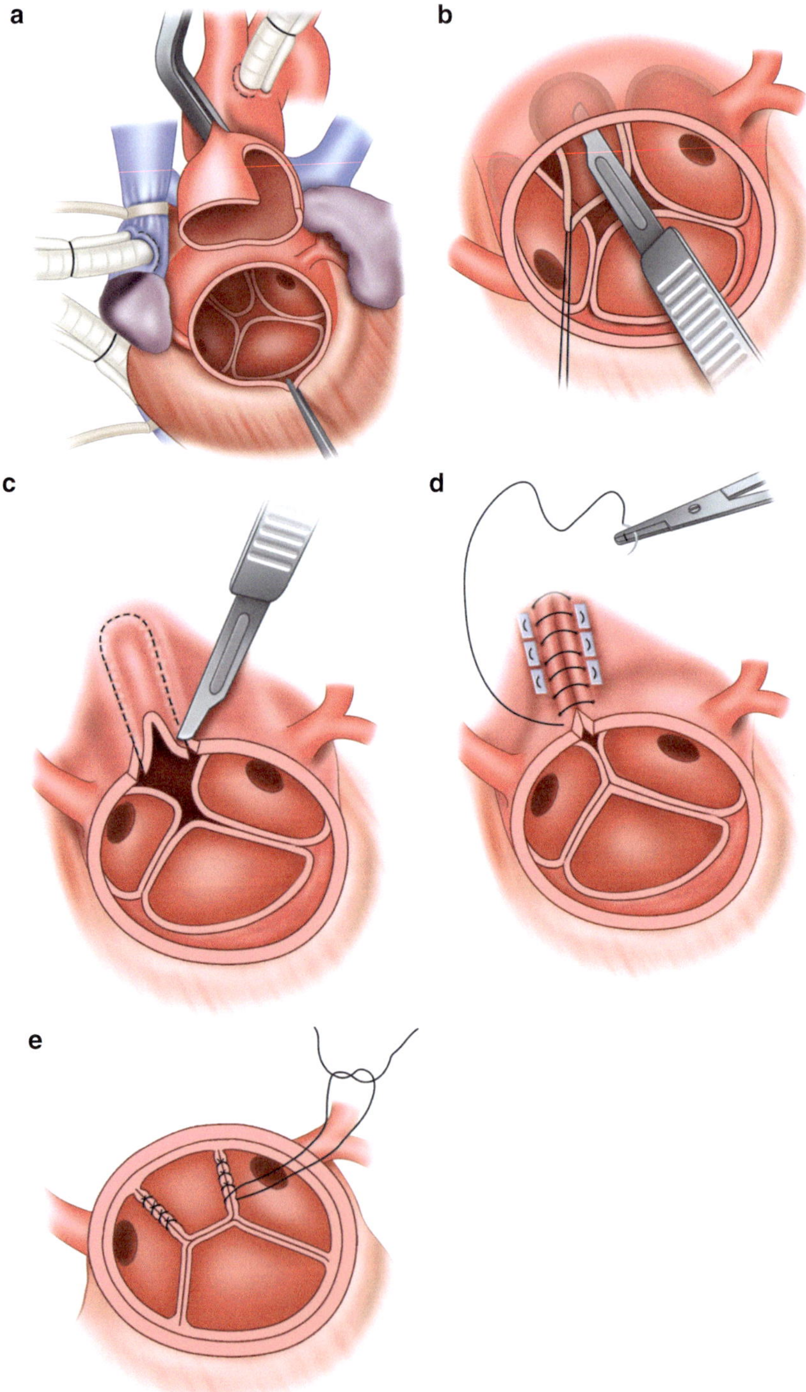
a
b
c
d
e

Fig. 31.4 Truncal Valve Repair. The common arterial trunk is transected showing an incompetent quadricuspid truncal valve and the prolapsed leaflet (**a**). The prolapsed leaflet (**b**) and the corresponding sinus of Valsalva truncal wall (**c**) are resected and the defect in the truncal wall closed, bringing the remaining leaflets together and tightening the annulus (**d**). Alternative techniques include suture valvuloplasty, performed by attaching the edges of the prolapsed leaflet to either one or both adjacent leaflets, thereby creating a functional tricuspid or bicuspid semilunar valve (**e**), often supplemented with a sub-commissural supporting suture

nitric oxide in conjunction with analgesia, sedation and paralysis to avoid pulmonary hypertensive crises. When these events occur, precipitating factors such as pain, acidosis, fever, infection, vasoconstrictors, overfilling or tamponade should be attended to in conjunction with intravenous paralysing and sedating agents and manual hyperventilation with pure oxygen.

Outcomes

Natural history studies, prior to the era of surgical intervention, show that untreated the vast majority of patients will succumb by the end of infancy and that the earlier intervention occurs, the greater the survival of all patients born with Truncus Arteriosus [6]. Single centre surgical outcomes for Truncus Arteriosus repair are excellent with early mortality in the modern era of typically of less than 10 % [17, 25, 26, 29, 33, 34] particularly if repair is performed in the neonatal period, with minimal use of mechanical support [25, 26, 45].

Though both single centre and multicentre studies show that coronary abnormalities [15, 22, 23], significant truncal valve regurgitation [20, 21, 23, 26, 27] or aortic arch interruption [15, 20, 21, 23, 33] to be strong predictors of peri-operative mortality, some centres have been able to the neutralise the risk of truncal valve surgery [28, 29, 31] or arch repair [29, 45] at the time of Truncus Arteriosus repair. The issue of coronary abnormalities is an intriguing one as many centres have not found this to be a risk but it is important to note that three series reported a concerning incidence of an intramural course of a coronary artery [15, 22, 37]. Though 22Q deletion does not appear to increase operative mortality, it can have important effects on duration of stay and long-term outcomes [35].

Long-term studies do show a small number deaths remote from the initial repair but late survival of 65–90 % can be expected [4, 14–26, 28–34, 36, 37]. Two issues tend to lead to re-intervention in patients who have had early primary repair, dysfunction of the right ventricular to pulmonary artery connection or native pulmonary artery stenosis and truncal vale dysfunction.

The choice of techniques to establish right ventricular to pulmonary artery continuity are multiple broadly based around non-autologous repairs with valved or valveless conduit or autologous repairs often supplemented with a monocusp technique on the anterior wall. Non-autologous valved conduits include homografts, both aortic and pulmonary, heterografts with a small bioprosthesis within a synthetic graft and xenografts conduits such as the bovine jugular vein graft.

Homografts perform well in terms of valve durability but inevitably require replacement, often due to dilation or stenosis within the conduit. Although it is an often-quoted belief that aortic homografts are less durable than pulmonary allografts because of their propensity to calcify, large reports of fail to bear this out in repair of Truncus Arteriosus [46, 47]. There is conflicting data regarding conduit size as a risk factor for re-intervention [47, 48] but it seems that right-sided re-intervention will remain an important long-term issue in patients with repaired Truncus Arteriosus. The potential for percutanous [48, 49] or percutanous valves [50] to delay the need for surgery is encouraging.

Heterografts with a small bioprosthesis within a synthetic graft were popular in the early era of Truncus Arteriosus Repair [10, 14] but these have been shown to have poor durability and are a strong risk factor for the need for early re-intervention [46], and are not commonly used in contemporary series. Valveless conduit reconstruction was reported in early series of repair [9, 51], but again has minimal use in contemporary series. Xenografts conduits such as the bovine jugular vein graft or Contegra® are an attractive option because of the off the shelf access to a variety of sizes but there has been much concern over stenosis of the distal anastomosis in Contegra® used in a variety of indications, which may limit there wide spread adoption [52].

The alternative technique of autologous repair has been previously been adopted with hesitation, given the increased early mortality reported in the initial reports [16, 44, 53] that led to concern about its use. However, more recent series have demonstrated that this is a safe procedure and may delay the need for re-intervention by not using a circumferential valve and limiting pulmonary artery distortion [15, 22, 30, 32, 54].

Re-intervention on the truncal valve can be challenging and often result in replacement. It is hoped that by the success of repair techniques in neonate and infants [55–57] will result in a lesser need for intervention on the truncal valve, later in life.

References

1. Ferencz C, Rubin JD, McCarter RJ, Clark EB. Maternal diabetes and cardiovascular malformations: predominance of double outlet right ventricle and truncus arteriosus. Teratology. 1990;41:319–26.
2. Goldmuntz E, Clark BJ, Mitchell LE, Jawad AF, Cuneo BF, Reed L, McDonald-McGinn D, Chien P, Feuer J, Zackai EH, Emanuel BS, Driscoll DA. Frequency of 22q11 deletions in patients with conotruncal defects. J Am Chem Soc. 1998;32:492–8.
3. Pierpont ME, Gobel JW, Moller JH, Edwards JE. Cardiac malformations in relatives of children with truncus arteriosus or interruption of the aortic arch. Am J Clin Pathol. 1988;61: 423–7.
4. Brizard CP, Cochrane A, Austin C, Nomura F, Karl TR. Management strategy and long-term outcome for truncus arteriosus. Eur J Cardiothorac Surg. 1997;11:687; discussion 695–6.
5. Calder L, Van Praagh R, Van Praagh S, Sears WP, Corwin R, Levy A, Keith JD, Paul MH. Truncus arteriosus communis. Clinical, angiocardiographic, and pathologic findings in 100 patients. Am Heart J. 1976;92:23–38.
6. Stark J, Gandhi D, de Leval M, Macartney F, Taylor JF. Surgical treatment of persistent truncus arteriosus in the first year of life. Br Heart J. 1978;40:1280–7.
7. Samánek M, Benesová D, Goetzová J, Hrycejová I. Distribution of age at death in children with congenital heart disease who died before the age of 15. Br Heart J. 1988;59:581–5.

8. McGoon DC, Rastelli GC, Ongley PA. An operation for the correction of truncus arteriosus. JAMA. 1968;205:69–73.
9. Behrendt DM, Dick M. Truncus repair with a valveless conduit in neonates. J Thorac Cardiovasc Surg. 1995;110:1148–50.
10. Ebert PA, Robinson SJ, Stanger P, Engle MA. Pulmonary artery conduits in infants younger than six months of age. J Thorac Cardiovasc Surg. 1976;72:351–6.
11. Marcelletti C, McGoon DC, Danielson GK, Wallace RB, Mair DD. Early and late results of surgical repair of truncus arteriosus. Circulation. 1977;55:636–41.
12. Marcelletti C, McGoon DC, Mair DD. The natural history of truncus arteriosus. Circulation. 1976;54:108–11.
13. Anderson RH, Baker EJ, MacCartney FJ, Rigby ML, Shinebourne EA, Tynan M. Paediatric cardiology. Philadelphia: Churchill Livingstone; 2002.
14. Ebert PA, Turley K, Stanger P, Hoffman JI, Heymann MA, Rudolph AM. Surgical treatment of truncus arteriosus in the first 6 months of life. Ann Surg. 1984;200:451–6.
15. Danton MH, Barron DJ, Stumper O, Wright JG, De Giovannni J, Silove ED, Brawn WJ. Repair of truncus arteriosus: a considered approach to right ventricular outflow tract reconstruction. Eur J Cardiothorac Surg. 2001;20:95–103; discussion 103–4.
16. Lacour-Gayet F, Serraf A, Komiya T, Sousa-Uva M, Bruniaux J, Touchot A, Roux D, Neuville P, Planché C. Truncus arteriosus repair: influence of techniques of right ventricular outflow tract reconstruction. J Thorac Cardiovasc Surg. 1996;111:849–56.
17. Imamura M, Drummond-Webb JJ, Sarris GE, Mee RB. Improving early and intermediate results of truncus arteriosus repair: a new technique of truncal valve repair. Ann Thorac Surg. 1999;67:1142–6.
18. Alexiou C, Keeton BR, Salmon AP, Monro JL. Repair of truncus arteriosus in early infancy with antibiotic sterilized aortic homografts. Ann Thorac Surg. 2001;71:S371–4.
19. Tlaskal T, Chaloupecky V, Hucin B, Gebauer R, Krupickova S, Reich O, Skovranek J, Tax P. Long-term results after correction of persistent truncus arteriosus in 83 patients. Eur J Cardiothorac Surg. 2010;37:1278–84.
20. Urban AE, Sinzobahamvya N, Brecher AM, Wetter J, Malorny S. Truncus arteriosus: ten-year experience with homograft repair in neonates and infants. Ann Thorac Surg. 1998;66:S183–8.
21. Brown JW, Ruzmetov M, Okada Y, Vijay P, Turrentine MW. Truncus arteriosus repair: outcomes, risk factors, reoperation and management. Eur J Cardiothorac Surg. 2001;20:221–7.
22. Raisky O, Ali WB, Bajolle F, Marini D, Metton O, Bonnet D, Sidi D, Vouhé PR. Common arterial trunk repair: with conduit or without? Eur J Cardiothorac Surg. 2009;36:675–82.
23. Hanley FL, Heinemann MK, Jonas RA, Mayer JE, Cook NR, Wessel DL, Castaneda AR. Repair of truncus arteriosus in the neonate. J Thorac Cardiovasc Surg. 1993;105:1047–56.
24. Pearl JM, Laks H, Drinkwater DC, Milgalter E, Orrin A-C, Giacobetti F, George B, Williams R. Repair of truncus arteriosus in infancy. Ann Thorac Surg. 1991;52:780–6.
25. O'Byrne ML, Yang W, Mercer-Rosa L, Parnell AS, Oster ME, Levenbrown Y, Tanel RE, Goldmuntz E. 22q11.2 Deletion syndrome is associated with increased perioperative events and more complicated postoperative course in infants undergoing infant operative correction of truncus arteriosus communis or interrupted aortic arch. J Thorac Cardiovasc Surg. 2014;148(4):1597–605.
26. Thompson LD, McElhinney DB, Reddy M, Petrossian E, Silverman NH, Hanley FL. Neonatal repair of truncus arteriosus: continuing improvement in outcomes. Ann Thorac Surg. 2001;72:391–5.
27. Konstantinov IE, Karamlou T, Blackstone EH, Mosca RS, Lofland GK, Caldarone CA, Williams WG, Mackie AS, McCrindle BW. Truncus arteriosus associated with interrupted aortic arch in 50 neonates: a Congenital Heart Surgeons Society Study. Ann Thorac Surg. 2006;81:214–22.
28. Bove EL, Lupinetti FM, Pridjian AK, Beekman RH, Callow LB, Snider AR, Rosenthal A. Results of a policy of primary repair of truncus arteriosus in the neonate. J Thorac Cardiovasc Surg. 1993;105:1057–65; discussion 1065–6.
29. Jahangiri M, Zurakowski D, Mayer JE, del Nido PJ, Jonas RA. Repair of the truncal valve and associated interrupted arch in neonates with truncus arteriosus. J Thorac Cardiovasc Surg. 2000;119:508–14.

30. Chen JM, Glickstein JS, Davies RR, Mercando ML, Hellenbrand WE, Mosca RS, Quaegebeur JM. The effect of repair technique on postoperative right-sided obstruction in patients with truncus arteriosus. J Thorac Cardiovasc Surg. 2005;129:559–68.
31. Hawkins JA, Kaza AK, Burch PT, Lambert LM, Holubkov R, Witte MK. Simple versus complex truncus arteriosus: neutralization of risk but with increased resource utilization. World J Pediatr Congenit Heart Surg. 2010;1:285–91.
32. Honjo O, Kotani Y, Akagi T, Osaki S, Kawada M, Ishino K, Sano S. Right ventricular outflow tract reconstruction in patients with persistent truncus arteriosus: a 15-year experience in a single Japanese center. Circ J. 2007;71:1776–80.
33. Sinzobahamvya N, Boscheinen M, Blaschczok HC, Kallenberg R, Photiadis J, Haun C, Hraška V, Asfour B. Survival and reintervention after neonatal repair of truncus arteriosus with valved conduit. Eur J Cardiothorac Surg. 2008;34:732–7.
34. Kalavrouziotis G, Purohit M, Ciotti G, Corno AF, Pozzi M. Truncus arteriosus communis: early and midterm results of early primary repair. Ann Thorac Surg. 2006;82:2200–6.
35. O'Byrne ML, Mercer-Rosa L, Zhao H, Zhang X, Yang W, Cassedy A, Fogel MA, Rychik J, Tanel RE, Marino BS, Paridon S, Goldmuntz E. Morbidity in children and adolescents after surgical correction of truncus arteriosus communis. Am Heart J. 2013;166:512–8.
36. Russell HM, Pasquali SK, Jacobs JP, Jacobs ML, O'Brien SM, Mavroudis C, Backer CL. Outcomes of repair of common arterial trunk with truncal valve surgery: a review of the society of thoracic surgeons congenital heart surgery database. Ann Thorac Surg. 2012;93:164–9; discussion 169.
37. Benjacholamas V, Namchaisiri J, Khongphatthanayothin A, Lertsapcharoen P. Bicuspidized pulmonary homograft for truncus arteriosus repair. Asian Cardiovasc Thorac Ann. 2008;16:189–93.
38. COLLETT RW, Edwards JE. Persistent truncus arteriosus; a classification according to anatomic types. Surg Clin North Am. 1949;29:1245–70.
39. Van Praagh R, Van Praagh S. The anatomy of common aorticopulmonary trunk (truncus arteriosus communis) and its embryologic implications. A study of 57 necropsy cases. Am J Clin Pathol. 1965;16:406–25.
40. Russell HM, Jacobs ML, Anderson RH, Mavroudis C, Spicer D, Corcrain E, Backer CL. A simplified categorization for common arterial trunk. J Thorac Cardiovasc Surg. 2011;141:645–53.
41. Jacobs ML. Congenital Heart Surgery Nomenclature and Database Project: truncus arteriosus. Ann Thorac Surg. 2000;69:S50–5.
42. Mair DD, Ritter DG, Davis GD, Wallace RB, Danielson GK, McGoon DC. Selection of patients with truncus arteriosus for surgical correction; anatomic and hemodynamic considerations. Circulation. 1974;49:144–51.
43. McElhinney DB, Hedrick HL, Bush DM, Pereira GR, Stafford PW, Gaynor JW, Spray TL, Wernovsky G. Necrotizing enterocolitis in neonates with congenital heart disease: risk factors and outcomes. Pediatrics. 2000;106:1080–7.
44. Barbero-Marcial M, Riso A, Atik E, Jatene A. A technique for correction of truncus arteriosus types I and II without extracardiac conduits. J Thorac Cardiovasc Surg. 1990;99:364–9.
45. Bohuta L, Hussein A, Fricke TA, d'Udekem Y, Bennett M, Brizard C, Konstantinov IE. Surgical repair of truncus arteriosus associated with interrupted aortic arch: long-term outcomes. Ann Thorac Surg. 2011;91:1473–7.
46. Reddy VM, Rajasinghe HA, McElhinney DB, Hanley FL. Performance of right ventricle to pulmonary artery conduits after repair of truncus arteriosus: a comparison of Dacron-housed porcine valves and cryopreserved allografts. Semin Thorac Cardiovasc Surg. 1995;7:133–8.
47. Vohra HA, Whistance RN, Chia AX, Janusauskas V, Nikolaidis N, Roubelakis A, Veldtman G, Roman K, Vettukattil JJ, Gnanapragasam J, Salmon AP, Monro JL, Haw MP. Long-term follow-up after primary complete repair of common arterial trunk with homograft: a 40-year experience. J Thorac Cardiovasc Surg. 2010;140:325–9.
48. Lund AM, Vogel M, Marshall AC, Emani SM, Pigula FA, Tworetzky W, McElhinney DB. Early reintervention on the pulmonary arteries and right ventricular outflow tract after neonatal or early infant repair of truncus arteriosus using homograft conduits. Am J Clin Pathol. 2011;108:106–13.

49. McElhinney DB, Rajasinghe HA, Mora BN, Reddy VM, Silverman NH, Hanley FL. Reinterventions after repair of common arterial trunk in neonates and young infants. J Am Chem Soc. 2000;35:1317–22.
50. Haas NA, Moysich A, Neudorf U, Mortezaeian H, Abdel-Wahab M, Schneider H, De Wolf D, Petit J, Narayanswami S, Laser KT, Sandica E. Percutaneous implantation of the Edwards SAPIEN(™) pulmonic valve: initial results in the first 22 patients. Clin Res Cardiol. 2013;102:119–28.
51. Spicer RL, Behrendt D, Crowley DC, Dick M, Rocchini AP, Uzark K, Rosenthal A, Sloan H. Repair of truncus arteriosus in neonates with the use of a valveless conduit. Circulation. 1984;70:I26–9.
52. Urso S, Rega F, Meuris B, Gewillig M, Eyskens B, Daenen W, Heying R, Meyns B. The Contegra conduit in the right ventricular outflow tract is an independent risk factor for graft replacement. Eur J Cardiothorac Surg. 2011;40:603–9.
53. Nakae S, Kasahara S, Kuroyama N, Lin ZB, Hiraishi S, Agata Y, Yoshimura H. Correction of truncus arteriosus with autologous arterial flap in neonates and small infants. Ann Thorac Surg. 1996;62:123–8; discussion 129.
54. Alfieris GM, Gangemi JJ, Schiralli MP, Swartz MF, Cholette JM. Modified repair of truncus arteriosus to maintain pulmonary artery architecture. Ann Thorac Surg. 2010;90:1038–9.
55. Mavroudis C, backer CL. Surgical management of severe truncal insufficiency: experience with truncal valve remodeling techniques. Ann Thorac Surg. 2001;72:396–400.
56. McElhinney DB, Reddy VM, Rajasinghe HA, Mora BN, Silverman NH, Hanley FL. Trends in the management of truncal valve insufficiency. Ann Thorac Surg. 1998;65:517–24.
57. Kaza AK, Burch PT, Pinto N, Minich LL, Tani LY, Hawkins JA. Durability of truncal valve repair. Ann Thorac Surg. 2010;90:1307–12; discussion 1312.

Chapter 32
Common Arterial Trunk with Interrupted Aortic Arch

Francois Lacour-Gayet

Abstract The surgical repair of Truncus Arteriosus Communis associated with an Interrupted Aortic Arch (TAC-IAA) is challenging. The association with a severe truncal valve regurgitation as well as the presence of pre-operative multiple organs failure is a major risk factor. The early mortality in the published series varies from 0 to 50 %. The two large multicentric studies of the CHSS in 2006 and the STS in 2013 show an early mortality of: 68 % (34/50) and – 21 % (12/58) respectively. Nevertheless, the results can be excellent in experienced centers using a modern one stage surgical technique, undertaken in the first weeks of life.

Keywords Common arterial trunk: Truncus arteriosus communis • Interrupted aortic arch • Congenital heart surgery • Neonates • 22q11 deletion

Introduction

Truncus arteriosus communis (TAC) with interrupted aortic arch (TAC-IAA) is a rare form of conotruncal anomaly. It represents 1/1000 of congenital heart diseases. Neonatal one stage repair has emerged as the optimal procedure. Surgical repair of TAC-IAA is the most challenging procedure in terms of mortality and morbidity as evaluated by the STS and the EACTS database 2014 (see Chap. 4).

F. Lacour-Gayet, MD
Department of Pediatric Cardiac Surgery, National Heart and Lung Institute,
Royal Brompton Hospital, Imperial College University, Sydney Street, London SW3 6NP, UK
e-mail: flacourgayet@mac.com

F. Lacour-Gayet et al. (eds.), *Surgery of Conotruncal Anomalies*,
DOI 10.1007/978-3-319-23057-3_32

Anatomy and Physiopathology

Collet and Edwards published the first anatomic classification of TAC [1]. The classification by Richard Van Praagh [2] was the first one describing truncus with IAA (Fig. 32.1). Depending on the level of the aortic arch interruption, a Type IV-A and a Type IV-B can be identified. Most often in TAC-IAA, the common trunk is of type I with the PDA in prolongation of the PA trunk; with an ascending aorta clearly seen (Fig. 32.1). When the TAC-IAA has a common trunk of type II (Pr Yen Ho specimen and drawings, Fig. 32.2), the pulmonary arteries arise laterally in high position and the PDA arises in between the PA branches like a sort of trifurcation. There is no ascending aorta, unless the trunk itself is the ascending aorta, as stated by Richard Van Praagh (personal exchanges). The large PDA could be taken for a transverse arch. Richard Van Praagh suggests calling this PDA a "ductal arch" (personal exchanges). This form is more difficult to repair.

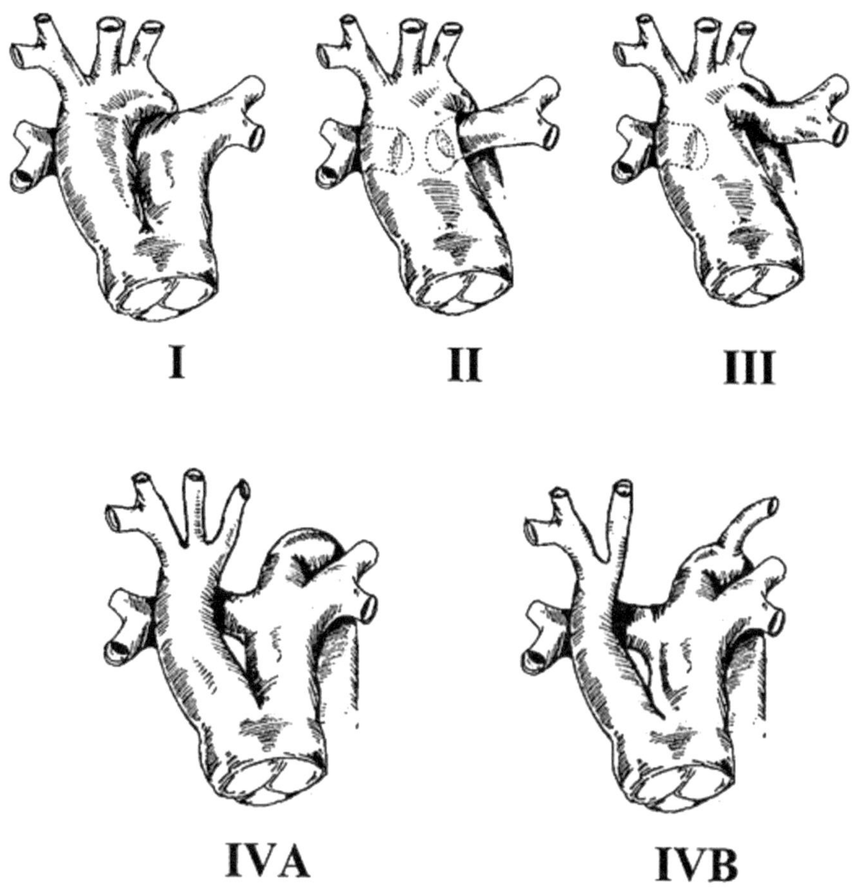

Fig. 32.1 Van Praagh classification of Truncus Arteriosus [2]. Truncus with Interrupted Arch is type IV. Depending on the level of IAA interruption, Type IV A and IV B can be described

The presence of an arterial duct is a singular characteristic of TAC-IAA.

Pulmonary branches stenosis or hypoplasia can be seen. The VSD is cono-ventricular (outlet) and usually large. A dextroposition of the common arterial trunk is frequent; when severe, the VSD may have to be enlarged, to prevent subaortic obstruction. Truncus without VSD (type B of Van Praagh [2]) seems not viable. The truncal valve could have all aspects; it is frequently quadri-sigmoid. TAC-IAA share equally with other truncus the risk of regurgitation of the truncal valve; a condition with severe prognosis. Coronary arteries can be abnormal. In rare cases the abnormal coronary patterns have an impact on surgery, like intra-mural course. The left coronary ostium is many times very close to the left PA ostium. The association with a di George syndrome with 22q11 deletion is usual.

The closure of the arterial duct (PDA) is a catastrophic event. Fetal diagnosis [3] and early diagnosis are crucial to start Prostaglandin infusion immediately after birth. Patients seen after PDA closure may be moribund with major multiple organs failure (renal failure, hepatic failure and necrotizing enterocolitis) and severe heart failure with massive increase of the pulmonary flow and worsening of the truncal regurgitation. Small birth weight ≪2.5 kg is not unusual.

Diagnosis and Imaging

The chest X-ray shows plethoric lungs with massive shunt and cardiomegaly. The thymus can be absent.

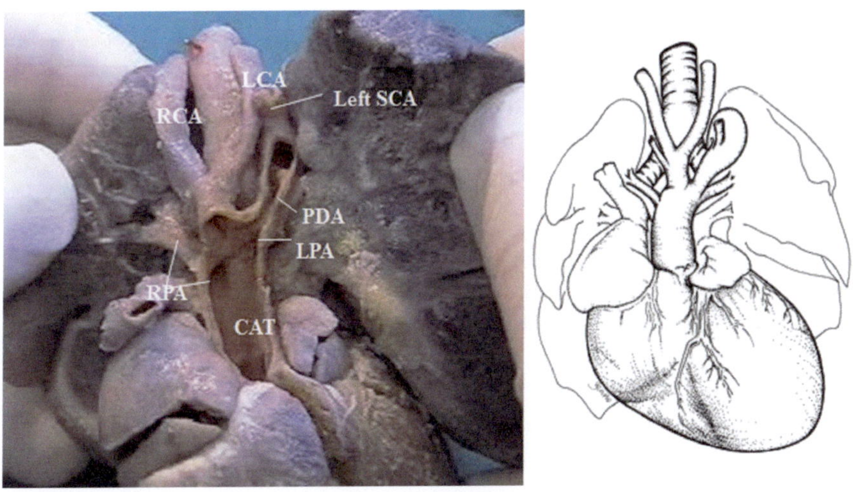

Fig. 32.2 TAC-IAA type IV B. Courtesy of Pr. Yen Ho, Cardiac Pathology Laboratory, Royal Brompton Hospital, London, UK. (*LCA* left carotid artery, *RCA* right carotid artery, *LSCA* left subclavian artery, *RPA* right PA, *LPA* left PA, *CAT* common arterial trunk.) An aberrant right subclavian artery arises from the descending aorta and is not seen on the specimen

Echocardiography, done immediately after birth, is usually sufficient to make an accurate diagnosis. It allows defining the presence and degree of a truncal valve regurgitation, the level of the arch interruption, the patency of the ductus arteriosus, the take off of the pulmonary arteries, the dextroposition of the truncal valve, the coronary anatomy, the presence of a thymus.

A catheterization is rarely performed as it could worsen the clinical status.

CT scan with 3D reconstruction would provide excellent images but are rarely performed due to the emergency of the surgical treatment. A head sonogram is necessary to exclude an intra-cranial bleeding that will contra-indicate a CPB.

Pre-operative Check-List

Weight
Truncal valve regurgitation
Level of IAA interruption
Diameter ductus arteriosus
Pulmonary arteries morphology, stenosis and take off (usually truncus type 1)
Extra cardiac damages (NEC, intra cranial bleeding, infection, etc.…)
Di George syndrome
Irradiated blood.

Surgery

The optimal procedure is neonatal one stage repair [4].

Indications

There are *contra-indications to one stage repair.* Some patients may be referred in very poor conditions with multiple organ failure due to delayed diagnosis. Other may have associated extra cardiac damages like NEC intra-cranial bleeding or ongoing infections. Newborns with low birth weight less than 2 kg, or so, remain extremely challenging.

Palliative Procedure

TAC-IAA could be palliated by a PA branches banding through sternotomy. The ductus arteriosus is kept open using prostaglandin infusion or alternatively the PDA could be stented either at the time of PA branch banding (hybrid stage 1) or later on.

The palliation allows to differ the repair around 2 months of life and over 3.5 kg, which gives time to rule out extracardiac damages.

5.3 One Stage Repair

5.3.1 Pre-operative management. The medical treatment includes ventilation with low FiO_2, prostaglandin infusion, high haematocrit, inotropic support to maintain optimal perfusion to the lower body.

5.3.2 Surgical technique for neonatal one stage repair of TAC-IAA.

The first successful repair of TAC-IAA was reported by Dwight C. McGoon [5] at the Mayo Clinic in 1971. Surgical series of one stage neonatal repair were published in the early 90s by Frank Hanley et al. [6] and Ed Bove et al. [7]. We previously published the technique described below [8, 9].

First the arch is reconstructed. As for interrupted arch repair, we avoid circulatory arrest and use antegrade cerebral perfusion [10]. The blood is irradiated when a di George syndrome is confirmed or suspected. A Goretex 3.5 mm is implanted on the brachio-cepahalic artery or right carotid and an aortic canula #8 is used. A second canula is placed through the PDA to perfuse the descending aorta. The CPB is run in hypothermia. The PA branches are snared at the beginning of the CPB. A left vent is placed. The descending aorta is widely mobilised. Once 25° is reached, the second canula is removed, the PDA is ligated, the neck vessels are snared and the descending aorta is cross clamped, with attention made to protect the left recurrent nerve. The flow is reduced around 50 ml/kg/min and the antegrade cerebral perfusion is started with monitoring of the right radial artery and NIRS. Cardioplegia is injected into the common trunk.

First the IAA is repaired. The common trunk is then divided at the level of take off of the ascending aorta (Fig. 32.2). Care is taken to preserve the pulmonary ostia as well as the left coronary trunk that could be very close. A large button containing the two pulmonary ostia is resected from the common trunk. The entirety of the ductus tissue is resected until a clean section of the descending aorta is obtained. The ascending aorta is incised on its left border up to the neck vessels (Fig. 32.3). An end to side anastomosis is performed between the terminal end of the ascending aorta and the mobilized descending aorta. The descending aorta is incised at least on 1 cm and then an ovale patch (homograft, bovine pericardium) (Fig. 32.4) is anastomosed so as to enlarge the arch and the ascending aorta to reach the diameter of the common trunk. Then the common trunk is anastomosed to the reconstructed ascending aorta. The cross clamp is moved on the ascending aorta, cross clamp and snares are released. Full flow is resumed at 32°.

Then *the TAC is repaired.* A lower infundibulotomy is performed. The large conventricular VSD is closed using a patch of Goretex or bovine pericardium, secured by running suture and separate pledgeted sutures on the superior border. A RV to PA valved conduit is implanted, using either a Contegra bovine jugular vein conduit (diameter 12 in neonates) or a pulmonary homograft. Considering the risk of mortality, it seems challenging to avoid a valved conduit [11, 12]

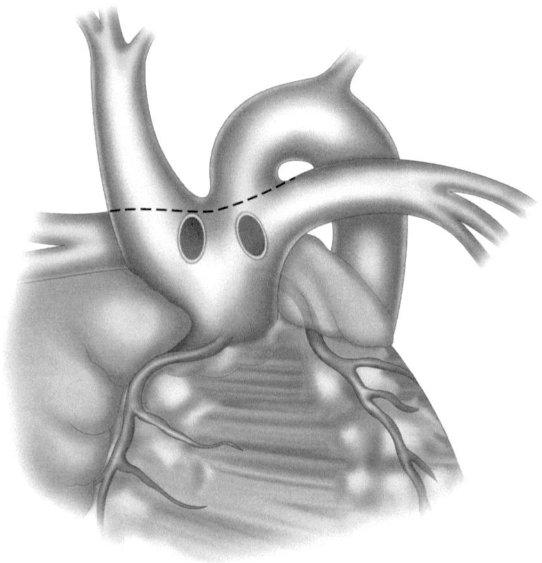

Fig. 32.3 The truncal root is divided at the level of the take off of the ascending aorta

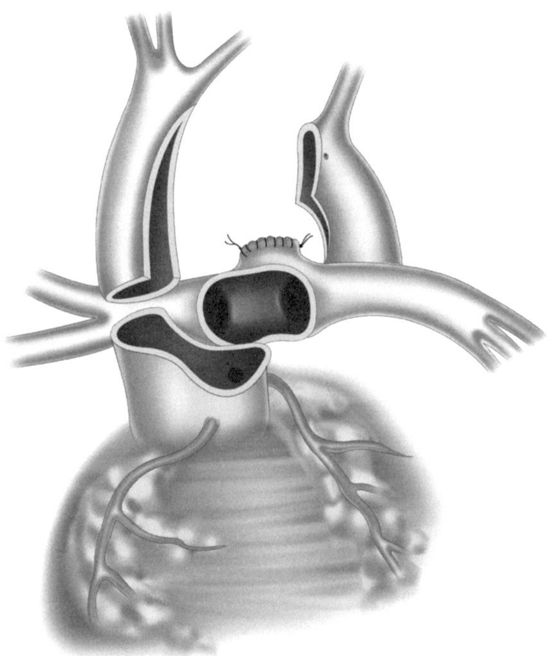

Fig. 32.4 The pulmonary trunk is harvested. All ductal tissue is resected and the IAA repaired [8, 9]

The truncal valve regurgitation should be treated only when severe. Different techniques were described, including resection one leaflet and reimplantation of a coronary ostium [13]. Repair is challenging in neonates. Truncal valve replacement with homograft has been attempted as salvage procedure.

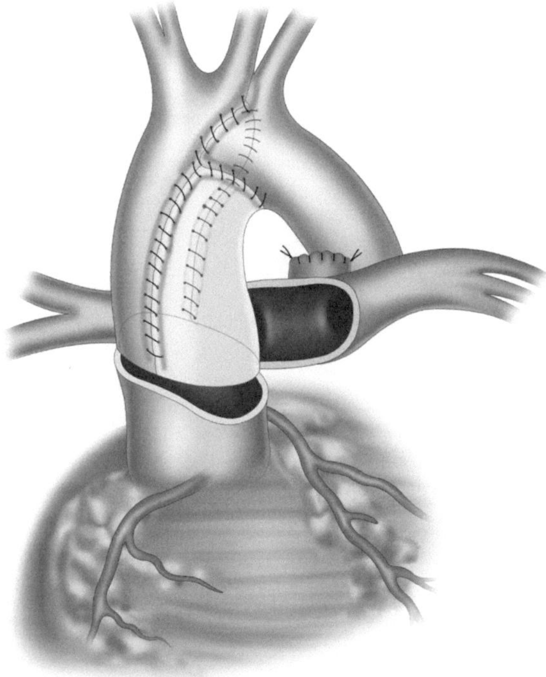

Fig. 32.5 The aortic arch and the ascending aorta are enlarged using a large patch (homograft or bovine pericardium). The continuity with the truncal root is reconstructed by direct anastomosis. A RV to PA valved conduit is then implanted (Contegra or homograft) [8, 9]

5.3.3 Post-operative course. Many times, the sternum is left open. Inotropes are infused. The prevention of pulmonary hypertension crisis is secured using: deep sedation, myorelaxant, Nitric Oxyde with monitoring of the PA pressure through a transthoracic line. The chest is usually closed within 3–4 days and the patient extubated when PA pressure is normalized without sedation. Older patients are placed on oral Sildenafil for several weeks.

Outcome

Most institutional reports [3, 14], are less than 10 patients (Table 32.1) The association with aortic arch interruption in patients with TAC is a marked risk factor for death [15, 16]. In the 50 cases of TAC-IAA reported by the CHSS multicentric study [3], the early mortality is 68 % It is 27 % for 58 TAC-IAA at the STS database for the period 2010–2013 (Chap. 5).

The risk factors for mortality are: severe truncal regurgitation [17] and multiple organ failure [13]. Palliation with PA branches banding and maintaining the duct open, with prostaglandin or stenting, is an interesting option [18]. Palliation repairing only the IAA is associated with poor results [3]. In any case, moribund infants seen late have very poor prognosis [8, 13]

The optimal RVOT reconstruction remains controversial. Using a valved conduit, either pulmonary homograft [9] or Contegra [16] bovine jugular conduit,

Table 32.1 Published series of TAC-IAA (Truncus Arteriosus Communis-Interrupted Aortic Arch)

Centers	Year	N TAC-IAA	Early deaths TAC-IAA
Bove et al., Ann Arbor, USA [7]	1993	5	20 % (1)
Lacour-Gayet et al., Paris, France [8]	1996	7	43 % (3)
Jahangiri et al., Boston, USA [17]	2000	9	0 % (0)
Hanley et al., Boston, USA [6]	2001	8	25 % (2)
Miyamoto et al., Bonn, Germany [14]	2005	10	50 % (5)
Konstantinov et al., CHSS [4]	2006	50	68 % (34)
Bohuta L et al., Melbourne, Australia [15]	2008	16	12.5 % (2)
STS Database, USA	2013	58	20.7 % (12)

seems a safe option given the operative risk. The Contegra is user friendly and easily available in small sizes [19–21]. Mid term results at 7 years on the CHSS [22] multicentric series of 101 TAC show satisfactory results. Some centers suggest avoiding a RV to PA valved conduit [12]. Trans-catheter implantation of pulmonary valve may reduce the incidence of surgical re-intervention on the RVOT (Chap. 14).

Late reoperations are frequent [4]; mainly to treat conduit dysfunction. Truncal valve repair for residual truncal valve regurgitation show encouraging results [23]. Stenosis of pulmonary arteries are treated by interventional cardiology.

Surgical repair of TAC-IAA is the most challenging procedure in terms of mortality and morbidity as documented by the STS and the EACTS database 2014 (see Chap. 4).

References

1. Collet RW, Edwards JE. Persistent truncus arteriosus; a classification according to anatomic types. Surg Clin North Am. 1949;29:1245–70.
2. Van Praagh R, Van Praagh S. The anatomy of common aorticopulmonary trunk (truncus arteriosus communis) and its embryologic implications. A study of 57 necropsy cases. Am J Cardiol. 1965;16:406–25.
3. Galindo A, Mendoza A, Arbues J, Grañeras A, Escribano D, Nieto O. Conotruncal anomalies in fetal life: accuracy of diagnosis, associated defects and outcome. Eur J Obstet Gynecol Reprod Biol. 2009;146(1):55–60.
4. Konstantinov IE, Karamlou T, Blackstone EH, Mosca RS, Lofland GK, Caldarone CA, Williams WG, Mackie AS, McCrindle BW. Truncus arteriosus associated with interrupted aortic arch in 50 neonates: a Congenital Heart Surgeons Society study. Ann Thorac Surg. 2006;81:214–22.
5. Gomes MM, McGoon DC. Truncus arteriosus with interruption of the aortic arch: report of a case successfully repaired. Mayo Clin Proc. 1971;46:40–3.
6. Hanley FL, Heinemann MK, Jonas RA, Mayer Jr JE, Cook NR, Wessel DL, Castaneda AR. Repair of truncus arteriosus in the neonate. J Thorac Cardiovasc Surg. 1993;105:1047–56.
7. Bove EL, Lupinetti FM, Pridjian AK, Beekman 3rd RH, Callow LB, Snider AR, Rosenthal A. Results of a policy of primary repair of truncus arteriosus in the neonate. J Thorac Cardiovasc Surg. 1993;105:1057–65.

8. Lacour-Gayet F, Serraf A, Galletti L, Bruniaux J, Belli E, Piot D, Touchot A, Petit J, Houyel L, Planche C. Biventricular repair of conotruncal anomalies associated with aortic arch obstruction: 103 patients. Circulation. 1997;4;96(9 Suppl):II-328–34.
9. Lacour-Gayet F, Goldberg S. Surgical repair of truncus arteriosus associated with interrupted aortic arch. EACTS Multimedia Manual Cardiothorac Surg. Oxford Journals. Volume 2008, Issue 0328. http://mmcts.oxfordjournals.org/content/2008/0328/mmcts.2006.002451.full.
10. Tchervenkov CI, Korkola SJ, Shum-Tim D. Surgical technique to avoid circulatory arrest and direct arch vessel cannulation during aortic arch reconstruction. Eur J Cardiothorac Surg. 2001;19:708–10.
11. Barbero-Marcial M, Riso A, Atik E, Jatene A. A technique for correction of truncus arteriosus types I and II without extracardiac conduits. Journal of Thoracic and Cardiovascular Surgery. 1990;99:364–9.
12. Raisky O, Ali WB, Bajolle F, Marini D, Metton O, Bonnet D, Sidi D, Vouhé PR. Common arterial trunk repair: with conduit or without? Eur J Cardiothorac Surg. 2009;36(4):675–82.
13. Mavroudis C, Backer CL. Surgical management of severe truncal insufficiency: experience with truncal valve remodeling techniques. Ann Thorac Surg. 2001;72:396–400.
14. Miyamoto T, Sinzobahamvya N, Kumpikaite D, Asfour B, Photiadis J, Brecher AM, Urban AE. Repair of truncus arteriosus and aortic arch interruption: outcome analysis. Ann Thorac Surg. 2005;79:2077–82.
15. Bohuta L, Hussein A, Fricke TA, d'Udekem Y, Bennett M, Brizard C. Konstantinov Surgical repair of truncus arteriosus associated with interrupted aortic arch: long-term outcomes. Ann Thorac Surg. 2011;91(5):1473–7.
16. Sinzobahamvya N, Boscheinen M, Blaschczok HC, Kallenberg R, Photiadis J, Haun C, Hraska V, Asfour B. Survival and reintervention after neonatal repair of truncus arteriosus with valved conduit. Eur J Cardiothorac Surg. 2008;34(4):732–7.
17. Jahangiri M, Zurakowski D, Mayer JE, del Nido PJ, Jonas RA. Repair of the truncal valve and associated interrupted arch in neonates with truncus arteriosus. J Thorac Cardiovasc Surg. 2000;119:508–14.
18. Weinstein S, Liveris A, Shenoy RU, Lacour-Gayet F. Bilateral pulmonary arterial banding for complex transposition of the great arteries. J Thorac Cardiovasc Surg. 2013;145(3):876–8.
19. Dave H, Mueggler O, Comber M, Enodien B, Nikolaou G, Bauersfeld U, Jenni R, Bettex D, Prêtre R. Risk factor analysis of 170 single-institutional contegra implantations in pulmonary position. Ann Thorac Surg. 2011;91:195–302; discussion 202–3.
20. Rastan AJ, Walther T, Daehnert I, Hambsch J, Mohr FW, Janousek J, Kostelka M. Bovine jugular vein conduit for right ventricular outflow tract reconstruction: evaluation of risk factors for mid-term outcome. Ann Thorac Surg. 2006;82:1308–15.
21. Lacour-Gayet F, Serraf A, Komiya T, Sousa-Uva M, Bruniaux J, Touchot A, Roux D, Neuville P, Planche C. Truncus arteriosus repair: influence of techniques of right ventricular outflow tract reconstruction. J Thorac Cardiovasc Surg. 1996;111:849–56.
22. Hickey EJ, McCrindle BW, Blackstone EH, Yeh Jr T, Pigula F, Clarke D, Tchervenkov CI, Hawkins J, CHSS Pulmonary Conduit Working Group. Jugular venous valved conduit (Contegra) matches allograft performance in infant truncus arteriosus repair. Eur J Cardiothorac Surg. 2008;33(5):890–8.
23. Russell HM, Pasquali SK, Jacobs JP, Jacobs ML, O'Brien SM, Mavroudis C, Backer CL. Outcomes of repair of common arterial trunk with truncal valve surgery: a review of the society of thoracic surgeons congenital heart surgery database. Ann Thorac Surg. 2012;93(1):164–9; discussion 169.

Chapter 33
Interrupted Aortic Arch

Roberto M. Di Donato and Francois Lacour-Gayet

Abstract Interrupted aortic arch (IAA), usually associated with a ventricular septal defect (VSD), is a rapidly fatal congenital heart anomaly with ductus-dependent systemic circulation. Three types of IAA – A, B and C – are classicaly recognized. Only type B is, but not exclusively, a true cono-truncal anomaly. The critical condition of these neonates dictates early referral and surgical treatment. Careful preoperative assessment, and particularly the identification of a severe left ventricular outflow tract obstruction (LVOTO, <4 mm), is crucial for a successful outcome. DiGeorge syndrome is another frequently associated feature with important clinical implications. Many surgical options are available. Staged repair was popular in the past, but primary repair through a median sternotomy (using either deep hypothermic circulatory arrest or moderately hypothermic antegrade selective cerebral perfusion) is currently the preferred approach. Aortic arch reconstruction is accomplished by end-to-side anastomosis with the ascending aorta, more or less associated with patch augmentation of the anastomosis. A severe LVOTO may require more aggressive procedures, e.g. Yasui or Ross-Konno operations. Current early mortality for repair of IAA with VSD ranges from 4 to 10 %. Fifteen-year survival is about 60 %. Recurrence of arch obstruction has been reported from 10 to 30 %, while recurrence of LVOTO has averaged 20 %. Anatomic features affect mortality and initial LVOT procedures, whereas characteristics of the arch repair affect arch reintervention.

Keywords Congenital heart disease • Interrupted aortic arch • Aortic arch reconstruction • Ventricular Outflow Obstruction • Congenital heart surgery • Yasui operation • Ross-Konno operation

R.M. Di Donato, MD (✉)
Pediatric Cardiac Surgery, Prince Sultan Cardiac Center, Riyadh, Saudi Arabia
e-mail: robdido@hotmail.com

F. Lacour-Gayet, MD
Department of Pediatric Cardiac Surgery, National Heart and Lung Institute,
Royal Brompton Hospital, Imperial College University, Sydney Street, London SW3 6NP, UK
e-mail: f.lacour-gayet@rbht.nhs.uk

F. Lacour-Gayet et al. (eds.), *Surgery of Conotruncal Anomalies*,
DOI 10.1007/978-3-319-23057-3_33

Introduction

Interrupted aortic arch (IAA) is defined as loss of luminal continuity between the ascending and descending aorta [1]: this may include either complete discontinuity between the two aortic ends or an impervious fibrous strand in the transverse arch or aortic isthmus. In most cases, IAA combines with a ventricular septal defect (VSD) and a patent ductus arteriosus (PDA) supplying blood to the descending thoracic aorta. It accounts for 1.5 % of all congenital heart anomalies and, untreated, leads to death within the first month of life in 75 % of the cases. In fact, IAA is a typical anomaly with ductus-dependent systemic circulation. These neonates usually present in severe heart failure and shock, with loss of femoral pulses, mildly reduced O_2 saturation in the lower body, rising metabolic acidosis and anuria. Cardiac failure ensues from combined pressure overload (for aortic arch obstruction and ductal closure) and volume overload (for large VSD shunt). Circulatory collapse occurs after ductal closure and concurrent fall of pulmonary resistance followed by flooding of pulmonary circulation at the expense of systemic perfusion in the lower body. Flow reversal is seen in the aortic branches distal to the interruption (left subclavian and common carotid arteries) but this is usually insufficient to supply the infra-diaphragmatic territory.

Anatomy

Three main types of IAA are unanimously recognized in relation to the site of the aortic arch interruption, as proposed by Celoria and Patton [2] (Fig. 33.1): *type A*, with interruption distal to the left subclavian artery; *type B*, with interruption

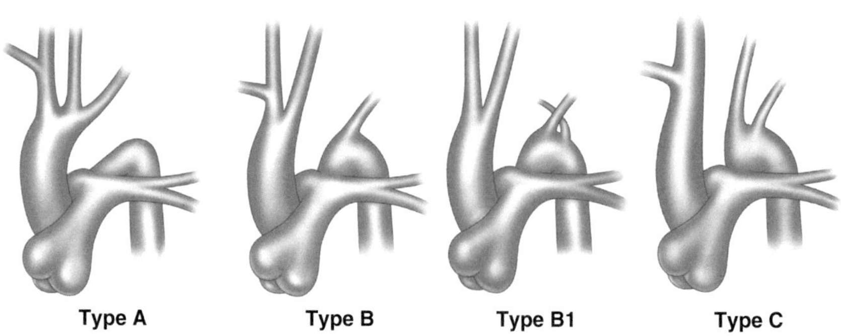

Fig. 33.1 Anatomic types of IAA, according to Celoria and Patton. Type A: Interruption distal to the left subclavian artery. Type B: Interruption between the left carotid and left subclavian arteries. Type B1: type B with aberrant right subclavian artery from descending aorta is frequent. Type C: Interruption between the innominate and the left common carotid arteries is exceptional. Similarly, there are type A1 and C1. In the latter the aorta gives only the right carotid and, due to the very small aortic annulus, this C1 form is usually associated with HLHS

between the left carotid and left subclavian arteries; and *type C*, with interruption between the right brachio-cephalic artery and the left carotid. The most common is type B (55–70 %), then type A (28–40 %) and type C (1–5 %) [3]. Sub-classifications have been introduced according to presence and site of an *aberrant right subclavian artery*, whether originating from the descending aorta and taking a retro-esophageal course (type A1, B1, C1) [4, 5] (Fig. 33.1). Type B1 is a real problem as the ascending aorta gives only the two carotids.

Etiopathogenesis of IAA

Different pathogenetic mechanisms have been suggested for patients with IAA type A and B [6]. Alterations in cardiac hemodynamics secondary to a large ventricular septal defect with or without LVOT obstruction may cause IAA type A [7, 8], whereas IAA type B seems strongly related to abnormal migration [9] of neural crest cells. Noteworthy, a higher prevalence of del 22q11 syndrome has been reported in children with IAA type B (50–80 %) [10, 11], whereas this chromosomal microdeletion is very rare (but not absent) in patients with IAA type A [10–12]. The pathogenetic mechanism of IAA type C is, instead, still uncertain, although intuitively more related to type B than A.

Probably only IAA type B should be classified as a true cono-truncal anomaly (CTA), according to Van Praagh's definition (Chap. 1); stating that CTAs include both a conal and a truncal anomaly. In IAA type B, the conal anomaly is due to the posterior displacement deviation of the conal septum [14], whereas the truncal anomaly is due to the hypoplasia of the ascending aorta and aortic annulus. IAA type B, and particularly B1, are frequently associated with 22q11 deletion syndrome like several cono-truncal anomalies, e.g. tetralogy of Fallot [13] and truncus arteriosus [13], etc… Therefore, for completeness of information, all three types of IAA are described in this chapter, although with more emphasis for IAA type B.

Associated Anomalies

Associated anomalies are seen in 98 % of these patients [3]. An isolated VSD is present in 72 % of the cases and usually is of the conoventricular/malalignment type, in subarterial position. Yet, all types of VSD may occur, including multiple VSDs in 2.7 % of the cases. In another 27 %, a VSD is part of a complex lesion. An intact ventricular septum is found in only 1 % of the patients [3].

Left ventricular outflow obstruction (LVOTO) is also common, mainly due to posterior deviation of the conal septum (Fig. 33.2) but also for other anatomical factors, e.g. a generalized narrowing of the LVOT, a prominent anterolateral muscle of the left ventricle [15] (*muscle of Moulaert*, Fig. 33.3), discrete fibrous subaortic stenosis, and aortic valve stenosis (hypoplastic aortic annulus and/or bicuspid aortic valve).

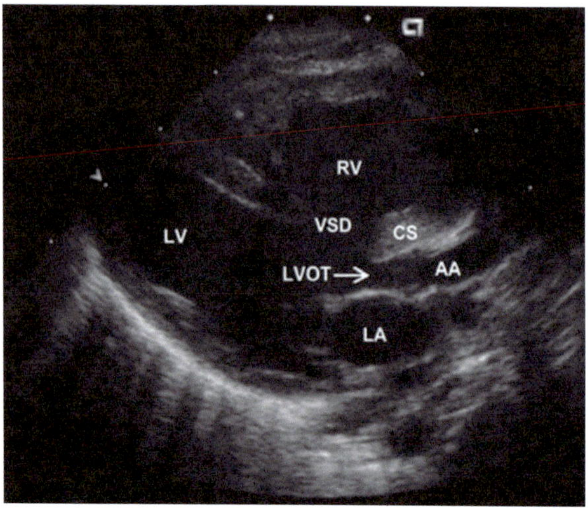

Fig. 33.2 Subaortic obstruction (LVOTO). 2D-echocardiographic appearance of subaortic obstruction in IAA. LVOTO is typically caused by posterior deviation of the conal septum. *Legends: RV* right ventricle, *LV* left ventricle, *VSD* ventricular septal defect, *LVOT* left ventricle outflow tract, *CS* conal septum, *AA* ascending aorta, *LA* left atrium

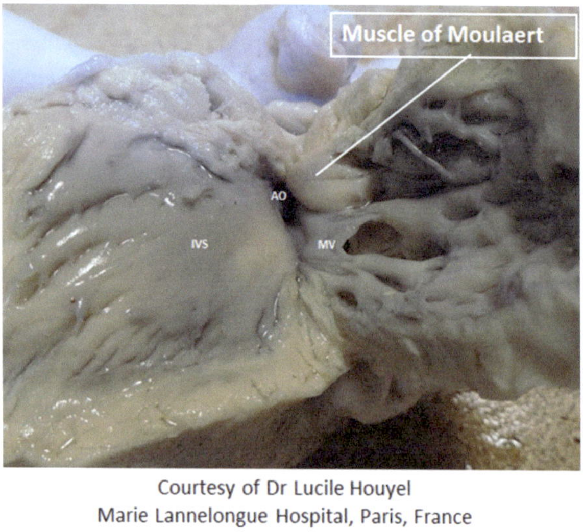

Fig. 33.3 Muscle of Moulaert (Courtesy of Dr Lucile Houyel, Marie Lannelongue, Paris). Legends. *AO* aorta, *MV* mitral valve, *IVS* interventricular septum

Typically, the ascending aorta is small, straight and bifurcated (the "V sign"); in contrast, the pulmonary trunk is considerably dilated. The finding of an aberrant right subclavian artery may elicit suspicion of a relevant LVOTO. Other concomitant aortic arch anomalies occur rarely including a right-sided ductus giving origin to the right subclavian artery, a right pulmonary artery originating from the ascending aorta and a right aortic arch.

There is a strong association of IAA (particularly type B) with chromosome 22q11 deletion, DiGeorge syndrome, characterized by different expressions of velocardiofacial syndrome, absence or hypoplasia of thymic tissue, hypocalcemia and immunodeficiency problems. Association with CHARGE syndrome has also been reported.

Diagnosis/Imaging

The main diagnostic tool in babies with IAA is 2D-echocardiography that usually provides all the essential morphologic data about the aortic arch and the intracardiac structures. 2D-echocardiography has proven increasingly useful also for intrauterine diagnosis. In the rare case of persistent diagnostic doubts, mainly regarding the aortic arch anatomy, CT angiography and gadolinium-enhanced 3D-MRI provide excellent imaging of the anomalous vascular structures. Currently, there is minimal if no role for cardiac catheterization with angiography in IAA diagnosis.

Preoperative Check List

(a) IAA anatomic type
(b) Diameter of ascending aorta
(c) Status of the PDA
(d) VSD location, diameter and number
(e) Measurement of LVOT diameter and of aortic annulus
(f) LV volume
(g) Status of pulmonary valve
(h) Presence of major associated cardiac anomalies
(i) DiGeorge syndrome or other chromosomic anomalies
(j) General factors (weight, prematurity, necrotizing enterocolitis, intra-cranial bleeding, etc.)
(k) Aristotle score

Indications

Having made the diagnosis of IAA, the following anatomical, haemodynamic and clinical features are relevant for proper planning of the surgical strategy.

Anatomy of the Aortic Arch

The type of IAA is central for the choice of surgical approach, keeping in mind that IAA type B is frequently associated with LVOTO [3]. Other relevant features include: sidedness of aortic arch, length of arch discontinuity and presence of an aberrant right subclavian artery from the upper descending thoracic aorta (more frequent in IAA type B and also indicative of LVOTO [3]). An aberrant right subclavian artery may also affect the pressure reading of a right radial arterial line.

Size of the Ascending Aorta

A severely hypoplastic ascending aorta, e.g. in IAA type B2 and C, may prompt a Norwood-type approach. A tentative cutoff diameter of ascending aorta for Norwood-type approach is $\leq$4.5 mm [14].

Status of the PDA

Although usually managed by prostaglandin infusion, impending PDA closure may dictate the timing of surgery.

Ventricular Septal Defect

The approach for VSD closure may vary according to number, size, type and location of the VSD/s. Noteworthy, the presence of a hypoplastic conal septum complicates the approach to the upper margin of a subarterial VSD through the tricuspid valve, therefore imposing a transpulmonary approach. The presence of multiple VSDs may suggest a staged approach.

Presence of Severe LVOTO

This is probably the single most important preoperative diagnostic factor. The presence of even a severe LVOTO in IAA is masked by the large left-to-right shunt at the VSD level. Therefore, the indication to its primary treatment cannot rely on haemodynamic evidence but only on morphologic findings. Disparate criteria for the diagnosis of LVOTO have been proposed, including: (a) degree of *posterior displacement of the conal septum* [14]; (b) hypoplasia of *aortic annulus* e.g. $\leq$4.5 mm [14] (alternatively, diameter of aortic valve cm/BSA $m^2 \leq 1$, aortic valve cross-sectional area cm^2/BSA $m^2 \leq 0.85$); (c) presence of a transaortic *echo gradient of >10 mmHg*; (d) presence of *obstructing tissue* in the subaortic area; (e) *transaortic inspection* of aortic valve and subaortic area at the time of surgery [16, 17]. The most sensible predictor of LVOTO, however, is (f) the *direct measurement of the LVOT*, either as cross-sectional area indexed to body surface area (<0.7 cm^2/m^2) [17] or as the antero-posterior LVOT-to-descending thoracic aorta (at the diaphragm level) diameter ratio measured in diastole (<1.0) [18], or, more simply, as an LVOT diameter<4 mm [19]. Tchervenkov suggests guidelines of great practical value to address LVOTO in IAA [19]:

- If the LVOT diameter (mm) is smaller than the baby's weight (kg), a radical approach for LVOTO is mandatory.
- If the LVOT diameter (mm) is greater than the baby's weight (kg) + 2 mm, no treatment for LVOTO is indicated.
- In between these two cases, survival may be possible but with significant residual LVOTO. Therefore, treatment of LVOTO in these cases is totally discretional.

Hypoplasia of the Left Ventricle

Association of IAA with hypoplastic left heart syndrome has been reported in sporadic cases [20].

Status of Pulmonary Valve and Artery

The size of the pulmonary root and, particularly, the competence of the pulmonary valve are relevant issues if a Yasui or a Ross-Konno operation are contemplated.

Presence of Major Associated Cardiac Anomalies

An aortopulmonary window has been reported in 4–5 % of the cases of IAA and is typically associated with absence of a VSD. Other complex congenital cardiac anomalies occasionally described in association with IAA include truncus arteriosus (10–18 %), transposition of the great arteries (4–6 %), Taussig-Bing heart (5 %) as well as single ventricle (3 %) [3]. The coexistence of major cardiovascular anomalies imposes specific adaptations of IAA treatment.

Associated DiGeorge Syndrome

Two forms of *DiGeorge syndrome* are recognized: (a) *complete form*, with absence of thymus gland, dysmorphic facial features, hypocalcaemia and low CD4+ T-lymphocyte count (<400 cells/mm); (b) *partial form*, with hypoplastic thymus, dysmorphic facial features, hypocalcaemia and no deficit of the CD4+ T-lymphocyte subpopulation. Hypocalcemia, in relation with absence or hypoplasia of the parathyroid glands, may be a critical issue. All blood products should be irradiated to remove donor lymphocytes, in order to prevent graft-vs-host disease.

General Factors

Patient presenting with low cardiac output and multi-organ failure may contraindicate surgery. Necrotizing enterocolitis [21] and intracranial bleeding [22] should always be ruled out: abdominal and transcranial sonograms are indicated in all IAA patients. Prematurity, low body weight and coexistence of complex extracardiac anomalies also considerably add to surgical risk.

Risk Assessment

Basic Aristotle score for IAA is 10.8. Comprehensive Aristotle Score may, then, be up to 20.8. Such a high surgical risk may suggest a *staged approach*, the latter provided that aortic arch reconstruction is amenable to a left thoracotomy approach.

Surgical Treatment

Timing

On admission to the hospital, diagnosis and clinical stabilization must be promptly pursued. Basic therapeutic measures include prostaglandin infusion (0.05–0.2 μg/kg/min), mechanical ventilation adjusted to maximize the pulmonary/systemic resistance ratio keeping the Qp/Qs around 1, moderate inotropic support (dopamine $\leq$ 5 μg/kg/min) and correction of metabolic acidosis. Clinical stabilization is usually achieved within 12–24 h, thereafter surgery should be undertaken within the first week of life.

Repair

IAA can be managed by either *staged* or *primary repair*. Both approaches, in turn, encompass a variety of surgical solutions [1].

Trans-Thoracic Off-Pump Arch Repair ± Pulmonary Artery Banding

The staged approach, more frequently used in the past, includes two or more steps. The first operation is carried out in the neonatal period through a left thoracotomy. It follows the same principles of aortic coarctectomy and consists of aortic arch repair, either by direct reconstruction (with or without patch augmentation), or by Goretex graft interposition, usually combined with placement of a pulmonary artery band. There are limiting factors to a trans-thoracic arch repair, including the degree of proximal arch and ascending aorta hypoplasia (making proximal aortic arch clamping difficult), the presence of an aberrant right subclavian artery (precluding the use of a right radial arterial line) and the diagnosis of severe LVOTO (incompatible with pulmonary artery banding). A proposed technique for dealing with proximal arch hypoplasia through a thoracotomy is the left carotid swing-down technique [23], possibly combined with a reverse subclavian flap. Complete repair is, then, accomplished at the age of 2–6 months [24].

Primary Repair

The single-stage repair of IAA and intracardiac defects in the neonatal period has become the preferred strategy in most centers [19]. In particular, this approach is always indicated when the proximal segment of the arch needs augmentation. Relevant technical issues are as follows.

Median Sternotomy Approach

When dealing with aortic arch surgery, right radial arterial monitoring and cerebral near-infrared spectroscopy, irrespectively of the type of approach for arch repair, are highly recommended to monitor the patency of the innominate artery during manipulations.

Through a standard median sternotomy, the great arteries are dissected free, encircling the pulmonary arteries, the aortic branches and the arterial duct. In critical patients, snaring of one branch pulmonary artery immediately after pericardial opening may help to control the torrential pulmonary blood flow.

Management of Cardiopulmonary Bypass

Arterial cannulation may be direct, and somewhat laterally placed, into the distal ascending aorta (ready to be advanced into the innominate artery if selective cerebral perfusion is adopted) or into the innominate artery itself, most commonly via a 3.5 mm Goretex graft. An additional cannula may be optionally inserted into the PDA for a more effective *perfusion of the lower body*, and/or into the proximal ascending aorta for *continuous coronary perfusion* during arch repair. Venous cannulation is preferably bicaval to facilitate intracardiac repair. A left atrial vent is also required. After starting cardiopulmonary bypass, the pulmonary arteries are snare-occluded and cooling of the patient to the desired temperature is commenced.

With regard to perfusion strategy, given the relatively short period of time required for arch repair (about 30 min), *deep hypothermic circulatory arrest* (*DHCA*) at 18 °C is safe and practical, as it provides a bloodless field. However, the related time constraint (safe DHCA period < 45 min) and the increasing recognition of the deleterious effects of DHCA on neurodevelopmental outcome [25] has recently induced many surgeons to adopt either *continuous antegrade cerebral perfusion* at 25–28 °C or *intermittent antegrade cerebral perfusion* at 18 °C. With these alternative techniques, the operative field is not bloodless and the improved long-term neurologic outcome has not been conclusively demonstrated yet [26]. By and large, the entire repair is performed during aortic cross-clamping with repeated shots of cardioplegia. Proper myocardial protection is achieved by strict adherence to established protocols.

Cardiac Repair

Using circulatory arrest strategy for arch repair, our preferred sequence of surgical steps consists of LVOTO relief, if needed, and VSD closure during cooling, followed by arch repair during deep hypothermic circulatory arrest.

Relief of Subaortic Stenosis

Most believe that LVOTO should rarely be addressed primarily, unless in very severe cases (LVOT diameter <3.5–4 mm), accepting the potential need for secondary treatment [27]. However, in the presence of a moderate subaortic stenosis, before closing the VSD, a *limited wedge resection* of the posteriorly deviated conal septum can be easily performed either through the tricuspid valve (Fig. 33.4), or the pulmonary [18]. During this manoeuvre, though, great care should be taken not to damage the underlying aortic

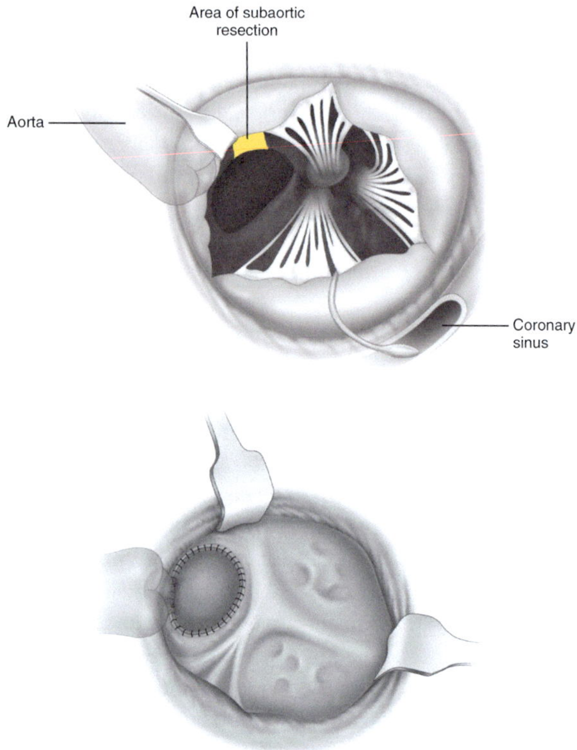

Fig. 33.4 Transatrial approach for VSD closure ± limited conal septum resection. If the conal septum is well developed, the upper edge of the VSD is easily exposed under the septal leaflet of the tricuspid valve, allowing the classical transatrial approach for VSD closure. Notice the anteriorly placed area for potential conal septal resection and its relationship with the underlying aortic valve

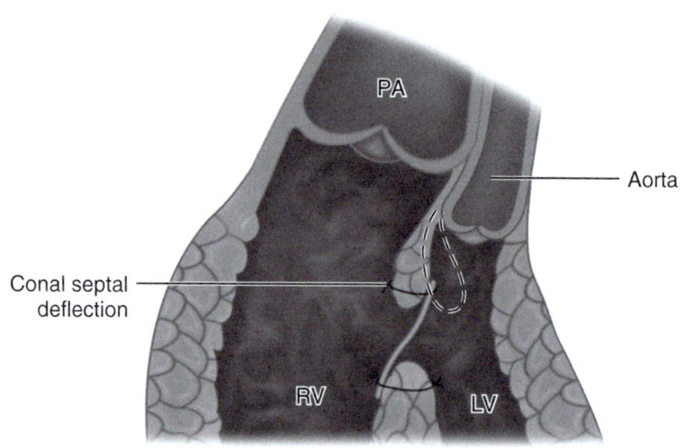

Fig. 33.5 Relief of subaortic stenosis by conal septum "deflection". Through either a transatrial or a transpulmonary approach, the apical portion of a downsized patch relative to the VSD area is anchored to the left side of the conal septum to produce deflection of the posteriorly deviated septum away from the LVOT

and/or the mitral valve. In some cases, the simple *anterior enlargement of the VSD* with partial detachment of the conal septum may be a valid and less risky surrogate of a radical full-thickness resection of the conal septum [22]. Alternatively, relief of LVOTO can also be achieved by anchoring an undersized VSD patch to the tip of the conal septum that, as a result, is *"deflected"* away from the LVOT [28] (Fig. 33.5).

VSD Patch Closure

The best approach to a typical subarterial VSD depends on the size of the conal septum: (a) *transatrial*, if the conal septum is well developed (Fig. 33.4); (b) *transpulmonary*, if the conal septum is deficient. In the latter case, sutures for the upper margin of the defect are put through the annulus of the overlying pulmonary valve cusps. Other types of VSD are managed by a transatrial approach. An atrial communication is closed before suturing the atriotomy.

Aortic Arch Repair Through Sternotomy

After identifying the left recurrent laryngeal nerve, the PDA is divided suturing its pulmonary stump, while the snares on the pulmonary arteries are released. Irrespectively of the perfusion strategy, the arch vessels are occluded at their origin by tourniquets or Yasargil clips and a Satinsky clamp is placed on the descending thoracic aorta, several millimiters distal to the ductal insertion (usually at the take-off of the second pair of intercostal arteries), to prevent back-bleeding and to facilitate the approximation of the two aortic ends. At this point, the proximal aortic cross clamp is removed, and so are the aortic cannula and the cardioplegia needle if circulatory arrest is used. The ductal tissue is completely resected and the distal aorta stump is fully mobilized. In the presence of an aberrant right subclavian artery, the vessel is usually divided. Occasionally, also the left subclavian artery must be divided to make a tension-free aortic anastomosis. A longitudinal aortotomy is carried out along the medial side of the distal ascending aorta up to the origin of the innominate artery (or the right common carotid artery in type B1). A direct end-to-side anastomosis (Fig. 33.6) of the

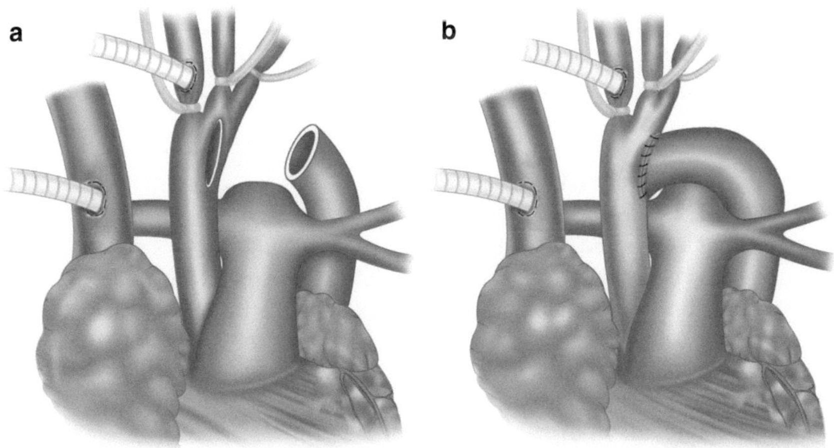

Fig. 33.6 Aortic arch reconstruction by direct end-to-side anastomosis. (**a**) After complete resection of ductal tissue and extensive dissection, (**b**) the descending aorta is directly anastomosed end-to-side to the terminal end of the ascending aorta

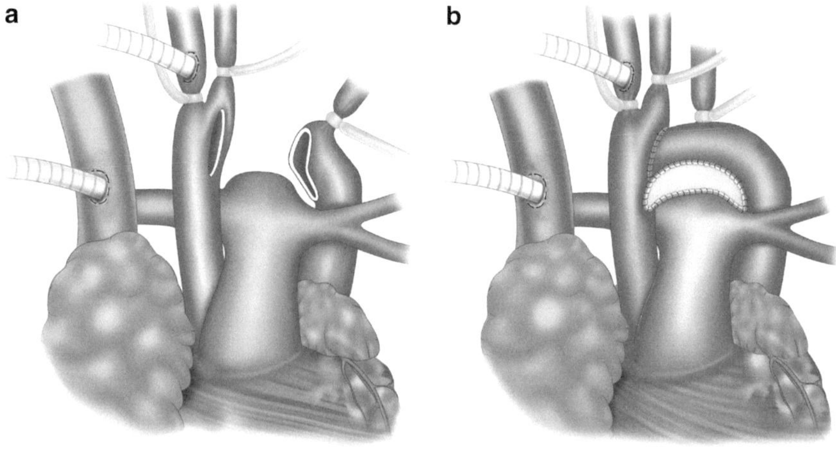

Fig. 33.7 Aortic arch reconstruction by end-to-side anastomosis and patch augmentation. (**a**) After complete resection of ductal tissue and full mobilization of the descending thoracic aorta, the two aortic ends are prepared for the anastomosis. (**b**) End-to-side anastomosis with patch augmentation

descending aorta to the postero-medial aspect of the distal ascending aorta is then performed, relegating the proximal native aortic arch to serve the left common carotid (in type B) or both the left common carotid and the left subclavian artery (in type A). In many cases, patch augmentation of this anastomosis is not needed [19, 29] Often, however, an elongated ovoid patch (Fig. 33.7). is preferably is used to augment the arch along its newly created inner curvature to reduce tension at the anastomosis and avoid re-coarctation and tracheo-bronchial compression [3, 19, 27, 30]. When diminutive in size, e.g. in IAA type B, the entire ascending aorta is opened longitudinally and incorporated in the aortic arch patch augmentation [31] (Fig. 33.8).

After arch repair, cardiopulmonary is re-started (releasing the neck vessels), the aortic cross-clamp is removed and the operation is completed in the routine fashion. Chest closure is frequently delayed.

Management of Severe LVOTO

When the diameter of the LVOT (in mm) is smaller than the baby's weight (in kg), as it frequently happens in IAA type B 1, an LVOT bypass procedure, e.g. a Yasui or a Norwood operation, should be adopted [19]. Alternatively, a Ross-Konno procedure may be considered.

Yasui Operation (Fig. 33.9)

This technique provides a bypass of the LVOTO and consists of a combination of Norwood and Rastelli operation. Through a right ventriculotomy, the left ventricle is baffled to the pulmonary artery via the large subarterial VSD. The pulmonary artery is transected and incorporated in a Norwood-type reconstruction of the aortic

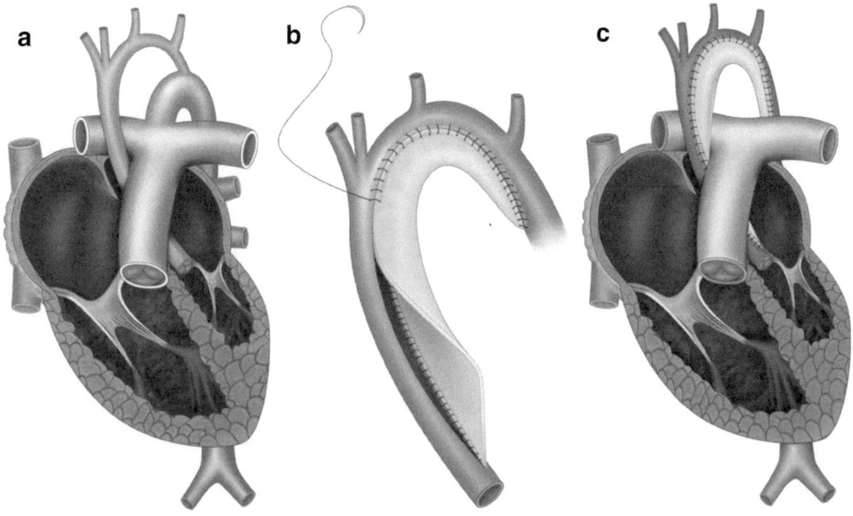

Fig. 33.8 Ascending aorta and aortic arch reconstruction by end-to-side anastomosis and extended patch augmentation. The entire ascending aorta above the sino-tubular junction is reconstructed by proximal extension of the patch used for aortic arch enlargement. (**a**) Very hypoplastic ascending aorta and aortic arch; (**b**) detail of the extended ascending aorta and aortic arch reconstruction; (**c**) final repair

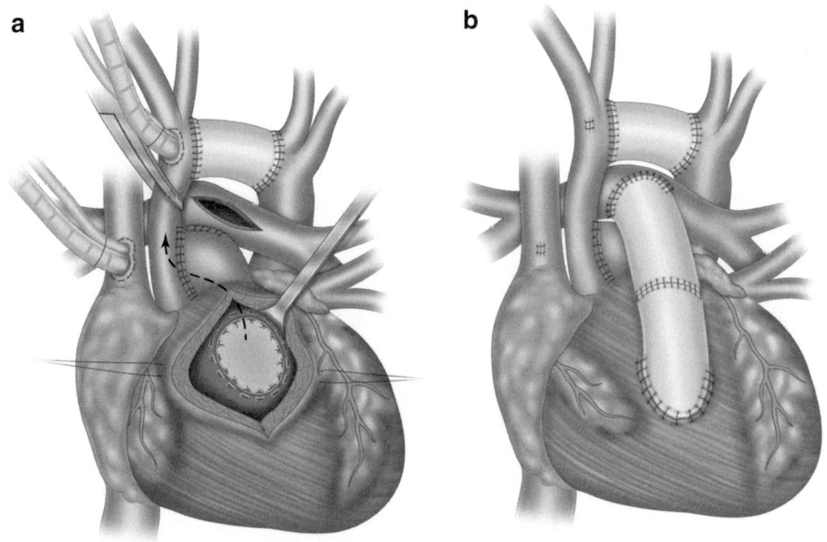

Fig. 33.9 Yasui operation (in case of LVOTO obstruction). (**a**) A Damus anastomosis is performed. The VSD is then baffled to the pulmonary valve orifice. (**b**) A valved conduit is implanted between the RV and the pulmonary artery. In many instances, the VSD could become restrictive with time and enlargement of the VSD during the procedure could be needed

arch. Finally, a right ventricle-to-pulmonary artery valved conduit is placed [32] The possibility of VSD narrowing with acquired LVOTO after a Yasui operation has been reported [33].

Norwood Operation

In particularly severe cases of LVOTO with borderline left ventricle and/or diminutive ascending aorta, a Norwood operation may be preferable in combination with a systemic-to-pulmonary artery or a Sano shunt. The following stages may include either a single ventricle or a two-ventricle repair track.

Ross-Konno Operation (Fig. 33.10)

The Ross-Konno operation allows an harmonious reconstruction of the LVOT. The entire conal septum is resected and the pulmonary autograt is implanted directly on the inferior edge of the VSD or using a patch. The coronary re-implantation and a right ventricle-to-pulmonary valved conduit implantation are similar to the routine Ross technique. Despite being technically challenging, the Ross-Konno procedure is an attractive solution for severe LVOTO in IAA [34].

Outcome

Early and Mid-term Survival

Current early mortality for repair of IAA with VSD ranges from 4 to 10 % [3, 35]. It can be as low as 4 % at 30 days for type A and 11 % for type B. Risk-adjusted 4-year survival after repair of IAA and VSD in a CHSS multi-institutional study on 174 patients was 63 % and 5-year survival for optimal repair of IAA with or without coexisting LVOTO was 93 % for type A, and 83 % for type B [27]. In a more recent CHSS multi-institutional study on 472 patients, early mortality continued to be significant, and the 6-month, 5-year, and 15-year survival rates were 83 %, 70 %, and 62 %, respectively, with better survival trend for patients with later date of birth [3]. Other studies report 5-year survival of 70–90 % [16, 23, 35, 36].

Incremental risk factors for premature death include: *date of operation*, *low birth weight*, *younger age at repair*, *condition of the patient* on entry into the operating room (in particular, low pH), *type B and C IAA*, *lack of augmentation of the arch*, *smaller size of the VSD* and *non-malaligned VSD*, *severe LVOTO*, *need for Norwood-type aortic reconstruction*, *major associated cardiac anomaly* (in particular, truncus arteriosus) [23, 35].

Outcome does not appear influenced by the type of repair (primary versus staged) [3, 35]. However, compared to the staged approach, primary repair provides the theoretical advantages of earlier normalization of physiology, a single operation, and avoidance of iatrogenic problems related to pulmonary banding.

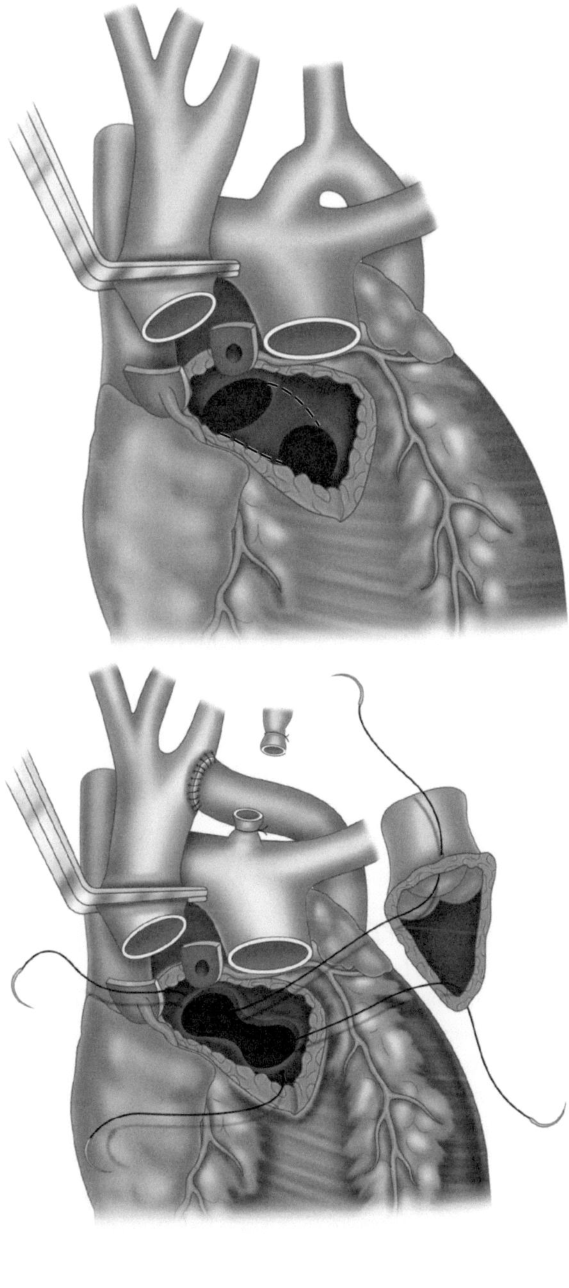

Fig. 33.10 Ross-Konno operation (in case of LVOTO obstruction). The complete excision of the conal septum allows a very wide LVOT reconstruction. The autograph is implanted directly on the inferior edge of the VSD or alternatively a patch could be used

Reoperations [37]

The long-term likelihood of undergoing a reoperation or a catheter-based reintervention after neonatal repair of IAA remains high, 40–65 % at 15 years [35, 36]. There are several late complications requiring surgical or interventional revision, as follows.

Arch Obstruction

Reported freedom from arch reintervention varies from 83 % at 12 years in one study [16] to 38 % at 16 years in another study [3]. The technique of direct anastomosis with patch augmentation has a protective effect against need for arch reintervention. In contrast, the use of an interposition graft is almost invariably doomed to re-intervention and risk of death during childhood [3]. Risk of re-intervention for residual or recurrent arch obstruction is also significantly higher in the presence of predisposing factors, e.g. use of PTFE material, inadequate excision of ductal tissues and complex associated anatomy [3]. Type B IAA is the most prone to arch reinterventions, probably related to lack of performing far-reaching mobilization of the descending aorta that is particularly needed in this IAA variant to accomplish a tension-free anastomosis.

Recurrent aortic arch stenosis is rarely treatable by balloon angioplasty, because of the very proximal location of the stenosis [23]. Surgical reconstruction of the aortic arch by sternotomy is the preferred approach.

LVOTO

The recurrence of significant residual LVOTO (peak gradient 25 mmHg) after IAA repair has been reported from 17 to 67 % [3, 18, 28]. LVOTO usually unfolds within months after surgery. In about 20 % of neonates undergoing IAA repair the LVOT is found inadequate and is addressed at the time of the first operation [3]. Initial LVOT procedure is more likely for those with type B IAA, bicuspid aortic valve and or anomalous right subclavian artery (and also single ventricle) [3]. In another 10–20 % evidence of LVOTO develops at midterm or late follow-up, even when the LVOT was adequate after initial operation [3]. At late follow-up, the 2006 CHSS study found that for the patients who had an initial LVOT procedure, there was a high early risk of death and a nearly constant risk of a second procedure. Risk factors for *early* LVOT intervention were low birth weight, single ventricle, and type B interruption. Risk factors for *late* LVOT intervention were anomalous right subclavian artery, bicuspid aortic valve and single ventricle. Risk factors for a *second LVOT procedure* were absence of a large VSD and initial balloon dilatation of the LVOT [3].

Reoperations for residual/recurrent LVOTO have generally been well tolerated, but often with residual gradients. *Balloon dilatation* can effectively address isolated aortic valve stenosis [3], but for the persistence of unresected conal muscle further surgery is needed to relieve the obstruction [28]. Most of these patients are treated by transaortic *myomectomy* of the obstructing subaortic muscle. In the more severe cases, a *Konno, Ross-Konno operation* or, even, a *secondary Yasui operation* may be indicated [19].

Other Residual Intracardiac Lesions

Other haemodynamically significant intracardiac lesions, apart from LVOTO, occurring after IAA/VSD repair may require a reoperation: (1) a large residual VSD; (2) isolated aortic valve stenosis, particularly in patients with a bicuspid aortic valve; (3) aortic valve regurgitation, as a result of conal septum resection or after a Yasui or Ross-Konno operation; (4) pulmonary valve regurgitation, in patients receiving transpulmonary VSD closure, especially if the sutures for the cranial portion of the VSD are put through the pulmonary annulus (this would also prevent the possibility of a secondary Ross-Konno procedure, if needed); (5) mitral valve regurgitation, also a result of conal septum resection.

Bronchial Compression [37]

Bronchial compression may be secondary to (1) insufficient mobilization of the descending aorta combined with a direct aortic anastomosis that is low and under tension, or to (2) the presence of residual heart lesions leading to cardiomegaly and dilatation of the left atrium, the pulmonary trunk and the aortic root. Postoperatively, these patients experience prolonged ventilator dependence or refractory left lower lobe collapse. Secondary relief of bronchial compression may be obtained by aortopexy with or without aortic elongation by a vascular interposition graft to attenuate aortic arch tension.

Pulmonary Artery Reintervention [37]

Freedom from any pulmonary artery reintervention is 78 %, 75 %, and 72 % at 1, 5, and 10 years, respectively [3]. Reintervention usually consists of balloon dilatation of the right pulmonary artery, often repeated, with or without stent placement and patch arterioplasty. Sometimes, both pulmonary arteries require treatment.

Conclusion

In conclusion, the rapid deterioration of neonates with IAA dictates early referral and treatment. Careful preoperative assessment, and particularly the identification of a severe LVOTO (<4 mm), is crucial for a successful outcome. Many surgical options are available, but primary repair is currently the preferred approach. Anatomic features affect mortality and initial LVOT procedures, whereas characteristics of the arch repair affect arch reintervention [3].

References

1. Backer CL, Mavroudis C. Congenital Heart Surgery Nomenclature and Database Project: patent ductus arteriosus, coarctation of the aorta, interrupted aortic arch. Ann Thorac Surg. 2000;69:S298–307.
2. Celoria GC, Patton RB. Congenital absence of the aortic arch. Am Heart J. 1959;58:407–13.
3. McCrindle BW, Tchervenkov CI, Konstantinov IE, Williams WG, Neirotti RA, Jacobs ML, Blackstone EH. Risk factors associated with mortality and interventions in 472 neonates with interrupted aortic arch: a Congenital Heart Surgeons Society study. J Thorac Cardiovasc Surg. 2005;129:343–50.
4. Dische MR, Tsai M, Baltaxe HA. Solitary interruption of the arch of the aorta. Clinicopathologic review of eight cases. Am J Cardiol. 1975;35:271–7.
5. Oppenheimer-Dekker A, Gittenberger-de Groot AC, Roozendaal H. The ductus arterious and associated cardiac anomalies in interruption of the aortic arch. Pediatr Cardiol. 1982;2:185–93.
6. Van Mierop LH, Kutsche LM. Interruption of the aortic arch and coarctation of the aorta: pathogenetic relations. Am J Cardiol. 1984;54:829–34.
7. Rudolph AM, Heymann MA, Spitznas U. Hemodynamic considerations in the development of narrowing of the aorta. Am J Cardiol. 1972;30:514–25.
8. Moore GW, Hutchins GM. Association of interrupted aortic arch with malformations producing reduced blood flow to the fourth aortic arches. Am J Cardiol. 1978;42:467–72.
9. Van Mierop LH, Kutsche LM. Cardiovascular anomalies in DiGeorge syndrome and importance of neural crest as a possible pathogenetic factor. Am J Cardiol. 1986;58:133–7.
10. Lewin MB, Lindsay EA, Jurecic V, Goytia V, Towbin JA, Baldini A. A genetic etiology for interruption of the aortic arch type B. Am J Cardiol. 1997;80:493–7.
11. Rauch A, Hofbeck M, Leipold G, Klinge J, Trautmann U, Kirsch M, Singer H, Pfeiffer RA. Incidence and significance of 22q11.2 hemizygosity in patients with interrupted aortic arch. Am J Med Genet. 1998;78:322–31.
12. Goldmuntz E, Clark BJ, Mitchell LE, Jawad AF, Cuneo BF, Reed L, McDonald-McGinn D, Chien P, Feuer J, Zackai EH, Emanuel BS, Driscoll DA. Frequency of 22q11 deletions in patients with conotruncal defects. J Am Coll Cardiol. 1998;32:492–8.
13. Marino B, Digilio MC, Persiani M, Di Donato R, Toscano A, Giannotti A, Dallapiccola B. Deletion 22q11 in patients with interrupted aortic arch. Am J Cardiol. 1999;84:360–1, A9.
14. Salem MM, Starnes VA, Wells WJ, Acherman RJ, Chang RK, Luciani GB, Wong PC. Predictors of left ventricular outflow obstruction following single-stage repair of interrupted aortic arch and ventricular septal defect. Am J Cardiol. 2000;86:1044–7, A11.
15. Moulaert AJ, Oppenheimer-Dekker A. Anterolateral muscle bundle of the left ventricle, bulboventricular flange and subaortic stenosis. Am J Cardiol. 1976;37:78–81.
16. Fulton JO, Mas C, Brizard CP, Cochrane AD, Karl TR. Does left ventricular outflow tract obstruction influence outcome of interrupted aortic arch repair? Annals of Thoracic Surgery. 1999;67:177–81.
17. Geva T, Hornberger LK, Sanders SP, Jonas RA, Ott DA, Colan SD. Echocardiographic predictors of left ventricular outflow tract obstruction after repair of interrupted aortic arch. J Am Coll Cardiol. 1993;22:1953–60.
18. Bove EL, Minich LL, Pridjian AK, Lupinetti FM, Snider AR, Dick M, Beekman III RH. The management of severe subaortic stenosis, ventricular septal defect, and aortic arch obstruction in the neonate. J Thorac Cardiovasc Surg. 1993;105:289–95.

19. Tchervenkov CI, Jacobs JP, Sharma K, Ungerleider RM. Interrupted aortic arch: surgical decision making. Semin Thorac Cardiovasc Surg Pediatr Card Surg Annu. 2005;8:92–102.
20. Devloo-Blancquaert A, Titus JL, Edwards JE, Vallaeys JH, De Gezelle HR, Coppens M. Interruption of aortic arch and hypoplastic left heart syndrome. Pediatr Cardiol. 1995;16: 304–8.
21. McElhinney DB, Hedrick HL, Bush DM, Pereira GR, Stafford PW, Gaynor JW, Spray TL, Wernovsky G. Necrotizing enterocolitis in neonates with congenital heart disease: risk factors and outcomes. Pediatrics. 2000;106:1080–7.
22. Serraf A, Lacour-Gayet F, Robotin M, Bruniaux J, Sousa-Uva M, Roussin R, Planche C. Repair of interrupted aortic arch: a ten-year experience. J Thorac Cardiovasc Surg. 1996;112: 1150–60.
23. Brown JW, Ruzmetov M, Okada Y, Vijay P, Rodefeld MD, Turrentine MW. Outcomes in patients with interrupted aortic arch and associated anomalies: a 20-year experience. Eur J Cardiothorac Surg. 2006;29:666–73.
24. Mainwaring RD, Lamberti JJ. Mid- to long-term results of the two-stage approach for type B interrupted aortic arch and ventricular septal defect. Ann Thorac Surg. 1997;64:1782–5.
25. Bellinger DC, Wypij D, Kuban KC, Rappaport LA, Hickey PR, Wernovsky G, Jonas RA, Newburger JW. Developmental and neurological status of children at 4 years of age after heart surgery with hypothermic circulatory arrest or low-flow cardiopulmonary bypass. Circulation. 1999;100:526–32.
26. Visconti KJ, Rimmer D, Gauvreau K, Del NP, Mayer Jr JE, Hagino I, Pigula FA. Regional low-flow perfusion versus circulatory arrest in neonates: one-year neurodevelopmental outcome. Ann Thorac Surg. 2006;82:2207–11.
27. Jonas RA, Quaegebeur JM, Kirklin JW, Blackstone EH, Daicoff G. Outcomes in patients with interrupted aortic arch and ventricular septal defect. A multiinstitutional study. Congenital Heart Surgeons Society. J Thorac Cardiovasc Surg. 1994;107:1099–109.
28. Luciani GB, Ackerman RJ, Chang AC, Wells WJ, Starnes VA. One-stage repair of interrupted aortic arch, ventricular septal defect, and subaortic obstruction in the neonate: a novel approach. J Thorac Cardiovasc Surg. 1996;111:348–58.
29. Morales DL, Scully PT, Braud BE, Booth JH, Graves DE, Heinle JS, McKenzie ED, Fraser Jr CD. Interrupted aortic arch repair: aortic arch advancement without a patch minimizes arch reinterventions. Ann Thorac Surg. 2006;82:1577–83.
30. Roussin R, Belli E, Lacour-Gayet F, Godart F, Rey C, Bruniaux J, Planche C, Serraf A. Aortic arch reconstruction with pulmonary autograft patch aortoplasty. J Thorac Cardiovasc Surg. 2002;123:443–8.
31. Tchervenkov CI, Tahta SA, Jutras LC, Beland MJ. Biventricular repair in neonates with hypoplastic left heart complex. Ann Thorac Surg. 1998;66:1350–7.
32. Nathan M, Rimmer D, del Nido PJ, Mayer JE, Bacha EA, Shin A, Regan W, Gonzalez R, Pigula F. Aortic atresia or severe left ventricular outflow tract obstruction with ventricular septal defect: results of primary biventricular repair in neonates. Ann Thorac Surg. 2006;82:2227–32.
33. Agematsu K, Naito Y, Aoki M, Fujiwara T. Takedown of Yasui procedure due to closed ventricular septal defect. J Card Surg. 2010;25:417–8.
34. Lacour-Gayet F, Sauer H, Ntalakoura K, Muller A, Razek V, Weil J, Haun C. Ross-Konno procedure in neonates: report of three patients. Ann Thorac Surg. 2004;77:2223–5.
35. Malhotra SP, Hanley FL. Routine continuous perfusion for aortic arch reconstruction in the neonate. Semin Thorac Cardiovasc Surg Pediatr Card Surg Annu. 2008;11:57–60.
36. Schreiber C, Eicken A, Vogt M, Gunther T, Wottke M, Thielmann M, Paek SU, Meisner H, Hess J, Lange R. Repair of interrupted aortic arch: results after more than 20 years. Ann Thorac Surg. 2000;70:1896–9.
37. Mishra PK. Management strategies for interrupted aortic arch with associated anomalies. Eur J Cardiothorac Surg. 2009;35:569–76.

Chapter 34
The Dilated Aortic Root in Adult Patients with Conotruncal Anomalies

Claudia Montanaro, Darryl F. Shore, and Michael A. Gatzoulis

Abstract This chapter addresses aortopathy in conotruncal disease and its impact on outcome including pregnancy. The aorta (and pulmonary artery) are often involved in conotruncal lesions with a combination of intrinsic abnormalities: further burned by hemodynamics. As these patients grow, we can anticipate progression of aortopathy, and associated risks including dissection.

Current data is limited, however, and existing guidelines failed to address this specific population and remain vague on timing of intervention. Monitoring of the aorta for patients with established aortopathy or with conotruncal lesions at risk of doing, so is clearly necessary. Level of monitoring, timing and type of therapy should be individualized for each patient, with property assessment of the patient's underlying congenital heart lesion, associated comorbidities, and the risk of surgery. Further research in this area of growth including pregnancy is clearly warranted.

Keywords Aortic root dilation • Adult congenital heart diseases • Grown-up congenital heart disease • Conotruncal anomalies • Aortic aneurysm • Aortic dissection • Pregnancy • Aortic root surgery • Long term follow up

Introduction

Conotruncal anomalies are a group of congenital heart defects (CHD) derived from embryological disarrangement of the ventricle outflow tracts and great vessels. Briefly, the outflow tract of the embryonic univentricular heart is also known as

C. Montanaro, MD • M.A. Gatzoulis, MD (✉)
Department of Cardiology, Royal Brompton Hospital, London, UK
e-mail: M.Gatzoulis@rbht.nhs.uk

D.F. Shore, MD
Heart Division, Royal Brompton Hospital, London, UK

Department of Cardiac Surgery, The National Heart & Lung Institute, London, UK

F. Lacour-Gayet et al. (eds.), *Surgery of Conotruncal Anomalies*,
DOI 10.1007/978-3-319-23057-3_34

conotruncus. There are different theories on how outflow tracts and great arteries develop; the most trustworthy among them is Van Mierop's [1]. He stated there are three pairs of ridges forming in the pulmonary, truncus and conus regions. The pairs of ridges fuse independently, and later on fuse with each other to complete the septation. His theory indicates that the truncus ridge forms first, generating the truncal septum. In the same time, aortopulmonary septum forms by invagination of the dorsal wall of the aortic sac between the fourth and the sixth aortic arch arteries. The truncal septum and the aortopulmonary septum then fuse into the final aortopulmonary septum. The helicoidal shape of the final septum divides the pulmonary artery from the anterior to lateral to posterior side, and the aorta in the opposite side. Any disarrangement in this process generates conotruncal disease.

There is a growing body of evidence documenting progressive aortic dilation in patients with both repaired and unrepaired congenital cardiac defects [2, 3], Several explanations might account for the increased incidence of aortopathy in adults with congenital heart disease (ACHD), including an ever increasing number of patients with CHD surviving into adulthood (up to 90 %), along with improved awareness of the conditions, matched with improvements in cardiac imaging, which, in turn provides unlimited and accurate assessment of aortic caliber, cardiac anatomy and function [4]. Furthermore, with advancing age, the aortic wall structure undergoes unfavorable changes, exacerbated by secondary effects due to adverse cardiovascular risk factors like systemic arterial hypertension, atherosclerosis, smoking, hypercholesterolemia, and diabetes, resulting in a decline in aortic elasticity and an increase in aortic circumference, ultimately leading to/or exaggerating aortic aneurismal formation [5]. As the life expectancy of ACHD continues to improve, cardiologists will continue to be challenged with evolving pathology, including aortopathy. Intriguingly, there are no guidelines at present specific to conotruncal lesions and how best to manage aortic dilatation in these patients.

Conotruncal cardiac defects include Tetralogy of Fallot (TOF), patient with double outlet right ventricle (DORV) as part of their diagnosis, truncus arteriosus (TA), transposition of the great arteries (TGA) and others (Table 34.1) [8].

Aortic Dilatation in Tetralogy of Fallot

Tetralogy of Fallot (TOF) is the most common form of cyanotic CHD comprising 10 % of all congenital heart disease [9]. Overall survival for TOF has dramatically increased in recent decades following repair, with at least 85 % of them surviving to a 36-year follow-up [10]. Progressive aortic dilatation is now recognized as a contributing factor to late morbidity in this patient group [11]; it occurs in between 15 and 48 % of patients [3, 12], Aortic root dilatation may lead to aortic regurgitation due to incomplete leaflet coaptation [13]; moreover, aortic dilatation imposes the risk of aortic dissection and rupture [14, 15], (Fig. 34.1). Aortic root disease has

Table 34.1 Commonest congenital heart disease lesions associated with aortic root abnormalities

Heart defect	Location of AoD	Incidence of AoD	Incidence of dissection	Recommendations for Ao replacement
Marfan syndrome	Sinuses of Valsalva (typical location)	35 % by 5 year [6] 68 % by 19 year [6]	4.3 % in childhood [7] 20 % in adolescence [7]	>50 mm accelerated aortic growth (>10 mm/year) Development of aortic regurgitation Need for mitral valve surgery
BAV	Ao root and ascending aorta	<19 year, isolated BAV 12 % marked AoD 25 % moderate AoD	Case reports in adolescents	>50 mm accelerated aortic growth (>10 mm/year) Need for aortic valve surgery with AoD >45 mm
TOF	Ao root and ascending aorta	<19 year, repaired TOF 87 % at sinus of Valsalva 63 % at ascending aorta	2 case reports in adults with repaired TOF	≥55 mm, especially when there is an indication for pulmonary valve implantation Development of aortic regurgitation with AoD >50 mm
CoA	Ascending aorta and site of previous surgical repair	Paediatric & adult population 9 % after surgical repair	Paediatric & adult population <1 % after surgical repair	~50 mm Accelerated aortic growth (>10 mm/year) Development of aortic regurgitation
Arterial switch	Neoaortic root dilatation	33.4 % after surgical repair	No reports	Severe neoaortic root dilatation (≥55 mm)

Abbreviations: *Ao* aortic, *AoD* aortic dilatation, *BAV* bicuspid aortic valve, *CoA* coarctation of the aorta, *TOF* Tetralogy of Fallot

been observed in repaired and non-repaired TOF suggesting more than one element may contribute to this detrimental process [3].

The underlying pathophysiology to progressive root dilatation was firstly attributed to increased blood flow through the aorta, due to right to left shunting, prior to anatomic repair [3]. This is supported by evidence that dilatation is greater in patients with pulmonary atresia, the extreme end of the morphological TOF spectrum, where volume load through the aorta is maximal [3]. Histologic intrinsic abnormalities have also been shown in young patients with TOF; Tan and colleagues [11] found histologic abnormalities of an intrinsic aortopathy (including cystic medial necrosis, elastic fragmentation, and elastic lamellae disruption) in pathologic specimens of

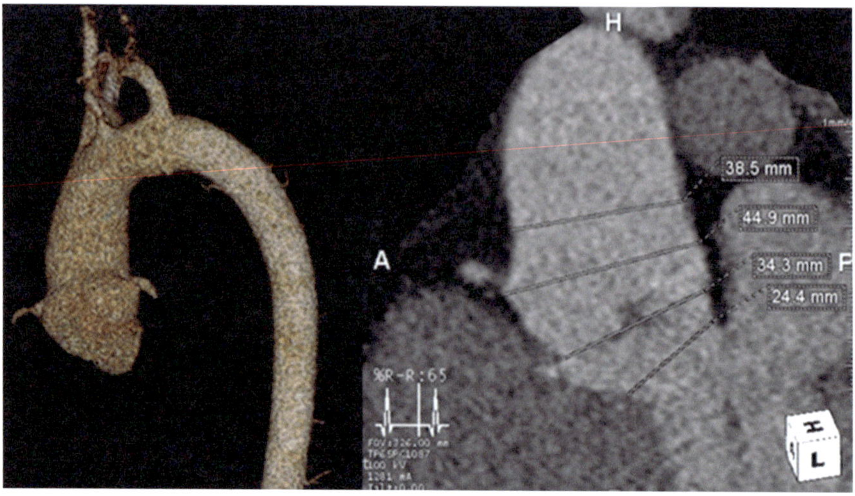

Fig. 34.1 A 40 year old man with diagnosis of tetralogy of Fallot repaired aged 3 and family history of aortopathy and fatal dissection, developed severe pulmonary regurgitation, moderately dilated Aortic Root. The patient, scheduled for surgical pulmonary valve replacement, underwent exo-stent reinforcement because of strong familiar history of aortic dissection

TOF, which were present as early as a few days after birth, amongst patients naive to surgery, suggesting a genetic component. Dilated aorta on fetuses with TOF has also been described by fetal echocardiography and also in histologic studies using either pathologic specimens or surgical biopsies in infants with unrepaired TOF [11]. Moreover, Niwa et al. [5] investigated the ultrastructure of great arteries in 15 TOF patients in his series patients, who were scheduled for heart surgery, showing at least grade 2 or 3 of elastin fragmentation. Moreover, a recent genetic study demonstrated specific polymorphisms predisposing the aortic wall to more or less stiffness: in particular, metalloproteinase-9, when present, modulates positively the aortic stiffness and the magnitude of aortic root dilation in repaired TOF [16].

Even if the anatomical culprit components are removed by surgical repair, abnormalities of smooth muscles, elastic fibers, collagen, and ground substance in the ascending aortic tunica media seem to persist in these patients [3, 11]. Rutz et al. [17] reported the incidence of aortic dilatation and reduced aortic distensibility in patients with repaired TOF compared to age- and sex-matched controls. Aortic wall stiffness was found to be increased in both children and adults with repaired TOF and was closely associated with aortic root dilatation [18]. The aortic diameters from the sinus to the level of the pulmonary artery bifurcation were larger, and the aortic distensibility was significantly reduced when compared to normal controls [17]. In fact, aortic root dilation has been described in children following TOF repair with a prevalence of 88 %, 87 %, 61 %, and 63 % at the annulus, sinus of Valsalva, sinotubular junction, and ascending aorta, respectively [19].

Interestingly, identified risk factors for progressive aortic dilatation in repaired TOF include male sex, longer time interval from palliation to repair, presence of pulmonary atresia and right aortic arch [3] (associated in up to 25 % of TOF patients [20]). It has been suggested that genetic element and mechanical wall stress (due to anatomical abnormalities) equally lead to irreversible changes of microstructure of aortic media tunic, causing a progressive tissue degeneration, further compromised by common risk factors for aortopathy (age, gender, physical activity, smoke, etc.). This is supported by the evidence of increased ascending aortic diameters and reduced ascending aortic distensibility, in all type of conotruncal disease, regardless of previous repair or palliation [17].

Currently, no guidelines for timing of aortic root surgery exist, nor a consensus on prophylactic b-blocker therapy for patients with TOF and aortic root dilatation. It would appear reasonable to consider these patients as "not congenital" patients, following general guidelines for aortic root dilatation. However TOF patients are different, and, as discussed, with a different and mixed aortic pathology. Their age is also younger and the vast majorities of them have already been subjected to surgeries during infancy and early childhood. Furthermore, limited literature suggests that the "normal population" cut off for aortic intervention may not apply to TOF patients. Despite the presence of aortic pathology in these patients, aortic dissection has only been reported in a few isolated cases with aortic diameter well above 53 mm and additional risk factors. In the only four TOF cases reported in the literature, the absolute diameter of the aorta was ≥7 cm in all at the time of dissection, except from one who had smaller aorta size (5.3 cm), whereas the patients age ranged between 18 and 60 years [6, 14, 15, 21] Therefore, uncertainty exists on timing of surgical intervention in this cohort of patients. Measurements of aortic stiffness, aortic curvature, and consideration of patient body size together with monitoring rates of progression may help us to further risk-stratify [14, 17]. Longitudinal studies on aortic dilatation in TOF, suggested an increase of 1.7 mm/year, in contrast to 0.03 mm/year in healthy controls [3]. Some authors claim that aortic root replacement should be considered in TOF patients when aortic diameter exceeds 55 mm, especially when patients are referred for surgical pulmonary replacement [3]. Additional, soft indications may include the development of aortic regurgitation with a root diameter of more than 50 mm, similar to patients with Marfan syndrome [3]. However, these are all arbitrary, and further studies are clearly required.

In cases of progressive aortic dilatation (defined as abnormal increase in aortic z-scores) imaging of the aorta should be performed on an annual basis [8]. This ideally should include a periodic cardiac MRI, as confirmation of annual transthoracic echocardiography.

It is clear that TOF, traditionally thought as a "right" heart lesion, involves the aorta; the latter needs to be monitored periodically as it may come to require surgical attention in a proportion of patients with TOF over their lifetime.

Aortic Dilatation in Truncus Arteriosus

Truncus arteriosus (TA) is an uncommon conotruncal anomaly consisting of a single artery (arterial trunk) coming off the ventricular mass. There is always a large ventricular septal defect. The pulmonary arteries in turn come off the ascending aorta, either through a common stem or independently. The truncal valve itself, is often dysplastic with three or more leaflets and may be regurgitant and/or stenotic from birth. The degree of valve deformity is one of the key determinants of outcome. Therapy is surgical, involving ventricular septal defect closure and conduit anastomosis between the right ventricle and the pulmonary arteries (which themselves may need a unifocalization procedure) [22]. Aortic arch interruption or coarctation may also be present requiring earlier surgical intervention.

Long-term follow-up data into adulthood after TA repair is very limited. A large retrospective review of TA surgery since 1975 by Rajasinghe et al. [7] reports long-term outcomes among 165 patients with TA who survived hospital admission for repair. During a median follow-up of 10.5 years, 107 patients had 133 conduit reoperations (median time to conduit redo surgery of 5.5 years from initial repair). In addition, 26 patients underwent 30 operations for truncal valve replacements. No patients from this young cohort had severe aortic dilatation to require aortic surgeries [7] (Fig. 34.2). Aortic and/or pulmonary arterial dilatation, however, has been reported in TA patients, including young adults, particularly amongst patients who did not have repair.

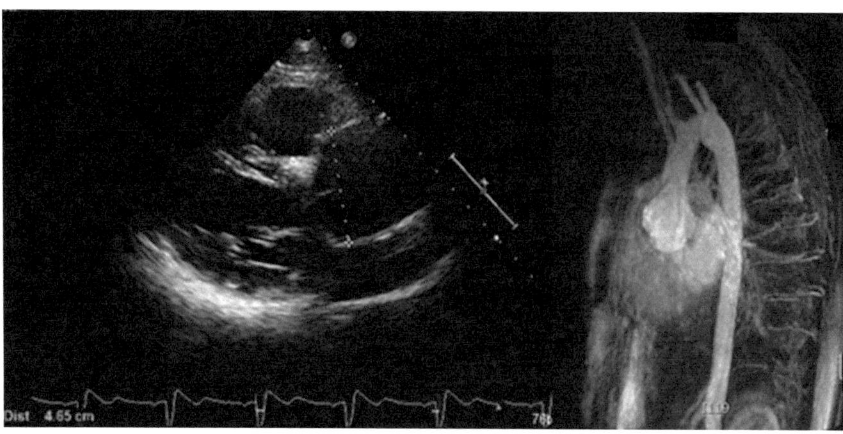

Fig. 34.2 A 29-year-old man with 22Q11.2 deletion and diagnosis of common arterial trunk, mild stenosis of left pulmonary artery, right aortic arch, left subclavian artery from descending aorta, underwent radical repair with valved biological conduit from right ventricle to pulmonary artery aged 1 month, balloon dilatation of right and left pulmonary arteries and later re-balloon dilatation of right pulmonary artery and stenting of left pulmonary artery. He developed severe proximal conduit stenosis subjected to replacement of homograft with 21 mm cryopreserved aortic homograft from right ventricle to pulmonary artery + repair of left pulmonary artery stenosis. Moderate aortic dilatation at follow up (max diameter 4.65 cm)

Aortic Dilatation in Transposition of the Great Arteries

Complete transposition of the great arteries (TGA) is the second commonest cyanotic heart defect, accounting for 5 % of all CHD [23]. In TGA, systemic and pulmonary circulations are in parallel, and this condition it is not compatible with long-term survival; therefore palliative procedures early followed by definitive surgery are essential. The atrial switch procedure was the standard repair in the 70s and 80s. Therefore, the arterial switch operation (ASO) became the treatment of choice, conveying anatomic correction of TGA, offering the advantage of a systemic left ventricle over the atrial repair (systemic right ventricle). Even though in aortic root dilatation in TGA is common the rate of enlargement seems to be low and, thus far clinically insignificant [24].

Histological abnormalities similar to those seen in Marfan syndrome and bicuspid aortic valve disease have been described in normal-sized ascending aortas of neonates with TGA undergoing ASO [5]. These findings may imply an inherent structural weakness of the aortic wall in these patients. In the first year of life, rapid dilatation of the new aorta has been observed, followed by normalization of the valve and sinus size. Aortic dilatation, by itself, was rarely associated with significant aortic insufficiency [25]. Furthermore, even in patients who underwent atrial switch surgery, dilatation of aortic annulus, sinus of Valsalva and reduced distensibility of the ascending aorta were also present, if compared to healthy controls [26].

Regarding progression of aortic root dilatation, data are somewhat conflicting; most studies nevertheless suggest that the rate of progression is slow [27]. Lim et al. [28] reported in a cohort of 220 patients freedom aortic root dilatation (aortic root Z-value >0) was 92.7 % at 1 year, 75.3 % at 5 years, 52.9 % at 10 years, 30.3 % at 15 years, 7.7 % at 20 years and 0.0 % at 23 years, respectively. This data was confirmed by Schwartz et al. [29] who, in a cohort of 335 patients who had undergone ASO for d-TGA (also including DORV with subpulmonary VSD), showed that at a median follow-up of 5 years 33 % of patients had aortic dilation (defined as a neo-aortic root z-score >3.0), only six of them had marked neo-aortic dilation (z-score 8.0). At 10-year follow-up, aortic dilatation was seen in 49 % of patients; only 5 % of the whole cohort required surgery for the neo-aortic root or valve. Schwarz at al [29] suggested that aortic root dilatation in this group of patients tended to plateau rather than progress with time. This observation has been supported by another retrospective single centre study with a cohort of 145 TGA patients, in which aortic dilatation appeared not to be progressive [24].

Development of severe neo-aortic root enlargement was associated with prior pulmonary artery (PA) banding, the presence of a VSD and Taussig-Bing anatomy [30]. Neoaortic root diameter was not related to neo-aortic valve regurgitation nor with associated heart defects [27]. There may also be a component to haemodynamic aortic dilatation in TGA patients. For example, sharper angulation of the aortic arch in patients with TGA has been associated with greater pulse wave reflection, dilatation of the ascending aorta, and aortic regurgitation late after ASO [31] (Fig. 34.3).

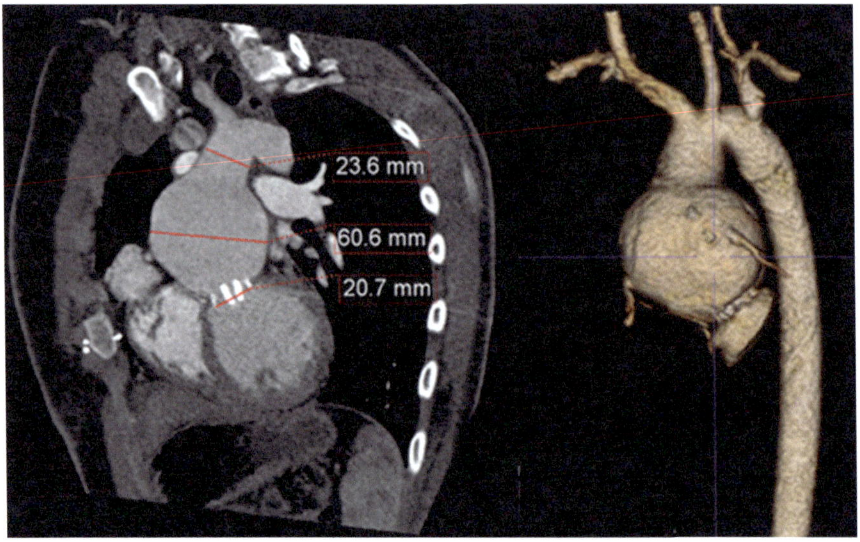

Fig. 34.3 A 18 year old man with diagnosis of Transposition of the great arteries with VSD, undergone pulmonary artery banding and left modified BT shunt, arterial switch and VSD closure, developed neo-aortic valve incompetence requiring valve replacement (21 mm, mechanic prosthesis has been implanted) and progressive dilatation of the neo aortic root (picture), has been referred to replacement of neo aortic root and aortic valve replacement (23 mm composite valve and graft)

Interestingly no cases of neoaortic dissection or rupture have been reported so far, although one should take into consideration the relative young age of patients with ASO (mid 80s); thus, the long-term clinical impact of aortopathy cannot be fully appreciated in these patients.

According to the current recommendations, annual follow-up is suggested for TGA patients undergoing ASO with root intervention in cases of severe neoaortic root dilatation (greater than 55 mm) [23, 32] We submit that optimal blood pressure is a target and periodic echocardiographic imaging to evaluate the anatomy and hemodynamics features is essential in these patients. Cardiac MRI and CT angiography should also be considered, especially if there is evidence of dilatation after ASO.

Aortic Dilatation in Double Outlet Right Ventricle

Double outlet is defined as more than 50 % of both great vessels arising from one ventricle. It is therefore part of a diagnosis, and not a diagnosis per se. The anatomic spectrum of CHD patients with DORV includes TOF, TGA (patients typically have Rastelli type of repair), simple VSD, non-committed VSD and complex/ univentricular heart not suitable for biventricular repair. The most common

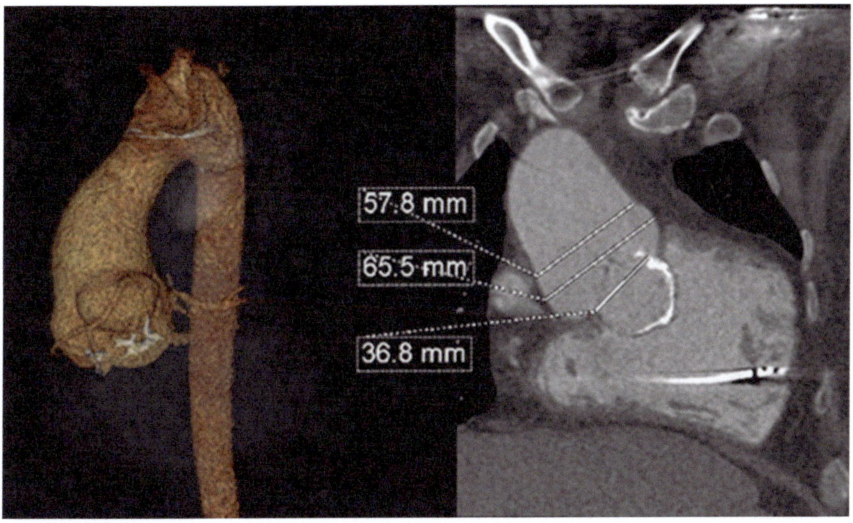

Fig. 34.4 A 50 year old man with diagnosis of double outlet right ventricle (DORV) Fallot type with VSD and PS, Right aortic arch, Coarctation of the aorta (CoA), Patent ductus arteriosus (PDA), undergone palliative shunts and eventually a biventricular repair (VSD patch, pulmonary valvotomy, subvalvular resection), repair of CoA and ligation of PDA. He developed moderate to severe pulmonary regurgitation and severe dilatation of the aortic root associated with moderate aortic regurgitation and is currently referred for aortic and pulmonary surgery. CRT-D was also implanted for primary prevention

diagnosis of DORV with CHD and associated aortopathy are TOF and TGA, already discussed.

In patients with single ventricle circulation and dilated aorta, aortic stiffness is increased and is an independent determinant of aortic dilatation [33], even if aortic root dilatation is a not common evolution in this cohort of patients (Fig. 34.4).

Patients with univentricular physiology had a complete mixed blood and the suggested procedure is Fontan palliation, typically performed between 18 months and 4 years of age. In the intermediate term, Fontan procedure is technically associated with low early mortality and lower reoperation rate, when compared to biventricular repair attempts [34].

Only few case reports have been published with regard to aortic or neoaortic root surgery after Fontan completion. Egan et al. [35] described the case of aortic dissection in a young man undergone modified external lateral tunnel Fontan palliation, who developed severe dilation of the aortic root (measuring 7.8 cm), severe aortic regurgitation, and moderate global right ventricular systolic dysfunction. Egan et al. were the only who described combination of aortic root replacement using a prosthesis in the Fontan circulation.

More rare is the double outlet left ventricle lesion di per se, and some case of aortic dilatation in patient after Fontan palliation have been reported [36, 37], In only one case Bental procedure has been performed [38].

Norwood Procedure

The first successful palliation of hypoplastic left heart syndrome (HLHS) was reported by Norwood et al. [39] in a series of infants who underwent surgery from 1979 to 1981. The Norwood operation is a staged palliative procedure to improve prospect for HLHS, which is incompatible with life. The procedure has been technically refined over the years, but the essential components remain (1) atrial septectomy, (2) anastomosis of the proximal pulmonary artery to the aorta with homograft augmentation of the aortic arch, and (3) aortopulmonary (modified Blalock-Taussig shunt) shunt or right ventricle–to–pulmonary artery shunt to provide for pulmonary blood flow. Ultimately patients undergo a Fontan operation, of necessity their systemic ventricle is of right ventricle morphology.

With improvement in late results for hypoplastic left heart syndrome and its variants, neoaortic aneurysmal dilation and neoaortic valvular dysfunction have been reported in these patients late after the Norwood operation [40]. Kanzaki et al. [41] described a patient who had left pulmonary artery compression and mild neoaortic regurgitation from a severely dilated neoaortic root (Z value, +8.7) 11 years after the Norwood operation and subsequent Fontan procedure. They performed successful valve-sparing neoaortic root replacement in this patient. Further and close follow-up of these patients with complex anatomy and neoaorta being forward from the pulmonary trunk is clearly warranted.

Pregnancy Evaluation

Aortic dissection is a well recognized complication of pregnancy. Women with congenital heart disease and in particular these with aortic involvement, whether congenital intrinsic or developing with time (relating to haemodynamic), should be counselled of the risk of aortic complication, including dissection and death during pregnancy [42, 43], Haemodynamic, hormonal and other pregnant related changes represent a burden and a risk on the aorta. Despite this, existing data suggest very low rates of aortic complication in patient with heart disease.

A systematic review of 2491 pregnancies in women with CHD by Drenthen et al. [44], for example, revealed no aortic complication. Veldtman et al. [45] reported 112 pregnancies in 42 patients with repaired TOF. There was no significant difference in aortic diameter between the patients with a history of pregnancy and those without. The most feared complication of an enlarged ascending aorta is clearly dissection. A relationship between aortic dissection (from all causes) and pregnancy was first reported in 1944 [46]. Chest pain occurring during pregnancy should raise the suspicion of aortic dissection. Although the majority of dissections occur due to proximal root dilatation, fatal dissection can also occur in patients with apparently normal root at baseline. Nevertheless, Immer et al. [47] in 2003 suggested that root diameter and rate of change were reliable predictors for proximal dissection; there are currently no equivalent predictors for distal aortic dissection (other than Marfan syndrome).

Women with pre-existing aortic pathology, whether congenital or acquired, should be supervised by a cardiologist and obstetrician throughout pregnancy and the peripartum [48, 49]. Serial transthoracic echocardiography should suffice for most. If concerns or new onset symptoms (such as chest or back pain) develop additional imaging such as MRI (safe after 1st trimester), CT and/or TOE may be required. It is good practice to establish the baseline aorta with a Cardiac MRI before conception and repeat this 1 year after successful pregnancy in women with pre-existing aortopathies. Physicians should remain alert of symptoms such acute onset of chest/back pain during pregnancy of women with or without heart disease, as these symptoms may suggest aortic dissection.

For women with pre-existing aortopathy and echocardiographic evidence of rapidly increasing aortic root diameters during pregnancy, delivery may have to be expedited. New aortic regurgitation may also be another indication of a developing "unstable" situation. If the fetus is viable, it has been suggested that the patient should be delivered promptly and then undergo urgent, or semi-urgent, aortic root surgery [50]. This is usually either a composite root and valve graft, or a valve–sparing aortic root replacement retaining the patient's own aortic valve. If pregnancy is at an earlier stage, root surgery may need to be undertaken with the fetus in situ. There are cardiopulmonary bypass techniques that can minimise fetal risk, even if it doesn't mean risk zero for fetus [51]. Different techniques take part during surgery, in order to avoid the feto-placental bed suffering: the normotensive high-flow, high pressure techniques and avoidance of full hypothermia can minimise the hypotensive ischaemic insult to the fetus [52].

Thanks to progresses of percutaneous approach, some lesions could be treated not-surgically. For example, distal dissections, assuming there is no extravasation of blood and no loss of arterial supply to a critical organ, may be suitable for endovascular stenting. Unfortunately, there are no data regarding this technique during pregnancy.

There is a possible, but not yet proven, beneficial effect of β-blocking agents to reduce the rate of aortic dilatation and improve survival [53], thus the use of cardioselective β-blockers is strongly advised [54]. Since β-blockers may be associated with growth retardation, fetal growth should be monitored closely.

From a delivery point of view, there is no randomised data suggesting whether vaginal delivery is superior to caesarean section, although the latter conveys better control and, perhaps less stress on the aorta.

Finally, the puerperium is a time of ongoing risk for the aortopathy patient. During this period, meticulous blood pressure control and further cardiac assessment should be performed. Patients with aortopathy should not be discharge dearly, and should have some imaging of the aorta before going home.

Acknowledgments Claudia Montanaro was supported by Italian School of Cardiology and by University Vita-Salute San Raffaele, Milan.

References

1. Van Mierop LSH. Morphological development of the heart. In: Berne RM, editor. Handbook of physiology, the cardiovascular system. Bethesda: American Physiology Society; 1979. p. 1–28.
2. Tzemos N, Therrien J, Yip J, Thanassoulis G, Tremblay S, Jamorski MT, Webb GD, Siu SC. Outcomes in adults with bicuspid aortic valves. JAMA. 2008;300(11):1317–25.
3. Niwa K, Siu SC, Webb GD, Gatzoulis MA. Progressive aortic root dilatation in adults late after repair of tetralogy of Fallot. Circulation. 2002;106(11):1374–8.
4. Grotenhuis HB, Ottenkamp J, de Bruijn L, Westenberg JJ, Vliegen HW, Kroft LJ, de Roos A. Aortic elasticity and size are associated with aortic regurgitation and left ventricular dysfunction in tetralogy of Fallot after pulmonary valve replacement. Heart. 2009;95(23):1931–6.
5. Niwa K, Perloff JK, Bhuta SM, Laks H, Drinkwater DC, Child JS, Miner PD. Structural abnormalities of great arterial walls in congenital heart disease: light and electron microscopic analyses. Circulation. 2001;103(3):393–400.
6. Konstantinov IE, et al. Aortic dissection and rupture in adolescents after tetralogy ofFallot repair. J Thorac Cardiovasc Surg. 2010;140(5):e71–3.
7. Rajasinghe HA, McElhinney DB, Reddy VM, Mora BN, Hanley FL. Long-term follow-up of truncus arteriosus repaired in infancy: a twenty-year experience. J Thorac Cardiovasc Surg. 1997;113:869–78.
8. Allen HD, Driscoll DJ, Shaddy RE, Feltes TF, editors. Heart disease in infants, children, and adolescents, including the fetus and young adult. 8th ed. 2013, Moss and Adams Editor, Lippincott Williams & Wilkins; pg 799–808
9. Therrien J, Webb G. Clinical update on adults with congenital heart disease. Lancet. 2003;362(9392):1305–13.
10. Nollert G, Fischlein T, Bouterwek S, Bohmer C, Klinner W, Reichart B. Long-term survival in patients with repair of tetralogy of Fallot: 36-year follow-up of 490 survivors of the first year after surgical repair. J Am Coll Cardiol. 1997;30(5):1374–83.
11. Tan JL, Davlouros PA, McCarthy KP, Gatzoulis MA, Ho SY. Intrinsic histological abnormalities of aortic root and ascending aorta in tetralogy of Fallot: evidence of causative mechanism for aortic dilatation and aortopathy. Circulation. 2005;112(7):961–8.
12. Jonsson H, Ivert T, Brodin LA. Echocardiographic findings in 83 patients 13–26 years after intracardiac repair of tetralogy of Fallot. Eur Heart J. 1995;16(9):1255–63.
13. Dodds 3rd GA, Warnes CA, Danielson GK. Aortic valve replacement after repair of pulmonary atresia and ventricular septal defect or tetralogy of Fallot. J Thorac Cardiovasc Surg. 1997;113(4):736–41.
14. Kim WH, Seo JW, Kim SJ, Song J, Lee J, Na CY. Aortic dissection late after repair of tetralogy of Fallot. Int J Cardiol. 2005;101(3):515–6.
15. Rathi VK, Doyle M, Williams RB, Yamrozik J, Shannon RP, Biederman RW. Massive aortic aneurysm and dissection in repaired tetralogy of Fallot; diagnosis by cardiovascular magnetic resonance imaging. Int J Cardiol. 2005;101(1):169–70.
16. Cheung YF, Hong WJ, Chan KW, Wong SJ. Modulating effects of matrix metalloproteinase-3 and -9 polymorphisms on aortic stiffness and aortic root dilation in patients after tetralogy of Fallot repair. Int J Cardiol. 2010;151:214–7.
17. Rutz T, Max F, Wahl A, Wustmann K, Khattab K, Pfammatter JP, Kadner A, Schwerzmann M. Distensibility and diameter of ascending aorta assessed by cardiac magnetic resonance imaging in adults with tetralogy of Fallot or complete transposition. Am J Cardiol. 2012;110(1):103–8.
18. Senzaki H, Iwamoto Y, Ishido H, et al. Arterial haemodynamics in patients after repair of tetralogy of Fallot: influence on left ventricular after load and aortic dilatation. Heart. 2008;94(1):70–4.

19. Chong WY, Wong WH, Chiu CS, Cheung YF. Aortic root dilation and aortic elastic properties in children after repair of tetralogy of Fallot. Am J Cardiol. 2006;97(6):905–9.
20. Rudolph A. Congenital diseases of the heart: clinical-physiological considerations, 3rd ed. Wiley-Blackwell, West-Sussex, UK; 2011. Chap 14.
21. Wijesekera VA, Kiess MC, Grewal J, Chow R, Raju R, Leipsic JA, Barlow AJ. Aortic dissection in a patient with a dilated aortic root following tetralogy of Fallot repair. Int J Cardiol. 2014;174:833–4.
22. Gatzoulis M, Swan L, Therrienm J, Pantel GA. Adult congenital heart disease, a practical guide. ed. BMJ book editor, UK; 1st 2005. p. 174–5.
23. Baumgartner H, Bonhoeffer P, De Groot NM, et al. ESC Guidelines for the management of grown-up congenital heart disease (new version 2010). Eur Heart J. 2010;31(23):2915–57.
24. Kempny A, Wustmann K, Borgia F, Dimopoulos K, Uebing A, Li W, Chen SS, Piorkowski A, Radley-Smith R, Yacoub MH, Gatzoulis MA, Shore DF, Swan L, Diller GP. Outcome in adult patients after arterial switch operation for transposition of the great arteries. Int J Cardiol. 2013;167(6):2588–93. doi:10.1016/j.ijcard.2012.06.066. Epub 2012 Aug 11.
25. Hutter PA, Thomeer BJ, Jansen P, Hitchcock JF, Faber JA, Meijboom EJ, Bennink GB. Fate of the aorticroot after arterial switch operation. Eur J Cardiothorac Surg. 2001;20(1):82–8.
26. Ladouceur M, Kachenoura N, Lefort M, Redheuil A, Bonnet D, Celermajer DS, Iserin L, Mousseaux E. Structure and function of the ascending aorta in palliated transposition of the great arteries. Int J Cardiol. 2013;165(3):458–62. doi:10.1016/j.ijcard.2011.08.847. Epub 2011 Sep 17.
27. Michalak KW, Moll JA, Moll M, Dryzek P, Moszura T, Kopala M, Mludzik K, Moll JJ. The neoaortic root in children with transposition of the great arteries after an arterial switch operation. Eur J Cardiothorac Surg. 2013;43(6):1101–8. doi:10.1093/ejcts/ezs709. Epub 2013 Jan 22.
28. Lim HG, Kim WH, Lee JR, Kim YJ. Long-term results of the arterial switch operation for ventriculo-arterial discordance. Eur J Cardiothorac Surg. 2013;43(2):325–34. doi:10.1093/ejcts/ezs264. Epub 2012 May 9.
29. Schwartz ML, Gauvreau K, delNido P, Mayer JE, Colan SD. Long-term predictors of aortic root dilation and aortic regurgitation after arterial switch operation. Circulation. 2004;110:II-128–32.
30. McMahon CJ, Ravekes WJ, Smith EO, Denfield SW, Pignatelli RH, Altman CA, Ayres NA. Risk factors for neo-aortic root enlargement and aortic regurgitation following arterial switch operation. Pediatr Cardiol. 2004;25(4):329–35.
31. Agnoletti G, Ou P, Celermajer DS, Boudjemline Y, Marini D, Bonnet D, Aggoun Y. Acute angulation of the aortic arch predisposes a patient to ascending aortic dilatation and aortic regurgitation late after the arterial switch operation for transposition of the great arteries. J Thorac Cardiovasc Surg. 2008;135(3):568–72.
32. Graham Jr TP, Bernard YD, Mellen BG, Celermajer D, Baumgartner H, Cetta F, Connolly HM, Davidson WR, Dellborg M, Foster E, Gersony WM, Gessner IH, Hurwitz RA, Kaemmerer H, Kugler JD, Murphy DJ, Noonan JA, Morris C, Perloff JK, Sanders SP, Sutherland JL. Long-term outcome in congenitally corrected transposition of the great arteries: a multi-institutional study. J Am Coll Cardiol. 2000;36(1):255–61.
33. Kojima T, Kuwata S, Kurishima C, Iwamoto Y, Saiki H, Ishido H, Masutani S, Senzaki H. Aortic root dilatation and aortic stiffness in patients with single ventricular circulation. Circ J. 2014;78(10):2507–11. Epub 2014 Aug 11.
34. Gatzoulis MA, Wenn GD, Daubeney PEF. Diagnosis and management of adult congenital heart disease. Philadelphia: Elsevier; 2011. p. 380–2, cap 50.
35. Egan M, Phillips A, Cook SC. Aortic dissection in the adult Fontan with aortic root enlargement. Pediatr Cardiol. 2009;30:562–3.
36. Erez E, Tam VK, Galliani C, Lashus A, Doublin NA, Peretti J. Valve-sparing aortic root replacement for patients with Fontan circulation. J Heart Valve Dis. 2012;21:175–80.

37. Pizarro C, Baffa JM, Derby CD, Krieger PA. Valve-sparing neo-aortic root replacement after Fontan completion for hypoplastic left heart syndrome. J Thorac Cardiovasc Surg. 2011;141:1083–4.
38. Spadotto V, Uemura H, Uebing A. Successful Bentall procedure in a patient with a Fontan circulation. Interact Cardiovasc Thorac Surg. 2014;19:520–2.
39. Norwood WI, Lang P, Casteneda AR, Campbell DN. Experience with operations for hypoplastic left heart syndrome. J Thorac Cardiovasc Surg. 1981;82(4):511–9.
40. Cohen MS, Marino BS, McElhinney DB, Robbers-Visser D, van der Woerd W, Gaynor JW, Spray TL, Wernovsky G. Neo-aortic root dilation and valve regurgitation up to 21 years after staged reconstruction for hypoplastic left heart syndrome. J Am Coll Cardiol. 2003;42:533–40.
41. Kanzaki T, Yamagishi M, Miyazaki T, Maeda Y, Yaku H. Valve-sparing neoaortic root replacement late after the norwood and Fontan procedures. Ann Thorac Surg. 2015;99:309–12.
42. Gelson E, Gatzoulis M, Steer PJ, Lupton M, Johnson M. Tetralogy of Fallot: maternal and neonatal outcomes. BJOG. 2008;115:398–402.
43. Pedersen LM, Pedersen TA, Ravn HB, Hjortdal VE. Outcomes of pregnancy in women with tetralogy of Fallot. Cardiol Young. 2008;18:423–9.
44. Drenthen W, Pieper PG, Roos-Hesselink JW, van Lottum WA, Voors AA, Mulder BJ, van Dijk AP, Vliegen HW, Yap SC, Moons P, Ebels T, van Veldhuisen DJ. Outcome of pregnancy in women with congenital heart disease: a literature review. J Am Coll Cardiol. 2007;49:2303–11.
45. Veldtman GR, Connolly HM, Grogan M, Ammash NM, Warnes CA. Outcomes of pregnancy in women with tetralogy of Fallot. J Am Coll Cardiol. 2004;44:174–80.
46. Schnitker MA, Bayer CA. Dissection aneurysm of the aorta in young individuals, particularly in association with pregnancy. Ann Intern Med. 1944;29:486–511.
47. Immer FF, Bansi AG, Immer-Bansi AS, et al. Aortic dissection in pregnancy: analysis of risk factors and outcome. Ann Thorac Surg. 2003;76(1):309–14.
48. Swan L. Artopathies, including Marfan syndrome and coartation. In: Steer PJ, Gatzoulis MA, Baker P, editors. Heart disease and pregnancy. London: Royal College of Obstetricians and Gynaecologists Press; 2006.
49. Rossiter JP, Repke JT, Morales AJ, Murphy EA, Pyeritz RE. A prospective longitudinal evaluation of pregnancy in the Marfan syndrome. Am J Obstet Gynecol. 1995;173(5):1599–606.
50. Zeebregts CJ, Schepens MA, Hameeteman TM, et al. Acute aortic dissection complicating pregnancy. Ann Thorac Surg. 1997;64:1345–8.
51. Parry AJ, Westaby S. Cardiopulmonary bypass during pregnancy. Ann Thorac Surg. 1996;61(6):1865–9.
52. Mahli A, Izdes S, Coskun D. Cardiac operations during pregnancy: review of factors influencing fetal outsome. An Thorac Surg. 2000;69:1622–6.
53. Gersony DR, McClaughlin MA, Jin Z, Gersony WM. The effect of beta-blocker therapy on clinical outcome in patients with Marfan's syndrome: a meta-analysis. Int J Cardiol. 2007;114:303–8.
54. Regitz-Zagrosek V, BlomstromLundqvist C, Borghi C, Cifkova R, Ferreira R, Foidart JM, et al. ESC Guidelines on the management of cardiovascular diseases during pregnancy: the Task Force on the Management of Cardiovascular Diseases during Pregnancy of the European Society of Cardiology (ESC). Eur Heart J. 2011;32:3147–97.

Chapter 35
Single Ventricle Repair for Conotruncal Anomalies

Constantine Mavroudis

Abstract Conotruncal heart defects are characterized by a defect in the conotruncal septum. Associated cardiac malformations are diverse and contribute to the complexity of treatment. Biventricular repair remains challenging, and as a result surgical management is controversial. Biventricular repair has advantages by establishing normal anatomy and physiology, however, it seems a high operative risk in certain more complex forms, and a univentricular heart repair is preferred in certain complex conotruncal anomalies.

Keywords Fontan • Double outlet right ventricle • Ventricular septal defect • Noncommitted VSD • VSD enlargement • Biventricular repair • Univentricular repair

Conotruncal heart defects include lesions such as truncus arteriosus, transposition of the great arteries (TGA), double outlet right ventricle (DORV), and tetralogy of Fallot (TOF) and are characterized by an abnormal development of the infundibulo-arterial structures. Malformations are diverse and treatment via biventricular repair remains challenging specifically for associated lesions such as hypoplasia of one of the ventricles, more than one ventricular septal defect (VSD), or severe atrioventricular valve anomalies. Surgical management of patients with DORV or TGA and straddling atrioventricular valves remains controversial. Biventricular repair has advantages by establishing normal anatomy and physiology, however, it seems a high operative risk in certain more complex forms, and a univentricular heart repair is preferred [1].

Double outlet right ventricle represents a complex spectrum of congenital cardiac malformations that morphologically lie between VSD with overriding aorta and TGA with VSD [2]. The frequently associated cardiac malformations seen with

C. Mavroudis, MD
Johns Hopkins University School of Medicine, Johns Hopkins Children's Heart Surgery, Florida Hospital for Children, 2501 N Orange Ave, Suite 540, Orlando, FL 32804, USA
e-mail: Constantine.Mavroudis.MD@flhosp.org

F. Lacour-Gayet et al. (eds.), *Surgery of Conotruncal Anomalies*,
DOI 10.1007/978-3-319-23057-3_35

DORV contribute to its overall complexity. Double outlet right ventricle is a type of ventriculo-arterial connection in which both great vessels arise entirely or predominantly from the right ventricle [2]. It is important to accurately categorize patients with DORV to determine the best course of treatment.

The aim of surgical treatment of DORV is complete anatomic repair [2]. This is defined as connection of the left ventricle to the aorta, the right ventricle to the pulmonary artery, and closure of the VSD. In general, the timing of surgical intervention depends on the symptomatic state of the patient and anatomic complexity. The anatomy determines the ultimate, corrective surgical approach, which in turn influences the optimal age for definitive repair. The clinical state of the patient before the age at which definitive repair is planned will determine the need for initial palliative procedures. In general, a complete repair is undertaken at as early an age as possible [2].

Anatomic repair of DORV can be contraindicated by the presence of ventricular hypoplasia, serious abnormalities of either atrioventricular valve, the presence of very remote and/or multiple VSDs, and the presence of irreversible pulmonary vascular disease [2]. An atrioventricular valve with a diameter more than two standard deviations smaller than the mean normal value for the patient's body surface area is usually attended by surgically important ventricular hypoplasia. In this situation successful anatomic repair is seldom possible. Severe straddling and/or overriding of either atrioventricular valve can render anatomic repair impossible. The presence of a single VSD far removed from either of the semilunar valves and the presence of multiple VSDs can make anatomic repair more challenging. The presence of borderline size right ventricular volume is a limiting factor for biventricular repair because the construction of the intracardiac right ventricular tunnel will reduce the right ventricular volume even more [2].

Some have suggested that with two functional ventricles of adequate size, a biventricular repair is preferable to single ventricle repair, thereby establishing normal anatomy and physiology [1, 3, 4]. Biventricular repair of DORV with remote VSD [5–7], is one of many situations in which the short and long-term survival afterward has been suboptimal [3, 6]. Hospital mortality exceeded 30 % and late mortality was 44 % [5, 8–10]. The history of intraventricular repair commenced with 100 % mortality owing to poor patient selection and the rate has been dropping ever since [11]. Ten to 20 % of patients with DORV have non-committed VSDs [5]. The challenge of the construction of the intraventricular tunnel is a result of (1) the VSD being distant from the aorta, often within the right ventricular inlet; (2) interference owing to anatomic structures, mostly the tricuspid valve; (3) the need for the intraventricular tunnel to somewhat surround the tricuspid valve so as to reach the aorta at the correct angle; (4) an obstructive subaortic conus may be present; (5) the right ventricular outflow tract is interposed along the intraventricular tunnel; and (6) other anomalies may exist. [5, 12] As a consequence, some authors have suggested that patients who require a valved conduit, complex intraventricular rerouting, non-committed VSD, left ventricular hypoplasia, or remote location of the aorta are better served by a Fontan procedure because it is technically simpler [1, 5, 10].

Delius et al. compared 34 patients undergoing biventricular repair with 16 patients who underwent single ventricle repair [3]. All patients had atrioventricular discordance, ventriculoarterial discordance, VSD, and pulmonary stenosis or atresia and the single ventricle repair patients had either an uncommitted VSD or a straddling atrioventricular valve. Follow up showed that patients after single ventricle repair had less need for reoperation owing to conduit replacement in the biventricular repair group, better survival in the single-ventricle repair group, and similar functional status [3]. The actuarial estimate of survival at 7 years of patients who had undergone biventricular repair was 68 % and for patients having undergone univentricular repair was 93.8 % (P=.048). In addition, freedom from reoperation at 7 years was 45.5 % in the biventricular group versus 100 % with the univentricular group (P=.014) [3].

Brown et al. performed intraventricular tunnel repair, use of conduit, arterial switch operation, or single ventricle repair in 124 DORV patients of all complexities and found that the modified Fontan procedure is the procedure of choice for patients in the complex group with anomalies such as straddling atrioventricular valves, atrioventricular septal defects, hypoplastic valve/ventricle, or a combination [4]. Further they found that although patients with noncomplex forms of DORV and non-committed VSD can undergo an intraventricular repair; in more than half of these patients, a cavopulmonary shunt or modified Fontan was chosen owing to associated atrial isomerism with some degree of ventricular imbalance. Further they found that regardless of the position of the VSD, results with intraventricular repair were disappointing [4].

Ruzmetov et al. reported on 47 patients with complex DORV who underwent a Fontan procedure between 1980 and 2007 [13]. Follow up ranged from 1 to 25 years with no early but six late deaths and functional status remained good. Their report showed good early- and mid-term results with the Fontan procedure as treatment for complex forms of DORV [13].

They noted that although patients with complex forms of DORV may ultimately be palliated by the modified Fontan operation, the mortality rate has been reported to be high; however, improvements with patient selection, perioperative management, and surgical techniques of the Fontan operation such as total cavopulmonary connection with a lateral tunnel plus/minus fenestration has resulted in improved results with both early and mid-term mortality [13]. Because staged reconstruction with an intermediate BCPA has further reduced overall mortality, Ruzmetov et al. prefer to create BCPA before the Fontan operation in most patients who have single-ventricle physiology to reduce morbidity and mortality [13]. However, the interval between construction of the BCPA and Fontan completion should not be too long, to avoid pulmonary arteriovenous malformations caused by a lack of hepatic factor. Although surgeons may choose from various Fontan modifications, Ruzmetov et al. prefer lateral tunnel Fontan pathway incorporating a portion of atrial wall as it allows for growth and endothelialization of the pathway [13]. Further, for patients with abnormalities of systemic and pulmonary venous connection, a lateral tunnel is sometimes not possible without risking obstruction to pulmonary venous blood flow. They use an extracardiac tube graft to avoid obstruction [13].

Kleinert et al. reviewed the records of 193 DORV patients, 117 were in group 1 (noncomplex: atrioventricular concordance/VSD/ balanced ventricles, no straddling atrioventricular valves, no major PA anomaly) and 76 in group 2 (complex: all remaining) [14]. Biventricular repair was undertaken in 148 patients, including 111 in group 1 and 37 of group 2. Early mortality was higher in group 2 patients undergoing biventricular repair (8 of 37 versus 4 of 111, $P<.005$) and higher than group 2 patients undergoing a Fontan procedure (none of 29, $P<.01$). A significantly higher proportion of group 2 patients (8 of 37 or 21.6 %; CI, 9.8 % to 38.3 %) died after a biventricular repair than in group 1 (4 of 111 or 3.6 %; CI, 1.0 % to 9.0 %; $P<.005$). There were no hospital deaths among the 29 group 2 or the two group 1 patients undergoing a cavopulmonary shunt or modified Fontan procedure. There were 9 late deaths, at a mean follow-up time of 4.7 ± 3.8 years, 1 of which had undergone a Fontan type procedure. Kleinert et al. concluded that the difference in early mortality between patients with complicating anatomic features undergoing biventricular repair and those undergoing some form of Fontan procedure strongly suggests that the Fontan is the procedure of choice, even more so among those with surgically inaccessible multiple VSDs [14].

Serraf et al. reported on 34 patients with DORV ($n=15$) or TGA ($n=19$) [1]. All but three patients had two ventricles of adequate size. Thirty patients underwent a biventricular repair and four had a univentricular repair. Biventricular repair was achieved by an arterial switch operation in 18 patients and by tunnel construction from the left ventricle to the aorta in 12. There were four early deaths and one late death, all occurring in the group having biventricular repair. Mean follow-up of 30.7 ± 19.4 months found all but one patient (univentricular repair) in New York Heart Association (NYHA) class I, without atrioventricular valve incompetence. Actuarial survival at 4 years was 85.3 ± 3 % [1].

Bradley et al. reviewed the CHSS records of 393 children with DORV presenting between 1980 and 2000 [15]. Biventricular repair was performed in 194 (55 %) and the Fontan operation in 182 (23 %) patients. For complex DORV, Rastelli-type repair increased early reintervention risk ($P=.04$) and late post-repair mortality ($P=.02$), and biventricular repair, especially Rastelli-type reconstruction, was associated with higher late mortality and reintervention than Fontan repair. Bradley et al. found that extending biventricular repair to borderline anatomic candidates with hypoplastic leftsided structures or a nonsubaortic VSD to be questionable. According to Bradley et al., innovative techniques and improved perioperative care have made biventricular repair achievable even in patients with complex forms of DORV, although it is with higher early mortality compared with single-ventricle repair [15]. They further noted that an adequately sized normal mitral valve and left ventricle are the main determinants of achieving a biventricular repair, whereas small left ventricle or abnormalities of the atrioventricular valve were associated with a greater tendency toward single-ventricle repair [15].

Discussion

The Fontan repair is a relatively uncomplicated operation with low initial mortality performed in patients with two ventricles. Early and midterm results are excellent [3, 13–15] and functional class is NYHA I to II in most series [16]. Modified Fontan procedures have been advocated when biventricular DORV repair has been either impractical or extremely complex [14]. Because short-term and medium-term outcome for Fontan procedures has improved over time [3, 17–19], this approach is promising for patients at increased operative risk for conventional biventricular repair [3]. The lateral tunnel has been widely adopted including an extracardiac tube or tunnel on the external surface of the right atrium and may decrease late development of atrial arrhythmias [3, 20–22]. Creating a limited right-to-left shunt by fenestration or an adjustable atrial septal defect also appears to improve short-term outcome. Finally, most survivors of the Fontan procedure do not require subsequent operations relating to valve-conduit replacement [3, 23]. In comparison with the potential risks of the VSD to aorta rerouting, the Fontan remains a satisfactory option [24].

Serraf et al. noted that a biventricular repair is used to create circulation with unobstructed intraventricular and extraventricular pathways [1]. At times, this involves intracardiac resections for enlargement of the VSD, construction of complex intracardiac baffles, and extensive atrioventricular valvar or subvalvar mobilization. These techniques are likely to extend crossclamp time, impact negatively on myocardial contractility, and threaten the conduction system in addition to subsequent difficult postoperative course and a high reoperation rate making the Fontan operation more attractive than the biventricular repair in certain populations. The single absolute limiting factor for biventricular repair is the respective size of each ventricle [1].

Bradley et al. continue by stating that in cases where there is a perceived benefit of a biventricular repair, increased risk of late death or reintervention compared with single-ventricle repairs favors the Fontan operation [15, 25]. Restriction or natural closure of the VSD in complex DORV can occur in a number of patients with DORV-nc-VSD treated with Fontan palliation. Consequently, some are in favor of performing a VSD enlargement at the time of Fontan completion in complex DORV (Fig. 35.1) [25, 26]. Surgeons at Boston Childrens Hospital [26] reported on 8 complex DORV patients presenting with severe left ventricle obstruction following Fontan. This study highlights the preventative need for VSD enlargement in DORV-nc-VSD repair. Enlarging the VSD superiorly at the time of the Fontan completion, when the VSD diameter is smaller than the aortic annulus is recommended to prevent natural VSD closure and to avoid heart block (Fig. 35.2) [25–27].

Is the early hazard of a "risky" biventricular repair mitigated by an important late benefit [15]? Are there certain anatomic characteristics that are consistently associated with a better outcome for either a biventricular or single ventricular approach? [15] Although there are no prospective randomized studies comparing these two treatment options one could extrapolate the results of each operation and project the long-term survival. The Fontan patient (Fig. 35.2) [27] may be operation-free for 20–40 years; whereas patients with biventricular repair face the possibility of pacemaker placement, right ventricle to conduit changes, and possible reoperations for left ventricular outflow tract obstruction.

It is important to remember the possible risks associated with the Fontan procedure owing to the physiology, in which the force driving pulmonary blood flow is

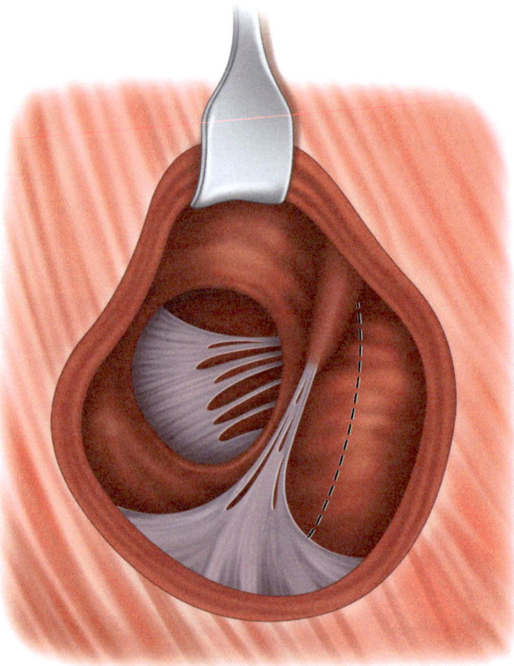

Fig. 35.1 Ventricular septal defect enlargement should also be performed at the time of the Fontan completion in complex double outlet right ventricle. The incision is carried out superiorly; the conduction tissue being located inferiorly in the double outlet right ventricle peri-membranous type ventricular septal defect

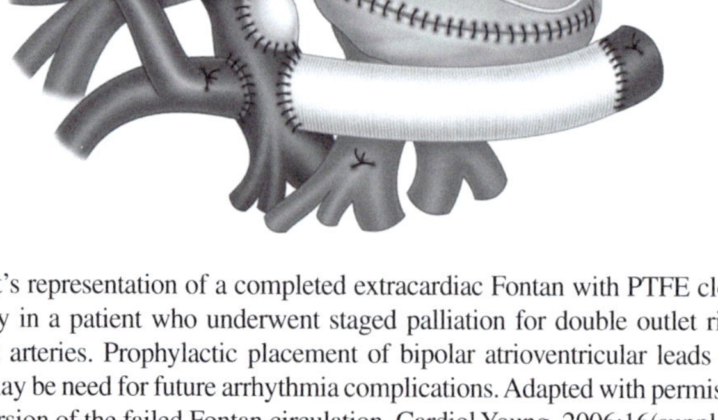

Fig. 35.2 Artist's representation of a completed extracardiac Fontan with PTFE closure of the main pulmonary artery in a patient who underwent staged palliation for double outlet right ventricle and transposed great arteries. Prophylactic placement of bipolar atrioventricular leads are shown in the event that they may be need for future arrhythmia complications. Adapted with permission from Backer CL, et al. Conversion of the failed Fontan circulation. Cardiol Young. 2006;16(suppl 1):85–91.[27]

largely a residue (in systemic venous pressure) of the main chamber's contractile force, imposes a gradually declining functional capacity and premature late death, even after the initial period of often excellent palliation [28]. Patients with single ventricle physiology, managed with Fontan operation, may face possible long-term problems, such as when as many as 50 % of Fontan patients will develop atrial tachycardia [29], which increases morbidity and mortality. Supraventricular arrhythmia occurs in most patients 20–30 years after Fontan operation [30]. Further, protein-losing enteropathy occurs in about 5–15 % [31] and plastic bronchitis, although rare, is significant and can lead to death [32]. Decreased cardiac output can decrease functional status (NYHA III or IV) and there is decreased exercise tolerance and abnormal hemodynamic response to stress, which ultimately has deleterious effects on the pulmonary circulation [28]. Finally, the longer the interval between surgery and follow-up, the worse the functional class (NYHA III/IV) of the Fontan [28].

To be sure, patients with DORV with non-committed VSD and two functional ventricles present treatment options that challenge short- and long-term survival, event-free survival, and eventual cardiac transplantation. The theoretical benefits of a 2-ventricle repair are attended by interventricular septal resection, complex interventricular tunneling, conduit placement, and heart block. Others [24] recommend avoidance of interventricular septal resection in favor of a VSD to pulmonary artery baffle and an arterial switch operation and have reported excellent results. However, even in well executed operations, ventricular dysfunction, conduit obstructions, and pacemaker therapy can often mute the well intended efforts of practitioners. On the other hand, the Fontan operation has better short- and long-term event-free survival but ominous long-term problems that generally require cardiac transplantation. The choices are difficult; the future may hold the answer if stem cells can cure ventricular dysfunction; if the key to conduit growth can be found, and if the immunologic mysteries of cardiac transplantation can be deciphered.

References

1. Serraf A, Nakamura T, Lacour-Gayet F, et al. Surgical approaches for double-outlet right ventricle or transposition of the great arteries associated with straddling atrioventricular valves. J Thorac Cardiovasc Surg. 1996;111:527–35.
2. Walters HL, Mavroudis C. Double-outlet ventricles. In: Mavroudis C, Backer CL, editors. Pediatric cardiac surgery. Chichester: Wiley-Blackwell; 2013.
3. Delius RE, Rademecker MA, de Leval MR, Elliott MJ, Stark J. Is a high-risk biventricular repair always preferable to conversion to a single ventricle repair? J Thorac Cardiovasc Surg. 1996;112(6):1561–8; discussion 1568–9.
4. Brown JW, Ruzmetov M, Okada Y, Vijay P, Turrentine MW. Surgical results in patients with double outlet right ventricle: a 20-year experience. Ann Thorac Surg. 2001;72:1630–5.
5. Barbero-Marcial M, Tanamati C, Atik E, Ebaid M. Intraventricular repair of double-outlet right ventricle with noncommitted ventricular septal defect: advantages of multiple patches. J Thorac Cardiovasc Surg. 1999;118(6):1056–67.
6. Lacour-Gayet F. Biventricular repair of double outlet right ventricle with noncommitted ventricular septal defect. Semin Thorac Cardiovasc Surg Pediatr Card Surg Annu. 2002;5:163–72.

7. Kitagawa T, Durham LA, Mosca RS, Bove EL. Surgery for congenital heart disease: techniques and results in the management of multiple ventricular septal defects. J Thorac Cardiovasc Surg. 1998;115:848–56.
8. Judson JP, Danielson GK, Puga FJ, Mair DD, McGoon DC. Double-outlet right ventricle: surgical results, 1970–1980. J Thorac Cardiovasc Surg. 1983;85:32–40.
9. Kirklin JW, Castaneda AR. Surgical correction of double-outlet right ventricle: early and late results. Circulation. 1983;68(Pt 2):144–7.
10. Russo P, Danielson GK, Puga FJ, McGoon DC, Humes R. Modified Fontan Procedure for biventricular hearts with complex forms of double-outlet right ventricle. Circulation. 1988;78(Suppl):III20–5.
11. Barrett Boyes BG, Kirklin JW. Surgical management of double outlet right and left ventricle. In: Godman MJ, editor. Pediatric cardiology, vol. 4. London: Churchill Livingstone; 1981.
12. Kirklin JW, Pacifico AD, Blackstone EH, Kirklin JK, Bargeron Jr LM. Current risks and protocols for operations for double-outlet right ventricle. Derivation from an 18 year experience. J Thorac Cardiovasc Surg. 1986;92(5):913–30.
13. Ruzmetov M, Rodefeld MD, Turrentine MW, Brown JW. Rational approach to surgical management of complex forms of double outlet right ventricle with modified Fontan operation. Congenit Heart Dis. 2008;3(6):397–403.
14. Kleinert S, Sano T, Weintraub RG, Mee RB, Karl TR, Wilkinson JL. Anatomic features and surgical strategies in double-outlet right ventricle. Circulation. 1997;96(4):1233–9.
15. Bradley TJ, Karamlou T, Kulik A, Mitrovic B, Vigneswaran T, Jaffer S, Glasgow PD, Williams WG, Van Arsdell GS, McCrindle BW. Determinants of repair type, reintervention, and mortality in 393 children with double-outlet right ventricle. J Thorac Cardiovasc Surg. 2007;134(4):967–973.e6.
16. Gentles TL, Gauvreau K, Mayer Jr JE, Fishberger SB, Burnett J, Colan SD, Newburger JW, Wernovsky G. Functional outcome after the Fontan operation: factors influencing late morbidity. J Thorac Cardiovasc Surg. 1997;114(3):392–403; discussion 404–5.
17. Pearl JM, Laks H, Drinkwater DC, Capouya ER, George BL, Williams RG. Modified Fontan procedure in patients less than 4 years of age. Circulation. 1992;86(Suppl II):II-100–5.
18. Bridges ND, Castaneda AR. The fenestrated Fontan procedure. Herz. 1992;17:242–5.
19. Jacobs ML, Norwood Jr WI. Fontan operation: influence of modifications on morbidity and mortality. Ann Thorac Surg. 1994;58:945–52.
20. Laschinger JC, Ringel RE, Brenner JI, McLaughlin JS. The extracardiac total cavopulmonary connection for definitive conversion to the Fontan circulation: summary of early experience and results. J Card Surg. 1993;8:524–33.
21. Balaji S, Gewillig M, Bull C, de Leval MR, Deanfield JE. Arrhythmias after the Fontan procedure: comparison of total cavopulmonary connection and atriopulmonary connection. Circulation. 1991;85(5 Suppl):III162–7.
22. Pearl JM, Laks H, Stein DG, Drinkwater DC, George BL, Williams RG. Total cavopulmonary anastomosis versus conventional modified Fontan procedure. Ann Thorac Surg. 1991;52:189–96.
23. deVivie E-R, Rupparth G. Long-term results after the Fontan procedure and its modifications. J Thorac Cardiovasc Surg. 1986;86:690–7.
24. Lacour-Gayet F, Haun C, Ntalakoura K, Belli E, Houyel L, Marcsek P, Wagner F, Weil J. Biventricular repair of double outlet right ventricle with non-committed ventricular septal defect (VSD) by VSD rerouting to the pulmonary artery and arterial switch. Eur J Cardiothorac Surg. 2002;21(6):1042–8.
25. Lacour-Gayet F. Management of older single functioning ventricles with outlet obstruction due to a restricted "VSD" in double inlet left ventricle and in complex double outlet right ventricle. Semin Thorac Cardiovasc Surg Pediatr Card Surg Annu. 2009;12:130–2.
26. Meadows J, Pigula F, Lock J, Marshall A. Transcatheter creation and enlargement of ventricular septal defects for relief of ventricular hypertension. J Thorac Cardiovasc Surg. 2007;133:912–8.

27. Backer CL, Deal BJ, Mavroudis C, Franklin WH, Stewart RD. Conversion of the failed Fontan circulation. Cardiol Young. 2006;16 Suppl 1:85–91.
28. Fontan F, Kirklin JW, Fernandez G, Costa F, Naftel DC, Tritto F, Blackstone EH. Outcome after a "perfect" Fontan operation. Circulation. 1990;81(5):1520–36.
29. Deal BJ, Mavroudis C, Backer CL. Arrhythmia management in the Fontan patient. Pediatr Cardiol. 2007;28(6):448–56.
30. Cetta F, Boston US, Dearani JA, Hagler DJ. Double outlet right ventricle: opinions regarding management. Curr Treat Options Cardiovasc Med. 2005;7(5):385–90.
31. Lin WS, Hwang MS, Chung HT, Chu JJ, Lai MW, Yang JS, Huang SC, Huang JL, Su WJ. Protein-losing enteropathy after the Fontan operation: clinical analysis of nine cases. Chang Gung Med J. 2006;29(5):505–12.
32. Goo HW, Jhang WK, Kim YH, Ko JK, Park IS, Park JJ, Yun TJ, Seo DM. CT findings of plastic bronchitis in children after a Fontan operation. Pediatr Radiol. 2008;38(9):989–93.

Chapter 36
Genetics of Conotruncal Anomalies

Brigitte Laforest and Stéphane Zaffran

Abstract Conotruncal (or outflow tract) defects are among the most common congenital heart diseases found at birth, and are the leading cause of mortality and morbidity in the first year of life. In the last 20 years, the progenitor cells that contribute to cardiac outflow tract development have received much attention. Thus, the role of neural crest and second heart field derivatives has been established during outflow tract development. Particularly, second heart field cells contribute to growth of the outflow tract by addition of cells from the splanchnic pharyngeal mesoderm, whereas neural crest cells populate the endocardial cushions within the outflow tract. It is now well accepted that defective neural crest or second heart field deployment results in a spectrum of conotruncal anomalies ranging from outflow tract alignment to septation defects. In addition, recent studies have improved our understanding of signaling pathways and transcriptional networks required for outflow tract development. In this chapter, we present an overview of cardiac development, with emphasis on the genetic causes of outflow tract anomalies and highlight relevant genetic data for cardiac development in humans as well as animal models.

Keywords Outflow tract • Conotruncal anomalies • Transcription factors • Tetralogy of Fallot • Cardiac neural crest cells

B. Laforest, PhD
Génétique Médicale & Génomique Fonctionnelle (GMGF), UMR_S910, Aix Marseille Université, Faculté de Médecine de la Timone, Marseille 13005, France

Inserm, U910, Marseille 13005, France

S. Zaffran, PhD (✉)
Medical Genetics & Functional Genomics, UMR_S910, Aix Marseille Université, Medical School of Marseille, Marseille, France

Laboratoire de Génétique Médicale et Génomique Fonctionnelle, Faculté de Médecin, 27 Bd Jean Moulin, Marseille 13005, France

Génétique Médicale & Génomique Fonctionnelle (GMGF), UMR_S910, Aix Marseille Université, Faculté de Médecine de la Timone, Marseille 13005, France

Inserm, U910, Marseille 13005, France
e-mail: stephane.zaffran@univ-amu.fr

F. Lacour-Gayet et al. (eds.), *Surgery of Conotruncal Anomalies*,
DOI 10.1007/978-3-319-23057-3_36

Introduction

Cardiac morphogenesis is a complex process that requires the precise and coordinate interactions between multiple cardiac and extra-cardiac cell types. Any perturbation in the cells that contribute to heart formation leads to cardiac defects. In humans, this is reflected by the high incidence of congenital heart diseases (CHDs), which is estimated to affect 1–2 % of all live births [1]. Conotruncal (also called cardiac outflow tract (OFT)) anomalies constitute one of the major categories of CHD, with a prevalence of 30 %, and can lead to significant mortality and morbidity both in children and adults if not repaired. Historically, knowledge of the embryogenesis of heart defects was difficult to achieve because of the lack of animal models. However, with the increased advances in gene targeting techniques, researchers have been able to improve our understanding of the etiology of these defects. The following sections will focus on early cardiac development and embryological origins of conotruncal defects such as tetralogy of Fallot (ToF), double outlet right ventricle (DORV), overriding aorta (OA), transposition of the great arteries (TGA) and persistent truncus arteriosus (PTA).

Overview of Early Heart Development

The heart is the first organ to form in vertebrates, where it plays an essential role in the distribution of nutrients and oxygen in the early embryo. In the embryo, myocardial progenitor cells are located in bilaterally paired cardiogenic fields in the splanchnic layer of anterior lateral mesoderm. At embryonic (E) day 7.5 in the mouse embryo (corresponding to the 3rd week of gestation in human), these cells form a "horseshoe-shaped" or "crescent-shaped" epithelium, the cardiac crescent, where myocardial markers are first detected (Fig. 36.1). By E8.0, these cells extend across the midline to form the early heart tube, composed of an outer myocardial layer and an inner endocardial layer separated by extracellular matrix, called cardiac jelly. Subsequently, the linear heart tube undergoes rightward looping to bring the atrial region of the early tube in a posterior position relative to the ventricles (Fig. 36.1). Concomitant with cardiac looping, the forming heart tube increases dramatically in length by addition of myocardial cells at its arterial and venous poles. In the mouse, the population of myocardial progenitors located in the splanchnic pharyngeal mesoderm that contributes to the growth of the embryonic heart tube has been termed the second heart field (SHF) [2, 3]. Several studies have shown that these cells contribute to the cardiac OFT, right ventricle and a major part of the atrial myocardium, whereas the left ventricle derives only from the cardiac crescent called the first heart field (FHF) [2, 3] (Fig. 36.1). As the heart tube grows, the cardiac chambers begin to form by activation of chamber genes and localized proliferation of myocardial cells. This may involve cell growth at the outer curvature of the cardiac tube, while oriented cell growth is probably important in shaping the chambers.

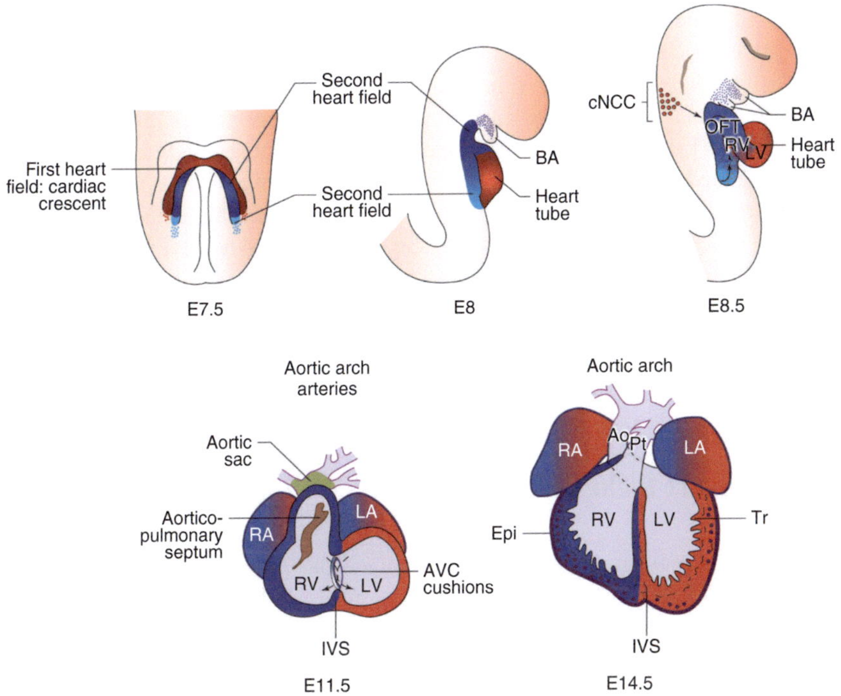

Fig. 36.1 Cardiac development in the mouse. Diagram showing stages of heart development and contribution of the first heart field (*FHF; red*) and second heart field (*SHF; blue*) to the heart. Frontal view is shown for embryonic day 7.5 (E7.5), E11.5 and E14.5 and lateral view for E8 and E8.5 stages. At E7.5, the first differentiated myocardial cells are observed in the cardiac crescent (FHF), with the SHF lying medial to it. At E8, a linear heart tube is formed by fusion of the cardiac crescent at the midline of the embryo. While the heart tube as begins to loop, SHF progenitor cells are added to its arterial and venous poles (E8.5). Subsequently, the SHF contributes to formation of the right ventricle, outflow tract (*OFT*) and both atria. The left ventricle derives exclusively from the FHF, which also contributes to atria formation. At E11.5, the articopulmonary septum is dividing the distal OFT into the aorta and the pulmonary trunk. The aortic sac branches into a series of aortic arch arteries. At E14.5, atrial and ventricular septa separate the atria and ventricles, respectively. *Ao* aorta, *AVC* atrioventricular canal, *BA* branchial arch, *cNCC* cardiac neural crest cells, *Epi* epicardium, *IVS* interventricular septum, *LA* left atrium, *LV* left ventricle, *Pt* pulmonary trunk, *RA* right atrium, *RV* right ventricle, *Tr* trabecules

Septation of the OFT is somewhat complicated and is briefly introduced here. Between E9.5 and E11.5, the endocardium of the OFT and atrioventricular canal generates mesenchymal cells that populate the cardiac jelly between the endocardium and myocardium (Fig. 36.1) [4]. The budges formed during this process are called endocardial cushions. Shaping of the cushions in the distal OFT (truncus) is accompanied by, and perhaps results from, the infiltration of cells originating from the neural crest [4]. The fusion of the endocardial cushions, which begins distally in the aortic sac, physically divides the OFT into the intra-pericardial component of the aorta and the pulmonary trunk. This process is called the aorticopulmonary septation. As the OFT septum forms, the proximal OFT (conus) is incorporated into the right ventricle. At the same time, the OFT shortens, undergoes rotation and shifts to a medial position above the presumptive interventricular septum to connect the future aorta and pulmonary trunk to their respective ventricles [5]. Hence, rotation of the OFT is a crucial event in proper OFT alignment, and reduced rotation has been correlated to DORV, OA, and other OFT remodeling defects in humans. In the atrioventricular canal, the cushions are remodeled to form the components of the mitral and tricuspid valve apparatus (Fig. 36.1). In the fetal heart (E14.5) the chambers are separated by the interventricular septum, whose muscular part derives from growth of the primitive ventricle. The ventricles are now connected to the pulmonary trunk and aorta, which ensure separate pulmonary and systemic circulation of the blood, respectively, after birth.

Second Heart Field Lineage

Three articles published in 2001 [6–8] changed our previous view that the early heart tube contains all ventricular and atrial chambers. Indeed, these studies revealed that the forming OFT elongates by addition of cells to the arterial pole, and furthermore identified the origin of these myocardial progenitor cells in the splanchnic mesoderm laying dorsally to the primitive heart tube (see [2]). This region of the mesoderm is now referred to the second heart field (SHF), of which cells express different transcription factors including Islet 1 (Isl1), Nkx2-5 and T-box 1 (Tbx1) [2]. Since the identification of this field, there has been accumulating evidence showing that the SHF is pre-patterned along the anterior-posterior axis [3]. Briefly, cells at the anterior domain of the SHF, express fibroblast growth factor (*Fgf8*/*Fgf10*) genes and activate Mef2c-AHF-enhancer, and contribute to the OFT and right ventricular myocardium, whereas the posterior SHF, marked by *Hoxb1* and *Hoxa1* genes expression, contributes to a large part of the atria and the myocardium at the base of the pulmonary trunk [3]. The contribution of posterior SHF cells to the atria and the inferior wall of the OFT, which subsequently gives rise to sub-pulmonary myocardium, has recently been confirmed by fate mapping analysis (Fig. 36.1).

During heart tube extension, the SHF receives multiple signals from surrounding cell types, including pharyngeal ectoderm and endoderm [3]. These signals have been shown to control proliferation and differentiation of SHF cells. It is now accepted that direct or indirect perturbations of SHF deployment may result in a spectrum of conotruncal defects ranging from OFT alignment to septation defects [9]. Increasing knowledge has been gained in the last couple of years about the signaling pathways playing critical roles in SHF deployment, and they have been reviewed in detail elsewhere [2, 3]. *In vitro* approaches indicate that during progressive colonization of the OFT, SHF cells are submitted to pro-proliferative FGF/Erk, canonical Wnt and Hedgehog signals in the pharyngeal region [10]. Following proliferation within the SHF, progenitor cells will be recruited to the arterial and venous poles where they are now exposed to signals, including bone morphogenetic proteins

(BMP), non-canonical Wnt and Notch proteins, which positively regulate their differentiation [11]. Using tissue marking technique, Waldo et al. (2005) demonstrated that the SHF, in addition to providing myocardium to the OFT, also differentiates into smooth muscle near the base of the remodeling aorta and pulmonary trunk [12]. Hence, impaired SHF proliferation and function can lead to severe conotruncal hypoplasia and concomitant CHDs.

Cardiac Neural Crest Cell Lineage

Neural crest cells are a multipotent and transient migratory embryonic lineage that originates from the dorsal neural tube. The region of neural crest migrating to the heart was identified nearly 30 years ago using chick-quail chimera and was called cardiac neural crest. This region was found to be critical for normal heart development [4]. Cardiac neural crest cells (NCCs) migrate through the primordial pharynx and over the pharyngeal arches three, four and six where they surround the aortic arch arteries, and are necessary for the smooth muscle layer of the great arteries. A subset of cardiac NCCs continues migrating from the pharynx to reach the distal cardiac OFT (truncus) where they participate to the formation of the aorticopulmonary septum. In addition, a recent study showed that preotic NCCs migrate beyond the OFT of the heart, where they give rise to coronary smooth muscle cells and mesenchymal like cells in the interventricular septum and papillary muscle of the right ventricle.

Neural crest ablation results in cardiovascular and non-cardiovascular defects. These phenotypes include hypoplasia or aplasia of the thymus, thyroids and parathyroids, defective development of the cardiac OFT, abnormal patterning of the great arteries and abnormal myocardial function [4, 13]. The effect of NCCs in OFT development is also shown in the mouse. Pax3 is a key regulator of neural crest and in the Splotch^{2H} mouse, where Pax3 function is affected, reduction of neural crest migration results in OFT defects. The OFT defects associated with defective neural crest cells include complete absence of OFT septation, or PTA, and OA.

NCCs respond to a variety of signaling factors, including the BMP/TGFβ, endothelin and PDGF signaling pathways during their induction, migration and population of various sites [10, 11]. The interaction between cardiac NCCs and the surrounding mesoderm is evident by examination of the neural crest ablation phenotype. Interestingly, operated chick embryos displayed cardiac looping defects prior to the colonization of the OFT by NCCs [14]. This looping defect is the result of a shortened OFT that occurs due to a failure in the addition of SHF cells to the elongating heart tube. Instead of migrating and subsequently differentiating into myocardium, SHF cells kept proliferating, suggesting interaction between the SHF and neural crest-derived cells in the pharynx. Recently, it was shown that FGF8 signaling is elevated in the pharynx of neural crest-ablated embryo concomitant with cardiac looping, likely indicating that FGF8 could be the potential factor. Finally, endodermal Sonic Hedgehog (Shh) signaling is required for cardiac NCCs to survive and populate the OFT cushions. Overall, these findings reveal a complex relationship between cardiac NCCs and the SHF, and any perturbation in the interaction between these two cell types results in conotruncal defects.

Conotruncal Anomalies

Over the last 20 years, tremendous advances in medical and surgical care of children have reduced the morbidity and mortality of many CHDs. As a result, an increasing number of adults living with complex CHDs that may be at risk of transmitting a congenital abnormality to their offsprings. The etiology of CHD is still largely unknown; however in recent years, separate environmental and genetic causes have been identified. The lack of genotype-phenotype correlation coupled with locus heterogeneity have limited gene discovery and only 15 % of cases of CHDs have been traced to a known cause to this day. Interestingly, new technologies in human genetics coupled with model organisms provided important insights into the signaling pathways and transcriptional networks regulating heart development and underlying CHD pathogenesis. As mentioned above, the arterial pole of the heart is composed of diverse cell types including myocardial, endocardial and cardiac NCCs. It is not surprising that one malformation may result from the contribution of defective NCCs migration and/or abnormal rotation of OFT myocardium and/or a defect in the deployment of SHF progenitor cells and/or endocardial cushion defect. This hypothesis has led to the concept of "one heart disease – several mechanisms – several genes" (Fig. 36.2).

Tetralogy of Fallot

Tetralogy of Fallot (ToF) is a CHD that involves four heart malformations characterized by pulmonary stenosis, right ventricular hypertrophy, overriding of the aorta (OA) and a ventricular septal defect. In addition, ToF may be present in association with other cardiac malformations such as pulmonary atresia, right sided aortic arch, atrioventricular septal defects, atrial septal defects, abnormal pulmonary venous return and coronary artery anomalies. An increasing number of genes have been linked to ToF in the last couple of years. Mutations have been identified in *JAG1*, *NKX2-5*, *GDF1*, *VEGF*, *GATA4*, *GATA5*, *GATA6* and ZFPM2/*FOG2* (Fig. 36.3; Table 36.1) [17–19, 26, 27, 29–32]. Approximately 10 % of patients with ToF have an interstitial deletion of chromosome 22 (del22q11.2) (Digeorge syndrome, velocardiofacial syndrome or 22q11.2 deletion syndrome), which appears to be the most frequent genetic defect associated with ToF [33]. Fifty percent of children with ToF caused by del22q11.2 have other cardiac anomalies such as absent pulmonary valve,

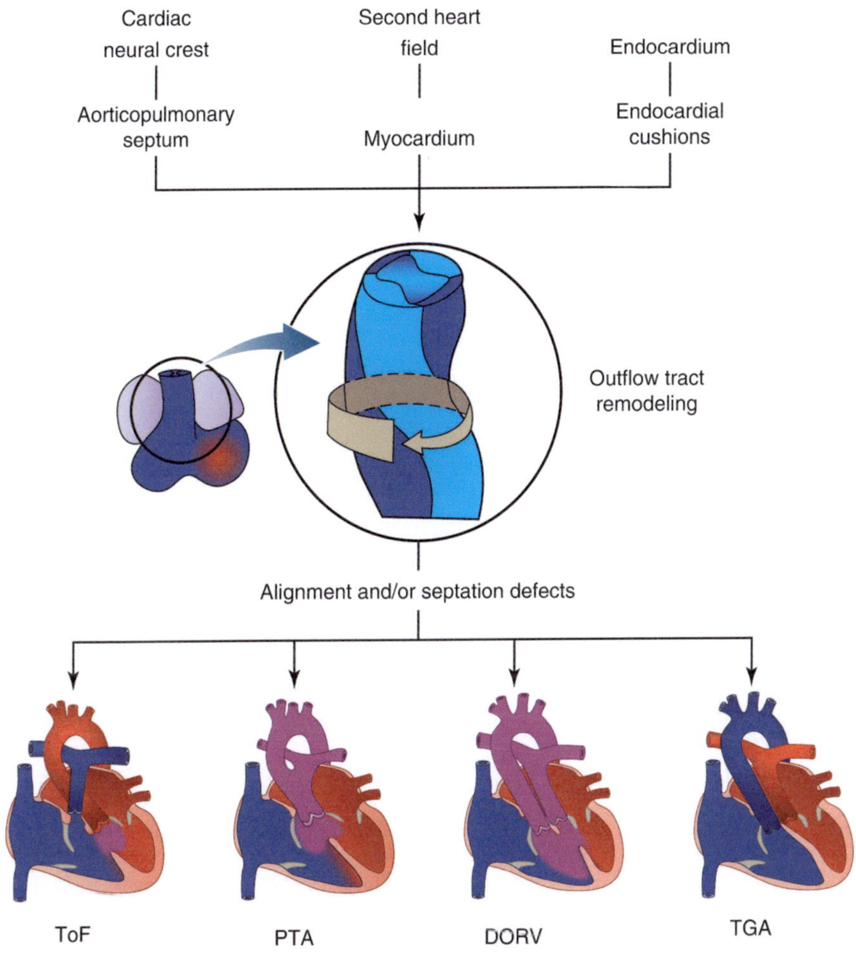

Fig. 36.2 One heart disease – several mechanisms – several genes. A malformation may be caused by different mechanisms. For example, persistent truncus arteriosus (*PTA*) results from defective second heart field development as well as impaired of cardiac neural crest cells migration, which involve multiple genes (*Tbx1*, *Pax3*, *Fgf8*, *Shh*, Bmp…). The result is a concept known as "one heart disease – several mechanisms – several genes". In addition, perturbation of these mechanisms may generate different anomalies of the outflow tract (conotruncal) region. *DORV* double outlet right ventricle, *TGA* transposition of the great arteries, *ToF* tetralogy of Fallot, *PTA* persistent truncus arteriosus

hypoplastic pulmonary arteries, and aortic arch defects. *TBX1* maps within the del22q11.2 regions and mutations in *TBX1* have been identified in some patients with features of Digeorge syndrome but without the classical del22q11.2 [24]. One recent study demonstrated that rare *TBX1* variants with functional consequences are present in a small proportion of non-syndromic ToF [34].

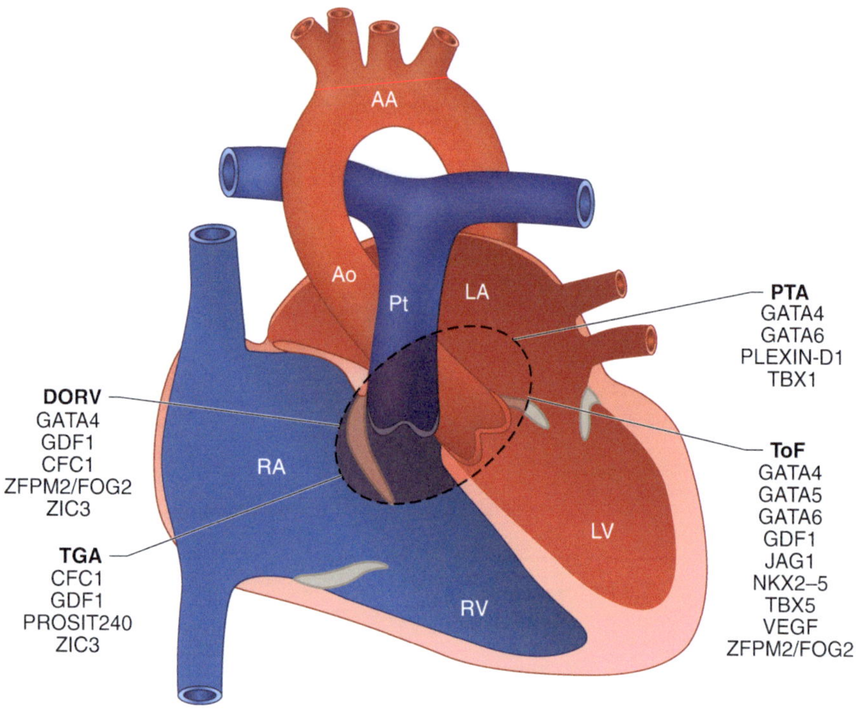

Fig. 36.3 Sites of structural malformations associated with conotruncal anomalies. Note that one congenital heart disease (CHD) may be cause by mutations in different genes and the same transcription factor may be associated to different conotruncal anomalies. *DORV* double outlet right ventricle, *TGA* transposition of the great arteries, *ToF* tetralogy of Fallot, *PTA* persistent truncus arteriosus

ToF is rarely reported in mouse models of OFT defects. This may be partially reflected by the fact that the four characteristic phenotypes of ToF are not found very frequently together. Moreover, a large number of mouse models lead to early embryonic lethality, which impedes the study of new genes that could be associated with ToF. Only two mouse models have been reported to date and these include targeted homozygous deletion of *Hoxa1* and *Hey2* [35, 36]. *Hoxa1* mutant mice have ToF in addition to bicuspid aortic valve, interruption of the aortic arch type B and aberrant subclavian artery, recapitulating the phenotypes observed in patients with homozygous mutations in *HOXA1* [35]. Interestingly, in their study, Makki and Cappechi (2012) suggested that the cardiovascular defects in *Hoxa1*$^{-/-}$ mice could be due to a role of this factor during NCC specification. In addition, all *Msx1/2* null mice have hallmarks of ToF as well as other conotruncal anomalies (PTA or DORV) [37].

Table 36.1 Human genetic mutations associated with cardiac phenotype

Gene	Locus	Protein	Phenotype	Refs.
CFC1	2q21	Cryptic protein	DORV, D-TGA	[15]
GATA4	8p23	Gata4 transcription factor	ToF, DORV, PTA	[16]
GATA5	20q13	Gata5 transcription factor	ToF	[17]
GATA6	18q11	Gata6 transcription factor	ToF, PTA	[18]
GDF1	19p13	Growth differentiation factor 1	ToF, DORV, D-TGA	[19]
JAG1	20p12	Jagged-1 ligand	ToF	[20]
NKX2-5	5q34	Homeobox containing transcription factor	ToF, DORV	[21]
PLEXIN-D1	3q22	Plexin-Semaphorin receptor	PTA	[22]
PROSIT240	12q24	Similar to TRAP240	D-TGA	[23]
TBX1	22q11	T-box transcription factor	PTA, ToF	[24]
TBX5	12q24	T-box transcription factor	ToF	[25]
VEGF	6p21	Vascular endothelial growth factor	ToF	[26]
ZFPM2/FOG2	8q23	Friend of GATA (Zinc finger protein)	ToF, DORV	[27]
ZIC3	Xq26	Zinc finger transcription factor	DORV, D-TGA	[28]

DORV double outlet right ventricle, *PTA* persistent truncus arteriosus, *D-TGA* transposition of the great arteries, *ToF* tetralogy of Fallot

Double Outlet Right Ventricle

Double outlet right ventricle (DORV), which occurs in 1–3 % of all CHDs, is a form of conotruncal anomalies where both the aorta and pulmonary trunk arise from the right ventricle and is always associated with a ventricular septal defect. DORV occurs in multiple forms, with variability of great arteries position and size. DORV is not considered as an OFT septation defect, but rather as an OFT alignment defect. The only genes known in humans are *CFC1, GATA4*, GDF1, ZFPM2/*FOG2* and *ZIC3* (Fig. 36.3; Table 36.1) [15, 19, 28, 38, 39].

There are no animal models of isolated DORV. However, a large number of mouse mutations cause DORV associated with additional aortic arch and ventricular septation defects [13]. Addition of SHF progenitor cells to the arterial pole is essential for the elongation of the OFT and its proper alignment. Hence, deletion of genes involved in SHF deployment results in abnormal right ventricular development and OFT defects, including *Isl1*, *Mef2c*, *Foxh1*, *Foxc1* and *Foxc2* (see [2]). In addition, several lines of evidence suggest that the SHF relies on different signaling pathways in order to mediate its effects, and members of the FGF signaling pathway are good candidates. Specifically, global deletion of *Fgf8* results in early embryonic lethality whereas embryos lacking *Fgf10* do not develop a cardiac phenotype, possibly due to compensation by *Fgf8* [40]. Moreover, *Fgf8* hypomorphs display a complex cardiac and OFT phenotypes, suggesting that this protein is required at different times and location for proper OFT morphogenesis [41, 42]. Using different

Cre lines to conditionally inactivate *Fgf8*, several studies have shown a requirement for *Fgf8* in migratory NCC survival and therefore OFT septation and a role in SHF survival and proliferation (see [3]). Furthermore, Park et al. showed that mesodermal *Fgf8* is required for the proper alignment of the OFT while endodermal FGF8 is involved in OFT septation [43].

Overriding Aorta

Overriding aorta (OA) is a CHD where the aortic valve is positioned directly over a ventricular septal defect. The result is that the aorta receives blood from both the right and left ventricles. OA is defined as an OFT alignment defect, and OA is found frequently associated with ToF and Alagille syndrome. Interestingly, the only difference between OA, DORV and TGA is the relative position of the aorta with that of the interventricular septum. In fact, the pathogenesis of OA, DORV and TGA may underlie a common mechanism as all three are the result of abnormal rotation of the OFT, leading to alignment defects [5]. To date, no genes have been linked to OA in humans and mouse models of isolated OA are rare. However, mouse models of *Bmpr2*, *β-catenin*, *Cited2*, *Ece1*, *Frs2*, *Hes1*, *Hey2*, *Ssp1*, *Tgfβ2* and *Rarα/Rarβ* mutants display OA in addition to other cardiovascular phenotype (reviewed in [13]). Specific deletion of *Frs2*, *Rarα/Rarβ*, *Tgfβ2* in the mesoderm revealed the OA phenotype, clearly suggesting a role of mesodermal cells in this pathogenesis. Specific deletion of *Bmpr2* in neural crest cells, using either the *Wnt1-Cre* or *SM22α-Cre*, leads to OA with varying degrees of severity, suggesting a role for *Bmpr2* in neural crest-derived cells in positioning of the ascending aorta [44]. As mentioned above, OA is also one of the cardiac abnormalities observed in Alagille syndrome, where mutations in *JAG1* and *NOTCH2* have been identified [20, 45]. In mice, OA is not seen upon deletion of *Jag1* or *Notch2* but mice heterozygous for *Jag1/Notch2* display fully penetrant OA phenotype, clearly suggesting a genetic interaction among these genes [46].

It is interesting to note that altered SHF development has been shown to result in OA. Using chick embryos, Ward et al. (2005) demonstrated that ablation of the right side of the SHF results in OA, confirming a role for the SHF in the appropriate alignment of the OFT [9].

Transposition of the Great Arteries

Transposition of the great arteries (TGA) is the most common cyanotic congenital heart anomalies present at birth, in which the two great arteries, the aorta and pulmonary trunk, are reversed. TGA represents 5 % of all cases of CHDs and 34 % of conotruncal anomalies [47]. TGA is very severe and if not repaired, is the leading cause of death in infants. Ventricular septal defects are often associated with TGA and their position and size are variable. In humans, only few genes have been identified, *CFC1*, *GDF1*, *PROSIT240* and *ZIC3* (Fig. 36.3; Table 36.1) [15, 19, 23, 48]. Moreover, global deletion of *Cfc1* and *Gdf1* in mice also results TGA, clearly identifying these genes as a genetic modifier of TGA in both mice and humans. Mutations in several mouse genes, such as *Pitx2* and *type IIB activin receptor*, result in TGA and other cardiac anomalies in addition to left-right asymmetry defects, suggesting a role for left-right asymmetry in the pathogenesis of TGA [5]. This hypothesis is further supported by the recent study of De Luca et al. (2011) demonstrating that TGA may be caused by mutations in laterality genes in humans [38].

Global inactivation of *Hspg2*, which is expressed in the extracellular matrix, leads to fully penetrant TGA phenotype with very low incidence of other cardiac defects, making this the closest genetic animal model to TGA to date [49]. In *Hspg2* null mice, the endocardial cushions of the distal OFT (truncus) become hyperplastic possibly due to increased cardiac NCC migration and this may prevent the proper orientation of the aorta and pulmonary trunk over the chambers culminating in TGA. In the last decade, an increasing number of mouse models displaying TGA have been published [13]. Of note, inactivation of *β-catenin* revealed a decreased expression of *Pitx2* in migrating NCCs that normally invade the OFT, causing TGA, PTA and DORV. Member of the non-caconical Wnt pathway, like Wnt5a and Wnt11, play essential role during OFT morphogenesis as global inactivation of *Wnt5a* and *Wnt11* also leads to multiple OFT defects including TGA.

Persistent Truncus Arteriosus

Persistent truncus arteriosus (PTA) is a cardiac defect consisting of a single outlet from the heart supplying the systemic, the coronary, and the pulmonary circulation. Nearly all cases are associated with a VSD and the truncal valve is often abnormal. The majority of children diagnosed with PTA have congestive heart failure in the first weeks of life and surgery must be performed to repair the defect. Approximately 30–35 % of patients with PTA have a microdeletion of chromosome 22 (see [33]). As for ToF, patients with PTA and del22q11.2 have a higher incidence of associated other cardiac anomalies such as interrupted aortic arch, discontinuity of the pulmonary arteries, and coronary artery anomalies. The *TBX1* gene is the major candidate in DiGeorge syndrome; while mutations in human patients with PTA have been difficult to identify, mutations in *TBX1* have been identified in patients without del22q11.2 deletion [24]. In addition, mutations in other genes, *GATA4*, *GATA6* and *PLEXIN-D1* have also been identified in patients with PTA (Fig. 36.3; Table 36.1) [22, 39, 50].

In humans, the full spectrum of del22q11.2 associated malformations is observed in a haplo-insufficient manner in contrast to mice, where deletion of *Tbx1* leads to fully penetrant PTA (see [33]). This likely suggests that neighboring genes may modify *Tbx1* function and/or that genetic deletions in humans may contribute to DiGeorge syndrome. In addition, *Tbx1* is not expressed by migrating neural crest cells but instead is expressed in the pharyngeal endoderm, ectoderm and SHF mesenchyme where it is thought to exert its function by influencing the expression of secreted growth factors [2]. *Pax3* is one of the earliest NCC markers, being transiently expressed in premigratory NCC and turned off before the emigration of these cells to other tissues. Global *Pax3* knockout leads to a significant reduction in migration of NCCs into the OFT resulting in PTA and mid-gestation lethality, however later deletion of *Pax3* in NCCs does not affect OFT development [51]. This likely indicates that Pax3 is not involved in the migration of NCCs to the heart but rather is required for early expansion of the NCC population. Semaphorin signaling also plays important roles in OFT septation. Of note, mice deficient for *semaphorin3c* (*sema3c*) develop PTAs and interrupted aortic arch while other neural crest derivatives remain unaffected [52]. Sema3c is expressed in the OFT myocardium, but is also expressed by cardiac NCCs as these cells colonize the endocardial cushions suggesting that reciprocal signaling between these two cell types is important during OFT septation. Indeed, neural crest cells express receptors for Sema3c, more specifically *neuropilin-1* (*Nrp1*) and *plexinA2* (*Plxna2*) and either *Nrp1* or *Plxna2*-null mice have PTA and interrupted aortic arch, suggesting that NCCs use guidance cues to reach the OFT. Interestingly, Gata6 has been shown to regulate *Sema3c* expression in the OFT and mutations in the *GATA6* gene have been reported in two different studies [50]. A large number of mutated genes in mice lead to PTA and the TGF/BMP, Notch, FGF, VEGF, WNT and SHH pathways are among some of the critical regulators involved in OFT septation. Overall, these studies strengthen the idea that reciprocal signaling between NCCs, pharyngeal endoderm, ectoderm and the SHF is critical for the proper establishment of OFT septation.

Chromosomal Disorders and Conotruncal Anomalies

Chromosomal aberrations are also present in 8–18 % of all CHD cases. The most common is Down syndrome (Trisomy 21) but cardiac malformations have also been identified in patients with Turner syndrome (monosomy X), Edward syndrome (Trisomy 18) and Patau syndrome (Trisomy 13). An important conclusion that was drawn from these studies is that the cardiac malformations associated with these syndromes are more likely the result of altered gene dosage rather than a global change in genomic content. In addition, conotruncal anomalies have been reported in abnormal chromosomal structural syndromes or single gene mutation syndromes including 22q11 deletion, Cri-Du-Chat (deletion 5p15.2), Cat eye syndrome (inversion duplication 22q11), Alagille syndrome (20p12), Noonan syndrome, Holt-Horam (12q24), CHARGE (8p12), Okihiro (20q13.2) and Kakubi syndrome (12q13.12) [53]. Therefore, children diagnosed with conotruncal defects should be evaluated for karyotype evaluation. Interestingly, chromosomal analysis and FISH testing for specific deletions are well accepted tools that are used these days to try and provide a family with a clear cause for the disease. However, many of these syndromes are associated with extra-cardiac malformations and some of them are caused by single gene mutations for which no testing is clinically available.

Acknowledgments Work in the authors' laboratory is supported by the Association Française contre les Myopathies (NMH-Decrypt Project), the Agence Nationale pour la Recherche (ANR-13-BSV2-0003-01), and the Institut National de la Santé et de la Recherche Médicale (S.Z.). B.L. received postdoctoral fellowship from the Fondation pour la Recherche Médicale (FRM) and the Agence Nationale pour la Recherche (ANR-13-BSV2-0003).

References

1. Hoffman JI, Kaplan S. The incidence of congenital heart disease. J Am Coll Cardiol. 2002;39(12):1890–900.
2. Buckingham M, Meilhac S, Zaffran S. Building the mammalian heart from two sources of myocardial cells. Nat Rev Genet. 2005;6(11):826–35.
3. Zaffran S, Kelly RG. New developments in the second heart field. Differentiation Res Biol Divers. 2012;84(1):17–24.
4. Kirby ML. Cardiac development. Oxford: Oxford University Press; 2007.
5. Bajolle F, Zaffran S, Kelly RG, Hadchouel J, Bonnet D, Brown NA, Buckingham ME. Rotation of the myocardial wall of the outflow tract is implicated in the normal positioning of the great arteries. Circ Res. 2006;98(3):421–8.
6. Kelly RG, Brown NA, Buckingham ME. The arterial pole of the mouse heart forms from Fgf10-expressing cells in pharyngeal mesoderm. Dev Cell. 2001;1(3):435–40.
7. Waldo KL, Kumiski DH, Wallis KT, Stadt HA, Hutson MR, Platt DH, Kirby ML. Conotruncal myocardium arises from a secondary heart field. Development. 2001;128(16):3179–88.
8. Mjaatvedt CH, Nakaoka T, Moreno-Rodriguez R, Norris RA, Kern MJ, Eisenberg CA, Turner D, Markwald RR. The outflow tract of the heart is recruited from a novel heart-forming field. Dev Biol. 2001;238(1):97–109.
9. Ward C, Stadt H, Hutson M, Kirby ML. Ablation of the secondary heart field leads to Tetralogy of Fallot and pulmonary atresia. Dev Biol. 2005;284(1):72–83.
10. Hutson MR, Zeng XL, Kim AJ, Antoon E, Harward S, Kirby ML. Arterial pole progenitors interpret opposing FGF/BMP signals to proliferate or differentiate. Development. 2010;137(18):3001–11.
11. Tirosh-Finkel L, Zeisel A, Brodt-Ivenshitz M, Shamai A, Yao Z, Seger R, Domany E, Tzahor E. BMP-mediated inhibition of FGF signaling promotes cardiomyocyte differentiation of anterior heart field progenitors. Development. 2010;137(18):2989–3000.
12. Waldo KL, Hutson MR, Ward CC, Zdanowicz M, Stadt HA, Kumiski D, Abu-Issa R, Kirby ML. Secondary heart field contributes myocardium and smooth muscle to the arterial pole of the developing heart. Dev Biol. 2005;281(1):78–90.
13. Neeb Z, Lajiness JD, Bolanis E, Conway SJ. Cardiac outflow tract anomalies. Wiley Interdiscip Rev Dev Biol. 2013;2(4):499–530.
14. Yelbuz TM, Waldo KL, Kumiski DH, Stadt HA, Wolfe RR, Leatherbury L, Kirby ML. Shortened outflow tract leads to altered cardiac looping after neural crest ablation. Circulation. 2002;106(4):504–10.
15. Goldmuntz E, Bamford R, Karkera JD, dela Cruz J, Roessler E, Muenke M. CFC1 mutations in patients with transposition of the great arteries and double-outlet right ventricle. Am J Hum Genet. 2002;70(3):776–80.
16. Garg V, Kathiriya IS, Barnes R, Schluterman MK, King IN, Butler CA, Rothrock CR, Eapen RS, Hirayama-Yamada K, Joo K, Matsuoka R, Cohen JC, Srivastava D. GATA4 mutations

cause human congenital heart defects and reveal an interaction with TBX5. Nature. 2003;424(6947):443–7.
17. Wei D, Bao H, Liu XY, Zhou N, Wang Q, Li RG, Xu YJ, Yang YQ. GATA5 loss-of-function mutations underlie Tetralogy of Fallot. Int J Med Sci. 2013;10(1):34–42.
18. Maitra M, Koenig SN, Srivastava D, Garg V. Identification of GATA6 sequence variants in patients with congenital heart defects. Pediatr Res. 2010;68(4):281–5.
19. Karkera JD, Lee JS, Roessler E, Banerjee-Basu S, Ouspenskaia MV, Mez J, Goldmuntz E, Bowers P, Towbin J, Belmont JW, Baxevanis AD, Schier AF, Muenke M. Loss-of-function mutations in growth differentiation factor-1 (GDF1) are associated with congenital heart defects in humans. Am J Hum Genet. 2007;81(5):987–94.
20. Spinner NB, Colliton RP, Crosnier C, Krantz ID, Hadchouel M, Meunier-Rotival M. Jagged1 mutations in Alagille syndrome. Hum Mutat. 2001;17(1):18–33.
21. Schott JJ, Benson DW, Basson CT, Pease W, Silberbach GM, Moak JP, Maron BJ, Seidman CE, Seidman JG. Congenital heart disease caused by mutations in the transcription factor NKX2-5. Science. 1998;281(5373):108–11.
22. Ta-Shma A, Pierri CL, Stepensky P, Shaag A, Zenvirt S, Elpeleg O, Rein AJ. Isolated truncus arteriosus associated with a mutation in the plexin-D1 gene. Am J Med Genet A. 2013;161A(12):3115–20.
23. Muncke N, Jung C, Rudiger H, Ulmer H, Roeth R, Hubert A, Goldmuntz E, Driscoll D, Goodship J, Schon K, Rappold G. Missense mutations and gene interruption in PROSIT240, a novel TRAP240-like gene, in patients with congenital heart defect (transposition of the great arteries). Circulation. 2003;108(23):2843–50.
24. Yagi H, Furutani Y, Hamada H, Sasaki T, Asakawa S, Minoshima S, Ichida F, Joo K, Kimura M, Imamura S, Kamatani N, Momma K, Takao A, Nakazawa M, Shimizu N, Matsuoka R. Role of TBX1 in human del22q11.2 syndrome. Lancet. 2003;362(9393):1366–73.
25. Basson CT, Bachinsky DR, Lin RC, Levi T, Elkins JA, Soults J, Grayzel D, Kroumpouzou E, Traill TA, Leblanc-Straceski J, Renault B, Kucherlapati R, Seidman JG, Seidman CE. Mutations in human TBX5 [corrected] cause limb and cardiac malformation in Holt-Oram syndrome. Nat Genet. 1997;15(1):30–5.
26. Lambrechts D, Devriendt K, Driscoll DA, Goldmuntz E, Gewillig M, Vlietinck R, Collen D, Carmeliet P. Low expression VEGF haplotype increases the risk for Tetralogy of Fallot: a family based association study. J Med Genet. 2005;42(6):519–22.
27. Pizzuti A, Sarkozy A, Newton AL, Conti E, Flex E, Digilio MC, Amati F, Gianni D, Tandoi C, Marino B, Crossley M, Dallapiccola B. Mutations of ZFPM2/FOG2 gene in sporadic cases of Tetralogy of Fallot. Hum Mutat. 2003;22(5):372–7.
28. D'Alessandro LC, Latney BC, Paluru PC, Goldmuntz E. The phenotypic spectrum of ZIC3 mutations includes isolated d-transposition of the great arteries and double outlet right ventricle. Am J Med Genet A. 2013;161A(4):792–802.
29. Eldadah ZA, Hamosh A, Biery NJ, Montgomery RA, Duke M, Elkins R, Dietz HC. Familial Tetralogy of Fallot caused by mutation in the jagged1 gene. Hum Mol Genet. 2001;10(2):163–9.
30. Goldmuntz E, Geiger E, Benson DW. NKX2.5 mutations in patients with Tetralogy of Fallot. Circulation. 2001;104(21):2565–8.
31. Nemer G, Fadlalah F, Usta J, Nemer M, Dbaibo G, Obeid M, Bitar F. A novel mutation in the GATA4 gene in patients with Tetralogy of Fallot. Hum Mutat. 2006;27(3):293–4.
32. Lin X, Huo Z, Liu X, Zhang Y, Li L, Zhao H, Yan B, Liu Y, Yang Y, Chen YH. A novel GATA6 mutation in patients with Tetralogy of Fallot or atrial septal defect. J Hum Genet. 2010;55(10):662–7.
33. Baldini A. Dissecting contiguous gene defects: TBX1. Curr Opin Genet Dev. 2005;15(3):279–84.
34. Griffin HR, Topf A, Glen E, Zweier C, Stuart AG, Parsons J, Peart I, Deanfield J, O'Sullivan J, Rauch A, Scambler P, Burn J, Cordell HJ, Keavney B, Goodship JA. Systematic survey of variants in TBX1 in non-syndromic Tetralogy of Fallot identifies a novel 57 base pair deletion

that reduces transcriptional activity but finds no evidence for association with common variants. Heart. 2010;96(20):1651–5.
35. Makki N, Capecchi MR. Cardiovascular defects in a mouse model of HOXA1 syndrome. Hum Mol Genet. 2012;21(1):26–31.
36. Donovan J, Kordylewska A, Jan YN, Utset MF. Tetralogy of Fallot and other congenital heart defects in Hey2 mutant mice. Curr Biol. 2002;12(18):1605–10.
37. Ishii M, Han J, Yen HY, Sucov HM, Chai Y, Maxson Jr RE. Combined deficiencies of Msx1 and Msx2 cause impaired patterning and survival of the cranial neural crest. Development. 2005;132(22):4937–50.
38. De Luca A, Sarkozy A, Ferese R, Consoli F, Lepri F, Dentici ML, Vergara P, De Zorzi A, Versacci P, Digilio MC, Marino B, Dallapiccola B. New mutations in ZFPM2/FOG2 gene in Tetralogy of Fallot and double outlet right ventricle. Clin Genet. 2011;80(2):184–90.
39. Pehlivan T, Pober BR, Brueckner M, Garrett S, Slaugh R, Van Rheeden R, Wilson DB, Watson MS, Hing AV. GATA4 haploinsufficiency in patients with interstitial deletion of chromosome region 8p23.1 and congenital heart disease. Am J Med Genet. 1999;83(3):201–6.
40. Watanabe Y, Miyagawa-Tomita S, Vincent SD, Kelly RG, Moon AM, Buckingham ME. Role of mesodermal FGF8 and FGF10 overlaps in the development of the arterial pole of the heart and pharyngeal arch arteries. Circ Res. 2010;106(3):495–503.
41. Abu-Issa R, Smyth G, Smoak I, Yamamura K, Meyers EN. Fgf8 is required for pharyngeal arch and cardiovascular development in the mouse. Development. 2002;129(19):4613–25.
42. Frank DU, Fotheringham LK, Brewer JA, Muglia LJ, Tristani-Firouzi M, Capecchi MR, Moon AM. An Fgf8 mouse mutant phenocopies human 22q11 deletion syndrome. Development. 2002;129(19):4591–603.
43. Park EJ, Ogden LA, Talbot A, Evans S, Cai CL, Black BL, Frank DU, Moon AM. Required, tissue-specific roles for Fgf8 in outflow tract formation and remodeling. Development. 2006;133(12):2419–33.
44. Beppu H, Malhotra R, Beppu Y, Lepore JJ, Parmacek MS, Bloch KD. BMP type II receptor regulates positioning of outflow tract and remodeling of atrioventricular cushion during cardiogenesis. Dev Biol. 2009;331(2):167–75.
45. McDaniell R, Warthen DM, Sanchez-Lara PA, Pai A, Krantz ID, Piccoli DA, Spinner NB. NOTCH2 mutations cause Alagille syndrome, a heterogeneous disorder of the notch signaling pathway. Am J Hum Genet. 2006;79(1):169–73.
46. McCright B, Lozier J, Gridley T. A mouse model of Alagille syndrome: Notch2 as a genetic modifier of Jag1 haploinsufficiency. Development. 2002;129(4):1075–82.
47. Martins P, Castela E. Transposition of the great arteries. Orphanet J Rare Dis. 2008;3:27.
48. Megarbane A, Salem N, Stephan E, Ashoush R, Lenoir D, Delague V, Kassab R, Loiselet J, Bouvagnet P. X-linked transposition of the great arteries and incomplete penetrance among males with a nonsense mutation in ZIC3. Eur J Hum Genet EJHG. 2000;8(9):704–8.
49. Gonzalez-Iriarte M, Carmona R, Perez-Pomares JM, Macias D, Costell M, Munoz-Chapuli R. Development of the coronary arteries in a murine model of transposition of great arteries. J Mol Cell Cardiol. 2003;35(7):795–802.
50. Kodo K, Nishizawa T, Furutani M, Arai S, Yamamura E, Joo K, Takahashi T, Matsuoka R, Yamagishi H. GATA6 mutations cause human cardiac outflow tract defects by disrupting semaphorin-plexin signaling. Proc Natl Acad Sci U S A. 2009;106(33):13933–8.
51. Olaopa M, Zhou HM, Snider P, Wang J, Schwartz RJ, Moon AM, Conway SJ. Pax3 is essential for normal cardiac neural crest morphogenesis but is not required during migration nor outflow tract septation. Dev Biol. 2011;356(2):308–22.
52. Feiner L, Webber AL, Brown CB, Lu MM, Jia L, Feinstein P, Mombaerts P, Epstein JA, Raper JA. Targeted disruption of semaphorin 3C leads to persistent truncus arteriosus and aortic arch interruption. Development. 2001;128(16):3061–70.
53. Fahed AC, Gelb BD, Seidman JG, Seidman CE. Genetics of congenital heart disease: the glass half empty. Circ Res. 2013;112(4):707–20.

Index

F. Lacour-Gayet et al. (eds.), *Surgery of Conotruncal Anomalies*,
DOI 10.1007/978-3-319-23057-3

Q

R

S

MIX
Papier aus verantwortungsvollen Quellen
Paper from responsible sources
FSC® C105338

If you have any concerns about our products,
you can contact us on
ProductSafety@springernature.com

In case Publisher is established outside the EU,
the EU authorized representative is:
Springer Nature Customer Service Center GmbH
Europaplatz 3, 69115 Heidelberg, Germany

Printed by Libri Plureos GmbH
in Hamburg, Germany